THE CASE MANAGER'S SURVIVAL GUIDE

WINNING STRATEGIES FOR CLINICAL PRACTICE

TONI G. CESTA, PhD, RN, FAAN

Director of Case Management
St. Vincent Catholic Medical Centers of New York
St. Vincent's Hospital
New York, New York
Principal, Case Manager Solutions, LLC
Tucson, Arizona

HUSSEIN A. TAHAN, MS, DNSc(C), RN, CNA

Director of Nursing, Cardiothoracic and Vascular Services
New York Presbyterian Hospital
Columbia Presbyterian Medical Center
New York, New York

SECOND EDITION

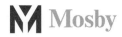 Mosby

An Affiliate of Elsevier Science
St. Louis   London   New York   Philadelphia   Sydney   Toronto

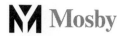

An Affiliate of Elsevier Science

11830 Westline Industrial Drive
St. Louis, Missouri 63146

Library of Congress Cataloging-in-Publication Data

Cesta, Toni G.
   The case manager's survival guide: winning strategies for clinical practice/Toni G.
Cesta, Hussein A. Tahan.—2nd ed.
     p. ; cm.
   Includes bibliographical references and index.
   ISBN 0-323-01688-X
   1. Primary nursing—Administration. 2. Hospitals—Case management services. I.
Tahan, Hussein A. II. Title.
   [DNLM: 1. Case Management—United States—Forms. 2. Managed Care
Programs—organization & administration—United States—Forms. 3. Nursing
Care—organization & administration—United States—Forms. WY 100 C422c 2002]
RT90.7.C47 2002
362.1'73'068—dc21

                                     2002032663

Acquisitions Editor: Yvonne Alexopoulos
Developmental Editor: Danielle M. Frazier
Publishing Services Manager: Patricia Tannian
Senior Project Manager: Suzanne C. Fannin
Senior Book Design Manager: Gail Morey Hudson
Cover Design: Jen Brockett

CE/MVB

Printed in the United States of America

Last digit is the print number: 9   8   7   6   5   4   3   2   1

THE CASE MANAGER'S SURVIVAL GUIDE
WINNING STRATEGIES FOR CLINICAL PRACTICE

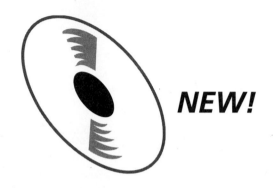

NEW!

CD-ROM *to accompany*
The Case Manager's Survival Guide
Winning Strategies for Clinical Practice, 2e

This valuable resource allows you to:

- Read the entire text, chapter-by-chapter

- Search the entire text by key word or phrase

- Customize and print Planning Guides, Multidisciplinary Action Plans, and Patient Guidelines and Pathways

- Visit the "Resource Center" where you'll find all of the Case Manager's Tip Boxes, Case Studies, Tables, Boxes, and Figures gathered for easy reference

See the inside back cover for your copy of
The Case Manager's Survival Guide CD-ROM!

Contributors

TONI DANDRY AIKEN, RN, BSN, JD
President, RN Development, Inc.
New Orleans, Louisiana

JULIE W. AUCOIN, DNS, RN,C
Faculty, North Carolina Central University
Durham, North Carolina

LYNN A. JANSEN, PhD, RN
Senior Ethicist and Assistant Research Professor
John J. Conley Department of Ethics
St. Vincent Catholic Medical Centers of New York
Manhattan Region
New York, New York

GERRI S. LAMB, PhD, RN, FAAN
Associate Dean, College of Nursing, University of Arizona
Tucson, Arizona

KATHLEEN A. LAMBERT, BSN, RN, JD
Attorney at Law
Tucson, Arizona

PAUL S. SHELTON, EdD
Outcomes Analyst, Health Systems Research Center
Carle Foundation
Urbana, Illinois

MARGUERITE C. WARD, MS, BSN, RN
Director, Quality Management, Cabrini Medical Center
New York, New York

DONNA ZAZWORSKY, MS, RN, CCM, FAAN
Director, Home Health and Outreach
St. Elizabeth of Hungary Clinic
Tucson, Arizona

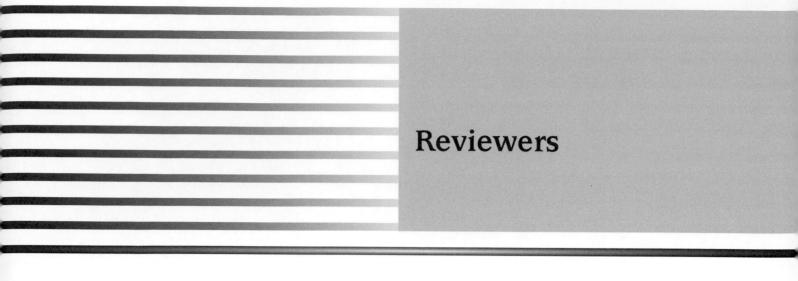

Reviewers

JUDITH A. HARRIS, MSN, NP-C, CRRN, CCM, LHCRM
Advanced Registered Nurse Practitioner
Seniors First Health Care Center
Tallahassee, Florida

RUTHIE ROBINSON, RN, MSN, CCRN, CEN
Faculty, Department of Nursing, Lamar University
Beaumont, Texas

Dedicated to

Our Families, Friends, and **Colleagues**

and to the

Case Managers of the Past, Present, and Future

With Our Heartfelt Thanks . . .

Foreword

Case managers fundamentally are care coordinators. Their role is related to helping people navigate through a confusing and fragmented system fraught with frustration and fear to ensure that they receive those services that are most safe and appropriate to their needs. Clients, patients, consumers, providers, payers, and, in fact, all segments of the healthcare delivery system urgently need well-prepared case managers. While rigorous research providing the evidence base for this assertion grows, the fact remains—there is an urgent need for competent, knowledgeable, and skilled case managers. The genesis of the vital role that case managers play comes from the simple yet enduring need for active coordination of care delivery within a complex system and often chaotic healthcare delivery environment. This role is one of creating a smooth path toward desired outcomes in healthcare.

It is easily assumed that the most important element of healthcare services is the diagnosis and designation of which healthcare services are needed to treat a condition. Although this is important, achieving quality outcomes is much more complex and involves follow-through care management. There is a larger reality to the labyrinth of the consumer interface with healthcare. Access to services is an issue. Costs pile up and may be prohibitive. Many conditions require intensive or extensive communication, education, continuity, and motivational and supportive supplementation. Such infrastructure services may be taken for granted, tend to be unacknowledged as to their importance, and often are not reimbursed. However, in their absence, care is fragmented, quality of care is lower, outcomes are poorer, and costs (ultimately) are higher. Case managers address these and other related issues that reside in the competing demands for cost containment, safer care, and high quality. Case managers use advanced expertise to solve problems in care delivery and healthcare systems and to advocate for the services needed by their clients. Because this requires complex decision-making skills, premier preparation is required for case managers. Fortunately, a premier and practical text has been available since 1998 to help case managers grow and develop knowledge and skill in the concepts, processes, and tools used in case management practice.

The Case Manager's Survival Guide: Winning Strategies for Clinical Practice has become a leading case management text in the field. The first edition, published in 1998, was widely popular as a reference and resource manual and as a textbook for case management curricula. I have used it ever since its publication in the Introduction to Case Management course that forms the foundation of the case management curriculum at the University of Iowa. This curriculum was a direct outgrowth of the vision of the late Kathy C. Kelly, PhD, RN, who, in 1993, felt that the traditional public health model, including the intervention of case management, was reemerging in healthcare as a viable option for addressing urgent healthcare delivery needs. My students have been highly complimentary of the book, citing its clear explanations, easy readability, and practical tips and tools. This, the second edition, has been eagerly awaited. Special features of the second edition include greater detail and depth in the content, an expanded number of chapters, an up-to-date reflection of the current state of case management practice, and a focus on the continuum of care in multiple environments and settings.

Now is an exciting time to be involved in case management. The recognition of the urgent need for care coordination and management makes case managers a most valuable asset in healthcare. Case managers and students of case management practice will find Cesta and Tahan's second edition of *The Case Manager's Survival Guide: Winning Strategies for Clinical Practice* a precious resource, one that they are likely to turn to again and again as they savor its knowledge and treasure its practical usefulness.

Diane L. Huber, PhD, RN, FAAN, CNAA
Associate Professor, College of Nursing, University of Iowa
Iowa City, Iowa

Preface

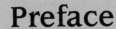

We are proud and delighted to bring to you the second edition of *The Case Manager's Survival Guide: Winning Strategies for Clinical Practice*. From its inception, this award-winning text and hands-on guide for case managers has been a labor of love.

Armed with the knowledge that the field of case management desperately needed a "how-to" book, we began writing the first edition in 1995. Our concept was to write a small pocket guide that case managers could carry with them on the job and refer to as needed. It ultimately turned out to be much more than that. So, 261 pages later, we published a comprehensive, informative, and practical yet theoretically based text in 1998.

In the last 5 years, the field of case management has grown significantly, and so it was time to update and add to the first edition. Topics such as disease management, ethics, utilization management, and transitional planning were not in the first edition. The chapters of the second edition, however, contain these topics, as well as updates and additional and new information.

It has been a labor of love because we both have devoted large portions of our professional as well as personal lives to the pursuit of the advancement of the field of case management, at the delivery, academic, and research levels. We could not have given up so much if we did not genuinely believe that case management is not just important but essential to the future of healthcare, from the perspectives of cost, quality, access, consumerism, nursing advancement, and outcomes of care.

We truly care about case management's future and the future of all case managers who struggle to master a complex and challenging specialty. *The Case Manager's Survival Guide* is our gift to you for your hard work and for the quality of care you bring to patients and families every day through the excellent contributions you make.

This second edition combines pragmatism with theory in a way that we have not seen published before. We sincerely hope that you will find it useful and informative.

Acknowledgment

The authors would like to acknowledge Lois Fink for her excellent work and contributions to the first edition of this book. Our thanks to Lois for helping to make *The Case Manager's Survival Guide* the quality text that it is.

Toni G. Cesta
Hussein A. Tahan

Contents

Detailed Contents

THE CASE MANAGER'S
SURVIVAL GUIDE
WINNING STRATEGIES FOR CLINICAL PRACTICE

1

Introduction to Case Management

If you have purchased or borrowed this book, you must be a **case manager,** or you are thinking of becoming one. If you are *already working* in the field, you are probably beginning to experience many of the conflicts and confusions that come with this role. If you are *thinking of becoming* a case manager, you are probably reading as much as you can about this delivery system and the role you will play in it.

Because **case management** is relatively new to many nurses, it may be difficult to find other nurses working with you or colleagues who have been case managers. Although there are tens of thousands of case managers across the country, there may not be many in your organization or your part of the country. This book is written with you in mind. Although its overall objective is to provide comprehensive information on the role of the case manager and on case management, its format is designed so that it is a ready reference for the on-the-job questions and issues you may face every day.

The case management process is often an intangible one—a behind-the-scenes process and outcomes role that is, at its worst, very stressful and, at its best, very rewarding. The role is complex and eclectic. Not for the meek or mild, it requires confidence and comprehension of a vast array of topics, many of which are reviewed in this book.

Although case management has become somewhat of a household word in healthcare, there is still a tremendous amount of confusion about what it is, how it applies to various settings, how its success can be measured, and what the role of the case manager is (Box 1-1). As a profession, we have yet to answer all of these questions consistently. There are core components of the model and of the case manager role that

---

BOX 1-1   Commonly Asked Questions About Case Management

1. What is it?
2. How does it apply to various healthcare settings?
3. How can its success be measured?
4. What is the role of the case manager?

---

can be taken and applied in a variety of ways. The objective is to find what works best for you and your organization without losing the essence of case management.

USING THIS GUIDE

The purpose of this book is to provide the hands-on information you will need to be an effective and successful case manager. This book contains a lot of information that can be used in the study of case management and in the implementation of case management models. To be a successful case manager you need to understand the role itself, but you also need to understand how case management fits into the bigger pictures of healthcare delivery, healthcare reform, and the future of healthcare. Pick up this book whenever you have a general or specific question. Use it as a ready reference as you develop your expertise in case management.

Broad topics are addressed, and their specific implementation techniques and strategies follow. It is important to understand both the concepts and their application. We suggest that you review both.

HEALTHCARE INDUSTRY IN CRISIS

The healthcare industry continues to be in crisis—a chronic crisis of epic proportion, unprecedented in its

---

BOX 1-2   Factors Affecting the Healthcare Industry

1. Changes in healthcare reimbursement
2. An aging patient population
3. Increasingly complex and chronic illnesses
4. HIV/AIDS epidemic
5. Technology: advances in medical equipment
6. Technology: advances in surgical procedures such as robotics and minimally invasive surgery
7. Information technology
8. Educated patients as consumers of healthcare

---

history, and brought about by many factors (Box 1-2). Both the **prospective payment system** and **managed care** infiltration have necessitated a reassessment of the industry's work, how it is organized, and how it is evaluated. The changing demographics of the patient population have forced us to reexamine our values and our expectations or expected outcomes of the work we perform (e.g., patient care). These changes have come about as a result of an aging patient population with a concomitant increase in chronic illnesses and a more educated patient as the consumer of healthcare. Technology, including medical informatics, has driven up the cost of healthcare. Complex, high-tech and minimally invasive surgery; expensive, life-prolonging treatments such as kidney dialysis; costly antibiotics; computerization; and the need for more and more durable medical equipment to support the care and recuperation of the elderly and the chronically ill have all contributed to escalating costs as we have never seen before.

The frenzy of activity going on in every healthcare setting across the country is an indicator of the need to bring massive and significant change to the industry. Many of the changes involve cost-cutting efforts that many criticize as compromising the quality of care. Managed care is one change that has been consistently criticized for its cost-cutting approach that has appeared to be less concerned with quality of care (Curtin, 1996; Kongstvedt, 2001). Other changes are intended to control both cost and quality. Case management is one such effort. It is designed to manage care, which results in a monitoring and control of resources and cost regarding management of the resources applied and the cost of the care. It is also designed to be an outcomes model, and it has as part of its methodology a close monitoring of the products of the care it manages and their effects on the patient and family. Case management is not equivalent to managed care. They are not interchangeable concepts or phrases. Whereas managed care is a system of cost-containment programs,

case management is a process of care delivery sometimes used within the managed care system.

HISTORY OF CASE MANAGEMENT

Case management is not a new concept. It has been around for more than 80 years (Box 1-3). As a means of providing care, it originated in the 1920s out of the fields of psychiatry and social work and focused on long-term, chronic illnesses that were managed in the outpatient, community-based settings. Case management processes were also used by visiting nurses in the 1930s. The original public health nursing models used community-based case management approaches in their care of patients (Knollmueller, 1989). As a care delivery system, case management is a relatively new concept to the acute care setting, having developed and flourished in the mid-1980s. Between the 1930s and the 1980s the model remained essentially in the community setting. It was not until the introduction of the prospective payment system that the model shifted to the acute care, hospital-based setting.

Definition of Case Management

Whether case management is being applied in the acute care, community, or long-term care setting, its underlying principles and goals are consistent. As a system for providing patient care, case management is designed to ensure that quality care is provided in the most cost-effective manner possible. This is accomplished by improving the processes of care delivery, making them more efficient and effective. Other strategies involved include the management of product and personnel resources. By better administration and control over the ways in which care is provided and the resources used, outcomes can be achieved while ensuring that quality is maintained or improved.

There are a variety of definitions of case management, including the following:

- A nursing care delivery system that supports cost-effective, patient-outcome-oriented care (Cohen and Cesta, 1997).
- A role and process that focuses on procuring, negotiating, and coordinating the care, services, and

---

BOX 1-3   Evolutionary Process of Case Management Application

1. 1920—Psychiatry and social work; outpatient settings
2. 1930—Public health nursing
3. 1950—Behavioral health across the continuum
4. 1985—Acute care
5. 1990—All healthcare settings

resources needed by individuals with complex issues throughout an episode or continuum (Bower and Falk, 1996).

- Case management is a system of healthcare delivery designed to facilitate achievement of expected patient outcomes within an appropriate length of stay. The goals of case management are the provision of quality healthcare along a continuum, decreased fragmentation of care across settings, enhancement of the client's quality of life, efficient utilization of patient care resources, and cost containment (American Nurses Association, 1988).
- A multidisciplinary clinical system that uses registered nurse (RN) case managers to coordinate the care for select patients across the continuum of a healthcare episode (Frink and Strassner, 1996).
- A collaborative process that assesses, plans, implements, coordinates, monitors, and evaluates the options and services required to meet an individual's health needs, using communication and available resources to promote quality, cost-effective outcomes (Commission for Case Manager Certification, 1996).
- A process of care delivery that aims at managing the clinical services needed by patients, ensuring appropriate resource utilization, enhancing the quality of care, and facilitating cost-effective patient care outcomes (Tahan, 1999, p. 270).

Case Management and the Role of Case Manager

It is difficult to separate the model of case management from the role of the case manager. Case management as a model provides the system, but it is the case manager who implements the model and makes it come alive. In other words, the model provides the foundation and organizational structure within which the case manager role is implemented. This may be the reason for the added confusion related to what case management really is and how it works. It is difficult to understand the model without understanding the role, and vice versa. Once the various adaptations of the role and the model are mixed and matched, things really get complicated. The best way to understand the role and the model is to think of them in terms of what the goals of case management are (Box 1-4).

Regardless of the setting in which case management is implemented, there are goals that can be identified that are consistent across the healthcare continuum (see Box 1-4). Whether it is a hospital, a nursing home, or a community care setting, the model attempts to address both cost and quality issues and to deliver care in ways that result in the most positive patient and organizational outcomes.

BOX 1-4   Goals of Case Management and the Case Manager's Role Functions

Overall Goals
1. Manage cost and quality
2. Achieve positive patient and organizational outcomes

Role Functions
1. Care coordination
2. Facilitation
3. Education
4. Advocacy
5. Brokerage of community services and resources
6. Transitional/discharge planning
7. Resource and utilization management
8. Outcomes management

The case manager accomplishes these goals by performing a number of complex role functions. These may include but are not limited to care coordination, facilitation, education, **advocacy, discharge planning,** resource management, and **outcomes management.** These functions remain consistent across care settings along the continuum.

Case Management as an Outcomes Model

Case management is not only a process model but also an outcomes model in that it provides a prospective approach for planning the ways in which care will be provided, the steps in the care process, and the desired outcomes of care. In other words, for each step in the process, there is also an expected **outcome** that can be predetermined and managed. All steps in the process are designed to move the patient toward the desired outcome.

CHANGES IN REIMBURSEMENT: THE DRIVING FORCE BEHIND CASE MANAGEMENT

It was not until the 1980s that case management truly came into its own. Before 1983, healthcare costs were not of major concern to the healthcare provider. Because most healthcare reimbursement was based on a **fee-for-service (FFS)** structure, there were no financial incentives to reduce costs. In fact, because the use of resources was financially rewarded by the system, overuse abounded. This overuse and misuse of healthcare resources, particularly those in the acute care setting, resulted in spiraling costs for the consumers of care (Box 1-5). Concurrently, the costs of pharmaceuticals, radiology, and supplies continued to escalate with minimal management of those costs. In the 1990s and beyond, healthcare in the United States is a trillion-dollar business.

BOX 1-5   Forces Driving the Move Toward Case Management

1. 1970s—Escalating healthcare costs
2. 1980s—Prospective payment system in acute care settings
3. 1990s—Managed care infiltration
4. 2000s—Prospective payment system in home care, outpatient care, rehabilitation services, and long-term care

---

It is therefore no great surprise that the healthcare system eventually broke down. Consumers and **third-party payers** were no longer willing to pay these high costs when the quality of the services they were receiving was barely keeping pace. In fact, it appeared to most consumers of healthcare that the quality of the services they were receiving was diminishing and that the value of the care was reduced. The costs were rising while the value was subsiding.

The mid-1980s were witness to a flurry of activities all designed to figure out how to improve the quality of healthcare while reducing the cost. The expected result was an increase in value. On the payer side, we first saw the introduction of the prospective payment system with the **diagnosis-related groups (DRGs)** as the reimbursement scheme. Shortly after that, the western United States saw an increase in the use of managed care and **health maintenance organizations (HMOs).** DRGs and managed care are discussed in Chapter 2. Employers saw the use of HMOs as a way to reduce the cost of providing healthcare insurance to their employees. Several states, including Minnesota, California, Arizona, and Tennessee, have since adopted broad-based managed care programs. By the turn of the twenty-first century, managed care reimbursement systems had permeated throughout the United States.

Unfortunately, many of the efforts resulting in changes in reimbursement and the introduction of managed care were perceived solely as cost cutting. Although much lip service was given to the notion of quality, effective and consistent outcome measures, as well as measures of quality of care, were lacking. What did exist were financial parameters that guided outcomes evaluation, such as length of stay and cost per case. Within 3 to 5 years, organizations began to recognize the need to incorporate quality into the agenda. Much of this came out of healthcare organizations themselves. Two major quality improvement models drove the quality initiatives. The first was total quality management and the use of **continuous quality improvement (CQI)** methods. The second was case management. Ultimately, both of these concepts became the framework for redesign efforts and patient-focused care.

CONTINUOUS QUALITY IMPROVEMENT AND CASE MANAGEMENT

CQI and case management are linked in philosophy and practice. CQI methods are used to drive case management processes and to monitor outcomes (Cesta, 1993). Case management is now recognized as a system for delivering care that coordinates interdisciplinary care services, plans care, identifies expected outcomes, and helps facilitate the patient and family toward those expected outcomes. The case manager is responsible for ensuring that the patient's needs are being met and that care is being provided in the most cost-effective setting or level of care.

CQI can address both system and practice issues, looking for opportunities for improvement that will result in reduced cost and improved quality of care. Without addressing and improving these processes, case management as a delivery system will not be effective. When implemented, case management affects the patient population served, as well as every part of the organization, every discipline, and every department. Therefore it is sometimes necessary to correct existing systems or interdisciplinary problems before the model can be successfully implemented. CQI can then be applied to measure and continuously monitor the progress and outcomes of the model.

NURSING CASE MANAGEMENT

Nursing case management evolved as a hospital-based care delivery system in 1985. Before that time there had been a number of other nursing care delivery systems, including functional, team, and primary nursing. It has been said that nursing case management incorporates elements of both team and primary nursing. In team nursing, a nurse team leader directs the care being provided by all the members of the nursing team, including RNs, licensed practical nurses, and nurse aides. The team leader generally does not provide direct patient care but directs the care being provided by the members of the team.

Move from Team to Primary Nursing

In the 1970s team nursing evolved to primary nursing. In primary nursing, the RN is responsible for providing all aspects of care to an assigned group of patients. With the assistance of a nurse aide, the RN carries out all direct and indirect nursing functions for the patient. One of the goals of primary nursing is the reduction in fragmentation of nursing care. The primary nurse provides all facets of care to the patient but works independently. It was anticipated that primary nursing would enhance the professionalism of nursing by upgrading the level of autonomy and independent practice.

Breakdown of Primary Nursing

With the advent of the prospective payment system in 1983, primary nursing became increasingly difficult to implement. Although it provided a structure for the RN to function autonomously and independently, it did not address the cost/quality issues affecting the healthcare delivery system in the 1980s. As **lengths of stay** began to shorten, care activities had to be accelerated. At the same time the nursing profession began to experience a nursing shortage, and various strategies were put into place to recruit and retain nurses. One of these was flexible (flex) time, including 12-hour shifts. Twelve-hour shifts provided the RN with more flexibility in terms of the work schedule. This might mean more time to spend raising a family, or it might mean time to return to school. In any case, nurses working 3 days a week, combined with accelerated hospital stays, resulted in increasing difficulty in maintaining a primary nursing model. Continuity of patient care was all but destroyed as nurses worked only 3 days a week. With shortened lengths of stay, it was possible that the nurse who began caring for the patient on admission might not be the same nurse caring for the patient on discharge. It was very expensive to staff nursing units to the extent necessary to maintain as much continuity as possible. In addition to the cost of personnel, primary nursing was not designed to manage care in shorter timeframes or place an emphasis on the management of resources. Care was not outcome focused, and the healthcare providers were fragmented.

Early Hospital-Based Case Management

Two hospitals attempted to respond to the changing times by addressing the changes in healthcare reimbursement, shortened lengths of stay, and dwindling hospital resources. Carondelet St. Mary's Hospital in Tucson, Arizona, and New England Medical Center in Boston, Massachusetts, were the first to recognize the need to redesign their nursing departments. Each introduced nursing case management models that incorporated elements of both team and primary nursing within a context of controlled resources and shortened lengths of stay. The early case management models were structured on using hospital-based nurse case managers to monitor the patient's progress toward discharge.

Carondelet's model was initially designed as an acute care case management model. The job title *Professional*

Nurse Case Manager described an RN with the minimum educational preparation of a bachelor's degree. The case manager assumed responsibility for managing patients toward expected outcomes along a **continuum of care.** Carondelet collected data for the first 4 years after implementation of the model and found that quality and cost were both improved. Job satisfaction improved for nurses, and their job stress decreased. In addition, patient satisfaction increased (Ethridge, 1991).

Perhaps the most compelling finding was that some patients with chronic illnesses were not hospitalized at all (Ethridge and Lamb, 1989). Those who were admitted had lower **acuity** levels. They were immediately linked to the healthcare system so that the length of stay at the beginning of the hospitalization was decreased. This resulted in lower costs for the hospital (Ethridge, 1991).

These findings resulted in the development of the first nursing HMO. The initial program, begun in 1989, focused on case managing patients from a senior-care HMO. The nurse case manager screened all patients admitted under the Senior Plan contract. The assessment included determining the necessary nursing services before discharge, monitoring of any community services being provided, and ensuring a continuation of care in the community if necessary. Because the fees were capitated, the case manager could match the patient's needs with the appropriate services.

New England Medical Center Hospitals (NEMCH) in Boston, Massachusetts, used RNs in positions of senior staff nurses to pilot the case manager role. The case managers carried a core group of patients for whom they provided direct patient care. They worked closely with physicians, social workers, utilization managers, and discharge planners. The core of the care delivery system was that outcomes should drive the care process. Several versions of critical pathways were developed for planning, managing, documenting, and evaluating patient care. During those early years the "tools of the trade" moved more and more toward care management tools that structured the care process and outcomes and were more interdisciplinary (Zander, 1996).

Both models were deemed successes by their organizations. Across the country other hospitals began turning to these two role models for ideas, direction, and support. This was a watershed moment in healthcare delivery. Unprecedented numbers of healthcare organizations began to think about or implement case management. Its position in the healthcare arena was secured.

Although case management initially addressed the changes necessary for organizations to survive prospective payment, it was even more effective in its management of cases under a managed care system. In both reimbursement systems, patient care must be managed and controlled, with a tight rein on the use of resources, the length of stay, and continuing care needs.

The majority of the models of the 1980s did little in terms of changing the role functions of the other members of the healthcare team. Whereas nursing provided the driving force for the movement toward hospital-based case management, the other disciplines were slower in recognizing the value of such a system. Additionally, serious downsizing was only just beginning in the industry. Corporate America had already begun its massive layoffs and downsizing initiatives. Thousands of people lost their jobs. Healthcare had not yet begun to feel the economic pinch as it was being felt in other businesses; therefore the incentive for merging and downsizing departments was not yet there.

Shortly after these early models, case management began to mature as more and more hospitals began to implement case management models. One could see a direct correlation between the degree of managed care infiltration and the use of case management. In nursing case management, the nurse essentially functions as the leader of the team, similar to the team nursing approach. The difference was that the team did not consist of nurses only. Now the team was an interdisciplinary one, and each healthcare provider had a say in terms of how a patient's care would be delivered and monitored.

Shortly after this popularity of the nursing case management models, other disciplines caught on and began to pursue the design and implementation of case management systems. This increased buy-in from other disciplines resulted in an outbreak of these models throughout the country, leading to the birth of interdisciplinary approaches in the design; hence dropping "nursing" from the label to better reflect the models because they no longer were nursing in nature. Today, case management departments most commonly report to the chief operations or medical officers of an organization rather than to nursing services. This shift in reporting structure has resulted in giving case management departments more credence and power in an organization.

EARLY COMMUNITY-BASED CASE MANAGEMENT

Case management, although more commonly thought of as an acute or hospital-based model, has its roots in the community. Long before hospitals were considered the center of the healthcare universe, case management was being used for a variety of purposes and to meet the needs of diverse populations of patients.

Case management finds its roots in public health nursing, social work, and behavioral health. We can find evidence of case management in the 1860s, where case management techniques were used in the settlement houses occupied by immigrants and the poor. "Patient care records" consisted of cards that catalogued the individual's and family's needs and/or follow-up needs, all aimed at ensuring that the patient/family received the services that they needed and that additional services would be provided as necessary (Tahan, 1998).

Another example of a case management application, also in the 1860s, was the first Board of Charities established in Massachusetts. Aimed toward the sick and the poor, public human services were coordinated with a primary goal of conserving public funds (Tahan, 1998). Even in the 1860s, cost containment was a concern as it related to the distribution of public funds to the poor. Social workers were the health professionals responsible for managing these processes.

In the early 1900s case management strategies were implemented by public health nurses at the Yale University School of Nursing. A collaborative effort was established between a clergyman and the superintendent of the school. The clergyman described the nurse's role and the requirements he sought in the following ways:
1. Knowledge and expertise
2. Communication skills
3. Cost containment
4. Collaboration with physicians
5. Appropriate allocation of resources
6. Responsibility for overall care of the patient and family
7. Provision of emotional and psychosocial support and the assurance of a dignified and peaceful death
8. Coordination and management of care
9. Facilitation of the delivery of patient care activities
10. Obtaining funds for special programs (Tahan, 1998)

Review a contemporary case manager's job description and you are likely to find the superintendent's expected role functions and requirements there.

Around the same time that public health nursing was embracing case management concepts and techniques, the field of social work was using care coordination techniques with a focus on linking patients and families to available resources. Social work began to emerge as the discipline focused on linking or brokering healthcare services for individuals. Conversely, the early nursing case management models included both coordination and care delivery functions. In many ways these differences remain in the approaches taken by both disciplines in the delivery of contemporary case management.

The 1950s was the decade in which behavioral health workers began to use case management tools and strategies. Targeted were World War II veterans who presented mental and emotional problems in addition to physical disabilities. *Continuum of care* was labeled for the first time, and in this context it related to the myriad of community health services these individuals required and accessed. Behavioral health case managers accessed, coordinated, and ensured that service needs were met on a continuous basis. These strategies can still be found today in many behavioral health models of care delivery.

The 1970s and 1980s

During the 1970s and 1980s the federal government provided funding to support the development of several demonstration projects focused on long-term care. Legislation was enacted at the state and federal levels to incorporate these projects into strategic planning policies. Reimbursement was established through **Medicare** and **Medicaid** waivers. Some of the better known projects included the Triage Program in Connecticut, the Wisconsin Community Care Organization, the On Look Project in San Francisco, the New York City Home Care Project, and the Long-Term Care Channeling Demonstration Project in San Francisco (Cohen and Cesta, 1994).

By the late 1980s, community-based case management programs were emerging in many parts of the country as a mechanism for managing patients and resources in capitated environments. One important example is the Carondelet Saint Mary's Model in Tucson, Arizona (Cohen and Cesta, 2001). These emerging and contemporary models returned case managed to its original roots, the community. Case management had now completed a circle that took over 100 years to circumnavigate.

The 1990s

As a result of the reemergence of community-based case management, the Centers for Medicare and Medicaid Services (CMS), formerly the Health Care Financing Administration (HCFA), funded five demonstration projects that used registered professional nurses in the role of community case managers to coordinate care for the Medicare beneficiaries. These projects were called *community nursing centers,* and they are as follows:

1. The Carle Clinic at the Carle Organization in Urbana, Illinois (Schraeder and Britt, 1997)
2. A School-Based Health Center at The University of Rochester in Rochester, New York (Walker and Chiverton, 1997)

3. The Silver Spring Community Nursing Center at the University of Wisconsin, Milwaukee (Lundeen, 1997)
4. The University Community Health Services Group Practice at Vanderbilt University in Nashville, Tennessee (Spitzer, 1997)
5. The Carondelet Health Care Corporation at Carondelet St. Mary's Hospital in Tucson, Arizona (Ethridge, 1997)

A special feature of these centers is that they relied on nurses as the main providers of care with physicians in consultative roles. These centers demonstrated the ability to affect both the process and outcomes of care. Examples of the services provided or arranged for and coordinated by the nurse case managers were health risk assessments; **authorization,** coordination, evaluation, and payment of services; services such as home care, transportation, respite care, and home-delivered meals; preventive and psychiatric mental health; health promotion activities such as exercise, nutrition, and lifestyle changes; **durable medical equipment;** and medical or minor surgical care.

HISTORY OF CRITICAL PATHWAYS

It has been almost 2 decades since the introduction of **case management plans** as a method of controlling cost and quality in healthcare. First known as **critical pathways,** these tools have grown in scope and sophistication over the years (Box 1-6). Critical pathways were originally designed and implemented by nursing departments as a paper-and-pencil system for outlining the course of events for treating patients in a particular DRG for each day of hospitalization (Zander, 1991; Nelson, 1994; Cohen and Cesta, 1997).

In a broader fashion, critical pathways outlined the key or critical steps in the treatment of the DRG in a one-page summary. Because DRGs are broad groupings or classifications of similar types of patients, the critical pathway also had to be broad and nonspecific in nature (Edelstein and Cesta, 1993). The original critical pathways were mainly focused on nursing interventions and tasks. The daily interventions such as blood work or

---

BOX 1-6   Elements of an Effective Case Management Plan

1. Interdisciplinary in nature
2. Outcomes based
3. Clinically specific
4. Care provider documentation included
5. Flexible enough to meet individual patient's care needs

other diagnostics and therapeutics were outlined generically and were applicable to a host of different patient types. Because of the generic nature of the plans, they did little to control the use of resources, types of medications, route of administration, or other factors related to cost and quality. Although they did suggest the appropriate number of hospital days to allocate to the DRG, they did little beyond that to control the kinds of product resources applied to the particular broad grouping of patients.

CASE MANAGEMENT PLANS TODAY

Critical pathways were a good first attempt at providing a framework for controlling cost and quality within the prospective payment system of the acute caresetting. Subsequent adaptations of the critical pathway concept began to use more specific and direct clinical content in a multidisciplinary format and multiple settings or levels of care. These more sophisticated case management plans are called **multidisciplinary action plans (MAPs),** clinical guidelines, practice guidelines, practice parameters, care maps, and so on. Today's case management plans are clinically specific, incorporate other disciplines, are outcome oriented, and may include care provider documentation. In addition to being more clinically specific, these plans are focused around specific clinical case types rather than DRGs. Thus the content applies to the clinical issue being planned out. This may be a medical problem, surgical procedure, or workup plan (Hampton, 1993; Tahan and Cesta, 1994; Cohen and Cesta, 1997). Chapter 12 contains more detailed information on the various adaptations of the current "tools of the trade" in case management. Appendixes A through G at the end of this book present examples of several different types of case management plans.

Benchmarking

Evolutionary changes involved much more specificity in terms of the content of the case management plan. **Benchmarking** is used as a strategy for understanding internal processes and performance levels; it provides a basis for understanding where the performance gaps are. It brings the best ideas that identify opportunities and helps the organization to rally around a consensus. In addition, it results in the implementation of better-quality products and services (Czarnecki, 1994).

The clinical content for the case management plans should be based on **benchmarks** such as those established by the following:

■ Professional societies
■ Professional journals
■ Health systems and hospital corporations
■ Texts and manuals
■ National **databases**

One or more of these benchmarks can be used to develop any one plan. In this way much of the subjectivity is taken out of the plan of care and instead the care is based on sound judgment, expert opinion, and research outcomes. With this step in the evolutionary process, the plans became much more clinically directive and began to provide a framework for controlling resource application for specific case types.

MULTIDISCIPLINARY CARE PLANNING

The next step in the evolutionary process was the introduction of plans that had a more multidisciplinary focus and that incorporated the plan of care for all disciplines represented (Goode and Blegan, 1993; Adler et al, 1995). The final step was the addition of expected outcomes of care that applied to the specific interventions on the plan. In other words, for each intervention there was an expected outcome for the patient to achieve before the patient could move on to the next phase of care (Sperry and Birdsall, 1994). Box 1-7 presents an example of expected outcomes.

CHOOSING A CASE MANAGEMENT TOOL

A variety of case management tools are available today. The tool chosen by any organization should be based on that organization's needs and goals. Some issues to

---

BOX 1-7   Expected Outcomes as They Might Appear on a Multidisciplinary Action Plan for Community-Acquired Pneumonia

Intermediate Outcomes (Also Known as Milestones or Trigger Points)
Convert from intravenous to oral antibiotics when the patient:
1. Has two consecutive oral temperatures of less than 100.4° F obtained at least 8 hours apart in the absence of antipyretics
2. Shows a decrease in leukocytosis to less than 12,000
3. Exhibits improved pulmonary signs/symptoms
4. Is able to tolerate oral medications

Discharge Outcomes
In less severe pneumonia, discharging the patient from the hospital may occur simultaneously or up to 24 hours after switch to oral antibiotics, providing there is no deterioration or other reason for continued hospitalization.

CASE MANAGER'S TIP 1-1

Choosing a Case Management Tool

When choosing a case management tool, be sure to address the following issues during the design and implementation process:

1. Format: Critical pathway versus MAP
2. Utility as a documentation system
3. Inclusion as a permanent part of the medical record
4. Interdisciplinary nature
5. Legal issues related to care providers' use of the tool
6. Fulfillment of the standards of accreditation and regulatory agencies (e.g., Joint Commission on Accreditation of Healthcare Organizations [JCAHO] requirements)

---

be addressed during the design and implementation process are summarized in Case Manager's Tip 1-1 and described in more detail in the following paragraphs.

Format: Critical Pathway Versus Multidisciplinary Action Plan

A critical pathway is generally formatted as a one-page summary of the tasks to be accomplished for a specific diagnosis or DRG. It does not include outcomes and is usually not used as a documentation tool. In addition, it is customarily not a part of the patient's medical record. MAPs, however, are more comprehensive in nature, are usually a part of the patient's permanent record, include outcomes, and are interdisciplinary.

Utility as a Documentation System for Nurses and Other Healthcare Providers

The MAP is intended to be used as a documentation tool. This is most often accomplished by using the MAP in conjunction with a documentation-by-exception system, whereby the expected patient outcomes are prospectively identified and then charted against the timeframes established. To date the majority of such documentation systems incorporate only nursing documentation. Some organizations have successfully included other disciplines such as social work, nutrition, and physical and occupational therapy. The format can be adjusted to include other disciplines such as physicians by including more narrative note space within the document and medical orders as a preprinted order set.

Inclusion as a Permanent Part of the Medical Record

If the MAP is to be used as a documentation tool, then it clearly must be included as part of the permanent medical record. Some organizations, out of fear of legal **liability,** opt not to include the MAP as a part of the record. It is believed that this reduces their liability. In reality, if the plan is the standard of care for the organization, then the organization is responsible for producing the standard should a legal issue arise (Hirshfeld, 1993); therefore it is discoverable and admissible in court regardless of whether it is a part of the medical record. If the MAP is used to guide the clinical care of a particular patient the hospital is being sued for, the court may demand that the MAP be made available. If the physician did indeed follow the MAP, then it will afford legal protection to the physician and the organization.

In any case, some organizations may choose to test the MAP outside the medical record first before sanctioning it. In situations such as this in which the MAP has not been approved by the hospital, patient consent may be necessary. Otherwise the use of two different standards of care cannot be justified.

Including the MAP as part of the medical record lends the medical record more weight and credibility than not including it. Including the MAP clearly gives the message that the organization stands behind it as the standard of care and believes that the MAP represents state-of-the-art care.

Interdisciplinary Nature, Incorporating All Disciplines in the Care Process, and Expected Outcomes

Early case management plans did not include all disciplines but had a heavy nursing focus and emphasis. As case management has evolved and matured, case management plans have become more multidisciplinary. Although it may be more difficult to include the documentation of all care providers, it should be easier to include all disciplines in the actual plan itself. Expected outcomes for each discipline can be prospectively identified and incorporated. The biggest advantage to creating an interdisciplinary plan is that it reduces duplication and fragmentation and provides proof of an integrated plan of care for accrediting and regulatory agencies. Opportunities to reduce redundancy become more obvious when the plans for each discipline can be reviewed and compared. This approach also enhances the use of existing personnel by ensuring that all are carrying out the care activities most appropriate to their disciplines. Areas in which this becomes obvious include patient education and discharge planning, where there is greater likelihood that duplication of effort may take place.

Because quality and length of stay are affected by the efforts of each and every member of the healthcare team, it only makes sense to include all of them in the planning process.

Legal Issues for Physicians, Nurses, and Other Providers

Many healthcare providers may feel anxiety related to the use of MAPs and other case management plans. This may be due to a lack of understanding related to the legal issues concerning these kinds of tools. Legal issues should be carefully discussed with the organization's risk management department after a thorough review of the literature is completed. Each organization must weigh the legal pros and cons and draw its own conclusions as to whether this is a concept that the physicians can adopt and embrace. Another strategy to reduce legal risk and curtail providers' hesitancy to using the MAPs is to review the stance taken by the various professional societies and associations, such as the American Medical Association and the American Nurses Association. Almost all professional societies are in favor of using MAPs in some form or another.

Fulfillment of JCAHO Requirements for Care Planning, Patient Teaching, and Discharge Planning

The standards for the Joint Commission on Accreditation of Healthcare Organizations (JCAHO) focus on the incorporation of all disciplines into the plan of care for those tasks that are interdisciplinary in nature (JCAHO, 2001). The MAP, by nature of its format and philosophy, is designed to ensure that all disciplines are represented and integrated in the plan.

PHYSICIAN SUPPORT

Physician support is a key component in the success or failure of any case management plan, no matter what format it takes. Although these plans were once feared as legally dangerous, physicians are beginning to realize some of their legal benefits. Conceptually, case management plans can meet physician, hospital, and patient needs in a number of ways.

Aid to Shortening Length of Stay

To maintain financial viability, acute care settings must shorten the number of inpatient hospital days. Whether the **reimbursement** system is negotiated managed care or the prospective payment system, length of stay can translate to financial success or failure for any hospital in today's healthcare environment.

Selling Tool for Managed Care/HMOs

An ability to demonstrate systems that control cost and quality is essential to any forward-thinking healthcare organization in the 1990s and beyond. Case management plans that are prospective and outcome oriented and outline both the appropriate length of stay and expected outcomes and the appropriate use of resources for a particular case type provide a structure for controlling cost and quality. These plans can be shared with managed care organizations before admission to demonstrate how the hospital manages a particular case type, or they can be used as a **concurrent review** tool to justify the length of stay and resource allocation.

Means of Legal Protection

Practice guidelines and case management plans can protect physicians from a risk liability perspective in that they outline what is appropriate to do, as well as what is not appropriate to do. They provide for a plan of care that is supported by the organization in which they work (West, 1994).

Aid to Regulatory Agency Compliance

For the JCAHO or other regulatory bodies, case management plans are recognized as an excellent vehicle for integration of care and maintaining and improving quality. By outlining the expected clinical outcomes and documenting deviations from those outcomes, the organization can identify opportunities for clinical process improvements (JCAHO, 2001).

Means of Providing a Competitive Edge

Clearly the organizations that maintain market-share advantage will be the ones that will remain competitive in the managed care environment. If "covered lives" is the name of the game, a competitive edge will lie with those organizations that have captured the greatest market share. This means that they will have negotiated managed care contracts that provide for maximum reimbursement and that have large patient populations.

Source of Practice Parameters

A variety of respected organizations have developed **practice guidelines** (see section entitled "Benchmarking" earlier in this chapter). Physicians, nurses, and other providers can refer to their own specialty organizations regarding state-of-the-art guidelines (Holzer, 1990).

BENEFITS OF CASE MANAGEMENT

Internally there are many reasons why case management plans spell success or failure (Case Manager's Tip 1-2).

Simplify Care

Case management plans provide a systematic format for all disciplines to use in the treatment of specific case

CASE MANAGER'S TIP 1-2

Benefits of Case Management Plans

When soliciting support for case management plans, focus on the ways in which they can help to ensure the healthcare organization's success. Case management plans help do the following:

1. Simplify and integrate care
2. Improve reimbursement
3. Objectify decision making
4. Contain cost
5. Prioritize resources
6. Ensure quality outcomes

types. All disciplines involved in the care of the specific group of patients represented are included in one interdisciplinary plan of care. In some cases, documentation is also included so that the entire course of events is seen in one documentation tool (Adler et al, 1995).

Improve Reimbursement

Because documentation is enhanced, there is greater opportunity for the medical record to be coded properly and for managed care organizations to authorize needed services. Proper **coding** and authorizations mean maximization of reimbursement.

Objectify Decision Making

Although a tremendous amount of subjectivity and judgment goes into the art of practicing medicine, there still remains a core of safe and appropriate clinical practice that is based on research and state-of-the-art recommendations. Case management plans provide a vehicle for communicating these clinical recommendations in an objective manner.

Contain Cost

Because case management plans provide a foundation for reducing variability in medical treatment, they serve as a tool for controlling cost. Care needs, both product and personnel, are prospectively determined so that the organization can predict its resource needs and reduce the need for a variety of different brands and types of the same product. This ultimately has an effect on cost. The plans outline the expected length of stay, thereby controlling the number of hospital days and resulting in cost savings to the hospital. Daily resource application is also outlined, which will translate to saved dollars for the organization (Edelstein and Cesta, 1993; Jijon and Jijon-Letort, 1995).

Prioritize Resources

Resource use is closely tied to cost containment. By properly using resources, costs are reduced. Other issues involve the appropriate use of existing resources, both product and personnel. Case management plans can provide a framework for identifying which members of the healthcare team will provide which services. So much of the misutilization and/or **overutilization** of healthcare resources occurs because of lack of communication between departments and disciplines. Through case management, the work to be done can be allocated to the most appropriate member of the team. Responsibilities are outlined prospectively rather than on a case-by-case basis. This reduces the opportunity for redundancy or for things to fall through the cracks and not be done at all. For example, discharge planning functions can be allocated to the most appropriate care provider, thereby using personnel most appropriately and as early in the process as possible (Tahan and Cesta, 1994).

INTERDISCIPLINARY TEAM

Case management has provided a structure for healthcare providers to develop teams that are truly interdisciplinary and collaborative. In the past, either various disciplines have controlled the team or the team was composed of only one discipline. For example, "patient care rounds" were generally physician dominated and focused on the medical plan. In team nursing, the team was composed of only nurses. The team leader was a nurse, members of the team were nurses, and so on. Discharge planning rounds were often interdisciplinary but were focused on the patient's discharge plan and social services.

CHANGE PROCESS

Case management as a delivery model crosses all boundaries within the organization. Therefore it is critical that the members involved in the development of the team represent all those affected. The roles most closely affiliated with that of the case manager are utilization management, transitional/discharge planning, and home care. During the design process, an interdisciplinary team representing these departments should be brought together to examine current practice and look for opportunities to redefine role functions within the organization.

Logically the membership should consist of those individuals who have the power and authority to make the necessary changes in the role functions of these departments. During the analysis phase, some disciplines may feel threatened or defensive about their current functions within the organization and may interpret the need to change as a criticism of their current job performance rather than as identifying opportunities to make the organization more productive and efficient.

This period while current processes are analyzed and critiqued may cause some anxiety. How well this group works through the process will greatly depend on the members' interpersonal relationships, their vision, and their ability to collaborate.

Using the techniques of CQI and performance improvement will help to facilitate this process (Cesta, 1993). CQI helps to place everyone on an equal playing field as processes are analyzed and changed (see Chapter 13). The team should first examine current practice by looking at what the various departments and disciplines are currently doing, where there may be overlap or redundancy, and where things may be falling through the cracks. Only then can opportunities for improvement be initiated. One useful tool for this technique is the flow diagram. The flow diagram provides the team with a visual representation of their current practice, where quality barriers may be, and where opportunities for improvement may lie (Figure 1-1).

The social worker and the case manager may be duplicating some discharge planning functions. There may be confusion between them in terms of who is doing what; specific tasks must then be negotiated as they arise. This results in confusion and delays because each episode requires an analysis, a discussion, and a resolution.

This executive-level team essentially designs the case management model after a thorough analysis has taken place. The role functions of each member of the team are clearly outlined and delineated prospectively before going further with the implementation process.

Once these role functions have been determined, the members of the interdisciplinary case management team can be assembled to carry out a number of important functions. The team members are those clinicians and others who are directly involved in the care process. The team first prospectively develops the case management plan. The plan, as discussed in Chapter 12, is collaboratively developed by the team to manage the case as efficiently and cost-effectively as possible. The team also individualizes the plan to the specific patient. Finally, the team implements the plan. The case manager serves as the thread that binds the interdisciplinary team together. The case manager does not lead the team but essentially guides the team and the patient/family toward the achievement of the expected outcomes as identified in the plan.

The members of the team are fluid and depend on the patient's location, clinical problem, and expected long-term needs. Core members of the team should always include the physician, nurse, case manager, social worker, discharge planner, and patient/family. Additional members depend on the picture presented. For example, orthopedic problems warrant the physical therapist's membership on the team; pulmonary problems necessitate the respiratory therapist. For the diabetic or other patient with metabolic problems, the nutritionist should be a member of the team. Clearly, members should be those healthcare providers who have some relevance to the case and who have something to contribute to the interdisciplinary plan of care.

In a time when containing costs has never been more important, a collaborative, interdisciplinary approach is critical to the success of any case management model. Without it, true case management can never take place.

MANAGED CARE

It has not been uncommon for the terms *case management* and *managed care* to sometimes be used interchangeably. However, there are specific differences between the terms. Although linked philosophically, managed care is a broader term that refers to an organized delivery of services by a select **panel of providers** (Rehberg, 1996; Kongstvedt, 2001). These services are managed under a prepayment arrangement between a provider of services and a managed care organization. Managed care is a system that provides the generalized structure and focus when managing the use, cost, quality, and effectiveness of healthcare services. HMOs and **preferred provider organizations (PPOs)** are the two most common types of managed care arrangements. They are essentially health insurance plans that link the patient to provider services, and their purpose is to improve the efficiency of the healthcare delivery system (Mullahy, 1995, 1998; Kongstvedt, 2001).

Because some physicians' only exposure to case managers has been through a managed care organization, they may see the two as synonymous. They may believe that case managers and case management means managed care. In reality, although case managers can be found in managed care organizations, they are also found in a wide variety of other practice settings (see Chapters 3 and 4).

Case management is a patient care delivery system. Perhaps the most profound difference between case management and managed care is the fact that managed care is a function of a healthcare reimbursement system, whereas case management is a structure for providing care within a managed care reimbursement system. Case management also applies to provider areas that are not reimbursed under managed care. *Managed care* is defined as a means of providing healthcare services within a defined network of providers. These providers are responsible for managing the care in a quality, cost-effective manner (Baldor, 1996).

The initial driving force for case management in the hospital setting was the prospective payment system

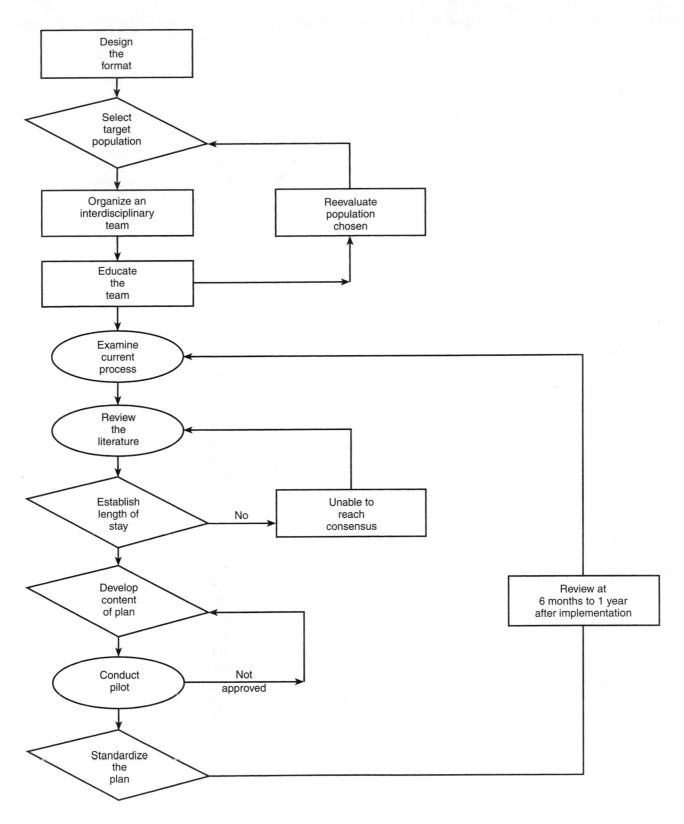

Key:
Box = Activities
Circle = Inputs to/outputs from
Diamond = Decision to be made (Yes/No)
Arrow = Direction of flow of activities

Figure 1-1 Flow diagram: developing a case management plan.

because of the dwindling reimbursement associated with the DRGs. As managed care continues to proliferate, it has become an even greater force in the movement toward case management. Under full capitation, the incentive is greatest (see Chapter 2). In between full capitation and FFS we now find a wide variety of combinations of insurers, reimbursement systems, and service settings. It may be 5 years or more before the dust settles nationally, systems are in place and integrated, and the continuum of care has been defined.

KEY POINTS

1. Case management originated as a community-based model in the late 1800s and early 1900s.
2. In the 1950s case management emerged in the field of behavioral health, in which the term "continuum of care" was first applied.
3. Case management applications in the 1980s evolved out of changes in the healthcare reimbursement system, specifically the prospective payment system.
4. Case management can be defined in a number of ways but is essentially a process and outcomes model designed to manage resources and maintain quality of care.
5. Case management tools such as pathways and guidelines can help facilitate the case manager role.
6. It is important for physicians to be part of the design, implementation, and evaluation processes related to case management.
7. Case management uses a team approach and incorporates elements of CQI.

REFERENCES

Adler SL, Bryk E, Cesta TG, et al: Collaboration: the solution to multidisciplinary care planning, *Orthop Nurs* 14(2):21-29, 1995.

American Nurses Association: *Task force on case management*, Kansas City, Mo, 1988, The Association.

Baldor RA: *Managed care made simple*, Cambridge, Mass, 1996, Blackwell Science.

Bower K, Falk C: Case management as a response to quality, cost, and access imperatives. In Cohen E, editor: *Nurse case management in the 21st century*, St Louis, 1996, Mosby.

Cesta TG: The link between continuous quality improvement and case management, *J Nurs Adm* 24(12):49-58, 1993.

Cohen EL, Cesta TG: Case management in the acute care setting: a model for health care reform, *J Case Manag* 3(3):110-116, 1994.

Cohen EL, Cesta TG: *Nursing case management: from concept to evaluation*, ed 2, St Louis, 1997, Mosby.

Cohen EL, Cesta TG: *Nursing case management: from essentials to advanced practice applications*, St Louis, 2001, Mosby.

Commission for Case Manager Certification: *CCM certification guide*, Rolling Meadows, Ill, 1996, The Commission.

Curtin L: The ethics of managed care—part 1: proposing a new ethos? *Nurs Manage* 27(8):18-19, 1996.

Czarnecki MT: *Benchmarking strategies for health care management*, Gaithersburg, Md, 1994, Aspen.

Edelstein EL, Cesta TG: Nursing case management: an innovative model of care for hospitalized patients with diabetes, *Diabetes Educ* 19(6):517-521, 1993.

Ethridge P: A nursing HMO: Carondelet St Mary's experience, *Nurs Manage* 22(7):22-27, 1991.

Ethridge, P: The Carondelet experience, *Nurs Manage* 28(3):26-28, 1997.

Ethridge P, Lamb GS: Professional nursing case management improves quality, access and costs, *Nurs Manage* 20(3):30-35, 1989.

Frink BB, Strassner L: Variance analysis. In Flarey DL, Blancett SS, editors: *Handbook of nursing case management*, Gaithersburg, Md, 1996, Aspen.

Goode CJ, Blegan MA: Developing a CareMap for patients with a cesarean birth: a multidisciplinary approach, *J Perinat Neonat Nurs* 7(2):40-49, 1993.

Hampton DC: Implementing a managed care framework through care maps, *J Nurs Adm* 23(5):21-27, 1993.

Hirshfeld E: Use of practice parameters as standards of care and in health care reform: a view from the American Medical Association, *J Qual Improve* 19(8):322-329, 1993.

Holzer JF: The advent of clinical standards for professional liability, *Qual Rev Bull* 16(2):71-79, 1990.

Jijon CR, Jijon-Letort FX: Perinatal predictors of duration and cost of hospitalization for premature infants, *Clin Pediatr* 34(2): 79-85, 1995.

Joint Commission on Accreditation of Healthcare Organizations: *The 2000 Joint Commission AMH accreditation manual for hospitals*, Oakbridge Terrace, Ill, 2001, JCAHO.

Knollmueller RN: Case management: what's in a name? *Nurs Manage* 20(10):38-42, 1989.

Kongstvedt P: *Essentials of managed health care*, ed 4, Gaithersburg, Md, 2001, Aspen.

Lundeen S: Community Nursing Center: issues for managed care, *Nurs Manage* 28(3):35-37, 1997.

Mullahy CM: *The case manager's handbook*, Gaithersburg, Md, 1995, Aspen.

Mullahy CM: *The case manager's handbook*, ed 2, Gaithersburg, Md, 1998, Aspen.

Nelson MS: Critical pathways in the emergency department, *J Emerg Nurs* 19(2):110-114, 1994.

Rehberg CA: Managed care contracts: a guide for clinical case managers, *Nurs Case Manag* 1(1):11-17, 1996.

Schraeder C, Britt T: The Carle Clinic, *Nurs Manage* 28(3):32-34, 1997.

Sperry S, Birdsall C: Outcomes of a pneumonia critical path, *Nurs Econ* 12(6):332-345, 1994.

Spitzer R: The Vanderbilt University experience, *Nurs Manage* 28(3):38-40, 1997.

Tahan HA: Case management: a heritage more than a century old, *Nurs Case Manag* 3(2):55-60, 1998.

Tahan HA: Clarifying case management: what is in a label? *Nurs Case Manag* 4(6):268-278, 1999.

Tahan HA, Cesta TG: Developing case management plans using a quality improvement model, *J Nurs Adm* 24(12):49-58, 1994.

Walker H, Chiverton P: The University of Rochester experience, *Nurs Manage* 28(3):29-31, 1997.

West JCC: The legal implications of medical practice guidelines, *J Health Hosp Law* 27(4):97-103, 1994.

Zander K: CareMaps: the core of cost and quality care, *New Definition* 6(3):3, 1991.

Zander K: The early years: the evolution of nursing case management. In Flarey DL, Blancett SS, editors: *Handbook of nursing case management*, Gaithersburg, Md, 1996, Aspen.

2 Financial Reimbursement Systems

ORIGINS OF THE PROSPECTIVE PAYMENT SYSTEM: AN OVERVIEW

The **prospective payment system** (PPS) and **diagnosis-related groups (DRGs)** were probably the strongest catalysts for the movement of **case management** from the community to the acute care setting. Under **fee-for-service (FFS)** plans there were no financial incentives for hospitals to reduce cost and length of stay. In the 1960s and 1970s public policy was focused on improving access to services. **Medicare, Medicaid,** and other entitlement programs were designed to make services available to the poor, the disabled, and the elderly.

By the early 1980s cost containment had become the driving issue. Healthcare policy had begun to shift from the issues of access and entitlements to quality, cost, and fiscal monitoring. The PPS was initiated to control hospital costs by providing a price-per-case **reimbursement.** The onus of responsibility was shifted to the provider to manage resource utilization as a set reimbursement would be allotted. The tool designed to determine the amount of reimbursement was the DRG. It was believed that the DRG would encourage physicians, nurses, ancillary departments, and administrators to work together to provide the most efficient care and to manage the patient through the system as efficiently as possible. It was also believed that the PPS would help to standardize care and improve the efficiency of the care process. In reality, although the DRG controlled the payment rate the hospital was to receive, it did not control the cost of care. Therefore despite these rather dramatic and strict reimbursement schemes, hospital costs continued to escalate. This resulted in the resurgence of the managed care reimbursement systems in the 1990s, especially **capitation.**

USE OF DOCUMENTATION

Under the PPS, it was believed that proper documentation could ensure that the DRG assignment would be timely and accurate and that the hospital would be reimbursed as quickly as possible. Therefore it became clear that much of the financial success of the hospital would depend on accurate and appropriate documentation. Some hospitals introduced a new position known as *DRG manager, DRG coordinator,* or *documentation specialist.* The DRG coordinator/manager was responsible for disseminating information related to the DRGs, particularly data regarding how the hospital was doing in terms of **length of stay,** cost of care, and case mix. The coordinator, based on analytical findings, could make recommendations regarding areas for improvement in length of stay or cost, where the hospital might be able to maximize revenues or work with the healthcare providers to help them enhance **coding** through improvements in their documentation.

In 1982 the Tax Equity and Fiscal Responsibility Act (TEFRA) enacted the DRGs (Richards, 1996). They were initially designed to set limits on Medicare reimbursement. The development of the methodology that would determine the reimbursement rates was intricate, complex, and laborious. The first generation of DRGs was based on the ICDA-8 (International Classification of Diseases, Adapted, Eighth Revision) and HICDA-2 (Hospital Adaptation of ICDA, Second Revision) diagnostic coding schemes. The second generation was based on the International Classification of Diseases, Ninth Revision, Clinical Modification **(ICD-9-CM)** codes. The "I-8" was a four-digit scheme used to measure the incidence of disease, injury, or illness (Commission on Professional and Hospital Activities, 1975). The "I-9," introduced in 1979, is a five-digit scheme and adds more specificity in terms of location and precision in the reporting of clinical conditions. For example, the I-8 described all fractures (e.g., fracture of the femur), whereas the I-9 added the actual location of the fracture (top or bottom). Tumors of the large intestine could be identified, as well as whether there was an associated obstruction.

DRGs

The DRGs are a patient classification scheme that provides a means of relating the type of patient a hospital treats (also known as its *case mix*) to the costs incurred by the hospital. The DRGs lump "like" patients together. Patients are considered alike if they demonstrate similar resource utilization and **length of stay.** Resource utilization is defined by the product or personnel resources used to care for that type of patient. Product resources refer to diagnostic and therapeutic interventions such as use of medications, laboratory tests, radiology, and so on. Personnel costs refer to the use of nursing hours per case or other personnel. Length of stay refers to the number of days that the patient remains in the hospital (also known as *bed days*).

Major Diagnostic Categories

The DRGs are categorized into major diagnostic categories (MDCs). The number of DRGs in each MDC varies from 1 to 20 or more. The MDCs are consistent with anatomical or pathophysiological groupings and/or the ways in which patients would be clinically managed. Examples include diseases of the central nervous system, diseases of bone and cartilage, and diseases and disorders of the kidney and urinary tract. The major diagnostic categories are broken down into either medical or surgical, meaning the presence or absence of a surgical procedure.

Relative Weights and Case Mix Index

Each DRG is assigned a **relative weight.** Weights are based on length of stay and cost. The assigned weight is relative to the number 1, meaning that the number 1 represents a DRG class using an average amount of resources. The assigned weight is intended to reflect the relative resource consumption associated with each DRG. The higher the relative weight, the greater the payment to the hospital. DRGs with relative weights above 1.00 represent those of greater **case mix complexity** and the use of greater amounts of resources. Those with a relative weight that falls below 1.00 represent lower resource use and lesser complexity.

The weight assigned to the DRG for the hospital is based on the **case mix index (CMI).** The CMI is the sum of all DRG-relative weights divided by the number of cases (patients) cared for over a period, usually

one calendar year. The higher the CMI, the higher the assumed case mix complexity of the hospital. Case mix is affected by the following:

- Severity of illness
- Prognosis
- Treatment difficulty
- Need for intervention
- Resource intensity
- Presence of complications and comorbidities

Hospital payment is calculated by multiplying the CMI with the hospital's assigned base rate. Each hospital is assigned a base rate for reimbursement by the federal government, that is, the Centers for Medicare and Medicaid Services (CMS). The base rate is determined based on the specific hospital (teaching, academic, community), geographical location, population served, cost of living in that area, and types of services provided. CMI and base rates are reviewed periodically by the CMS and adjustments made as needed based on actuarial data.

Measuring the Elements in Case Mix

Severity of illness and prognosis reflect the complexity of services or the types of services provided. **Severity of illness** is made up of objective, clinical indicators of the patient's illness that reflect the need for hospitalization (Box 2-1). Prognosis indicates the patient's likelihood of recovering and to what extent. Treatment difficulty, need for intervention, and resource intensity comprise the **intensity of service** or the number of services per patient day or hospital stay (Box 2-2). The case mix influences hospital costs. It is not the number of patients that affects the costs incurred by the hospital but rather the types of patients and their use of resources. Table 2-1 presents some examples of the components of a Medicare DRG.

Assigning the DRG

Assignment of a DRG is made based on the documentation in the medical record. For the proper information

---

BOX 2-1   Severity of Illness Criteria

1. Clinical findings: chief complaints and working diagnosis identified on physical examination, direct observation, and patient interview
2. Vital signs: temperature, pulse, respiratory rate, and blood pressure
3. Imaging: diagnostic radiology, ultrasound, magnetic resonance imaging, and nuclear medicine results
4. Electrocardiogram (ECG)
5. Hematology, chemistry, and microbiology results
6. Other (clinical parameters not identified above)

BOX 2-2   Intensity of Service Criteria

1. Physician evaluation
2. Monitoring (those clinical elements requiring direct observation and monitoring)
3. Treatments/medications
4. Scheduled procedures
5. Presence of comorbidities

TABLE 2-1   Examples of the Components of a Medicare DRG (HCFA, 1995)

DRG	Description	Relative Weight	Mean LOS	Outlier
001	Craniotomy age >17 except for trauma	3.1565	13.5	32
90	Simple pneumonia and pleurisy age >17 without CC	0.6924	5.7	15

CC, Complication comorbidity; *LOS,* length of stay.

to be obtained the record must be comprehensive and complete. The documentation must be timely, legible, thorough, and proper.

The DRG assignment is made after discharge. Once that assignment has been made, the hospital receives one lump-sum payment based on the relative weight (Case Manager's Tip 2-1). Some DRGs are given a higher relative weight based on existing complications or comorbidities. **Complications** are defined as conditions occurring during the hospitalization that prolong the length of stay at least 1 day in 75% of the cases. **Comorbidities** are **preexisting conditions** that increase the length of stay about 1 day in 75% of the cases.

Outliers

Patients with atypically long or short lengths of stay are referred to as **outliers.** All other patients are considered

 CASE MANAGER'S TIP 2-1

Elements of DRGs
1. The DRG is assigned after discharge.
2. Payment to the hospital is made once the DRG has been assigned.
3. One lump-sum payment is made for:
   - DRGs with complications or comorbidities
   - Cost outlier payments

to be inliers. The placement of a patient as an outlier depends on the trim points for the DRG. Each DRG has a high length-of-stay trim. Some DRGs also have a short length-of-stay trim. Trim points are based on medical and statistical criteria and represent the lowest and highest average lengths of stay for the DRG (see components of a DRG, earlier in this chapter). Patients may also fall into a cost outlier category. These are patients who have fallen within the appropriate length of stay but who have used an exceptional amount of resources. This may be determined by a flat amount (such as $500) or by determining that the charges exceed the rate by at least 50%.

Managing the DRGs

In 1985 the PPS was advanced to allow some states to designate reimbursement rates for Medicaid and all other **third-party payers.** Based on hospitals' experiences with the Medicare DRGs and the advent of the system at the state level, strong incentives appeared for the control of hospital resources. Regardless of the cost incurred for caring for a particular case type, the hospital would still be reimbursed a fixed amount of money based on the coded DRG.

It was recognized rather quickly that the registered nurse (RN) could play a vital role in managing these dwindling healthcare dollars. The RN's role became increasingly important in terms of the following:
- Coordination of tests, treatments, and procedures
- Confirmation of physician orders
- Accurate documentation
- Timely admissions
- Necessary patient and family teaching
- Timely discharges

In the past, much of the care process had a life of its own, running its course to completion. There were few financial incentives to control the healthcare process; in fact, there were disincentives. In an FFS environment, longer lengths of stay and greater use of product resources translated into greater revenue and financial success for the hospital. The PPS changed all that. It became important to maximize the patient's hospital stay by coordinating the flow of patient care activities. This meant coordination of the patient's tests, treatments, and procedures so that delays could be avoided. Additional strategies included the confirmation of physician orders and/or questioning of their appropriateness when necessary. Getting the patient into the hospital on time and out of the hospital on time were other strategies for maximization.

Finally, documentation in the medical record, although always important, carried even greater weight under this system. Because reimbursement is contingent on the diagnoses and surgical procedures, charting must be complete and accurate. In some hospitals the utilization manager monitors the medical record documentation to ensure that it is accurate, timely, and reflective of what is currently happening in the case. Under case management this is often a role assigned to the case manager.

DRG Assignment

After discharge, the medical record coders review the patient's record. The DRG assignment requires a thorough accounting of the following:

- Principal diagnosis
- Secondary diagnosis
- Operating room procedures
- Complications
- Comorbidities
- Age
- Discharge status

The **principal diagnosis** (or primary diagnosis) is the condition determined to have been chiefly responsible for the admission to the hospital. The major diagnosis is that which consumed the most hospital resources. The principal diagnosis and the major diagnosis are not necessarily the same. The secondary diagnosis is the next priority in terms of resource consumption. **Principal procedures** are those performed to treat the chief complaint or complication rather than those performed for diagnostic purposes. If more than one procedure is performed, then the one most closely related to the principal diagnosis will become the principal procedure. Any other surgical procedures are considered as secondary. Operating room procedures other than those performed for diagnostic purposes are also considered as principal procedures. Complications and comorbidities, as defined previously, are also considered. Age is a determining factor for about one fifth of the DRGs. Age 65 is a demarcation line for some. For a small number of DRGs, the patient's **discharge status** is considered. Discharge status refers to the final patient destination after discharge, such as nursing home, home, or home with services.

In some cases the DRG is used for **per diem** rate setting. States with these rate-setting programs use the DRGs to adjust per diem rates. In addition, there are some DRG-exempt categories in some states. These may include the following:

- HIV/AIDS
- Psychiatry
- Pediatrics (if children's hospital)
- Other specialty hospitals (such as cancer hospitals)

Payments are calculated by multiplying the relative weight by the current reimbursement rate. The relative weight is determined by the final DRG coding. Short

---

BOX 2-3   Calculating Payments*

Example 1: Average Relative Weight
Payment = Relative weight × Current inlier rate
Payment = 1.0 × $1,000.00
Payment = $1,000.00

Example 2: Light Relative Weight
Payment = Relative weight × Current inlier rate
Payment = 0.5 × $1,000.00
Payment = $500.00

Example 3: Heavy Relative Weight
Payment = Relative weight × Current inlier rate
Payment = 22 × $1,000.00
Payment = $22,000.00

Example 4: Short-Stay Payments Before the Short-Trim Point
Short-trim point = 2 Days
Average length of stay = 5 Days
Relative weight = 1.0
Current inlier payment = $1,000.00
Each day's payment = 1.0 × 1,000.00/5 Days
Each day = $200.00
Patient stays in hospital 1 day
Payment = $200.00 × 150%
Payment = $300.00
Revenue loss = $700.00

Example 5: Outlier Payments Above the High-Trim Point
Outlier point = Day 20
Average length of stay = 10 Days
Relative weight = 2.0
Current inlier payment = $1,000.00
Payment = $2,000.00
Each day = $200.00
Patient stays 2 days
Payment = DRG payment + $200.00 × 60%
Payment = $2,000.00 + $120.00
Final payment = $2,120.00

*Figures are for example only; they do not reflect actual hospital reimbursements. $1,000.00 is used arbitrarily as the current inlier rate for the purpose of this illustration.

---

stays, or patients discharged below the short trim point, are paid at 150% of the daily rate. Outliers, those above the high trim point, are paid 60% of the daily rate for each day above (Box 2-3).

IMPACT OF DRGS ON THE HEALTHCARE INDUSTRY

In addition to the move toward case management after the institution of the DRG system, other changes have occurred in response to this reimbursement system.

Increased Number of Outpatient Procedures

For some low–relative-weight DRGs it is more financially lucrative for the hospital to treat patients on an outpatient basis. Generally the adjusted per diem rate will reimburse less than the DRG reimbursement but more than the short trim outlier payment. This financial incentive led many hospitals to open ambulatory or day surgery facilities, outpatient dialysis, and same-day surgery programs.

Reduced Length of Stay via Preoperative Testing, Home Healthcare, and Discharge Planning

The industry quickly realized that the management of the length of stay on the preadmission and postdischarge sides was extremely important. No longer could the focus be on the inpatient days only. Preoperative or preadmission testing departments were created to respond to these changes. The expense to the hospital and the reimbursement were greater if the hospital did as many tests before admission as possible. Conversely, the better the **discharge planning** process, as well as the availability of community-based programs, the sooner the patient could be discharged to a less-costly care setting.

USE OF DRGs TODAY

Today we find a mixture of reimbursement systems and schemes. Although more and more patients are being reimbursed under managed care contracts, which is the subject of the next section, others remain under either state or federal reimbursement systems. These systems continue to use the DRG as a measuring stick for either flat rates of reimbursement for the hospital stay or in negotiating discounted rates.

APCs: MEDICARE'S OUTPATIENT PROSPECTIVE PAYMENT SYSTEM

Years after the implementation of the inpatient PPS, the CMS, formerly the Health Care Financing Administration (HCFA), turned its attention to other care delivery settings across the continuum. It was only logical that great attention would be paid to ambulatory and outpatient settings, including ambulatory surgery, emergency departments (EDs), and clinics. As healthcare delivery shifted away from the acute care setting, more and more complex (and therefore more expensive) services were being provided in outpatient settings.

The Balanced Budget Act of 1997 (see p. 28) instructed CMS to develop and implement a PPS for hospital outpatient services. The September 1998 Federal Register published, in review form, the proposed form for the outpatient prospective payment system (OPPS), including the implementation regulations. Finally, in 1999, the Balanced Budget Refinement Act (BBRA) was passed and the OPPS was a go.

As a follow-up to the previous publication in the Federal Register, the final regulations were published in the April 2000 edition, including an expected implementation date of July 1, 2000. With such an ambitious implementation date, it was no surprise when CMS extended the deadline by 1 month to August 1, 2000.

APCs

The **ambulatory payment classification (APC) system** is an encounter-based patient classification system. The system approaches outpatient reimbursement from the same philosophical vantage point as the inpatient PPS. Similar groupings of patients are identified, and predetermined reimbursement amounts are allotted (Case Manager's Tip 2-2). The system attempts to predict the amount and type of resources used for a variety of types of ambulatory visits.

The initial program identified 451 ambulatory payment classification groups. Table 2-2 outlines the categories of APCs and the number of APCs in each category. The groups and payment rates are based on categories of services that are similar in cost and

 CASE MANAGER'S TIP 2-2

Comparing APCs and DRGs
1. APCs follow the same methodology as DRGs.
2. Similar groupings of patient types are prospectively identified with corresponding reimbursement amounts.
3. Unlike DRGs, a single outpatient encounter can result in the payment of one or more APCs.

TABLE 2-2 APC Groupings

Category	Number of APCs
Significant procedures	240
Medical visits	7
Ancillary	39
New technology	15
Transitional pass-through	132
Extensive pharmaceuticals	17
Partial hospitalization	1
Total	451

resource utilization. **Current Procedural Terminology** (CPT)-4 or Health Care Financing Administrators Common Procedure Coding System (HCPCS) codes are *mapped,* or identified with, an APC (see p. 29 for more detail on CPT codes). Each APC has an associated status indicator. The status indicator defines if and how a service will be paid. Some status indicators are paid under an APC, whereas others are not. In total, 936 new codes have been added; 645 of these are codes for billing pass-through and new technology items.

CMS has also identified certain procedures as "inpatient only." These are mainly surgeries that CMS has identified as requiring more services than can be provided in an outpatient setting. Hospitals must be very careful to ensure that patients are placed in the appropriate setting so that revenue is not lost (see Chapter 5).

Procedure APCs include surgical and nonsurgical procedures (see Table 2-2). Included under nonsurgical procedures are nuclear medicine, magnetic resonance imaging (MRI), radiation therapy, and psychotherapy.

Pass-through items include drugs, biologicals, and devices that can be claimed for reimbursement in addition to the APC payment if they meet certain criteria as set by CMS. Examples of these items would be pacemaker devices, cataract lenses, and cardiac catheterization lead wires.

In addition, certain services are packaged. Packaged services include the following:
- Operating room
- Recovery and treatment rooms
- Anesthesia
- Observation services
- Medical/surgical supplies
- Drugs and pharmaceuticals (with exceptions)
- Donor tissue
- Implantable devices

Exceptions to packaged services include the following:
- Drugs, pharmaceuticals, biologicals, and/or devices that are eligible for transitional pass-through payments
- Other specific services defined by CMS:
  - Corneal tissue acquisition
  - Casting, splinting, and strapping
  - Blood and blood products
  - Certain other high-cost drugs

It is important to note that, unlike the inpatient PPS in which only one DRG can be assigned to a hospital stay, under an OPPS, an outpatient visit may consist of multiple APCs. The total reimbursement equals the sum of the individual payments for each service. Therefore a single outpatient visit might include APC- as well as non–APC-related payments. The total of all of these will determine the final reimbursement.

BOX 2-4 Included Services

- Emergency department visits
- Clinic visits
- Surgical procedures
- Radiology
- Chemotherapy
- Most ancillary services
- Partial hospitalization program services

The Scope of the OPPS

OPPS applies to acute care hospitals and includes hospitals that are currently exempt from an inpatient PPS. Also included are partial hospitalization services provided by community mental health centers (CMHCs). Cancer centers that are exempted from the inpatient PPS are not exempt from OPPS, but they are held permanently harmless for payment reductions. Simply stated, this means that they must implement the same infrastructure for mapping and billing under the OPPS, but should their reimbursement be negatively affected, the reimbursement will be supplemented. Similarly, small rural hospitals of less than 100 beds will be held harmless, but only through 2003.

Box 2-4 lists the services included in the OPPS. Additionally, there are services that are excluded from OPPS (Box 2-5).

Clinics, Emergency Departments, and Critical Care Services

Clinic visits, ED visits, and critical care are assigned to one of seven Medical APC groups. Assignment into the APC is based on 31 Evaluation and Management (E & M) CPT-4 codes. Hospital-based clinics have three APCs, identified as low, medium, and high. Assignment into one of these would be based on the CPT-4 code identified. The ED also has three categories, identified as low, medium, and high, and these would also be identified based on the CPT-4 code. Critical care has one CPT (CPT 99291).

BOX 2-5 Excluded Services

- Ambulance services
- Rehabilitation therapy services
- Laboratory services paid under a fee schedule
- End-stage renal disease (routine dialysis services) and Epoetin (EPO)
- Services provided by critical access hospitals
- Durable medical equipment
- Orthotic/prosthetic devices
- Screening mammography

Observation Services

Under the new system, observation is no longer reimbursed separately but would be included as part of the APC payment, either ED or ambulatory surgery. Exceptions to this are congestive heart failure, asthma, and chest pain. Patients admitted to observation with one of these diagnoses are mapped to their own APC.

Mapping

Hospitals are required to develop their own internal system for "mapping" provided services to the different levels of resource utilization represented by the APC groupings. The process includes each hospital's own identification of which CPT-4 codes they would map into either the low, medium, or high APC groupings and then to derive computerized systems for linking the coding to the APC and, finally, to the billing.

HOME CARE PROSPECTIVE PAYMENT SYSTEM

On October 1, 2000, CMS implemented prospective payment for home care visits. Unlike inpatient PPS, home care's system would be based on a prospective nursing assessment completed at the time the patient was entered for home care services. Home care, like acute care before it, was no longer paid based on a visit. Care would be reimbursed for an episode of care or 60 days. The dollar amount reimbursed would be fixed regardless of the number of visits the patient received. The final dollar amount reimbursed is based on the **Outcome and Assessment Information Set (OASIS)** (Case Manager's Tip 2-3).

OASIS

Scores in the OASIS are based on three categories. The first category is clinical and consists of four items, the second category is functional and consists of five items, and the third category includes service utilization

 CASE MANAGER'S TIP 2-3

Understanding Home Care Prospective Payment System

1. Home Care PPS is the only prospective payment system that relies on a nursing assessment as the driver for reimbursement.
2. The Outcome and Assessment Information Set (OASIS) data must be accurate because this is what drives reimbursement.
3. HHRGs are similar to DRGs and APCs.

and consists of four items. The final score results in the assignment of 1 of 80 resource groups called **home health resource groups (HHRGs).** Like the DRGs, each HHRG has a dollar amount attached to it.

Initial Claims

Home care agencies can make an initial claim for payment known as an *advance request for payment (ARP)* at the time the initial OASIS assessment is completed. This initial payment equals 60% of the designated HHRG. One of home care's first challenges following the implementation of this new system was to be sure that claims were processed as quickly as possible after the first assessment (no greater than 48 hours). A rapid turnaround time would better ensure that cash flow problems did not occur.

The dollar amount reimbursed for the HHRG is calculated based on several factors. The payment rate corresponds to the level of home health services for that HHRG. The national payment rate for a 60-day episode of home healthcare services is standard and is then adjusted based on several factors. The standard amount is for all home health services, excluding **durable medical equipment,** and osteoporosis drugs will continue to be paid by a fee schedule. It is inclusive of the per-visit amounts for all disciplines, as well as nonroutine medical supplies and the cost of managing the OASIS process. The national payment rate is proportioned at 77.668% for labor and 22.332% for nonlabor. It is expected that the national rate ($2,037.04) will be adjusted at predetermined times to allow for changes in the cost of goods and services necessary to provide home health services. Adjustments will be made to this rate on a periodic basis.

Final Payment

The final claim is paid at the end of the episode and must include all line-item visit information that was rendered during the 60-day period

Adjustments

The national payment rate is adjusted for the case mix and the wage index area of the patient. The case mix payment rate is based on the level of home health services for the particular HHRG. Finally, an adjustment is made for the wage index for the area in which the patient lives. This is split by labor and nonlabor in the percentages previously mentioned (see Example on next page).

Partial Episode Payments

Similar to a short-trim point in the DRG system, CMS has allowed for situations in which the 60 days for home care

Example

Standard Prospective Payment Rate	$2,037.04
Case Mix Payment Rate for C0F050	×0.5265%
Case Mix Adjusted PPS Payment Amount	$1,072.50
Wage Index Adjustments	
Case Mix Adjusted PPS Payment Amount	$1,072.50
Labor Percentage of PPS Payment Rate	×0.77668%
Labor Portion	$832.99

The labor portion is then multiplied by the Wage Index Factor:

	$832.99
Wage Index Factor	×1.1 (example)
Adjusted Labor Portion	$916.29
Nonlabor Portion	
Case Mix Adjusted Amount	$1,072.50
Nonlabor Percentage	×0.2233%
Adjusted Nonlabor Portion	$239.49
Labor Portion	$916.29
Nonlabor Portion	+239.49
Total Case Mix and Wage Adjusted	
PPS Rate	$1,155.78

services are interrupted. These Partial Episode Payments (PEPs) occur under only two circumstances. The first would be when a patient elects to transfer from one home health agency to another. The second would be when a patient is discharged and then returns to the same agency within the 60-day period. The PEP would only apply if the transfer or discharge/return was not related to a significant change in the patient's condition. The reimbursable amount is prorated based on the number of days the patient was seen. For example, if the patient was seen for 15 of the 60 days, the PEP would be calculated as 15/60 multiplied by the full original payment amount.

Significant Change in Condition Payment

For circumstances in which the patient's condition results in a new OASIS, a new HHRG, and a new set of physician orders, CMS has established a special payment rate. The change must not have been originally expected and must signify an interruption in the 60-day episode and the plan of care. As in the PEP, a prorated amount would be determined. Of the 60 days, a partial amount would be paid at the original

Example

Original HHRG	20 days of 60 days	$1,155.78×0.33=	$381.40
SCIC HHRG	40 days of 60 days	$2,200.00×0.66=	$1,452.00
		(new HHRG reimbursement)	
		Total Reimbursement =	$1,833.40

HHRG level, and an additional payment would be made at the significant change in condition payment (SCIC) level.

Low-Utilization Payment

A low-utilization payment adjustment (LUPA) would be made for patients who require minimal visits during their 60-day episode. For patients who receive four or fewer visits during their 60-day encounter period, the home health agency will be paid based on the national standard per visit amount by discipline. These amounts are adjusted based on wage area index but not on case mix.

Outlier Payments

Finally, when unusual variations occur in the amount of medically necessary home health services, an outlier payment may be considered. These unusual variations are determined based on two principles: (1) that the cost of services should exceed the payment and (2) that the outlier payment should cover less than the total amount of cost above the outlier threshold.

The amount of the outlier payment is limited to 5% of the total PPS payment. The fixed dollar loss amount is now 1.13 times the standard episode amount.

Example

Standard Prospective Payment Rate	$2,037.04
Fixed Dollar Loss Amount	$2,037.04×1.13=$2,301.86
Case Mix Adjusted PPS Payment Amount	+1,072.50
Outlier Threshold Total Amount	$3,374.36

Important Points to Consider

Under the home care PPS, the old paradigm of more visits, more incurred cost, more Medicare reimbursement is now extinct. Under PPS it is essential to coordinate the clinical and financial aspects of the agency. In other words, it is imperative that the patient receive the appropriate number of visits by the appropriate clinicians but that those visits not be in excess of the patient's true clinical needs.

In addition, the OASIS data must be accurate and timely because this is what drives reimbursement. Going forward, home care agencies, like hospitals before them, will need to identify their costs on an HHRG basis. This data will serve as the benchmark for identifying areas of profit and loss for the agency and lead to new product lines, elimination of old ones, or improvement in resource utilization for existing patient groups.

Home health agencies need to implement strategies similar to those applied in the acute care setting. For example, implementation of clinical **practice guidelines** will help to prospectively identify the expected resources to be applied to various case types and to standardize the care for that group of patients. Strategies such as this will better ensure that patients receive just the right amount of resources: not too much and not too little. Case managers will be deployed to manage high-risk populations who have a greater likelihood of falling outside the norms of the clinical practice guidelines. Because of the variation in these high-risk groups, it can be assumed that they will have a greater likelihood of using excess resources if not proactively managed.

Identification of these high-risk groups will have to be made based on high-risk assessment strategies so that patients can be immediately identified and the case manager can be deployed as quickly as possible. The OASIS data may provide the foundation for much of the data that will be necessary to identify patients at greater risk for poor outcomes or greater resource utilization.

INPATIENT REHABILITATION FACILITY PROSPECTIVE PAYMENT SYSTEM

Among its other mandates, the Balanced Budget Act of 1997 mandated prospective payment for inpatient or acute rehabilitation effective January 1, 2002. This new reimbursement scheme replaces the prior reimbursement structure as directed by TEFRA in 1982. TEFRA mandated the CMS regulations for Medicare reimbursement, Medicare **health maintenance organizations (HMOs),** and risk contracts.

Reimbursement is based on patient assessment forms completed on admission to and discharge from the acute rehabilitation unit (Case Manager's Tip 2-4). The assessment form, the **Inpatient Rehabilitation Facilities Patient Assessment Instrument (IRF-PAI),** contains 54 data items and takes approximately 45 minutes to complete.

The admission assessment reference date is calendar day 3 of stay. Completion date is calendar day 4. The

 CASE MANAGER'S TIP 2-4

Elements of the Acute Inpatient Rehabilitation Prospective Payment System

1. Acute rehabilitation uses case mix groups (CMGs) that function just like the DRGs and APCs.
2. This classification is based on the data in the Inpatient Rehabilitation Facilities Patient Assessment Instrument (IRF-PAI).

discharge assessment reference date is day of discharge or death. Completion date is calendar day 4 after discharge/death.

The IRF-PAI

The PAI is used to classify patients into distinct groups based on clinical characteristics and expected resource needs. Patients are classified as follows:
- First, patients are assigned to 1 of 21 **rehabilitation impairment categories (RICs).**
- Second, patients are classified into 1 of 100 distinct **case mix groups (CMGs).**

Completion of the PAI requires a skilled assessor. It cannot be completed by clerical staff but must be completed by a qualified clinician such as a physician, RN, or physical or occupational therapist. Therefore many organizations use RN case managers to complete the PAI, which contains physician, nursing therapy, and other care elements. In this way the case manager can complete the PAI and perform other case management functions so critical to financial survival under this system, such as monitoring of **resource utilization,** cost per case, and length of stay.

Each CMG has a relative weight that determines the base payment rate the IRF will receive. Included in the payment rates are the operating costs and capital costs of furnishing covered inpatient rehabilitation hospital services, including routine, ancillary, and capital costs. Not included are the costs of bad debts or approved educational activities.

Payment Adjustments

Payment may be adjusted for the following reasons:
- Labor share percentage, area wage index, disproportionate share, and rural factors
- Comorbidities present during the patient's stay

Although the admission assessment will be used to place a patient into a CMG, the discharge assessment is used to determine the relevant weighting factors associated with any existing comorbidities.

The short-stay category contains only one CMG. For patients who have expired there are the following four CMGs:
- Orthopedic, short-stay
- Orthopedic, regular stay
- Nonorthopedic, short-stay
- Nonorthopedic, regular stay

Method of Payment

A standardized amount per discharge is adjusted based on case mix, disproportionate share hospital (DSH), and a rural hospital add-on of 15.89%. Other adjustments include high-cost outlier payments. Transfer cases are

Example

CMG Relative Weights for RIC 03: Nontraumatic Brain Injury

CMG	Description	CMG Weight	Payment	Comorbidity Add-On	Payment with Comorbidity Add-On
0301	M=33-0 and C=22-35	0.6399	$3,855	12.6%	$4,342
0302	M=33-0 and C=5-21	0.8393	$5,056	12.6%	$5,695
0303	M=46-34	0.9467	$5,703	12.6%	$6,424
0304	M=56-47	1.2605	$7,593	12.6%	$8,553
0305	M=78-57	1.7517	$10,552	12.6%	$11,886

C, Cognitive; M, motor.

reimbursed at a per diem rate. Interrupted stays, defined as cases in which the beneficiary returns to the inpatient rehabilitation facility by midnight of the third day after a discharge, are reimbursed as a single discharge. Payment is based on the CMG classification determined from the initial PAI assessment.

Three-Step Process

Calculating the reimbursement encompasses a three-step process. First the patient is assigned to an RIC. Within the RIC, the patient is assigned to a CMG. Within the CMG, the patient is designated as either having or not having a relevant comorbidity. Relevant comorbidities are represented by codes.

The 21 RICs represent the primary cause of the rehabilitation stay. The RICs are clinically homogeneous. See the example at the top of the page.

Conversion Factor

As in the inpatient DRG system, each CMG is assigned a relative weight. Weights represent the variance in the cost per discharge and resource utilization among payment groups. Basic payment in 2001 was $6,024, and from that, each CMG payment was based on the relative weight multiplied by the payment amount.

Short-Stay Cases

There is one relative weight for short-stay cases. Short-stay cases are defined as patients with a length of stay of less than or equal to 3 days who do not meet the definition of a transfer case; for example, patients who leave against medical advice or patients who

are unable to tolerate intensive rehabilitation services. See the example below.

Expired Patients

Relative weights have also been identified for patients who have expired.

Wage Index

The hospital location will determine the classified wage index. The rate excludes 100% of wages for teaching physicians, interns and residents, and nonphysician anesthesiologists. The wage adjustment is to the labor-related portion of the payment only. The labor portion is 71.301%, and the nonlabor portion is 28.699% of the rate.

The disproportionate patient percentage (DPP) is calculated as Medicare supplemental security income (SSI) days (as a percentage of total Medicare days) plus Medicaid days (as a percentage of total days).

Outlier Cases

Additional payments are made for high-cost patients. These are calculated based on 80% of the case loss exceeding a deductible. Loss is determined by charges multiplied by the overall facility-specific ratio of cost-to-charges (RCC) minus the IRF PPS payment. The deductible, also known as the *threshold,* is $7,066 multiplied by the wage index, multiplied by the DSH adjustment. Outlier payments can be attributed to 3% to 5% of total program payments.

Transfer Cases

Transfer cases are those with a length of stay less than the arithmetic mean length of stay for the relevant

Example

CMG Relative Weight for Short-Stay Cases

CMG	Description	CMG Weight	Payment Add-On	Comorbidity	Payment with Comorbidity Add-On
5001	Short-stay cases (LOS≤3 days)	0.1908	$1,149	0.0%	$1,149

LOS, Length of stay.

CMG. Transfer cases would include those that were discharged to another inpatient site of care, such as an inpatient hospital, long-term care hospital, rehabilitation facility, or nursing home that accepts Medicare and/or Medicaid. Discharges to home health, outpatient therapy, or day programs are not considered as transfer cases.

Payment is based on a per diem inlier payment, which is divided by the mean length of stay for the CMG, multiplied by the number of actual days, plus an outlier payment. Unlike inpatient prospective payment systems, the first day is reimbursed only one per diem.

LONG-TERM CARE REIMBURSEMENT (SKILLED NURSING FACILITY)

Under the Balanced Budget Act of 1997, CMS implemented a PPS for services provided to nursing home residents during a Medicare Part A–covered stay. Implemented on July 1, 1998, PPS rates reimburse for routine, ancillary, and capital-related costs.

Residents of the nursing home are assessed on a schedule at certain points during their stay (on the fifth, fourteenth, thirtieth, sixtieth, and ninetieth days after admission to the skilled nursing facility [SNF]). Unlike inpatient rehabilitation, SNFs have a window in which to perform each assessment. As an example, a Day 14 assessment can have a reference date of Days 6, 7, 8, 9, 10, 11, 12, 13, or 14. Additional assessments would be required when a resident experiences a significant change in status or care needs.

The **Minimum Data Set (MDS)** is the assessment tool used in the SNF setting. The MDS collects comprehensive information, which includes the patient diagnosis, activities of daily living (ADLs) capabilities, cognition, and minutes per day of rehabilitation services received. The exception to this is the Day 5 assessment, which requests information regarding estimated rehabilitation minutes.

Based on the data captured in the MDS, the patient is placed into one of 44 **Resource Utilization Group** III (RUG-III) categories (Case Manager's Tip 2-5). Each MDS assigned is "locked-in" within 7 days of completion of the MDS and cannot be changed. Each RUG is assigned

 CASE MANAGER'S TIP *2-5*

Long-Term Care Reimbursement
1. The Resource Utilization Group III (RUG III) determines the reimbursement amount.
2. The RUG is selected based on the data in the Minimum Data Set (MDS).

TABLE 2-3 The RUG III System

Clinical Hierarchy	Activities of Daily Living	Problem/Service Split	Number of RUG Groups
Automatically Deemed Medicare Covered			
Rehabilitation Ultra-high Very high High Medium Low	14 Levels	Not used	14 RUGs
Extensive services	Not used	Various types of services	3 RUGs
Special care	3 Levels	Not used	3 RUGs
Clinically complex	3 Levels	Signs of depression	6 RUGs
Medicare Covered Based on Skilled Nursing Facility Guidelines			
Impaired cognition	2 Levels	Nursing rehabilitation	4 RUGs
Behavioral problems	2 Levels	Nursing rehabilitation	4 RUGs
Reduced physical function	5 Levels	Nursing rehabilitation	10 RUGs

a case mix weight, which is used to adjust the federal portion of the SNF's reimbursement for that resident.

The RUG-III system (Table 2-3) classifies patients into seven major clinical hierarchies and 44 groups. The RUG-III grouper, a computer software program, will classify the patient into the group with the highest payment. The seven major hierarchies are rehabilitation, extensive services, special care, clinically complex, impaired cognition, behavioral problems, and reduced physical function. A patient who classifies into a lower category may be covered if the coverage guidelines of the SNF are met.

GOVERNMENT PROGRAMS
Medicare

In 1966 the federal government enacted Title XVIII of the Social Security Act. Known as the *Medicare program,* it was designed to finance medical care for persons age 65 years and older and disabled persons who are entitled to Social Security benefits (Case Manager's Tip 2-6). Medicare also covers individuals with end-stage renal disease. Disabled individuals and those under age 65 with end-stage renal disease make up approximately 12% of Medicare beneficiaries.

The Medicare program is a federal program under the administrative oversight of CMS. CMS is a branch of the United States Department of Health and Human Services (DHHS).

CASE MANAGER'S TIP 2-6

Government Programs—Medicare

1. Medicare finances healthcare for the following:
   a. Persons over 65
   b. Disabled persons
2. Part A covers hospitalization.
3. Part B is a voluntary program covering physician services and emergency visits, among others.

Medicare's Dual Structure

Medicare consists of two parts. Part A is a hospital or acute care insurance program. Included in Part A are the following:

- Inpatient hospital
- Skilled nursing
- Home health
- Hospice
- Administrative expenses

Part A is financed by special payroll taxes collected under the Social Security program. Employer and employee share equally in financing this portion of the Social Security income known as the *hospital insurance trust fund*. The amount an individual contributes to this fund is distinctly identified on an employee's pay stub. This mandatory tax is paid by all working individuals, including those who are self-employed.

OBRA-93

The Omnibus Budget Reconciliation Act of 1993 (OBRA-93) eliminated the maximum taxable earnings base so that as of 1993, all earnings are now subject to Medicare tax. Despite OBRA, there still remains concern that the Hospital Insurance Trust Fund may eventually run out of money. Debates continue to focus on precisely when this may happen and as to whether the Fund should be financially supplemented in some other way. Some politicians have suggested that the minimum age to receive Medicare be increased to age 70.

Overview of Services

A maximum of 90 days of inpatient hospital care is allowed per benefit period. Once the 90 days are exhausted, there is a lifetime reserve of 60 hospital inpatient days. A benefit period is a spell of illness beginning with hospitalization and ending when a **beneficiary** has not been an inpatient in a hospital or SNF for 60 consecutive days. There is no limit to the number of benefit periods.

The beneficiary pays a **deductible** for each benefit period and **copayments** based on the duration of services.

Medicare pays for up to 100 days of care in a Medicare-certified SNF, provided that the beneficiary has been hospitalized for at least 3 consecutive days, not including the day of discharge. Admission to the SNF must occur within 30 days of hospital discharge.

Medicare pays for home healthcare when a person is homebound and requires intermittent or part-time skilled nursing care or rehabilitation care. There are no time or visit limits. For terminally ill patients, Medicare pays for care provided by a Medicare-certified hospice.

Supplementary Medical Insurance Part B

The **Supplementary Medical Insurance (SMI)** program is a voluntary program financed partly by general tax revenues and partly by required premium contributions. The main services covered by SMI include the following:

- Physician services
- Hospital outpatient services such as outpatient surgery, diagnostic tests, and radiology and pathology services
- ED visits
- Outpatient rehabilitation services
- Renal dialysis
- Prosthetics
- Medical equipment and supplies
  Services not covered by SMI include the following:
- Vision care and eyeglasses
- Outpatient prescription drugs
- Routine physical examinations
- Preventive services
  Exceptions for Part B Enrollees are as follows:
- Screening Pap smears
- Mammography
- Flu shots and vaccinations against pneumonia

Managed Medicare

In September of 1982, the laws treating Medicare HMOs were passed as part of TEFRA. The regulations became effective in 1985. In 1982 CMS funded several demonstration contracts to test the concepts of risk HMOs. These were known as the *Medicare competition demonstration projects*. These operated under a variety of waivers as part of the Social Security Act. By 1985 there were about 300,000 members enrolled out of a total of about 30 million Medicare beneficiaries. By 1995 nearly 3 million Medicare members had enrolled in TEFRA-risk HMOs.

TEFRA also modified the HMO contracting rules to permit CMS to contract with a new type of entity known as the *comprehensive medical plan (CMP)*. A CMP is defined as an entity that is state licensed, provides healthcare on a prepaid capitated basis, provides care through physicians who are employees or partners of the entity, assumes full financial risk on a prospective basis, and meets the Public Health Service Act requirements against insolvency. Today these differences between HMOs and CMPs no longer exist.

Requirements to Obtain a TEFRA Contract

A nonrural plan must have a minimum of 5,000 prepaid members, and rural plans a minimum of 1,500 members. At all times during the contract, membership cannot exceed 50% combined Medicare and Medicaid.

The entity must be able to render (or contract for) all Medicare services available in the service area. In addition, it must use certified Medicare providers and be able to provide 24-hour emergency services. Other requirements include provisions for emergency **claims** both within and out of network. All services must be accessible within reasonable promptness.

The HMO must provide all of the Medicare Part A and Part B services that a recipient would receive as available in his or her area. The HMO may provide additional services not traditionally covered under Medicare as additional and covered services or as optional supplemental services that the patient may choose to subscribe to (Case Manager's Tip 2-7). In some instances, additional benefits must be purchased as a condition of enrollment. For example, preventive care, not traditionally covered under Medicare but covered by HMOs, would be financed by mandatory **premiums.** Some HMOs opt to provide additional services beyond the traditional scope of Medicare at no cost to the patient.

Benefits to Enrollees

Medicare beneficiary enrollment in HMOs has been slow. Portions of the country see greater enrollment than others. Correlations can be found between highly **managed care** penetrated areas and the percent of Medicare **enrollees** who have opted for HMO plans. It should also be noted that not all areas offer HMO products to Medicare recipients. Some of the attractions of enrolling include lower out-of-pocket expenses. Some waive the plan premium, which includes the Medicare **coinsurance** and deductible payments. Most provide additional non-Medicare benefits such as prescription

CASE MANAGER'S TIP 2-7

Government Programs—Managed Medicare

1. Managed Medicare is an option afforded to Medicare enrollees.
2. The HMO must provide all the Medicare Part A and Part B services that a recipient would normally receive in his or her area.

drugs (to a capped amount per year), eyeglasses, and hearing aids.

Resistance to **enrollment** often has to do with an older person's longstanding relationship with his or her physician. In general, managed care concepts are not familiar to the senior population and therefore some may not realize that the HMO may offer higher coverage at a lower cost.

Medicaid

The Medicaid program is referred to as *Title XIX* of the Social Security Act and finances healthcare for the indigent. Started in 1966, the program is jointly financed by the federal and state governments (Case Manager's Tip 2-8). The federal government provides matching funds to the states based on the per-capita income in each state. Federal matching, known as the *Federal Medical Assistance Percentage (FMAP),* cannot be less than 50% or greater than 83% of total state Medicaid costs. Wealthier states have a smaller share of their costs reimbursed by the federal government, and federal outlays have no set limit. The federal government must match whatever the individual state provides.

The federal government also shares in the state's expenditures for administration of the program. Most administrative costs are matched at 50%. Each state administers its own Medicaid program. Eligibility criteria, covered services, and payments to providers vary from state to state.

Federal law mandates that every state provide some specific healthcare services. The mandated services include the following:

- Hospital inpatient care
- Hospital outpatient services
- Physician's services
- Laboratory and x-ray services
- SNF care
- Home health services for those eligible for SNF services
- Prenatal care
- Family planning services and supplies
- Rural health clinic services
- Medical services for dependent children under age 21
- Nurse-midwife services
- Certain federally qualified ambulatory and health center services

CASE MANAGER'S TIP 2-8

Government Programs—Medicaid

Medicaid finances healthcare for the indigent and is funded through the tax structure.

In addition to the mandated services, each state has the option of providing the following additional services:

- Prescription drugs
- Optometrist services
- Eyeglasses
- Dental care

States may impose nominal deductibles and copayments on some Medicaid recipients for certain services. Some services are exempt from copayment. These include emergency services, family planning services and supplies, and hospice care.

Eligibility Criteria

Eligibility criteria are based on income and assets. These criteria vary from state to state. Certain individuals are automatically covered if they are already receiving SSI, which includes many of the elderly, the blind and disabled, and families with children receiving support under an "aid to families with dependent children" program.

From the inception of the Medicaid program, there have been problems. The population of Medicaid recipients is composed of mainly women and children under age 18. This population of individuals requires a narrow range of healthcare services, mainly including obstetrical, prenatal, and well-child care. Members of this population have specific problems unique to their social situation, such as transportation issues, and they are more likely to be vulnerable to impoverished lifestyles, especially in urban areas. This type of lifestyle exposes them to violence, inferior living conditions, substance abuse, and other social problems related to poverty and inadequate living situations.

In addition, many healthcare providers have been reticent to care for the Medicaid population because of the low payment rates. This results in additional access issues. Many Medicaid recipients continue to use emergency rooms as their major source of primary care. This is referred to as the *Medicaid syndrome* and further results in additional expenditures in the ambulatory and inpatient settings (Hurley, Freund, and Paul, 1993).

Managed Medicaid

Traditionally, managed care organizations (MCOs) have not embraced Medicaid. HMOs that moved into this arena in the 1980s tended to provide services to select and small populations to have some greater amount of assurance that they might not experience excessive financial losses. Nevertheless, in recent years many states have turned their attention to managed care for their Medicaid populations (Case Manager's Tip 2-9). For example, Arizona enacted legislation that would

CASE MANAGER'S TIP 2-9

Government Programs—Managed Medicaid
1. An option for Medicaid recipients
2. Although Medicaid is mandatory in some states, it is still optional in others.

provide healthcare to the poor using what were described as alternative healthcare systems that used strategies such as cost containment, improved patient access, and quality care in managed care settings. Arizona was the first state to implement such a statewide program. Other states, such as New York and Virginia, used an incremental approach to enrolling Medicaid beneficiaries.

It was expected that organized services using modalities such as managed care would serve to address some of the inherent problems associated with the Medicaid program, such as overutilization of emergency rooms and issues of access. Focus was placed on primary care as a mechanism for managing cost and resource utilization. Inherent problems occurred as a result of the population itself. Medicaid participants can be transitory, entering and leaving the program as their income eligibility changes over time. The population generally cannot afford the traditional copayments and penalties for using out-of-network services associated with participation in managed care, thus raising the overall cost for the MCO. An inability to control resource utilization through economic incentives provided unusual challenges to MCOs.

It is unknown whether provider satisfaction is improved through participation in managed care. In addition, it has appeared that overall reductions in ED use have not been achieved. On a positive note, there tends to be more use of primary care physicians as opposed to specialists. This comes more as a result of changes in physicians' practice patterns and less as a result of changes in the behavior of the patients themselves.

In the future, HMOs will need to adjust their administration of these plans to the Medicaid population, who presents with challenges unique and different from the *commercial* populations. These individuals, with complex medical and social needs, require different approaches to those traditionally employed from healthy populations in commercial products.

Balanced Budget Act of 1997

The Balanced Budget Act of 1997 (BBA) was signed into law in August of 1997 by President Clinton. Titled Public Law 105-33, it enacted the most extensive changes to the Medicare and Medicaid programs since their inception in the 1960s. These changes will do the following:

- Extend the life of the Medicare Trust Fund and reduce Medicare spending
- Increase healthcare options available to seniors
- Improve benefits for staying healthy (prevention)
- Fight Medicare fraud and abuse
- Look at ways to help Medicare work well in the future

In addition to the significant changes the Act made to the government healthcare programs, it also enacted changes to the Child Health Insurance Program (CHIP) (Title XXI). CHIP expands block grants to states, increasing their Medicaid eligibility for low-income and uninsured children. Through CHIP, states are given the autonomy to set up their own programs. States must match the federal grant monies for each 3-year period that they are awarded. The success of CHIP will depend to a great extent on the ability of the states to identify and enroll eligible children. Therefore primary care and outreach become critical to its success. It is predicted that states that do not provide for adequate outreach and therefore do not enroll adequate numbers of children into CHIP may be at risk for some of the grant funding to be rescinded.

The BBA and the Case Manager

Case managers should stay current in all issues related to not only the BBA but all changes in healthcare legislation. In this chapter many of the most important changes in the Act have been reviewed as they relate to the new reimbursement structures implemented in the new prospective payment systems. Additional information on the BBA, as well as any of the payment structures discussed in this chapter, can be obtained through the Centers for Medicare and Medicaid Services Web site: http://www.hcfa.gov/rregs/bbaupdat.htm. The most current information available can always be found at this and similar sites (Case Manager's Tip 2-10).

CPT Codes and ICD-9-CM Codes

Case managers need to be familiar with both the ICD-9-CM and the CPT code systems. ICD-9-CM

(American Medical Association, 1996), is used for coding inpatient medical records. In addition, CPT is also used. CPT is a listing of descriptive terms and identifying codes for reporting medical services and procedures performed by physicians. The terminology provides a uniform language that accurately describes medical, surgical, and diagnostic services. By using this coding system, there is a reliable nationwide communication system among physicians, patients, and third-party payers. CPT codes define medical, surgical, and diagnostic procedures. ICD-9-CM codes are used for medical interventions.

THIRD-PARTY PAYERS/MANAGED CARE ORGANIZATIONS

Like it or not, the healthcare system has taken on a brand new shape. Most healthcare institutions are scurrying to learn how to reduce their costs without reducing their quality.

Managed care has taken on many meanings over the past several years. It has grown to mean different things to different people. Business executives, financial controllers, healthcare providers, and payers are viewing managed care as a means of reducing skyrocketing healthcare costs (Case Manager's Tip 2-11). Healthcare institutions may view it as the mechanism for negotiating better discounted rates for the care of their patients, but only if they can attract a larger volume of patients to their institution. To the physician base it probably seems like an external control over their previously unstandardized methods and treatment modalities. It is probably the patient who views managed care as a protective mechanism that helps keep healthcare costs down while maintaining quality services. However, this may not be as such, considering consumers' concerns about the occurring denials of services by MCOs.

Before a discussion can take place about managed care, it is important to understand and be well versed in

CASE MANAGER'S TIP 2-10

Balanced Budget Act

Case managers can stay current on the Balanced Budget Act (BBA) and other CMS updates by logging on to http://www.hcfa.gov/rregs/bbaupdat.htm or http://www.hcfa.gov to access current information related to reimbursement.

CASE MANAGER'S TIP 2-11

Diversity of Managed Care Plans and Services

Managed care is both a type of health insurance and a type of healthcare delivery system; that is, it focuses on both delivery and reimbursement of healthcare services. The intensity of the managed care services provided varies widely based on the type of health plan and the type of reimbursement method applied. The involvement of case management also differs based on the degree and complexity of the managed services offered to the consumers or demanded by the payers.

CASE MANAGER'S TIP 2-12

Understanding Types of Health Insurance and Terminology

It is important for a case manager to understand the basic types of health insurance plans and the related terminology to better serve the patient and to help provide the appropriate healthcare services in accordance with a patient's insurance benefits.

---

health insurance in general (Case Manager's Tip 2-12). Health insurance is the protection one seeks to provide **benefits** for an illness or injury. A person, group, or employer pays a price (called a *premium* in managed care terminology) for protection from the potential expenses that could be incurred during an illness or injury. Lack of insurance coverage can mean going without needed healthcare, having to settle for lower-quality healthcare, or having to *pay out of pocket*—your own pocket—for healthcare. The insurance company gambles that it will take in much more in the way of premiums than it will pay out to the insured as a result of illnesses. The contract a person negotiates states the nature of the *benefits* or the *coverage* that is available. It also lists the conditions under which the insurer will cover expenses, either in part or, less commonly, in full. *Deductibles* and copayments are those expenses the insured will be responsible for before and after the insurance **carrier** pays its portion of any medical bills.

The prominent types of health insurance are *group* and *individual* coverage. Group insurance is usually provided by an employer or professional organization to which one belongs. Employee group coverage is usually offered to spouses and dependents in addition to the employee. These policies vary from place to place and from one insurance company to another. Commercial or for-profit insurance companies dominate the group type of coverage. Individual health insurance is sometimes referred to as *personal* insurance. These policies also vary from provider to provider, and their premiums are often more expensive than group policies. Individuals may purchase individual insurance to supplement their group policy in areas that they identify as gaps in benefits (Enteen, 1992).

Currently the fastest-growing coverage option in the healthcare industry is the ***prepaid health plan***—commonly known as HMOs and **preferred provider organizations (PPOs).** In addition, government-paid coverage (i.e., Medicare, Medicaid, and veteran coverage) has recently undergone much scrutiny regarding its continued financial viability. These policies usually offer coverage for hospital expenses, surgical expenses, physician's expenses, and major medical (major illness or injury expenses). A person can also elect to pay larger premiums to supplement the basic plan for items not covered, such as home care benefits or durable medical equipment (Enteen, 1992).

It is important to discuss each type of insurance plan in more detail before moving on to an explanation of managed care. Each type of insurance plan has its advantages and disadvantages, and each is in such a state of flux that it is difficult to keep current and accurate on the various benefits. Definitions of each type of insurance as it is currently offered follow, but it is important to remember that managed care reform can affect these definitions at any time.

HMOs Versus PPOs

Because HMOs and PPOs are the most commonly confused managed care products, it is helpful to detail them more fully. An HMO is a state licensed entity that agrees by contract to provide medical services on a prepaid, capitated basis. It is an **indemnity** plan that delivers comprehensive, coordinated medical services to an enrolled membership in a defined geographical location on a prepaid basis. There are four main models of HMOs: **group model, individual practice association (IPA), network model** (health plan), and **staff model.** Different variations of these models are also available in certain locations of the country. Today there are more HMO models than the four traditional types just mentioned. Examples are open access, closed access, or mixed-type models.

Group Model HMO

A group model HMO contracts with multispecialty physicians organized in a partnership, corporation, or association. The physicians are not employed directly by the HMO but are employed directly by the group practice. The plan compensates the medical group for services they have contracted at a negotiated rate, and the group is then responsible for compensating its physicians and for contracting with healthcare providers for their patients. The HMO and the group thus share in the risk. Physicians in the group practice may be allowed to see HMO and non-HMO patients, although they are primarily available to provide services to the HMO patients.

There are two types of group model HMOs: captive group and independent group. The captive group exists solely to provide services to the HMO's beneficiaries. In most cases the HMO creates the group for that purpose and provides it with administrative services and oversight. An example of this HMO type is the Permanente Medical Group of the Kaiser Foundation Health Plan (Kongstvedt, 2001). In the independent group model HMO, the group is already in existence, and the HMO contracts with it to provide physician services to its members. The group is responsible for all administrative functions and the operations of the group practice. An example of this type is the Geisinger Health Plan in Danville, Pennsylvania (Kongstvedt, 2001).

Individual/Independent Practice Association

An HMO can also contract with an IPA to provide healthcare services for a negotiated fee. The IPA then contracts with physicians who practice in their individual or group practices. These physicians usually care for HMO and non-HMO patients and keep control and responsibility over the way their offices are run. The IPA compensates the physicians on a **fee schedule** or an FFS basis. Generally, IPAs recruit physicians of different specialties to participate in their plans. This makes their services more desirable and cost-efficient because they are able to provide a wide array of services within the IPA. In turn, this diversity in services makes the IPA more attractive to an HMO. IPA model HMOs are either exclusive or nonexclusive. They are exclusive in providing services to the HMO's beneficiaries if they were created by the HMO. If they were already in existence and contracted with the HMO, they often are not limited in their clients to the HMO's beneficiaries.

Network Model HMO

If the HMO contracts with more than one physician group practice, it is referred to as a *network health plan*. In this arrangement the physicians do not necessarily provide care exclusively to the HMO. The network model HMO, similar to the group practice, consists of physicians from a multitude of specialties. An example of this type is Health Insurance Plan of Greater New York. If an HMO contracts with groups of **primary care providers,** this forms a primary care network HMO. Other variations of the network model HMO are closed and open panels. A closed network panel is usually limited to contracts with a small group of already existing group practices, whereas in an open network panel, participation in the group practice is open to interested physicians who meet the HMO **credentialing** criteria (Kongstvedt, 2001).

Staff Model HMO

The last HMO model is the staff model. In this type the physicians are employed by the HMO to provide healthcare services to its beneficiaries. The physicians are paid a salary and are offered various incentive programs based on their performance and productivity. Physicians in this model are also of different specialties so that the HMO is able to meet the needs of its beneficiaries. Administrative functions of this model are the responsibility of the HMO. For rare services or specialties, the HMO may contract with independent specialty groups available in the community. The staff model HMO is also known as a *closed model* because participation of physicians is limited to those employed by the HMO. An interesting feature of the staff model HMO is that the HMO exerts a great degree of control over the physicians' practice.

HMOs in general are a good example of the **gatekeeper** model, in which a primary care provider is responsible for authorizing all specialist referrals. This serves to control costs and resource consumption.

PPOs

PPOs are generally neither state licensed nor federally qualified. They function as brokers by offering discounted healthcare services either directly to employers or to third-party payers. Under a PPO agreement, a limited number of providers are contracted as part of the network. The PPO provides this limitation in the size of the **panel of providers,** almost similar to an **incentive,** in return for the agreement of participating providers/physicians to abide by its utilization and resource management practices. Typically, capitation and other risk-bearing payment arrangements with providers are not used in PPOs compared with HMOs, where such payment structures are usually the norm.

Members of PPOs are encouraged to use the physicians and services of the PPO; however, they are permitted to go outside the network for their healthcare if necessary. In this case, members are held responsible for a copayment or higher levels of cost sharing compared with staying within the network. Those members who do elect to use out-of-network services may be reimbursed at a lower rate than those who remain within the network. Therefore there is incentive for subscribers to remain in the network because those providers will be offering their services at a discounted rate as part of the PPO. Those cost savings are passed on to the consumer. There is a further incentive to employers to contract with a PPO as a means of reducing overall healthcare costs for their employees. PPOs have become more popular than HMOs because their enrollees are less restricted regarding their choice of providers. Table 2-4 summarizes important differences between the two types of healthcare plans: HMOs and PPOs.

TABLE 2-4 Summary of HMO and PPO Characteristics

Types	Flexibility	Premiums	Reimbursement	Rates	Provider Risks
HMO	Must remain in network; less choice of providers	Prepaid; capitated	Not reimbursed out of network	Usually capitated; for-profit or not-for-profit	High incentive to control costs; high risk sharing
PPO	Less restrictive; more choice of providers	Fee-for-service; not prepaid	Covers services out of network	Not usually capitated	Low incentive to control costs; less financial risk sharing

MANAGED CARE AND ITS STAGES OF DEVELOPMENT/MATURATION

There had been an evolution of the healthcare market as it matured into the managed care environment. Managed care can be defined as a system of healthcare delivery aimed at managing and balancing the cost, risk, and quality of access to healthcare. It is both an industry and a process. Ultimately, managed care is nothing more than a range or spectrum of activities designed to control the means by which healthcare is delivered. It is used by HMOs and PPOs to improve the delivery of services and contain costs (Mullahy, 1998; Kongstvedt, 2001). This so-called evolution has been mapped out and studied by many economists, consulting firms, and healthcare experts and futurists. For example, the University Hospital Consortium and American Practice Management, Incorporated Management Consultants (1992) categorized the healthcare market and its evolution to managed care into four stages of development. Today, this categorization has expanded to include a fifth stage. Box 2-6 summarizes the various stages of evolution.

Stage I of this market refers to the "now historical" perspective of healthcare when hospitals, physicians, employers, and HMOs were operating under a more *unstructured* FFS payment system. At this stage, more options were available to the client and more flexibility within this framework was permissible. The penetration of the HMO market was barely noticeable during this stage—about 5% to 10%. An example of an HMO at this point of development was the Health Insurance Plan (HIP) of New York, or the oldest HMO, Kaiser Permanente, in California.

Characteristics of the environment of care in this stage were duplication and fragmentation of services and less pressure on hospitals to discharge their patients early or reduce length of stay. Competition was based on technology. Case managers' roles in this stage were just beginning in the acute care settings, particularly with nurses assuming the role.

Stage II of this market is referred to as the *loose framework/alliance*. Many areas of the country are

---

BOX 2-6   Stages of Evolution of the Health Care Market

Stage I: Unstructured
Independent hospitals
Independent physicians
Independent purchases, not price sensitive

Stage II: Loose Framework
HMO/PPO enrollment rise
Excess inpatient capacity
Hospitals/physicians under pressure
Provider networks form

Stage III: Consolidation
A few large HMOs/PPOs emerge
Provider margins erode
Hospitals form systems
Hospital systems align with physicians to form integrated systems

Stage IV: Managed Competition
Employer coalitions purchase health services
Integrated systems manage patient populations
Continued consolidation of provider systems and health plans

Stage V: Integrated Delivery Partnerships
Fully capitated market
Partnerships between providers, purchasers, and payers
Providers assume risk for the full continuum of care
Population health management

Modified from University Hospital Consortium and American Practice Management, Incorporated Management Consultants: *Stages of market evolution,* Chicago, 1992, University Hospital Consortium.

---

currently in this stage and struggling with it. HMOs and PPOs are beginning to emerge in greater numbers (10% to 30% of the market), and enrollment has skyrocketed. They are no longer unnoticeable in the healthcare market of today. As a result of their large enrollments, they now have the leverage to negotiate pricing and the ability to contract at lower reimbursement rates. During Stage II, the motivation is to lower the cost of providing healthcare so that the value of the money received is not eroded. Several types of HMOs are developing. In the past, HMOs were organized to employ their own *staff* physicians and service providers and pay them a salary. Soon after, *groups* began to emerge in which a number of physicians and other providers established partnerships and shared their profits. These groups usually practiced out of a common facility or location. Next came the independent practitioners who formed associations and contracted to be part of a group endeavor while still practicing out of their own offices. The last type of HMO to emerge was the *network,* in which large areas are covered, perhaps crossing various states or regions or even the entire United States. Networks are most popular among large conglomerates who want to obtain the benefits of HMOs for their employees with the same consistency at any of their sites.

This stage of development witnessed increased focus on eliminating delays, duplication, and unnecessary use of resources, as well as other activities to streamline the delivery of care processes. As the interest in cost effectiveness increased, the use of case managers also arose with a focus on care coordination across the **continuum of care.** Healthcare executives began to integrate utilization and case management practices with a major focus on transitional planning and expediting the patient's journey across the different levels of care settings.

After these states of development, the market moves into **Stage III, consolidation.** While HMOs are forming networks, hospitals are simultaneously forming systems and networks themselves. Managed care penetration increases to 30% to 50% of the market. This now sets up the beginnings of a competitive market in which hospitals are aggressively recruiting physicians and practitioners. These groups of physicians and providers are more commonly becoming known as PPOs. The payment system is based on a per case, per diem, capitation through the PPO. A contract is developed that outlines the cost per covered life in the plan. PPOs are now outgrowing the HMO market primarily as a result of their ability to offer greater savings for employers at a time when employers are extremely concerned about the cost of their employees' health benefits.

Case management programs in this stage became more popular and available in the majority of healthcare organizations and in different settings. These programs were necessary to curtail the rising cost of healthcare and increased risk on the part of the provider. Case management was viewed as the most desired strategy for cost-effectiveness and efficient service delivery. However, these programs took a new and improved structure: an initial integrative approach to case management with merged **utilization management,** clinical management, and **transitional planning**

functions. In addition, case managers in the payer-based system (i.e., MCOs) assumed the gatekeeper and utilization management role.

Many parts of the country, primarily the West Coast, have lived through Stage III and have now embarked on **Stage IV, managed competition.** This is the phase in which capitation prevails (50% to 80%). In this market, purchasers contract with hospital/physician networks to provide a comprehensive healthcare package to their clients. These integrated systems contract with the purchasers to accept the financial risk for managing their **utilization** of services (utilization management). In other words, they bear the burden of controlling their costs to deliver healthcare. The next level of this system is capitation, where a set fee is given to provide comprehensive care to a given population. This puts an even greater burden on the ability to provide quality care while controlling cost. The managed organization is no longer taking the risk with its premiums; the risk has now shifted to the provider of the healthcare services within the network or physician care group.

This phase of managed care is the most uncomfortable of all because this is where survival of the fittest comes into play. Competition is at its peak during this phase because MCOs are searching for membership from the most frugal yet quality-driven establishments. **Report cards** are now the judgment mechanism of any MCO and can be the demise of any physician or hospital not meeting the standards of cost containment as set up by the MCOs. An example of capitation is as follows: 1,000 HMO members sign up for a healthcare network as part of a full-risk contract. The network will reimburse approximately $400 per member per month to cover all of their healthcare needs regardless of how much or how little they access the healthcare system. It is the burden of the healthcare network to provide adequate resources to cover their healthcare needs at low cost.

The integrative approaches to case management services in this stage become the norm. Department consolidation also occurs. In Stage III it was possible for healthcare organizations, particularly hospitals, to still have either discharge planning, utilization management, or quality management as separate from case management. However, in Stage IV this lack of integration becomes no longer viable and is seen as a cost-ineffective practice. Because of the development of **integrated delivery systems** (IDSs), collaborative strategies in case management across the continuum of care and across different sites and settings are developed, strengthening the role of the case manager and its importance. Moreover, case management takes a new focus here to meet the demands of the managed care environment: population risk assessment, categorization, and management with special interest in disease prevention and health maintenance and promotion.

Stage V, *integrated delivery partnerships,* occurs when the market of managed care expands to include most of the population in such an arrangement of health insurance (>80%). IDSs (discussed in the next section) mature in size, focus, and method of operation. They also become more popular in almost every geographical location, even though not every market may have reached this stage of development. The environment of healthcare in this stage is characterized by full capitation as the reimbursement method; partnerships between providers, purchasers, and payers; and population health management. Another important characteristic is that the providers assume risk for the full continuum of care.

These characteristics and advanced developments impact the practice of case management in a way that new strategies and innovations are developed, such as telephonic or **Internet**-based case management services. These approaches tend to also focus on the population served and its needs rather than just the individual patient or person. Therefore proactive programs in demand management and risk reduction are more evident in this stage compared with Stage IV. Furthermore, both the provider and payer groups adopt these strategies and use them in their marketing efforts.

INTEGRATED DELIVERY SYSTEMS AS A RESPONSE TO MANAGED CARE

IDSs became more popular in the mid-1990s as a response to the mature managed care environment. Today they are present mostly in heavily penetrated managed care markets. The driving forces behind the development of IDSs are as follows:

- The healthcare reform climate
- Managed care contracts and the need to increase competitiveness and negotiating power
- Need to expand market share
- Desire to increase efficiency, productivity, and profitability
- Shift in reimbursement methods away from FFS to capitation
- Increasing activism of employers in seeking control over healthcare costs and spending
- Managed care technology advances
- Sophistication of the utilization management practices of MCOs
- Risk-sharing contracts between the payer and provider
- Shift to a managed health rather than managed illness approach to care

- Employers' desire to be owners and voting participants in the healthcare delivery system rather than only vendors and providers (Hastings, Luce, and Wynstra, 1995)

There is little agreement in the literature and among healthcare providers on how to define IDSs. However, according to Kongstvedt, an IDS can be defined as one or more "type of provider coming together in some type of legal structure to manage health care and, in most cases, to contract with payer organizations" (2001, p. 31). The main goal of an IDS is to improve efficiency in the delivery of healthcare services. Reflecting back on the past decade, we can see that some IDSs have succeeded, but others have failed and completely vanished.

There are no standard rules for the size or type of an IDS. Some are large and others are small; however, larger IDSs are known to gain increased leverage in negotiating contracts with an MCO. Successful IDSs are noted to include an acute care hospital, physician group practices, long-term care facilities, a home care agency, and managed care contracts with major payers. As for the type of an IDS, there are not formal structures. IDSs can be one of the following:

- Systems in which only physicians are integrated: physician practice integration
- Systems in which physicians are integrated with healthcare facilities: physician-hospital integration
- Systems that include insurance agencies (i.e., a payer structure: provider-payer integration) (Kongstvedt, 2001)

Regardless of the type of integration a healthcare institution may be involved in, case management services and departments play an important role in the integration of services to meet the primary goal for the formed IDS: efficiency of service delivery.

Physician Integration

Managed care and healthcare reform resulted in increased reliance on primary care physicians as providers of healthcare services. This shift left specialty care physicians in a bind and worried about the survival of their practice because they were no longer in demand. As a result, specialists and primary care providers pursued integrated group practices that witnessed the creation of IPAs with multispecialty providers. IPAs and physician networks discussed in the previous section are examples of IDSs that are built around physician integration. Other types of physician-integrated IDSs are primary care groups, specialist provider groups, and **management service organizations** (MSOs). These types of groups function similar to IPAs; however, MSOs are different. The main focus of

MSOs is managed care contract negotiation for IPAs and physician networks.

Physician-Hospital Integration

Specialty hospitals experienced the same concerns as specialist physicians. They were afraid that their referral source and base would dwindle; therefore they began to establish relationships with primary care physicians and expanded their scope of services and providers. As a result, hospitals were found to develop new collaborative or partnership agreements with other physician groups, such as those listed in the Physician Integration section. Other types of integration are **physician-hospital organizations** (PHOs), particularly for the purpose of managed care contracting power; MSOs, in which hospitals sponsored the physician practices; and physician-hospital integration through direct employment of physicians. The MSOs were a natural development or growth of PHOs. Both PHOs and MSOs are similar in their focus on managed care contracting; however, MSOs include additional hospital administrative services.

Managed care contracts negotiation was the main incentive behind physician-hospital integration efforts. In these ventures, hospitals assisted physicians in the management of their practices (i.e., provided practice management services) and assumed the administrative responsibilities for billing and collections, **utilization review** and management, and **quality assurance** activities. In these structures the hospital received a fee as a compensation for the services provided. The fee had to be at market value; otherwise, the MSO could incur legal problems.

Provider-Payer Integration

Provider-payer integration is different from the other two types of integration. Physician and physician-hospital modes of integration are unidimensional (i.e., provider-based). However, provider-payer integration is bidimensional because it merges the provider (physician and hospital) and payer sides of healthcare delivery. This type of integration is the most complex and challenging to manage. Picking the right partner is a leading success factor of this venture. Issues of concern in the provider-payer integration venture are as follows:

- Governance structure: Would the party with more capital assume ownership and control?
- Allocation of risk and profit.
- Acquisition versus start-up: Should a provider partner with an already existing payer or establish a new one? If a new one is established, one should be aware of its cost implications.
- Management: Who will run the new entity on a day-to-day basis?

- Exclusivity that is too expensive and complicated: Would the parties agree to only deal with each other on all managed care projects?
- Government regulations: The new entity must comply with all the related laws and governmental review (Hastings et al, 1995).

Government-Related Insurance Structures

Government provision of medical insurance is the final source when reviewing the options for the population at large. Both federal and state governments provide medical insurance benefits. The Medicare program under the federal government provides mandatory basic hospitalization benefits for most U.S. citizens over the age of 65 years and some other special classes of individuals, such as the disabled. This coverage is referred to as *Medicare Part A,* and it can be supplemented by *Medicare Part B,* which provides for payment of doctor bills. These plans are not all-inclusive enough for most senior citizens. Recently there have been growing cutbacks to Medicare; therefore it is prudent for any citizen over 65 years of age to supplement Medicare with another insurance plan. Many HMOs/PPOs are now expanding their plans to offer managed care Medicare and managed care Medicaid components.

At the state level, insurance benefits are also offered. These are commonly referred to as the *Medicaid program of benefits for the indigent.* They are no longer associated with the stigma of the term *welfare* because more and more citizens must apply for public assistance to cover their medical bills after they have exhausted their income and assets. Medicaid is a pool of funds used to provide insurance benefits for those who cannot afford health insurance. The amount of funds set aside for this purpose is most often a direct result of the economic status of a particular state. The amount of funding is undergoing a great deal of turmoil as many states are tightening their pocketbooks in anticipation of the full impact of managed care in a capitated environment.

A few examples of differing reimbursements for physician services are outlined in dollars in Figure 2-1. This is only a representative partial listing of potential physician fees and does not represent all practices or the many varieties of reimbursement schedules.

OTHER HEALTH BENEFIT PLANS
Workers' Compensation

An additional type of government provision that can vary from state to state is the workers' compensation guidelines. **Workers' compensation** cases are different from group medical insurance in that the insurers and

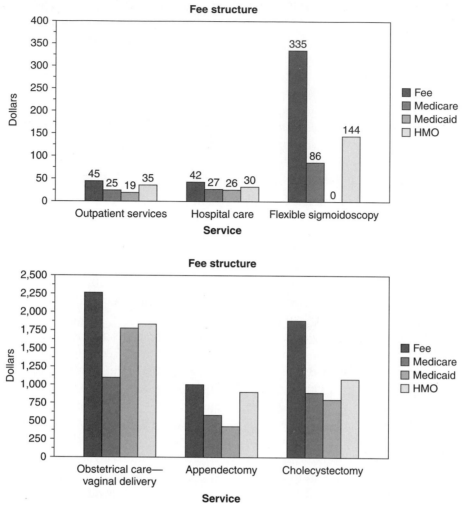

Figure 2-1 Differing reimbursements for physician services.

employers are mandated by legislature guidelines to reimburse for both medical costs and lost wages. It is imperative that a case manager working with workers' compensation claims be familiar with the state's laws, especially as they reflect the claimant's return to work.

Case Manager's Role in Workers' Compensation Cases

The case manager must be aware that there is a two-pronged effort in workers' compensation cases. That is, the insurance carrier is not only interested in the timely results of medical care but also wants to minimize the outlay of lost wages. Therefore getting the employee back to work as soon as possible, even with a modified work schedule and duties, becomes an additional motivational pressure on the case manager. At times the case manager may have difficulty balancing medical health and the timely return to the workforce. The case manager may be faced with the dilemma of a tight timeframe to return someone to work if the salary losses are a greater expense to the insurer than the medical care expenses.

Case managers specializing in the field of workers' compensation must be well versed in orthopedic injuries because these injuries dominate compensation cases. They must also be knowledgeable enough in rehabilitative medicine to recommend the resources necessary to assist a patient in increasing functionality. It is the goal of the case manager to return an employee to the previous state of well-being or the optimum level of improvement obtainable. The case manager achieves this by ensuring that the appropriate treatment plan is in effect and progressing, along with verifying compliance by the employee. It is also important for the case manager to know the employee/claimant well enough to prevent the person from engaging in any untoward activities that would hinder or sabotage the progress or ultimate recovery.

Automobile Insurance

As with workers' compensation guidelines, automobile policies and/or no-fault policies vary from state to state. Many rules depend on the location of the accident, where the person resides, or where the person's employment headquarters is located.

Case management usually becomes involved in motor vehicle accident cases when catastrophic injury has occurred. Case managers become very involved in the discharge planning and coordination, such as transfer from acute level of care to rehabilitative settings or decisions involving a chronic injury requiring adaptive equipment, home care, or home modifications.

Disability Insurance

Disability plans are usually referred to as *short-term, long-term,* or *total disability.* Each type of plan varies in its amounts of salary replacement and length of time covered. Disability plans will require a case management review. Usually a case manager will become involved as the length of time for disability coverage is winding down. It will be the creativity of a case manager's skills that will determine if the financial plan and the medical plan will balance to the benefit of the insured and the employer.

Long-Term Care

This is a relatively new type of insurance offered. The policy holder has a variety of possibilities for nursing care coverage. Such care as skilled nursing, subacute care, custodial nursing care, extended home care, respite care, or nursing home provisions can be covered. The insurance company usually case manages a claim to confirm the need for services and approves benefit coverage accordingly.

PROACTIVE TACTICS TO COUNTERACT THE EFFECTS OF MANAGED CARE

Most strategies are incorporating a two-pronged approach to tackle all of the major areas that the MCOs seem to be concentrating on. One approach could fall under the overall *operational management.* This is the area in which efforts are initiated to control costs and to become more accountable for costs. Work redesigns and changes in the work delivery systems are becoming commonplace in organizations that are taking a more proactive approach. A more active performance and reward system is becoming evident and attempts are being made to integrate physician best practice with a functional integration system so that quality standards of care can be maintained at the lowest cost possible.

The second approach, and the area in which case management has the most direct impact on its overall success, is *clinical management.* Nursing case management was the first tool used to oversee the patient's journey through the healthcare system. Without a clear system of managing the patient services and resources

in the least costly way, particularly in an environment of increased capitation, funds will quickly be wiped out. Capitation clearly requires control over resources, utilization management, length-of-stay reduction, disease management, and clinical process improvement. All of these listed areas can be incorporated into the case management role (see Chapters 4 through 7).

The emergence of the case manager using the clinical pathway was a major step toward a more cost-effective, efficient method of delivering care. By identifying variances to care, the case manager began to identify ways to continuously improve the delivery of care while not compromising quality. The use of clinical paths was the beginning initiative to control and reduce length of stay. An effective case management program can make a significant difference in managing and coordinating the clinical resources available for the patient (Case Manager's Tip 2-13) (Flarey and Blancett, 1996).

Integrating case management into managing a patient group or a specific disease entity is the next level of resource and clinical management. This strategy uses a multidisciplinary approach to care and requires input from the medical, clinical, ancillary, financial, and administrative teams. Many facilities have developed multidisciplinary teams to meet frequently on units and review the care of the patients to ensure that quality is being maintained while utilization of services is appropriate and cost-efficient. Similarly, length-of-stay committees have been launched to discuss problem cases, high-cost patients or certain areas of overutilization, and more efficient methods of providing services at lower cost. Future strategies must expand efforts beyond the hospital walls to include community services and community-based initiatives of case management (Case Manager's Tip 2-14).

Differentiating between case management and managed care can be somewhat confusing at times because the terms are used interchangeably in many arenas.

 CASE MANAGER'S TIP 2-13

Case Management Caveat

Case management must not be the catchall for fixing all that ails a facility.

 CASE MANAGER'S TIP 2-14

Case Management's Focus

The focus must always go beyond illness to include wellness, maintenance, and preventive case management.

In general terms, managed care is the umbrella for several initiatives of cost containment that include case management. Case management is a variation of the components that comprise managed care (i.e., managing cost, quality, and effectiveness of services) (Cohen and Cesta, 1997). Case management is a process that incorporates the components of managed care when attending to the needs of patient care. It can be used in any form of patient delivery system, such as team, functional, primary, or alternative nursing care.

Continuous monitoring of care rendered to a patient is maintained through interdisciplinary team meetings and analysis of variances from the outlined plan. Case management is effective because it coordinates, integrates, and evaluates the outcomes of the processes of care (Cohen and Cesta, 1997).

To have an effect on managed care, case managers must take an active role in watching for quality outcomes. **Benchmarking** research used by managed care companies will be an important tool that a case

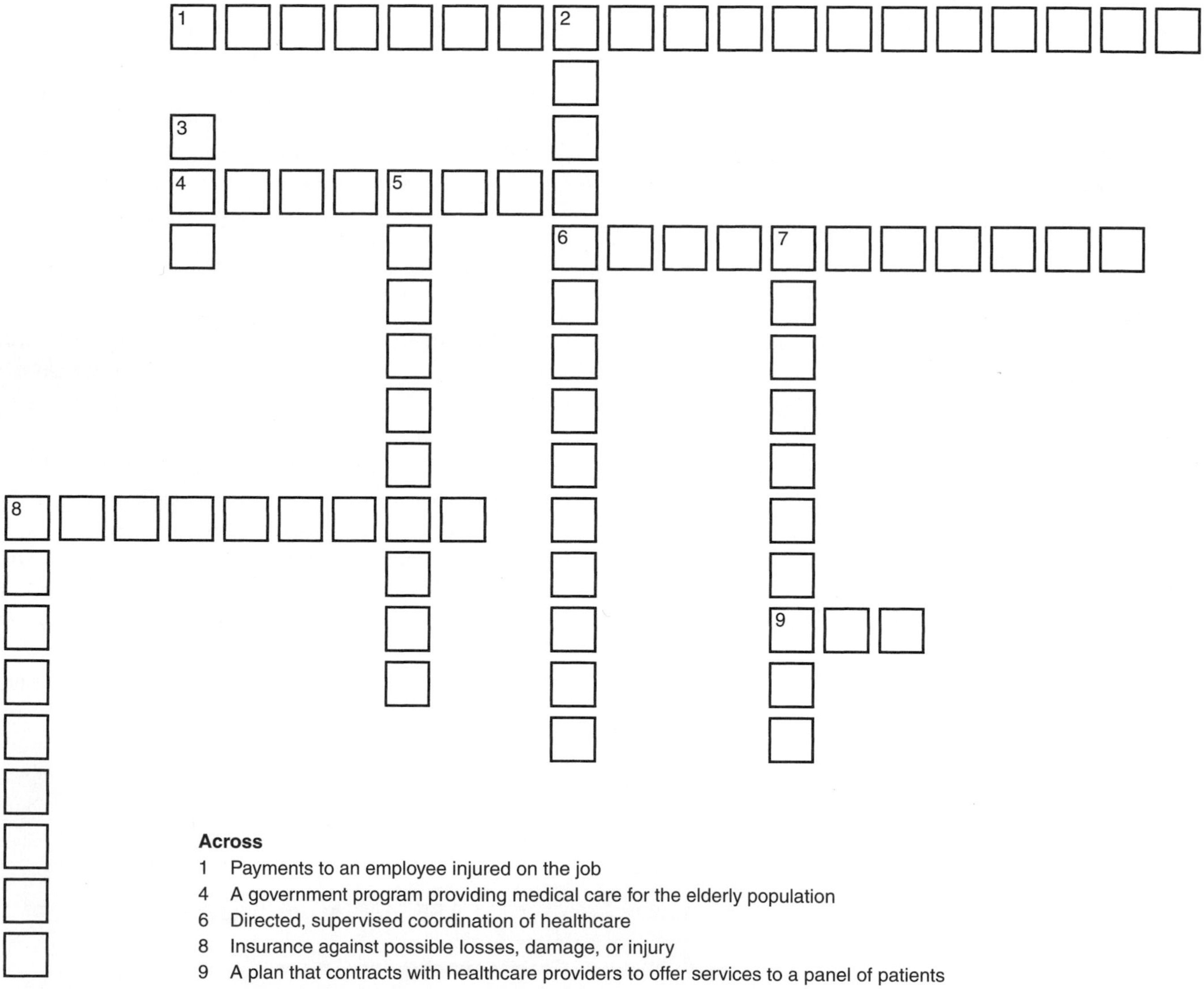

Across

1 Payments to an employee injured on the job
4 A government program providing medical care for the elderly population
6 Directed, supervised coordination of healthcare
8 Insurance against possible losses, damage, or injury
9 A plan that contracts with healthcare providers to offer services to a panel of patients

Down

2 A model to manage costs of healthcare and quality services that optimizes outcomes
3 Comprehensive medical services to enrolled membership on a prepaid basis
5 A set amount of money paid based on covered lives
7 A primary care physician who refers patients to specialists as needed
8 The protection one seeks to provide benefits for an illness or injury

Figure 2-2 Crossword puzzle: a review of managed care terminology.
Crossword puzzle answer key: *Across:* 1, workers' compensation; 4, Medicare; 6, managed care; 8, indemnity; 9, PPO. *Down:* 2, case management; 3, HMO; 5, capitation; 7, gatekeeper; 8, insurance.

manager must incorporate into the role because it will become clear that adequacy of care will be measured by outcomes. Case managers must demonstrate that they have the flexibility to ensure that care is delivered in a high-quality and cost-effective manner. They will undoubtedly play a vital role in the future of our healthcare industry and the survival of quality healthcare provided to its people.

 KEY POINTS

1. The prospective payment system was one of the forces leading acute care settings toward the adoption of case management models.
2. Case mix helps hospitals to determine their costs, as well as their types of patients and use of resources.
3. In addition to acute care settings, prospective payment methodologies can now be found in ambulatory care, home care, and long-term care.
4. Medicare and managed Medicare are government programs providing healthcare to those age 65 years and over and the disabled.
5. Medicaid and managed Medicaid are state-run healthcare programs for the indigent.
6. Regardless of the reimbursement system under which the patient is eligible, the length of stay will continue to need to remain short, and the use of resources will need to be monitored and controlled.
7. Health insurance is the protection one seeks to provide benefits for an illness or injury.
8. The insurance contract states the nature of the benefits or the coverage available to the insured.
9. The HMO delivers comprehensive medical services to an enrolled membership on a prepaid basis.
10. The PPO offers a more limited number of providers and encourages the use of physicians and services within the network, but patients are permitted to go outside the network for decreased reimbursement.

11. The evolution of the healthcare market has four stages of development in the managed care environment.
12. Work redesigns are becoming commonplace in organizations taking a proactive approach to managed care.
13. Managing patient services and resources in the least costly way while maintaining quality will be the primary goal of case management as it relates to managed care.
14. Managed care is the umbrella for several cost-containment initiatives that include but are not limited to case management. The crossword puzzle shown in Figure 2-2 will help you review some of the key terms related to financial reimbursement systems.

REFERENCES

American Medical Association: *CPT '97,* Reston, Va, 1996, St Anthony's Press.

Blancett SS, Flarey DL: *Case studies in nursing case management: health care delivery in a world of managed care,* Gaithersburg, Md, 1996, Aspen.

Cohen EL, Cesta TG: *Nursing case management: from concept to evaluation,* ed 2, St Louis, 1997, Mosby.

Commission on Professional and Hospital Activities: *The international classification of diseases,* rev 8, 2 vols, Ann Arbor, Mich, 1975, The Commission (adapted for use in the United States).

Enteen R: *Health insurance: how to get it, keep it, or improve what you've got,* New York, 1992, Paragon House.

Flarey DL, Blancett SS: *Handbook of nursing case management,* Gaithersburg, Md, 1996, Aspen.

Hastings DA, Luce GM, Wynstra NA: *Fundamentals of health law,* Washington, DC, 1995, National Health Lawyers Association.

Hurley R, Freund D, Paul J: *Medicaid managed care: lessons for policy and program design,* Ann Arbor, Mich, 1993, Health Administration Press.

Kongstvedt P: *Essentials of managed health care,* Gaithersburg, Md, 2001, Aspen.

Mullahy CM: *The case management handbook,* ed 2, Gaithersburg, Md, 1998, Aspen.

Richards S: A closer look at case management, *J Health Qual* 18(4): 8-11, 1996.

University Hospital Consortium and American Practice Management, Incorporated Management Consultants: *Stages of market evolution,* Chicago, 1992, University Hospital Consortium.

3

Case Management Models

Case management is a malleable and easily adapted model that applies to a variety of care delivery locations and systems. It is because of this flexibility that the model has been designed and implemented in various ways that respond to and meet the needs of the organizations applying it. Although **case management** has been used in the community setting for the longest period, it is now commonly seen as an integrated care delivery model in the acute care setting and other sites along the **continuum of care** (e.g., skilled nursing facilities and long-term care facilities). More and more organizations are recognizing the model's ability to manage resources while maintaining or improving quality.

Clearly the most effective models are those that provide a mechanism for managing patients across the continuum of care, thereby providing a seamless, integrated care process. In a **managed care** environment this is most easily done because of the integrated services inherent in a managed care system. The notion of managing patients in a variety of care settings is more difficult in payer systems in which there are no incentives for various settings to communicate and/or share resources. Managed care is traditionally viewed as a system that provides the generalized structure and focus when managing the use, cost, quality, and effectiveness of healthcare services. Managed care is the umbrella for cost-containment efforts such as case management. Case management is a process model. It is based on and contains elements of the managed care theme.

Many healthcare organizations have opted to first implement case management in the acute care setting. This accomplishes a number of things. First, it allows the organization to design, implement, and perfect its case management system in a more easily controlled environment, the hospital. Although it provides greater challenges in terms of the clinical management of patients in the acute care setting, it is still a place where team members are part of a team that is "within the walls." In fact, the term *within the walls* has been used to aggregate those case management models that manage patients' care during the acute care portion of the illness. Among the many applications of the within-the-walls models are a host of types using the members of the team in various role functions. In most cases the registered nurse (RN) is used as the **case manager.** It is the placement of the RN in the organizational structure and the associated role functions that differentiate the various models.

Case management is difficult to encapsulate because it describes many different approaches, including a patient care delivery system, a professional practice model, a defined group of activities performed by healthcare providers in a particular setting, and services provided by private practitioners (Goodwin, 1994).

TYPES OF CASE MANAGEMENT

Case management services can be provided in a variety of ways and care sites. There are basically four types: primary, medical/social, private, and **nursing case management.** Box 3-1 summarizes the types and the sites in which they typically occur.

Primary Care Case Management

In primary care case management the physician functions as the case manager. As case manager, the physician is responsible for coordinating and managing patient care services. Some managed care organizations (MCOs) are using nurse practitioners as primary care case managers. Nurse practitioners are able to take on this role because of their ability to function independently or under a collaborative agreement with a physician. The primary care case manager is the

BOX 3-1   Case Management Models and Sites in Which They are Used

Primary Care Case Management
1. Health maintenance organizations (HMOs)
2. Preferred provider organizations (PPOs)
3. Physician hospital organizations (PHOs)
4. Private practice

Medical/Social Case Management
1. Acute care
2. Outpatient settings (including clinics and community health programs)

Private Case Management
1. Direct referral for a variety of services and sites

Nursing Case Management
1. Ambulatory care
2. Acute care
3. Home care
4. Long-term care
5. Rehabilitation
6. Managed care

gatekeeper who plans, approves, and negotiates care for the patient.

In MCOs the case manager triages patients and determines their future needs and resource allocation. For example, the primary care case manager evaluating a newly diagnosed asthmatic patient will determine whether the patient needs to be seen by a specialist, in an emergency department (ED) setting, or in a doctor's office. This particular managed care function serves to control expenses by limiting the use of more expensive interventions and ensuring that they are provided in the most appropriate level of care/setting.

Medical/Social Case Management

This type of case management focuses on the long-term care of patient populations at risk for hospitalization. The needs may be either medical or social in nature, and the case manager may be a physician, social worker, or RN. In some instances the case manager will follow the patient regardless of the setting in which services are being rendered.

Private Case Management

Private case management is used for patients who fall outside the traditional patient care programs. In this type of case management an RN will either be self-employed, an independent practitioner, or work on a case-by-case

basis for an MCO or other **third-party payer.** The private case manager is contracted for services as needed. The case manager coordinates and manages the care for the patient regardless of the setting.

Because the case manager is independent of the organization, some believe that private case managers can provide the greatest level of completely unbiased services to the patient and family. The case manager functioning under this model is not advocating for anyone but the patient. This area is perhaps the newest addition to the case management arena. Many of the private case managers hired in the 1980s were master's prepared RNs or social workers (Knollmueller, 1989). In the 1990s this trend continued with case managers who were usually clinical nurse specialists (CNSs) or social workers. Often they were paid privately by the client or subcontracted by a third-party payer. The private case manager may coordinate services for the client, advocate on behalf of the client and/or provide counseling (Clark, 1996), and manage the patient's benefits based on the insurance/health plan.

Nursing Case Management

This approach to case management uses the RN as the case manager. The RN functions as the facilitator, coordinator, evaluator, and manager of patient care services and expected outcomes.

HOSPITAL-BASED/ACUTE CARE MODELS

Acute care models are those used in hospitals, EDs, and other acute care settings (Case Manager's Tip 3-1).

Primary Nurse Case Management

This model uses the staff nurse or primary nurse in the position of case manager. In addition to being responsible for hands-on, direct nursing care, the primary nurse case manager is also responsible for the indirect nursing functions that have often been the responsibility of other members of the healthcare team. Direct nursing functions include activities such as physical assessments, medication administration, vital sign monitoring, intravenous administration, wound

 CASE MANAGER'S TIP 3-1

Acute Care Case Management
Hospital-based or acute care models are also referred to as *episodic* case management. These models are applied to patients during an episode of illness that is short term.

management, and patient/family education. Indirect functions include facilitation and coordination of services, brokerage of community services, transitional/discharge planning, monitoring of utilization of resources, **outcomes management, variance** analysis, and others. In this model many of the functions that would have been traditionally handed off to other departments or disciplines are collapsed under the staff nurse case manager role.

Traditionally, the staff nurse's role has been focused on the acute care, clinical, hands-on component of the patient's illness. Some **discharge planning** may have been included in the job responsibilities, such as referrals to visiting nurse services. Other functions, such as **utilization,** continuing care placement, or patient/family education, might have been shared by others on the team. For example, **utilization management** would have been the responsibility of the utilization review nurse. Discharge planning and placement issues might have been managed by the social worker or the dedicated discharge planner. Patient/family education might have been shared with CNSs such as the enterostomal CNS, the pain management specialist, or the medical-surgical CNS. These professionals were often called on to provide specific clinical expertise to augment that being provided by the staff nurse.

Functions such as **outcomes monitoring** and variance analysis were not core components of the traditional primary nursing models. Both outcomes management and variance identification have evolved as byproducts yet important elements of case management. Traditional nursing care plans did not include expected outcomes or identification of variations from the expected outcomes. In this model, the staff nurse is expected to take responsibility for these role functions.

In some versions of the staff nurse model, the staff nurse may be given the responsibility for some of these additional role functions. However, some organizations kept role functions such as utilization management in the core department. The underlying principle of the staff nurse case manager model is that the staff nurse takes ultimate responsibility and accountability for the patient's hospital course and continuing stay needs.

The early primary nurse models were intended to place the RN in the position of being ultimately accountable for all aspects of the patient's care. The primary nursing models of the 1970s developed in response to nursing's evolution toward greater autonomy and professionalism. These responsibilities included those mentioned previously as related to the direct, hands-on care. In addition, responsibilities may have included discharge planning. Utilization management

responsibilities have not been traditional elements of the primary nurse role. Unfortunately, these models were unable to manage the cost and quality issues of the 1990s (Lynn-McHale, Fitzpatrick, and Shaffer, 1993).

In the primary nurse or staff nurse case management models, different levels of responsibility are placed on the staff nurse, depending on the level of integration of other departments. For example, in a fully integrated hospital the staff nurse may be responsible for direct care and all related indirect nursing functions, including transitional/discharge planning, utilization management, variance analysis, and outcomes/**quality improvement.** In other cases, levels of responsibility may vary. Utilization management is the most common exception to this list, with some basic utilization functions often retained by a central department. Some of the functions may include telephone communication with MCOs or other insurers, continued stay revenues, or denials.

Despite the degree of responsibility delegated to the staff nurse, a tremendous amount of education must take place to prepare the staff nurse or primary nurse to assume these added responsibilities. The staff nurse may be responsible not only for providing care to a caseload of patients on the unit but also for managing the care of patients in other parts of the hospital, regardless of location (Davis, 1996).

The staff/primary nurse case manager model may also serve as a framework for a clinical ladder, which may be composed of several positions of increasing responsibility with the case manager as the top level. This may mean that the case manager oversees more comprehensive or complicated patients. *In this model, all patients must be case managed.* This is because of the reduction of other services and personnel, which means that these job responsibilities must be absorbed by the staff nurse (Case Manager's Tip 3-2).

Advanced Practice Case Management

The advanced practice case manager is an RN with an advanced practice degree; either a CNS or a nurse practitioner. The advanced practice nurse brings additional dimensions to the case manager role and a level of

 CASE MANAGER'S TIP 3-2

Primary Nurse Case Management

In the primary nurse case management model, *all* patients must be case managed because of the reduction of other services and personnel.

educational preparation not held by the majority of staff nurses. The master's prepared nurse's educational preparation has a wellness or health focus that is clinically specialized and care-continuum–based (Koerner, 1991). These nurses are also educated to bring their advanced educational skills and focus on patient/family education to the daily care of their patients (American Nurses Association, 1988).

This case management model removes the case manager from direct patient care. The case manager becomes concerned with the continuum of care and moves the patient from one phase or level of care to the next, regardless of who is providing the specific care along the way. This facilitation/coordination role may also include discharge planning and/or utilization management responsibilities, depending on how the organization has been redesigned. Members of the team continually consult with each other, and the CNS case manager provides the coordination and facilitation role to the process. It is this cadre of additional and advanced skills that makes the advanced practice nurse a prime candidate for case management (Hamric, 1992).

To use existing personnel more efficiently, the organization may convert already existing CNS positions to case managers. In this case the current role functions of the CNS must be reevaluated. For example, mandatory Joint Commission on Accreditation of Healthcare Organizations (JCAHO) continuing education functions may need to be redeployed to other staff developers. By doing so, the CNS case manager is truly freed up to perform advanced practice role functions, which may have been impossible when other job responsibilities were added onto the role.

CNS case managers can be either unit-based or diagnosis (hospital)-based. In either case they should be assigned based on their clinical specialty. If the clinical care units are specialty-oriented, with cohorted, like-type patients, then a unit-based approach may work. If not, the case manager may need to be diagnosis-based to remain within the clinical specialty, regardless of the patient's physical location.

The removal of case managers from direct patient care means that they have more time to dedicate to advanced case management functions such as outcomes management and research. They are also educated to perform these role functions. Their clinical expertise, advanced preparation including research, and a continuum of care focus are benefits that they bring to the role of case manager (Norris and Hill, 1991). The CNS case manager position allows the CNS to function in a way that is more purely a clinical specialist role than when a host of staff-development responsibilities

are collapsed onto the role (Wells, Erickson, and Spinella, 1996). Because of their advanced clinical expertise, it is sometimes easier for the CNS to develop relationships with physicians that extend beyond the acute care setting. The advanced practice case manager, as part of the interdisciplinary team, may work with the team in the ambulatory setting, seeing patients after discharge from the hospital. The opportunity for the patient/family to develop a longstanding relationship with the case manager may mean greater compliance with their care regimen and more positive clinical outcomes over a longer period.

Nurse practitioners bring even more skills to the case manager role. With their ability to prescribe and discharge the patient from the hospital, the care process can be facilitated and less fragmented. The ambulatory care setting may be the most valuable place to use the nurse practitioner, particularly for those patients with chronic illnesses who are frequently accessing the healthcare system (Case Manager's Tip 3-3). The nurse practitioner's holistic approach with a focus on education and wellness may translate to reduced hospital admissions and a better quality of life for the patient in the community.

There are some commonalities and some differences between the two advanced practice roles of CNS and nurse practitioner. Case management models that integrate the two roles have been suggested (Schroer, 1991).

Commonalties between the roles include patient education, graduate-level preparation, practice, care coordination, referral, specialty practice, and autonomy. In contrast, the nurse practitioner has more of a focus on primary care, including the physical examination, history, and prescribing of medications. The title is protected by state regulations, and there can be reimbursement to primary care. The CNS is more inpatient focused and uses health promotion as a secondary consideration (Schroer, 1991).

Currently, nurse practitioners work in primary care, outpatient clinics, **health maintenance organizations (HMOs),** and other specialty areas. CNSs work in inpatient settings (Diers, 1993) or home care settings. The differences and similarities described may suggest the use of the CNS case manager in the acute care setting

 CASE MANAGER'S TIP 3-3

Advanced Practice Case Management
The ambulatory care setting may be the most valuable place to use the advanced practice case manager, particularly for chronically ill patients who access the healthcare system frequently.

and the use of the nurse practitioner case manager in the ambulatory setting.

Utilization Review Nursing Case Management

In this version of case management, some institutions have eliminated the traditional **utilization review** nurse and converted these positions to case managers. The first step in this process is the transition from utilization review to utilization management. This step is both philosophical and operational. Utilization review has been a retrospective process that attempted to correct problems after they occurred. The utilization review nurse would read and review medical records to determine appropriateness for hospitalization based on the physician's and other healthcare provider's documentation. In some cases the utilization review nurse would intervene when delay occurred in the care process. For example, a delay in completion of a computed tomography (CT) scan might result in the utilization review nurse making a call to radiology to determine the cause of the delay. In these cases the nurse identified a delay once it had occurred and then tried to remedy the situation. In any case, the delay had already happened. Other functions included review of services for medical necessity and assurance that services were being provided in the most appropriate setting and at an acceptable quality standard level.

Implementation of utilization case management means that the utilization management/review functions must be picked up by the case manager. One method of implementing this model has come as a result of the hospital's simply taking existing personnel and redeploying them as case managers. Responsibilities remain essentially the same without a reengineering of other departments/disciplines. In other cases the clinical case manager is given added responsibilities that include utilization management, after which the original positions are eliminated. Another approach may be to blend the discharge planning and utilization management functions together. All versions have the goal of eliminating redundant, currently existing positions and making the care process more efficient by streamlining the process and reducing the number of steps in the completion of tasks.

If financially feasible, maintaining a small utilization management core department is beneficial. Most institutions kept few centralized utilization management staff positions as part of the case management department, while converting the remainder of the positions to case managers. Such change resulted in complete elimination of utilization management as an independent department. The blending of all of the

utilization functions onto the case manager role may mean that the case manager gets completely absorbed in these functions and has less time to devote to the clinical dimensions of the role. Issues such as denial of **benefits** may remain within the purview of the utilization management core department. Retrospective insurance reviews may also be the responsibility of this department to reduce fragmentation and delays in the care process. The case manager should take over those functions that are most closely related to the patient's current hospitalization, including admission and continued stay reviews. As many cases as possible should be concurrently reviewed. These **concurrent reviews** are performed by the case manager every 3 days—or more frequently in the case of critical care areas or patients with much shorter **length of stay.** Among the functions performed during the concurrent review process are evaluations for severity of illness and **intensity of service.** Evaluation of **severity of illness** includes an evaluation of the patient's significant symptoms, any deviations from normal levels, or unstable or abnormal vital signs or laboratory values. Intensity of service includes evaluation of the plan of treatment, interventions, and expected outcomes. **Retrospective reviews** can be handled by the utilization management core staff.

Including concurrent reviews as part of the case management process can help expedite the plan more quickly. The case manager has the most comprehensive knowledge and understanding of the case and is observing it in its totality rather than in a fragmented approach. Payer interactions can also be facilitated through such an integrated approach. Benefits identification and eligibility are becoming more cumbersome processes as the number of MCOs continues to rise. Each organization brings with it a host of different benefits. Even within one MCO, similar patients will be entitled to different benefits. Negotiating these benefits for the patient while in the hospital and after discharge can mean a smoother transition for the patient from the acute care to the community setting. This comes as a result of fewer "hand-offs" of the work from one provider to another.

Caution must be taken in the implementation of such a model so as not to overload the case manager. It is highly recommended that the tasks identified previously as part of a centralized core utilization management department remain so, or the true case management focus will be lost in performing insurance reviews, dealing with **denials,** and so on (Case Manager's Tip 3-4).

Social Work Case Management

Social workers have used the title *case manager* for many years. In fact, after the RN, social workers are the other professionals most often seen in the role of case manager (Rantz and Bopp, 1996). The social worker, if functioning as the case manager, can focus on the patient's social, financial, and discharge planning needs. The social worker as case manager is effective in the outpatient setting, where many of the patient's needs are related more to financial or social issues and less to clinical ones. In the hospital setting, a dyad of RN case manager and social worker can be an effective way to manage cases based on needs. If the prevailing issues are clinical or educational in nature, the RN may be more appropriate for case management. If the patient's needs are more social or financial, the social worker may be more appropriate to provide the necessary services.

In the dyad model the RN and social worker case managers assess the patient on admission to the hospital; based on that assessment, it is determined which practitioner may be more appropriate to manage the case. In some cases it may be necessary for both disciplines to case manage the same patient.

The case manager's initial assessment would be a clinical or biological review of systems, reason for hospitalization, relevant previous medical history, clinical issues that may affect discharge, and educational needs. The social worker would be focused on the social support and psychological segments of the patient's overall clinical picture. A social assessment includes an evaluation of the patient's lifestyle, activities, interests, and support system. Family support, living environment, and the patient's ability to return to the preadmission environment would be assessed by the social worker. The psychological assessment would consist of an evaluation of the patient's mental status; use of alcohol, tobacco, and drugs; and previous history of mental disorders.

When implementing this model, it is extremely valuable for both disciplines to sit down together and outline what their case management inclusion or selection criteria will be (Box 3-2). Through techniques such as case conferencing, an ongoing evaluation can be made as to the patient's progress toward the expected

 CASE MANAGER'S TIP 3-4

Utilization Review Nursing Case Management

In the utilization review nursing case management model, it is easy for the case manager to become overloaded. Keeping the case manager's tasks part of a centralized core utilization management department can help prevent the true case management focus from being lost.

outcomes and as to whether additional providers may need to be added to the case.

This type of model, although extremely patient focused and beneficial to the patient and family, may be too costly for the organization to support. If so, the RN case manager can call the social worker on a referral basis for cases needing more comprehensive social work–type interventions (Case Manager's Tip 3-5).

In an RN/social worker dyad model, another effective strategy can be the use of specific referral criteria

---

BOX 3-2   Neonatal Case Management Team Role Responsibilities

Social Work

1. Psychosocial assessment, including evaluation of family situation/home/financial support, other high-risk social factors. Clarify medical coverage. Advocate; refer for such coverage. Refer for appropriate entitlements. Advocate for patients with various systems.
2. Evaluation of coping with illness/hospitalization; evaluation of family support systems; provision of emotional support.
3. Referral to community support agencies/mental health services as indicated.
4. Coordination of child abuse/neglect cases, including substance abuse cases.
5. Act as part of the neonatal intensive care unit (NICU) team in providing coordinated services to families with children in the NICU.

Shareable Skills/Tasks for Team

1. Attend regular interdisciplinary NICU rounds to share information.
2. Share in decision making with family.
3. Identify system barriers and solutions.
4. Provide patient/team continuity.
5. Collaborate with utilization management.
6. Optimize patient's adjustment to NICU.

Case Manager

1. Case management plan of care; length of stay.
2. Track data.
3. Follow clinical status.
4. Coordinate/facilitate plan of care.
5. Provide consultation regarding clinical issues.
6. Monitor outcomes.
7. Track clinical resource utilization with team.
8. Provide discharge teaching (e.g., cardiopulmonary resuscitation [CPR], medications).
9. Provide discharge planning, including equipment and home care referrals.
10. Posthospital follow-up.
11. Make transportation arrangements.

CASE MANAGER'S TIP 3-5

Social Work Case Management

Social work case management is beneficial to patients and families yet may be too costly for the organization to support. One solution is for the nurse case manager to call the social worker on a referral basis for cases that need more comprehensive interventions.

adapted to various clinical settings. Working as a team, the nurse and social worker can meet the needs of high-risk patients identified through the use of prospectively determined criteria that reflect the specific issues identified in discreet clinical settings. If you work in a hospital or clinic setting in which a variety of types of patients are treated, it may be helpful to outline the referral criteria by clinical specialty. The examples in Table 3-1 will serve as guides only. Each organization must develop its own unique set of criteria to meet its clinical needs, as well as remain appropriate to the specific case management departmental design.

For example, the criteria for referring a social worker to a patient in the ED will vary significantly from the needs of a patient on a maternal/child unit. By using this type of criteria, both disciplines can be deployed to specific patients as needed, and in a timely fashion. In all instances, the division of responsibilities should address the unique skill sets and knowledge base of each discipline. Clinical needs should be addressed by the RN case manager, whereas social/financial needs are best addressed by the social worker. In this way each discipline's knowledge and time are optimized.

Admitting Department Case Management

Early acute care case management models did not give great attention to the two fundamental routes of entry to the hospital, the ED and the admitting department. Acute care settings now recognize the importance of gatekeeping these hospital admission points to manage and

TABLE 3-1   Guidelines for Referrals

RN Case Managers/Social Workers	
Medical/Surgical Inpatient Adult Services	
RN Case Manager	**Social Worker**
Performs admission and concurrent utilization management, including insurance calls	Patient/family difficulty coping with new diagnosis (e.g., cancer, ventilator dependency, difficulty understanding/accepting decision making with long-term discharge planning options)
Coordinates/facilitates plans of care	Psychiatric, cognitive, or behavioral factors that may impede delivery of care and discharge planning process
Facilitates daily rounds and team meetings	
Assesses all patients for psychosocial needs	
Does discharge planning, including equipment, home care, rehabilitation, and long-term care facilities	Inadequate supports that may impact on compliance with continuing care needs (**PLEASE NOTE:** Social workers can provide case managers with information to give to patients and families regarding entitlements)
Orders transportation	
Completes discharge forms	
Oversees clinical guidelines	Ethical or legal concerns (e.g., patient, family, team conflicts related to medical plan of care, guardianship cases, or end-of-life issues around Advance Directives, DNR order)
Tracks data (e.g., variances in patient care and systems standards)	
Provides alternate level of care notification	Suspicion or evidence of domestic violence, elder abuse or neglect, child abuse or neglect, rape, sexual assault; known to PSA
Issues HINN letters	Substance abuse counseling referrals when patient requests or is viewed as amenable to intervention
	Unidentified patient(s) is seriously ill, and there is difficulty locating significant others
	Patients signing out against medical advice
	Homelessness (e.g., new onset, patient is unable to return to prior living situation)
	Long-term nursing facility placements for patients with complex family or financial situations

DNR, Do not resuscitate; *HINN,* hospital-issued notice of noncoverage; *PSA,* Protective Services for Adults.

TABLE 3-1 Guidelines for Referrals—cont'd

Inpatient Case Management Model For AIDS Patients		
Shared Responsibilities		
RN Case Manager	**RN Case Manager/Social Worker**	**Social Worker**
Completes discharge planning forms	Assesses each patient	Participates in daily rounds and team meetings
Performs admissions and concurrent utilization management, including insurance calls	Identifies and communicates with prior and future providers of medical and psychosocial services	Collaborates with community agencies, CBO's IDC providers round on complex psychosocial problems
Tracks data (e.g., variances in patient care and systems standards)	Assists physicians in completing discharge forms	Initiates referrals to AIDS community services and immigration advocacy groups
Facilitates daily rounds and team meetings		Provides crisis intervention; advocacy; counseling around impact of illness on the patient/significant other, bereavement, and sexual assault; child protection; substance abuse patient education
Makes referrals to home health services		
Orders transportation, equipment, supplies		
Provides alternate level of care notifications		Facilitates discussion around healthcare proxies, guardianship, DNR orders
Issues HINN letters		Provides financial assessments and referrals to entitlement programs
		Maintains contact with each patient through patient's first follow-up medical provider appointment postdischarge
		Refers patients to long-term and subacute placement

CBO, Community-based organization; *IDC*, infectious disease clinic.

control the types of patients approved for admission. Before managed care, the need for putting such controls in place was much less obvious and clearly less important.

Case management in the admitting department provides for a gatekeeping function at one of the two primary routes of entry to the hospital. Patients are screened through the use of clinical indicators. Through this process, the patient's severity of illness and the intensity of service requirements are compared with the services being requested by the admitting physician. When the patient's needs do not meet the admission criteria (see Chapters 5 and 6), the case manager contacts the physician to discuss care alternatives to the acute care setting.

The case manager may suggest to the physician the use of an alternative level of care/setting such as ambulatory surgery or an observation unit. It is important that the case manager never deny an admission without providing the physician with alternative settings along

the continuum that would more appropriately meet the patient's clinical needs and ensure reimbursement.

The case manager also screens all admissions for which the admitting physician is requesting preoperative days. Using established criteria, the case manager will either approve or disapprove the request. If approval cannot be granted because reimbursement cannot be obtained, the case manager will communicate this to the admitting physician. If the case manager and the physician feel that a patient cannot adequately prepare himself or herself for surgery, such as completing a bowel prep, then despite the lack of reimbursement, the approval will be granted. The patient's intensity of service should be the primary indicator determining whether a preoperative day is necessary.

The admitting department case manager also screens all patients being transferred into the hospital to ensure that the transfer is appropriate and meets all

Medicare guidelines. The basic rule of thumb for acute to acute transfers is that the receiving hospital should have the capacity to provide the higher level of service that the patient requires, and that cannot be provided in the transferring hospital. An example of this would be cardiac surgery. The patient may have been admitted to the sending hospital for a cardiac catheterization or on an emergency basis (e.g., acute chest pain). The sending hospital may not have open heart surgery services available, and therefore the patient must be transferred to receive this higher level of service.

Once admission to the hospital has been agreed to, the admitting case manager is responsible for communicating his or her approval to the admitting department. Generally the clerical staff in the admitting department then obtain a **preauthorization** or **precertification** from the insurance company. When the insurance company is requesting clinical information before giving its precertification, the case manager is often the appropriate person to provide that link between the clinicians, the admitting department, and the insurance company.

The admitting case manager reviews all same-day admissions before the scheduled day of surgery to ensure that preauthorization has been obtained. Additionally, the admitting case manager may be responsible for reviewing all "short-stay" medical records. These would be the medical records of patients who have been in the hospital for 24 hours or less and who were not placed in an observation status. The case manager would review the record to assess whether the care rendered and documented met acute care criteria. If the record does not support an inpatient level of reimbursement, the case manager has the authority to revert the hospital bill to the ED services only. In this way an insurance denial is avoided and the hospital is at least assured that it will receive the ED level of **reimbursement** in a timely manner (Case Manager's Tip 3-6).

Preadmission Testing Case Management

In some organizations the admitting case management functions may be integrated with the preadmission testing process. During the preadmission process the case

manager may interview and "intake" preoperative patients. During this interview process the case manager would evaluate the patient for any preadmission issues that might affect the hospitalization or posthospitalization process. Part of this assessment should include exploring discharge planning options with the patient/family. When appropriate, the patient should be referred to the social worker who will be responsible for the patient after admission and the inpatient case manager. The case manager may also collaborate with the attending physician when postdischarge needs can be clearly anticipated. For example, an elderly patient who is scheduled for a hip replacement will most likely need either subacute or home care rehabilitation after surgery. The preadmission case manager can begin to discuss options with the patient, family/caregiver, and physician and can also explore these options with the insurance company. All intake information should be communicated to the inpatient case manager so that a smooth transition can take place for the patient. The case manager should document a "preadmit" note in the patient's record that would include postdischarge needs and options.

Perioperative Services Case Management

Perioperative case management is designed to provide case management services to surgical patients. The process begins at the preadmission phase, continues postdischarge, includes surgery and postanesthesia recovery, and terminates at the postoperative period. The perioperative case manager provides an important link between the members of the surgical team and the patient. During the preoperative phase the case manager assesses the patient to be sure that the patient is ready for surgery. Readiness may be defined by the following checklist:

- All preoperative tests completed
- Medical clearance obtained
- **Informed consent** obtained
- Patient scheduled for surgery
- Authorization for surgery obtained

If any elements on the checklist are not completed and/or are problematic, the case manager can adjust the operating room (OR) schedule so that the patient is not left on the schedule, cancelled, and then another patient placed in that slot. For example, before surgery the patient may refuse to sign consent or may become unstable and unable to go to surgery the next day.

Perioperative case managers can also review same-day surgical admissions to ensure that the minimal requirements for surgery have been completed. They use the American Surgical Association (ASA) classification system (Box 3-3) as the review criteria in addition

 CASE MANAGER'S TIP *3-6*

Admitting Department and Emergency Department Case Management

Admitting department and emergency department case management models are key to any case management program design because they represent routes of entry to the hospital.

BOX 3-3   American Surgical Association Classifications

- **ASA Class I:** Patient with no systemic disease; takes no prescription or illicit drugs; pathology limited to surgical site, with no systemic implications.
- **ASA Class II:** Patient with mild systemic disease (e.g., diabetes controlled by diet or oral medications; controlled hypertension; smoker without respiratory symptoms).
- **ASA Class III:** Patient with severe systemic disease that limits activity but is not incapacitating (e.g., diabetic patient on daily insulin; poorly controlled hypertension).
- **ASA Class IV:** Patient with an incapacitating systemic disease that is a constant threat to life (e.g., diabetic patient with history of repeated episodes of ketoacidosis and/or hypoglycemia; patient with severe uncontrolled hypertension; patient with coronary artery disease and frequent episodes of chest pain).

---

to any other utilization management criteria as indicated by the organization or the managed care companies. For example, for ASA I and II categories a history and physical must be completed, as well as a complete blood cell count (CBC), electrocardiogram (ECG), chest x-ray examination, and PT/PTT when indicated. For ASA III and IV, all of these must be completed, the patient must be assessed by an anesthesiologist, and any additional tests as indicated by the patient's primary care physician must be completed. For example, a patient with hypertension may need additional testing before the medical clearance will be approved.

The perioperative case manager maintains a vital link between the patient, the surgeon, and the OR schedule. Potential delays or cancellations are identified earlier, and adjustments are made to the OR schedule so that OR time can be optimized every day. By identifying potential problems early, the patient can be reassessed and possibly go for the surgery later on the day scheduled rather than the surgery being cancelled, resulting in a potential denial of payment by a third-party payer.

COMMUNITY-BASED CASE MANAGEMENT MODELS

Community-based case management encompasses any of the case management functions that are being performed outside the acute care setting. Community-based case management, whether in the home care arena, the clinic setting, or the chronic care setting, is designed to support patients and families in achieving the optimal level of wellness by accessing and using community services. Community-based case management incorporates a focus on the continuum of care.

In some instances the community-based case manager provides episodic case management. For example, the home care case manager manages the care of a patient through a specific episode of illness, after which his or her span of responsibility concludes. The community-based case manager, working out of a clinic setting for a patient in a capitated, at-risk contract, may follow this patient from **enrollment** to **disenrollment**, passing the case management "baton" to the episodic case manager (e.g., the acute care or home care case manager [Box 3-4]).

Home Care Case Management

Case management in the home setting is designed with the same goals in mind as case management in the acute care setting. The role of home care in the success of case management is critical, especially because of the ability to care for increasingly complex and chronically ill patients. The implementation of chronic care management and disease management programs have provided a unique opportunity for home care case management to reduce the need for acute care services, therefore allowing healthcare providers and executives to curtail cost and reduce the hospital's length of stay. The continuum approach to case management programs and managed care have also spurred alternative approaches to the provision of healthcare services, such as subacute care, transitional living centers, infusion centers, day treatment centers, and especially sophisticated home care services that handle individuals requiring higher and alternative levels of care and **acuity** (Case Manager's Tip 3-7). The goals of home care case management are as follows:

- Optimizing the delivery of care across the continuum
- Keeping patients in less costly care settings
- Facilitating a proactive approach to patient care delivery and management
- Preventing deterioration in patients' conditions
- Reducing patients' risk and the need for acute care services

The demand for case managers to coordinate and integrate healthcare services in the home setting has

---

BOX 3-4   The Case Manager's Span of Accountability

Staff RN: admission to discharge
Acute care case manager: preadmission to postdischarge
Community case manager: enrollment to disenrollment

CASE MANAGER'S TIP 3-7

Home Care Case Management

Home care case management targets patients with chronic illness and seriously complex medical and psychosocial conditions and those who need immediate postacute care services.

---

increased exponentially over the past decade. This has resulted from the growth of managed care, increasing **capitation,** implementation of the home care **prospective payment system** by the federal government for Medicare and Medicaid beneficiaries, **demand management** programs, **integrated delivery systems,** and the payers' expectations that the providers do more for less. The case manager in the home environment directs the members of the interdisciplinary healthcare team (Box 3-5) toward the achievement of the best-quality care at the lowest possible cost (Case Manager's Tip 3-8). The home care case manager also makes visits to patients in their homes to ensure that they are receiving the appropriate services and that the expected outcomes are being met. During the home visit the case manager may decide to refer the patient to the physician or other healthcare providers as deemed necessary.

The home care case manager receives referrals from the hospital-based case manager. The home care case manager can obtain important information on

---

BOX 3-5 Members of the Home Care Case Management Team

Core Members
- Physician
- Nurses
- Case manager
- Physical therapist
- Occupational therapist
- Speech therapist
- Social worker
- Home health aide
- Home companion/homemaker
- Administrator

Ad Hoc Members
- Acute care case manager/discharge planner
- Health education specialist
- Clinical nurse specialist
- Home care intake coordinator
- Consulting/specialty physicians

 ## CASE MANAGER'S TIP 3-8

Home Care Case Management Services

Case managers in the home care setting are responsible for coordinating and integrating care for patients with complex therapeutic modalities and treatment plans such as the following:
- Nonhealing wounds and wound care management
- Infusion therapy
- Speech therapy
- Physical and occupational therapy; activities of daily living (ADLs)
- Mechanical ventilation and oxygen therapy
- Polypharmacy
- Tube feedings
- Psychosocial counseling and social services for the patient and family
- Pain management and palliative care

---

the patient's condition and related care by visiting the patient in the hospital and/or attending the hospital patient planning or discharge planning rounds. If a face-to-face exchange of information is not practical or possible, then the home care and hospital case managers must develop good systems for the sharing and exchange of information. Information to be shared should include the patient's medical history, physical symptoms and functional abilities or other findings, financial information including entitlements, and relevant psychosocial issues, including family support mechanisms (Brueckner and Glover, 1993).

Patients receiving home care services are not acute enough for hospitalization and are not ambulatory enough for daily visits to a clinic setting or physician's office. In most cases the cost of home care is a fraction of what a hospital stay would cost. In addition to monitoring the patient's progress during this phase of illness, the case manager will also ensure that the necessary services are being delivered in the home setting and that the patient's optimal level of wellness is being met. Under **fee-for-service (FFS)** reimbursement, there was no financial incentive for the home care agency to control the number of home visits. Just as hospital visits were relatively unlimited before the prospective payment system, the home care agencies are only now beginning to face reductions in resources and reimbursement for visits. Under capitated managed care and the prospective payment structure, the number of home visits are the most strictly controlled.

The criteria for selecting patients for the provision of home care case management services are similar to those of traditional home care services and defined by the conditions of participation in Medicare and/or Medicaid programs. In order for the patients to receive home care case management services, they must meet the following criteria:

- Homebound
- In need of skilled services (i.e., care provided by a licensed professional such an RN, social worker, or physical therapist)
- Under the supervision of a physician
- Show the medical necessity of services
- In need of intermittent or part-time services

Aliotta and Andre (1997) identified criteria for case managers to use for identifying high-risk seniors enrolled in a managed care health plan. They thought that the enrollee would benefit from home care case management services. Case managers used a screening questionnaire for this purpose. They also obtained referrals based on these criteria from other healthcare providers, including physicians. These criteria are broad in focus, which makes them applicable to any patient population and payer. Examples of these criteria are as follows:

- Diagnosis-specific indications (i.e., medical condition), such as spinal cord injury, traumatic brain injury, acquired immunodeficiency syndrome (AIDS), chronic obstructive pulmonary disease, premature neonate, high-risk pregnancy, and heart failure
- Behavioral and functional indicators, such as nonadherence to medical regimen, impairment in activities of daily living (ADLs) (e.g., bathing, dressing, toileting), lack of medical follow-up
- Healthcare resource utilization indicators, such as frequent readmissions to acute care settings, high clinic encounters, polypharmacy, complex wound care management, presence of multiple tubes (e.g., gastrostomy tube, Foley catheter, and drains), and frequent use of ED services
- Cost indicators, such as managed care health plans, capitation, benefits still available

Research has shown that a variety of factors may influence home care nurses' decisions regarding management of their clients, including the appropriate number of visits or the necessity for referrals to social service or other agencies (Feldman et al, 1993). Home care agencies have developed home care protocols similar to those previously developed for hospital care (e.g., pathways and **multidisciplinary action plans [MAPs]**). These prospectively developed tools become the case manager's frame of reference as they outline the appropriate number of visits for a particular disease entity or surgical procedure. Expected outcomes for each discipline are predetermined so that the number of patient care visits correlates with the expected outcomes. As a

 CASE MANAGER'S TIP *3-9*

Home Care Case Management
Home care case managers can help ensure that patients achieve expected outcomes without duplication or redundant use of resources by coordinating services and monitoring the patient's progress closely.

result, allotted visits are not arbitrary but can be validated, and the patient's progress toward these expected outcomes can be benchmarked. The termination point for the case is also clearly defined, and the expectations of the staff in terms of when to close the case are delineated. Cases kept open beyond the appropriate length of time become very costly to the home care agency. By prospectively identifying the criteria for case closure based on outcomes, the care provider no longer has to make a subjective decision regarding when to close the case. Closing cases in a timely fashion allows resources to be appropriated to those cases that truly need extended services beyond the norm.

Home care case managers can be assigned by disease entity or broader clinical specialty. Chronic illnesses, such as diabetes, asthma, human immunodeficiency virus (HIV) and AIDS, or congestive heart failure, may require case management services in the home after an episode of acute exacerbation of the disease. Rehabilitation after joint replacement is another clinical grouping for which case management may work well. These patients will require the services of more than one discipline, such as nursing and physical therapy. By coordinating these services and monitoring the patient's progress closely, the case manager can ensure that the patient is moving toward those outcomes as efficiently as possible without duplication or redundant utilization of resources (Case Manager's Tip 3-9).

Community-Based Nursing Case Management

Community-based case management models are focused on primary care and primary prevention. They are therefore predominantly focused on healthy individuals in the community who are at risk or who have the potential for needing healthcare services. These models can provide integrated services found nowhere else. Comprehensive, coordinated, community-based programs can interrelate the client's health, social, educational, employment, and recreational needs.

Community nursing centers are defined as those in which the key management positions are filled by RNs. These centers can range in size from a staff of one to

115 RNs, with an average of eight per agency (Barger and Rosenfeld, 1993). Some centers use a case management model and philosophy to guide the care delivery process. In nurse case management models, the practice may be an autonomous nursing one. Two thirds of the RNs employed in nursing centers are certified for advanced nursing practice (Barger and Rosenfeld, 1993). Nurse practitioners are able to provide primary care as the client's first contact with a healthcare provider. The remaining practitioners are generally master's prepared social workers. Referrals are made to on-site and off-site physicians and other off-site healthcare providers. Other resource referrals may be on or off site.

The goal of community-based case management is to support and empower individuals to maximize their optimal level of wellness through the use of community resources (Case Manager's Tip 3-10). Health promotion may be incorporated into activities such as day care classes, youth and adult recreation programs, support groups, meals for elders, community development activities, and adult education programs.

Both formal and informal mechanisms can be used to provide case management services. These might include nonscheduled walk-in clinics, scheduled appointments, home visits, or telephone consults. All are focused on continuous rather than episodic care (Trella, 1996).

The community-based case manager can provide other important services to the patient, such as continuing the educational program initiated in the hospital setting. Patients in the hospital may not retain the information they learned as a result of anxiety or pain and may therefore benefit greatly from reinforcement on returning to the community. The community-based case manager discusses topics the patient has been taught in the hospital and continues the educational process through repetition, reinforcement, or continuation of teaching related to the specific topic.

The ongoing education and support provided by the community-based case manager may mean that exacerbations of the patient's disease and/or readmissions can be reduced. Many programs are focused around specific disease entities such as diabetes, chemical dependency, or HIV. These programs are geared to already diagnosed individuals whose goal is to maintain their optimal level of wellness in the community for as long as possible.

Community-Based Social Work Case Management

Community-based social workers may perform a variety of functions. Generally, a social work model is predicated on some form of referral process whereby the social worker is referred cases that are deemed to be at high risk. High-risk criteria for a community-based social work referral might include such things as the need for psychosocial counseling/support, family counseling, financial counseling, and stress management. Social workers in the community may be referred patients through a physician, a clinic, or through self-referral.

In some high-risk cases, a patient may be case managed by both a nurse and a social worker in the community. The need for both disciplines is determined based on the patient's high-risk needs. Those with both psychosocial and clinical needs may therefore be case managed by both a nurse and a social worker. In this way, the neediest patients receive the care and support of the disciplines best able to meet those needs.

Social workers in the community may provide short-term psychosocial interventions or long-term support, depending on the needs of the patient and family. For example, a family with a child who has cystic fibrosis may need years of psychosocial intervention and support. The social worker may maintain a therapeutic relationship with that child and family for a very long time.

Subacute Care Case Management

The subacute setting is among the fastest growing care delivery settings within the continuum of care. The reasons for this growth are obvious. Just 10 years ago it was not uncommon to find patients recovering in acute care beds for weeks on end while receiving nothing more than an intravenous (IV) antibiotic, wound care, or ventilator weaning. Because of the high cost of managing these types of patients in acute care beds, MCOs began to expect that patients meeting the clinical criteria of subacute would be transferred to subacute units, whether in hospitals, nursing homes, or freestanding facilities.

Subacute care is considered restorative, meaning that it is expected that the patient's condition will improve as a result of the care rendered. The level of care is somewhere between acute care and traditional nursing

 CASE MANAGER'S TIP 3-10

Community-Based Case Management

By providing ongoing education and support to patients, the case manager can help ensure that the goal of community-based case management is met: to support and empower individuals to reach their optimal level of wellness through the use of community resources.

home care. Care rendered may be less invasive and less diagnostically oriented as compared with acute care. In comparison with traditional nursing home care it is more intensive and of shorter duration. The average length of stay is generally between 7 and 30 days. Admission criteria would be specific to the program of care, such as neurologic, rehabilitation, or orthopedic, and the patient would have to demonstrate clear outcome potential.

In the subacute setting the physician would visit 1 to 3 times per week. Average nursing care is 4.5 to 8 hours of direct nursing care per patient day, with a high use of nurse aides. To qualify for subacute rehabilitation, typically a patient must be able to tolerate a minimum of 1 to $1\frac{1}{2}$ hours of therapy per day. Patients are expected to be discharged home after the course of treatment.

Case managers who discharge patients to subacute settings must be familiar with the criteria for the levels of service in the subacute setting. The three categories include (1) short-term rehabilitative or restorative, (2) short-term complex medical or recuperative, and (3) long-term, chronic, or preventive maintenance (Table 3-2).

The hospital-based case manager should always consider transferring a patient to a subacute level of care/setting when the acute care outcomes have been met and the patient's care can be rendered in a less intensive setting.

The case manager in the subacute setting coordinates the services of the interdisciplinary team that would include physicians, therapists, nurses, and other professionals such as nutritionists. The case manager is responsible for ensuring that the patient is moving toward expected outcomes of care, whether restorative, recuperative, or end of life. In some instances the patient may be discharged home to continue with home care services, or the patient may need to be moved to a skilled nursing facility level of service. By closely monitoring the patient's progress toward expected outcomes, the case manager can assess that the patient is receiving the appropriate level of service, and if not, the case manager should work with the interdisciplinary team to transition the patient to the appropriate level or to home if outcomes have been met.

Nursing Home/Long-Term Care Case Management

Patients with any diagnosis can be admitted to a skilled nursing facility level of service. Care is considered to be either chronic or supportive. The average length of stay is approximately $1\frac{1}{2}$ years. Physician visits are about once a month, and patients receive about $1\frac{1}{2}$ to 3 hours of nursing care per patient day. Rehabilitation services provided to the nursing home resident are limited in scope and when provided are usually less than 30 minutes per day. Patients leave this level of service either when admitted to a hospital or at the time of their death.

As in the subacute setting, the long-term care case manager can provide a vital link between the members of the interdisciplinary team.

Emergency Department Case Management

As a commonly used route of entry to the hospital, acute care case management models should not neglect to staff this important hospital department. As does the admitting department case manager, the ED case manager provides an important gatekeeping function for the hospital. The ED case manager is responsible for facilitating the patient's hospitalization from preadmission

TABLE 3-2　Conditions Typically Considered Subacute

Short-Term Complex Medical	Short-Term Rehabilitative	Long-Term (Chronic)
Postsurgical recovery	Cerebrovascular accident	Coma
Respiratory management	Stroke	Multiple trauma
Pulmonary management	Brain injury	Ventilator dependency
Oncology	Spinal injury	Head injury
AIDS care	Amputation	
Wound care	Arthritis	
Tracheostomy/suctioning	Total hip/knee replacements	
Total parenteral nutrition	Other neurologic/orthopedic	
Intravenous therapies/administration	conditions	
Terminal care		
Dialysis		
Complication as a result of prematurity		

through discharge from the ED. The case manager interfaces with physicians, nurses, social workers, and other members of the team to expedite medically appropriate, cost-effective care.

The ED case manager manages different groupings of patients. These include the treat-and-release patients; patients admitted to the hospital; patients who can be discharged from the hospital but will require follow-up services, such as home care, in the community; observation patients; and inappropriate admissions such as social admissions.

Treat-and-Release Patients

This group of ED patients will receive all necessary services during their short-term treatment time in the ED and will be discharged without the need for follow-up home care or other community services beyond the routine follow-up physician or clinic appointment. The ED case manager can assist these patients to receive the care they require in the most expeditious way possible. Patients who typically fall into this category include asthmatics or those with other chronic illnesses and patients with injuries or viruses, colds, and the like. Because of the common misuse of EDs in the United States, many of the treat-and-release patients could have received the care they needed in their primary care physician's office or an urgent center.

The case manager facilitates the initiation of diagnostic services, treatment plans, and therapeutic treatments while the patient is in the ED. The case manager identifies any delays in service and either expedites the process by eliminating barriers or collaborates with other members of the interdisciplinary team to resolve the problem.

Patients Admitted from the Emergency Department

The case manager works with the interdisciplinary team to facilitate diagnostic testing in the ED and to ensure that the treatment plan is initiated immediately once a diagnosis has been rendered. For example, a pneumonia patient who is being admitted to the hospital should have his or her antibiotic therapy initiated while still in the ED once the diagnosis has been established. By initiating the treatment in the ED, hours can be shaved off the length of stay and quality of care is enhanced.

The case manager also works with the team to ensure that the patient is transferred to the inpatient bed as quickly as possible. Patients who are out of their managed care network may choose to be transferred to a hospital within their network. The case manager plays an important role in identifying these patients and discussing their options with them. Patients can only be transferred by their own request and if stable. So as to not violate any Emergency Medical Treatment and Active Labor Act (EMTALA) regulations, the case manager should only inform the patient that if they are admitted they may risk some financial responsibility for the hospital bill. The case manager should make it very clear to the patient that they have every right to remain and that they will receive appropriate care, but that there may be some financial risk associated with this decision.

Case managers working in EDs must have a working knowledge of EMTALA and its requirements. EMTALA (also known as COBRA, Section 1867, or the Federal Antidumping Act), governs the delivery of all hospital-based emergency medical care in the United States. It is an antidiscrimination statute.

Two sections in EMTALA relate directly to the initial interactions of EDs with managed care patients, or the "Appropriate Medical Screening Examination" (MSE) requirement, and the "No Delay on Account of Insurance" provision.

The Appropriate Medical Screening Examination provision states the following:

If any individual comes to the emergency department and a request is made on the individual's behalf for examination and treatment, the hospital must provide an appropriate medical screening exam within the capability of the hospital's emergency department, including **ancillary services** routinely available to the emergency department, to determine whether or not an emergency medical condition exists (42 USC 1395dd[a]).

For the case manager in the ED, this simply means that all patients who come to the ED must be given an appropriate medical screening. Patients cannot be turned away for any reason. Case managers should be sensitive to this provision and should never be pressured to transfer a patient to another facility unless by the patient's request and only after an appropriate medical screening.

The No Delay on Account of Insurance provision states the following:

A hospital may not delay provision of an appropriate medical screening examination or necessary stabilizing treatment ... in order to inquire about the individual's method of payment or insurance status (42 USC 1395dd[h]).

It should never be the policy of an ED to demand that a patient receive authorization from his or her managed care company before screening takes place. The ED case manager should never interfere in this process. In any event, a managed care company cannot deny authorization for an ED visit under any circumstances unless once triaged it is determined that the presenting condition is not an emergency condition. Under those circumstances, the patient's care may be delayed while authorization is being obtained. The patient may be referred to his or her urgent care center for further treatment of the non-emergent complaint.

If the patient requires hospitalization and is out of network, the ED should have a written procedure for informing the patient of the potential "financial risk" of being admitted to the out-of-network hospital. The patient should be clearly told that he or she may certainly stay at the out-of-network hospital if he or she so chooses and that the patient will receive all needed services if that is his or her decision. At the same time, the patient should know that this decision may result in his or her suffering some financial burden such as a **deductible** or a **copayment,** depending on the patient's coverage. If the patient chooses to transfer to an in-network hospital, the patient must sign a release indicating that he or she is transferring at his or her own request. The patient's plan should be billed for the transportation to the in-network hospital. Under no circumstances can a patient be transferred unless he or she is medically stable. Transfer would also be appropriate under circumstances in which the patient needed transfer to receive a higher level of service than was available in the first hospital.

Emergency Medical Conditions

Under EMTALA, the definition of an emergency medical condition (EMC) is much broader than typical medical usage. An EMC is any condition that is a danger to the health and safety of the patient or unborn fetus, or may result in a risk or impairment or dysfunction to the smallest bodily organ or part if not treated in the foreseeable future, and includes the following range of conditions:

■ Undiagnosed, acute pain, sufficient to impair normal functioning
■ Pregnancy with contractions present (legally defined as unstable)
■ Symptoms of substance abuse such as alcohol ingestion
■ Psychiatric disturbances such as severe depression, insomnia, suicide attempt or ideation, dissociative state, and inability to comprehend danger or to care for oneself

The ED case manager plays an important educational role for the hospital and an advocacy role for the patient and should remain cognizant and up-to-date on EMTALA at all times.

The ED case manager performs an intake assessment on admitted patients and communicates this assessment to the inpatient case manager. The assessment should include a discharge planning assessment and referral to the social worker if necessary. The case manager should provide any clinical information needed by the third-party payer during the admission process.

Discharged Patients with Services

The case manager in the ED is responsible for coordinating any needed follow-up services for patients returning to the community. In some instances, this intervention may prevent an unnecessary or nonreimbursable admission. The case manager will coordinate the discharge plan with the team and ensure that the services are covered by the patient's third-party payer. Once this has been completed, the case manager will facilitate and coordinate those services with the community agency. Typically, patients who fall into this category will need home care services. On occasion a patient may be transferred to a long-term care facility directly from the ED. In all instances the case manager should follow established criteria to ensure that the patient is receiving the appropriate level of service.

Observation Patients

Under Medicare, observation is an outpatient category in which the patient needs observation of a condition or following a procedure for less than 24 hours. Patients may be observed in a specific observation unit or scattered within the hospital. If the patient is placed in an inpatient bed, the patient's status remains outpatient and the bill should reflect that this level of care was provided. The hospital may bill the third party for the ED visit and for up to 24 hours after the time of transfer from the ED. Under the **ambulatory payment classification (APC) system,** the observation portion of the stay will be bundled with the ED APC and an enhanced rate should be reimbursed.

The ED case manager should work directly with the attending medical staff in the ED and assist them in the identification of patients appropriate for observation. The InterQual and Milliman and Robertson criteria both provide the clinical parameters of the observation status.

Inappropriate Admissions

When it is clear that a patient does not require admission, the case manager should assist the care team in identifying an alternative care regimen appropriate to the needs of the patient. For example, a patient may require admission to a long-term care or subacute setting or may require home care services. Working with the patient, the family and the care team, the case manager can facilitate the movement of the patient to the appropriate level of service and prevent a hospital denial of payment.

SYSTEM MODELS

The system models are designed to provide case management services along the continuum. A *continuum of care* is defined as an integrated, client-oriented system of care composed of both services and integrating mechanisms that guides and tracks clients over time through a comprehensive array of health, mental health, and social services spanning all levels of intensity of care (Evashwick, 1987). The continuum contains seven access points to healthcare, as described in Box 3-6.

BOX 3-6   Healthcare Access Points and Types of Care Offered

Primary Care
1. Clinics
2. Health fairs
3. Screening programs
4. Health education programs
5. Demand management programs

Ambulatory Care
1. Physician offices
2. Clinics
3. Diagnostic centers
4. Day surgery

Acute Care
1. Hospitals
2. Medical centers
3. Emergency departments

Tertiary Care
1. Teaching hospitals
2. Acute rehabilitation
3. Specialty physicians

Home Care
1. Visiting nursing services
2. Home medical equipment, including IV therapy
3. Community care programs

Long-Term Care
1. Nursing homes
2. Subacute care facilities
3. Long-term rehabilitation centers
4. Adult homes
5. Skilled nursing facilities

Palliative/Hospice Care
1. Home hospice programs
2. Hospital-based programs
3. End-stage group homes

The case manager is assigned to the case at one of the seven access points, depending on where the patient enters the healthcare system. In most cases the case manager is responsible for the patient no matter where the patient is along the healthcare continuum. This may mean that the primary case manager communicates with the case manager in the setting in which the patient currently is. For example, if a community-based case manager is following the patient, the responsibility for the case may be relinquished to the hospital-based case manager should the patient be admitted. The community-based case manager would share relevant information with the hospital-based case manager and might visit the patient. The ultimate responsibility for the management of the case while the patient is in the hospital would be the hospital-based case manager's.

In organizations in which the service line crosses the continuum and there are multiple service programs, patient referrals and continuity of care are not necessarily automatic. In fact, the more complex the organization, the greater the need for client referral and tracking mechanisms (Evashwick, 1987). Continuity can be maintained by the case manager for clients at any point along the continuum (Case Manager's Tip 3-11).

CHRONIC CARE CASE MANAGEMENT

Chronic conditions are those the patient is expected to have for years or possibly for the rest of his or her life. These individuals may access and use a variety of healthcare services in a multitude of settings during the course of their illness. It is the use of these various services and settings for the chronically ill that places them at risk for receiving less-than-adequate, duplicative, fragmented, or delayed healthcare services. Typical target populations for chronic care case management include the frail elderly, survivors of strokes, accident victims, the mentally ill, and children and infants with congenital abnormalities (Evashwick, 1987).

Patients with chronic illnesses may access a wide range of services from acute care to social services, mental health, home care, or subacute care. It is during

 CASE MANAGER'S TIP 3-11

System Model of Case Management
In organizations in which the service line crosses the continuum and there are multiple service programs, the case manager can help maintain continuity for clients at any point along the continuum by providing referral and tracking services.

CASE MANAGER'S TIP 3-12

Chronic Care Case Management

The case manager can coordinate the wide range of services needed by chronically ill patients so that care, financing, and information are integrated. This provides a foundation for planning and managing care across settings.

BOX 3-7   Conditions Typically Considered Subacute

Emphasis on subacute care as a cost-saving mechanism is increasing. The conditions that typically are included in this category include the following:
1. Short-term complex medical problems
2. Short-term rehabilitative conditions
3. Long-term (chronic) conditions

---

these transitions that the greatest opportunity for problems may arise. Case management integrates these wide-ranging services so that care delivery, financing, and information are integrated. It provides a foundation for planning and managing care across settings (Case Manager's Tip 3-12). The focus is more than just providing the patient with access to the various services; it is also geared toward integrating these systems to provide a coordinated, continuing care approach.

The patient population at greatest risk for chronic care needs is the elderly, particularly the frail elderly. This group is at high risk for complex health needs, potential for physical or social complications, and continued use of costly healthcare resources. A multidisciplinary approach such as that provided by a case management model has been documented to reduce cost and improve outcomes for this population (Trella, 1993). The application of case management to this population may mean providing adult day care programs with transportation. The children of aging parents may be able to maintain their parents in the community if they have access to an adult day care program that provides a flexible structure so that they can drop parents off on their way to work and pick them up in the evening. Other necessary services may be meal preparation, delivery services, housekeeping, or shopping services (Mullahy, 1995).

LONG-TERM CARE CASE MANAGEMENT

Long-term care settings such as the nursing home, rehabilitation facility, or skilled nursing facility are settings in which case management can serve the purpose of slowing the deterioration process and functional status of the resident. In long-term care settings, care has been task oriented (Smith, 1991), with different practitioners providing different services to the resident. Today's typical nursing home patient is sicker, requires more complex medical and nursing care, and will live longer.

Increasing focus is also being placed on other subacute care settings as managed care drives the need for less

expensive care settings appropriate to the needs of the patient (Stahl, 1996). Conditions that usually are considered subacute are listed in Box 3-7.

Short-term complex medical problems would include problems such as wound care, respiratory management, total parenteral nutrition, dialysis, intravenous therapies, and postsurgical recovery. The goal in case managing this group of patients is recuperative. The expected outcome is to bring the patient to the optimal level of wellness.

Short-term rehabilitative subacute care focuses on clinical issues such as stroke, amputation, total hip/knee replacement, and brain injury. The case management goal for this clinical group is restorative, to bring the patient as close to the preinjury condition as possible.

Long-term (chronic) case management is preventive maintenance, assisting the patient to maintain the level of functioning without deterioration for as long as possible. Long-term chronic conditions include coma, ventilator dependence, and head injury.

In response to these changes, nursing homes are adapting and undergoing modifications to the way they provided care in the past. Case management has been used as a mechanism not only for improving patient outcomes in long-term care settings but also for improving job satisfaction of care providers in these settings (Deckard, Hicks, and Rountree, 1986). With the introduction of a case management model, a healthcare provider can coordinate the services provided by nursing assistants, RNs, physical and occupational therapists, and nutritionists. Integrating these services and identifying interdisciplinary expected outcomes allow the resident's functional status to be closely monitored and managed. Care is managed using an interdisciplinary approach, and therefore goals can be more specific, realistic, and measurable. Furthermore, the move away from a task-oriented approach means that goals are patient-focused instead of staff-focused (Smith, 1991).

The case manager in the long-term care setting may not be an RN if there is a lack of RN staff in the facility. In some cases it may be necessary to use the licensed practical or licensed vocational nurse in the role of case

CASE MANAGER'S TIP 3-13

Long-Term Care Case Management
To manage the care and expected outcomes of long-term care clients, focus the case management plan on nursing needs, therapies, activities of daily living, and personal care.

manager. The case manager provides for ongoing monitoring and evaluation of the resident's progress. Progress is measured against an assessment of the patient's medical problems, functional capabilities, social supports, and psychosocial well-being (Zawadski and Eng, 1988).

Case management plans (see Chapter 12) can be used to manage the care and expected outcomes. Plans should focus on such things as nursing needs, therapies, ADLs, and personal care (Case Manager's Tip 3-13). The chronicity of the residents may mean that the case management plans are reviewed at a maximum of every 3 months or whenever the resident's condition or change in progress warrants a review. The case manager provides an ongoing evaluation process and liaisons between the resident, the physician, the family, and other members of the healthcare team.

MANAGED CARE MODELS AND CASE MANAGEMENT

Managed care is a broad, expansive term covering a wide variety of services. Its main objective is to contain costs by controlling utilization and coordinating care. It is used as the generic term for insurance plans offering managed healthcare services to an enrolled population on a prepaid basis such as capitation (per-member-per-month fixed rate). Access, cost, and quality are controlled by care gatekeepers. The gatekeeper is usually a physician in primary care. This physician, after assessing the patient, will determine whether the patient needs additional services such as a specialty physician or other service controlled by the MCO. There are many types of MCOs, but the most common is the HMO. The four basic models are the **group model HMO,** the **staff model HMO,** the **individual practice association (IPA) model HMO,** and the **network model HMO** (see Chapter 2).

In the various managed care models case managers are employed to carry out a variety of functions. Broadly speaking, the case management functions can be classified as either financial case management or clinical case management. The financial case manager functions in what might traditionally be classified

as utilization management. This case manager is in communication with the hospital case manager or utilization manager determining the patient's admission eligibility; continued stay; or discharge disposition, including eligibility of postdischarge services. The case manager in this role advocates on behalf of the MCO and may have a caseload of hundreds or thousands of patients. This role is based on a lower intensity–higher volume approach (Sampson, 1994).

Some MCOs supplement the patients being followed by a financial case manager with a more clinically focused case manager. These case managers tend to have a somewhat smaller caseload (Sampson, 1994). Their focus is more high intensity–low volume in nature. They may be assigned by degree of risk stratification (i.e., low, moderate, or high-risk patient population) as identified by the MCO. These may include such things as catastrophic illness or injury, high-user or high-volume members, chronic or disabling conditions, or cases with high annual cost projections ($25,000 to $50,000) (Hicks, Stallmeyer, and Coleman, 1993). It is hoped that assisting in the management of these patients will prevent unnecessary admissions to the hospital and minimize misutilization of healthcare resources (Case Manager's Tip 3-14).

MCOs vary in how they employ the services of case managers. Some have developed case management departments and hired salaried case managers to assume the financial and clinical roles discussed previously. Others have contracted with independent case management entities for these services (Mullahy, 1998) (e.g., outsourced this function). Still others have a hybrid arrangement in which most case management activities are performed by the MCO while **workers' compensation** and long-term disability cases are subcontracted to an independent or private case management provider. However, it is unlikely for a large MCO to outsource this important function. Regardless of the arrangement, the role of the case manager remains basically the same.

Some MCOs are focusing on the management of their older members. The elderly are at greater risk in

 CASE MANAGER'S TIP 3-14

Managed Care Case Management
Managed care case managers usually function either as financial case managers (utilization managers), who may have a caseload of hundreds or even thousands, or as more clinically focused case managers, who have fewer cases but of higher intensity.

terms of cost, chronicity, and frequency of care needs. It is hoped that case managing this population will enhance the health status of older adults while containing their use of healthcare resources (Pacala et al, 1995). MCOs have employed special strategies for managing the care of this population, such as telephonic case management and triage services.

Telephonic Case Management

Member services in MCOs (HMOs and **preferred provider organizations [PPOs]** alike) take place mostly via telephone communication. However, other methods of communication such as paper mailings still exist to some degree, and new ones such as the use of the **Internet** for electronic mailings are being developed and implemented (Case Manager's Tip 3-15). Regardless of the method employed, communication between the payer, the provider, and the members is an important subject in managed care and case management. The focus on the continuum of care in case management and disease management practices and in demand management programs sponsored by MCOs has led to an expansion in the role of the case manager. New additions include responsibility for interventions or functions that are based on the telecommunication advances such as **telephone triage** and **telephonic case management.**

Telephonic case management is defined as the delivery of healthcare services to patients and/or their families or caregivers over the telephone or through correspondence, fax, e-mail, or other forms of electronic transfer (Siefker et al, 1998). It is a patient and family encounter with a healthcare provider, in this case a case manager, applying the case management process (see Chapter 4) to appropriately meet the patient's needs.

 CASE MANAGER'S TIP 3-15

Communication Between MCOs and the Members
The greatest volume of interactions between MCOs and their members occurs in the form of telephone communications. However, other forms of communication do occur, such as routine paper mailings of the insurance identification cards, member newsletters, and other individualized forms of communication such as claims-related information. It is becoming more popular today for MCOs and their members to use electronic media such as e-mail, online discussion groups, and list serves for certain types of general communications that do not jeopardize an individual's right to privacy and confidentiality.

BOX 3-8   Benefits of Telephonic Case Management

- Patient's risk identification, stratification, and management
- Cost reduction
- Empowerment of patients and families for assuming responsibility toward self-care and health management
- Provision of timely interventions and real-time information
- Enhanced and ease of access to healthcare services, providers, and payers
- Patients are more likely to adhere to medical regimen
- One case manager could manage greater number of patients/enrollees
- Timely referral of patient/family to other providers, case managers, or community resources
- Provision of timely counseling and support for patient/family in troubleshooting problems
- Enhanced working relationships with patients, providers, and payers

---

It also is considered a cost-effective and proactive strategy for preventing catastrophic health outcomes and high expenses associated with major illness events. Box 3-8 contains additional benefits to telephonic case management.

Telephonic case management services exist across the continuum of care, particularly in the following settings:
- MCOs
- Physician offices and group practices
- Major medical centers, especially in pediatric services
- EDs
- Advice or call centers
- Community agencies

Although health advice lines have been in existence for quite some time, they did not become popular for the delivery of case management services until recently. This newer form of case management, known as telephonic case management, is the result of the pressures on managed care for cost containment and improved and timely access to healthcare services. However, MCOs incorporated telephonic case management services as an additional benefit to their members in the form of telephone triage. This service, when provided by the payer, focuses on the financial management (utilization management and resource allocation) aspect of case management. Today, the clinical aspect of case management is as popular as financial management. However, this is generally a focus of the provider rather than the payer.

Case managers provide telephonic case management services in a variety of forms and around the clock. The managed care case manager focuses on triage services and utilization management. The clinical case manager focuses on the coordination and integration of clinical services as they are needed by patients. Both types of case managers use **algorithms,** guidelines, or **protocols** for the delivery of case management services. These guidelines provide the case manager with prospectively developed plans of care that incorporate decision-making steps in the form of decision trees. For example, a mother may call the telephone triage line for an advice regarding her 3-year-old child, who is suffering from a high fever.

The case manager engaged in this telephone conversation will bring up the pediatric fever algorithm on his or her personal computer. The case manager will use this algorithm to guide the assessment and evaluation of the child's signs and symptoms so that he or she can determine the urgency of the child's medical/health condition and the type of advice or intervention he or she will be providing. Depending on how urgent the situation is, the case manager will advise the mother to (1) give the child a dose of Tylenol, (2) continue to observe the child and bring the child to the pediatrician's office, or (3) bring the child to the nearest ED.

In this example, the case manager would provide clinical case management advice and triage the patient to access the appropriate level of care/setting for further healthcare services. Other types of interventions are based on the type of call received. Telephone calls made to the MCO case manager are mostly related to problems with **claims,** clarifications of benefits, authorizations of services, or triage. Those made to clinical case management programs usually focus on the provision of advice, patient and family education, counseling, health risk management, self-care management skills building, and in some instances triage or brokerage of services. In both types of interventions, case managers apply a process of assessment of the situation/need, analysis of the situation using a related algorithm/protocol, prioritizing/determining the urgency of the situation and planning care, implementing care strategies, and evaluation of the outcomes (Blanchfield, Schwarzentraub, and Reisinger, 1997).

In telephone triage, case managers use their findings of the assessment they complete for each caller to categorize the call (i.e., the patient's condition) into one of three triage categories: emergent, urgent, or nonurgent (Rutenberg, 2000; Van Dinter, 2000).

1. **Emergent:** Patients must be seen immediately. Examples are conditions of airway compromise, cardiovascular collapse, wounds or lacerations, strokes, and sensory changes. The case manager refers patients with these conditions to the ED or may call emergency medical services for that purpose.

2. **Urgent:** Patients may be seen within 8 to 24 hours. Examples are vomiting after minor head injury, signs of infection, soft tissue injury, and increasing edema. The case manager suggests to these patients to see their primary care physician within 8 hours.

3. **Nonurgent:** Patients may be seen routinely or treated at home with appropriate follow-up. Examples are minor bruises or abrasions, persistent cough, and cold symptoms. The case manager may provide such callers with advice and recommend that if symptoms do not improve within 2 to 3 days that they see their primary care providers.

In deciding on the triage category, the case manager considers the patient's age, gender, past medical history, medication intake, and **access to care** (Rutenberg, 2000). When uncertain of a caller's situation, case managers may consult with a physician or nurse practitioner or may refer the patient/caller to them (Van Dinter, 2000).

Independent/Private Case Management

Independent/private case management entails the provision of case management services by case managers who are either self-employed or are salaried employees in a privately owned case management firm. They are known as "external" case management services. The terms *independent* and *private* refer to the absence of oversight by an MCO or a healthcare organization such as a home care agency or an acute care hospital (Case Manager's Tip 3-16). An insurance company or a healthcare facility usually subcontracts with independent case managers for the provision of case management services, particularly for long- and short-term disability cases. However, a patient or a family member may subcontract case management services from a private case manager for assistance in the coordination of cost-effective and appropriate care, for example, to the chronically ill elderly member of the family (Case Manager's Tip 3-17). Because the structure and services are almost the same in both independent and private case management, their descriptions in this section will be combined.

Independent/private case management focuses on enabling the patient to make the necessary transitions along the healthcare continuum and to successfully navigate the healthcare delivery system. It also focuses on monitoring resource utilization, managing costs and

CASE MANAGER'S TIP 3-16

Independent and Private Case Management

Although they provide similar services, the terms *independent case management* and *private case management* are not the same and should not be used interchangeably.

Independent case management refers to firms that are not a formal part of an insurance company or a healthcare facility. They exist solely for the provision of case management services based on a contractual agreement between the independent case management firm and the healthcare organization.

Private case management refers to the services provided by an independent case manager privately contracted or hired by a patient or a family member.

CASE MANAGER'S TIP 3-17

Dual Advocacy Role

Independent/private case managers function in a dual advocacy role that sometimes generates conflict. They are expected to deliver care that is efficient and cost-effective in a manner that is satisfactory for both the patient and the hiring insurance company or healthcare facility.

health benefits, and ensuring the provision of quality care and services. Healthcare organizations and MCOs are more likely to subcontract with an independent/private case management firm in the areas of rehabilitation and disability case management than for other clinical services. Subcontracting of such services is considered more cost-effective and thought to increase patient and family satisfaction. In these arrangements, case managers manage the care of their patients as representatives of the insurance company or healthcare facility unless they are hired directly by the patient or family, in which case they represent the patient.

The goals of independent/private case management are similar to other case management programs/models, particularly the insurance-based models. They include the coordination and facilitation of complex medical services; ensuring the provision of timely, quality, and appropriate services; cost-effectiveness; reduction of fragmentation or duplication of services; and providing the patient/family with a one-to-one personalized relationship with a case manager.

Independent/private case managers may not always receive referrals for their patients at an early stage of illness, trauma, or disability. On the contrary, most often they receive a referral after a patient has been ill or disabled for an extended period, which causes the illness to be considered chronic rather than acute and the focus of care to be rehabilitation and restoration of function rather than curative.

Although in independent case management the insurance company or healthcare facility hires the case managers, they are required to obtain certifications for services from the MCO before they are provided to the patient. Therefore independent case managers are usually seen interacting with the managed care–based case manager on an ongoing basis. They even provide concurrent and periodic review of the patient's condition, progress, and treatment plan to the managed care–based case manager. Usually these reviews are set to occur at a predefined time interval and are discussed. Ongoing authorizations of services are also required every 30 days regardless of whether new services are implemented. The same expectations apply for private case management unless the patient/family who made the arrangement for care is paying privately (self-paying) for the services.

Workers' Compensation

Case management approaches to workers' compensation have been implemented to curtail the increased cost and reduce the potential for legal **litigation.** They are even more important today because of the shift in workers' compensation insurance to a managed care structure in the form of HMOs and PPOs and their related utilization management practices. The application of case management in workers' compensation provides another example of the value of case management services and evidence that such models exist across the continuum of care.

Workers' compensation, also known as "workers' comp," is a type of insurance employers are mandated by law to offer to their employees in the event of an on-the-job injury (Case Manager's Tip 3-18). It is a no-fault system of benefits for employees who sustain occupational injury or illness (DiBenedetto, 2001). According to DiBenedetto, a person must sustain the injury or illness while on the job and must incur medical costs, rehabilitation costs, lost wages, or disfigurement to qualify for workers' compensation benefits. Employers are mandated by law to provide their employees with three types of benefits: **indemnity** cash benefits in lieu of lost wages, reimbursement for necessary medical expenses, and survivors' death benefits (Powell, 2000).

Workers' compensation claims are the result of trauma or job-related illness. Case management is an

CASE MANAGER'S TIP 3-18

Worker's Compensation Law

It is mandatory that employers provide their employees with a worker's compensation insurance benefit that covers on-the-job injury. This is in accordance with state law, and the mandates vary from state to state. There are some exclusions to this mandate depending on employer size and types of workers.

effective strategy used to expedite the return of injured employees to work. Case management services must be directed toward bringing the injured employee to maximal medical improvement and physical functioning and eventually back to work. Case managers are essential for meeting these goals. They assume the responsibility for coordinating medical care and rehabilitation services. They also facilitate the resolution of legal issues by acting as liaisons between the injured employee, legal representatives (lawyers), occupational health department, claims adjusters, and employer. Case managers achieve these goals by following the injured employee from the time the injury occurs until a safe, maximal, modified, or optimal return to work takes place (DiBenedetto, 1999). During this time they collaborate with rehabilitation professionals in the development, implementation, monitoring, and evaluation of the employee's plan of care and return-to-work plan.

The main focus of case management services in the field of workers' compensation is return to work. The case manager develops and achieves the return-to-work plan through the application of the case management process and in collaboration with the injured employee, the employer, and the physician(s) and other healthcare providers involved in the employee's care. Return-to-work plans are of three types (Case Manager's Tip 3-19): full, modified, or temporary. Full plans aim at returning the injured employee to a full work assignment and schedule similar to that which existed before the injury.

 CASE MANAGER'S TIP 3-19

Return-to-Work Plans

Case managers involved in the design and implementation of return to work plans must ensure compliance with relevant laws and regulations such as the Americans with Disabilities Act, Family Medical Leave Act, and Occupational Safety and Health Administration.

BOX 3-9 Sample Modifications of Return-to-Work Plans

- Decreased work hours
- Temporary job sharing
- Reducing responsibilities and tasks
- Acquisition and use of assistive equipment or other tools
- Technology modifications

Modified plans are those adjusted to meet the injured employee's abilities and physical limitations resulting from the injury. Case managers implement these plans to expedite the employee's return to work (Box 3-9). Temporary plans are those that are adjusted for a limited period during the time the injured employee is still undergoing rehabilitation. These plans include limitations in job functions based on the medical and functional condition of the employee. Before the employee returns to work with this temporary plan, human resources or occupational health services must approve the work schedule and assignment (DiBenedetto, 1998).

Case managers are effective in achieving these plans if they build trusting and humanistic relationships with the injured employee. They must treat their patients with courtesy, dignity, and respect. These relationships are important particularly because injured employees tend to disengage themselves from the work environment. This act of disengagement presents case managers with a greater challenge when facilitating an employee's timely return to work. The process may be delayed if the case manager is not successful in reengaging the injured employee with the work environment, and this cannot be achieved unless the case manager is able to build an effective relationship with the employee (Vierling, 1999).

Disability and Rehabilitation Case Management

The application of case management models for disability and rehabilitation management resulted from escalating costs of medical care, rising premiums, and other costs related to lost time from work and litigation of workers' compensation cases. It also became of greater demand because of the use of managed care insurance health plans by employers and the increased number of patients with complex, traumatic, and catastrophic injuries that required intensive short- or long-term disability and rehabilitation services. Employers usually refer their workers' compensation cases for comprehensive case management services because of their desire to control cost and improve the quality and continuity of care provided for this population.

Disability case management is defined as a process of managing occupational and nonoccupational diseases with the aim of returning the disabled person to a productive work schedule and employment (Powell and Ignatavicius, 2001). Occupational diseases are the result of injury on the job or illness caused by the work environment. Nonoccupational diseases are health conditions (e.g., trauma caused by an automobile accident) that are not related to the work environment but result in short- or long-term disability that prevents return to work for a period of time and sometimes indefinitely (DiBenedetto, 1998). The disability case management process involves the application of the concepts and strategies of workers' compensation case management and the rehabilitation treatment modality. Case managers in disability case management models focus on limiting the disability by coordinating and facilitating immediate medical interventions once an injury or illness occurs and by facilitating the referral process to rehabilitation providers and specialists. The ultimate goal of care and services is to return the patients to work and to restore optimal level of functioning and independence as soon as possible.

Disability case managers possess special training and expertise in the management of short- and long-term financial, psychological, sexual, physical, social, and vocational consequences of an illness or injury. Successful rehabilitation and cost-effectiveness result from the use of case managers who are specialized in the care of catastrophic injuries and disability insurance and claims management. Many employers and disability insurance companies employ the services of this type of case manager as soon as a catastrophic injury occurs because the earlier the case management services start, the better the financial and medical care outcomes (Hosack, 1998).

Because of the benefits of disability and rehabilitation case management services, we find case managers today working in almost every catastrophic injury specialty center. The focus of case management in these centers is similar to that of external case managers (i.e., private and independent) in the following areas:

- Developing care and projecting short- and long-term outcomes
- Planning the return-to-work plan
- Encouraging family involvement in the care of the injured person
- Coordinating necessary services and durable medical equipment
- Planning transitions
- Managing benefits and claims

- Communicating with the employer, insurance company, occupational health and risk management staff, medical and rehabilitation care team, and lawyers
- Ensuring compliance with the law

DESIGNING CASE MANAGEMENT MODELS

Whether introduced in the inpatient, outpatient, or any other setting across the continuum of care, case management models can be adapted to meet the goals of quality patient care in a fiscally responsible manner. Selection of the most appropriate model will depend on the needs of the organization, the available resources, and the expected goals and outcomes. When designing a case management model, healthcare executives must consider the following:

1. **Operationalization of the model at the patient level.** It must be easy to implement the model at the individual patient level, and patients must be able to realize its impact on their care and outcomes. Some models have been designed in a global, abstract, conceptual sense without any effort to explain how they apply to the individual patient. This leaves the healthcare providers and the case management staff in a struggle, trying to make sense of the model. To eliminate confusion, the conceptual framework of the model must be first redefined at the individual patient or patient care unit level before it is implemented.

2. **System-wide perspective.** Refrain from implementing a model that does not apply to all services and to the care of the different patient populations served. It is appropriate and acceptable to slightly modify the model to meet the needs of the different services; however, the basic concepts of the model must be maintained regardless of the patient population (e.g., the presence of a case manager in every service or a case manager/social worker dyad). Another example is the integrative role of the case manager; if it is integrated in one specialty, you may need to integrate it in others. However, an acceptable variation is the criteria used to identify patients who benefit from case management services.

3. **Redesign of the administrative, clinical, financial, and quality management processes.** Because the implementation of case management models means a change in the patient care delivery processes (i.e., clinical management), it behooves the healthcare executives who design and apply these models to redesign the other processes and align them with case management. The processes affected the most are those related to the role of the case manager: transitional/discharge planning, resource allocation

and utilization management, and quality and outcomes measurement. This redesign is important because it determines and ensures cost effectiveness and efficiency in the delivery of patient care.

4. **Sources of accountability and empowerment.** A clear definition of the case manager's role with identified role boundaries, scope of responsibility, and power is an important factor for success in case management. Case managers who are arbitrarily placed in their roles are set up to fail. Communicating the accountability and responsibility of case managers to all of the departments and staff in an organization is essential for promoting the case manager's power. One way of achieving this is by explicitly identifying the presence of case management as a department, and case managers as a staff, on the table of organization for every staff member to see.

5. **Integration of service delivery.** Cost savings are achieved by examining the number of departments an organization has and evaluating how each is impacted by the creation of the case management model/department. Almost always this results in merging and consolidation of departments. If an organization does not merge efforts, fragmentation and duplication will continue to exist and cost savings will not be accomplished. The departments affected the most by case management are social work, utilization review, discharge planning, and **quality management.** Some level of integration must be done as a result of case management (Box 3-10).

6. **Measurement systems.** Before implementing case management models, it is advisable to have a measurement system in place. The system must include the outcomes to be measured and must identify the process of data collection, aggregation, analysis, and reporting. A prospective approach to evaluating the effectiveness of the model assists in keeping all involved focused. It also prevents mistakes or unnecessary efforts from being made. The outcomes to be measured must always be driven by the goals and expectations of the model. One should maximize data collection from already existing automated systems, such as electronic medical records and data repositories, cost accounting systems, admitting, discharge, and transfer systems, and so on.

SETTING UP THE CASE MANAGEMENT PROGRAM

The following can be used when setting up a program in any setting across the continuum. As you move

---

BOX 3-10 Integration of Departments in Case Management Model Design

Integration of departments (e.g., utilization management, discharge/transitional planning and social work, clinical care management, and quality management) in the design and implementation of case management may be of three levels:

1. **Simple:** No integration at all and the focus of case management is on any one core activity. Most organizations focus on either clinical care management or utilization management. This type of model fragments care delivery, is expensive, and presents a potential for overuse or underuse of resources.

2. **Moderate:** Partial integration that focuses on merging two of the core activities. The most commonly integrated core activities are either clinical care management and transitional planning or clinical care management and utilization management. This level of integration results in better outcomes of cost effectiveness and efficiency in care delivery.

3. **Complex:** Full integration that includes all of the core activities. This type of integration is the most forward-thinking approach and results in best outcomes of cost effectiveness and efficiency in care delivery. However, one must balance the case manager's responsibilities and the patient caseload.

---

forward with your design and implementation, be sure you have addressed each of these points. Keep a running list for yourself and/or the committee working on the project to ensure that all relevant questions have been addressed. Each point can be addressed in any order, but be sure that each question is answered before the implementation of the program (Case Manager's Tip 3-20).

 CASE MANAGER'S TIP 3-20

Issues to Consider When Creating the Case Management Department
- Cost implications/budget
- Staff (professional/secretarial/clerical support)
- Equipment and supplies
- Table of organization
- Hours of operation
- Reporting structure
- Relationships to other departments
- Policies and procedures
- Information technology/systems
- Educating the organization

Creating the Department

Cost Implications/Budget

Develop a business plan. The plan should include both personnel and nonpersonnel costs needed to run the department. Consider all staff needed, including professional staff and support staff such as secretarial and clerical staff.

Also consider equipment needed, such as fax machines, photocopiers, and computers. Cost this out as part of the business plan. Set up a budget with the annualized cost of running the department.

Staff (Professional/Secretarial/Clerical Support)

Staffing should be based on the role functions to be performed. For example, RN case manager to patient ratios will be driven by the functions the RN is performing. If the RN case manager is performing clinical coordination/facilitation, **transitional planning,** and utilization/quality management functions, an appropriate caseload in the hospital setting would be 1:20. The number of case managers needed can then be calculated based on the bed capacity of the hospital.

Other staffing ratios should also be driven by the size of the organization and the functions to be performed.

Equipment and Supplies

The time to budget for equipment and supplies is before the implementation while the budgetary costs are being determined. Consider all functions being performed and the hardware and software needed to support those functions. Also consider the management needs and report writing capability when selecting a software package. Other supplies that should be budgeted for include stationery, paper, telephone lines, transportation, and conferences.

Table of Organization/Reporting Structure

Develop a table of organization for the department with a clearly differentiated reporting structure. Also consider where the department will fit into the organization and to whom the director of the department will report. Of significant importance is the case manager. The table of organization must clearly state where the case manager's position is and to whom he or she reports. This statement is essential for empowering those who assume the case manager's role.

Hours of Operation

The hours of operation of the department may be driven by budgetary constraints. Decisions will need to be made as to whether the department will operate 7 days a week or will function 5 or 6 days. Perhaps you will consider having the ED staff working longer shifts (such as 12 hours) while the inpatient staff work 8-hour shifts. Consider the clinical needs of the organization and the goals of the department when making these decisions. If there is a considerable amount of activity on the weekends, operations on the weekends must be planned for.

Relationships to Other Departments

The department may have either formal or informal relationships to other departments in the organization. Consideration should be given to how these relationships will be defined. You may want to consider an oversight committee that would be composed of leadership staff from related departments, such as admitting, medical records, patient accounts/billing, radiology, pharmacy, and so on.

Policies and Procedures

A policy and procedure manual should be developed and should include all policies and procedures needed to define the functions of the staff. For example, if utilization management is one of the functions of the department, then all appropriate utilization review policies should be included. Consider any JCAHO requirements when developing the manual. Include the table of organization and the staff job descriptions, training, and competencies in the manual. Also important to have on hand for use by case managers is a resource manual that has contact information readily available, particularly for community resources, volunteer agencies, charity and shelter services, transportation services, and skilled nursing/long-term facilities.

Information Technology/Systems

If the budget permits, select computer hardware that is state of the art and that will support the functions you are performing both now and in the future. For example, if one of the goals of the department is to eventually become paperless, be sure that your system will support this goal. In terms of case management software products, try to view and test several products before making your selection. Be sure that the software can store and manipulate all of the data needed, especially variance data, for reporting purposes for the department.

Educating the Organization

Before implementation, set up a series of educational programs. Programs should be conducted for case management staff at an in-depth level and for other staff on a less detailed level. Provide additional focused education to the medical staff and administrative staff as needed. Educational programs should be geared toward the needs of the different nursing, medical, and allied health staff.

Developing the Case Manager's Role

The following issues should be considered when designing the role of the case manager (Case Manager's Tip 3-21).

Role Functions

Careful consideration must be taken when defining the role functions of the case manager. Depending on the role functions selected, other departments may need to be restructured or eliminated. Consider all of the functions discussed in this chapter and match these to the goals and objectives of the department and the organization. If staff members from restructured or eliminated departments are used as case managers, they should be provided with special training. In addition, conducting teambuilding sessions for these staff members is advisable to work out any concerns they may have.

Integration with Other Departments/Disciplines

In some instances, other departments may become integrated with the case management department. Typically these may include social work and/or quality management. A physician staff member may also need to be integrated, such as a physician advisor. All related departments should be consulted as these decisions are being made, and appropriate staff should be trained accordingly.

 CASE MANAGER'S TIP 3-21

Issues to Consider When Developing the Case Manager's Role
- Role functions
- Integration with other departments/disciplines
- Job descriptions
- Management versus union
- Service line versus unit-based
- Reporting structure
- Staffing patterns
- Caseloads
- Hours of operation
- Clinical practice guidelines
- Variances/delays
- Documentation
- Orientation
- Goals and objectives
- Cost
- Quality

Job Descriptions

Job descriptions should be completed before the implementation of the department. As staff are interviewed and hired for these new positions, they should have an opportunity to review the job description and expectations for the position for which they are interviewing. Be sure to include all job functions, skills, performance expectations, and expected outcomes of the position. A job clarification exercise is usually helpful in determining who is best suited to assume responsibility for what functions.

Management Versus Union

If your organization is unionized, a decision will need to be made as to whether the case manager position will be in or out of the union. There are pros and cons to each position, but the ultimate decision will probably be dependent on the structure of your organization and its relationship with the union. It may be difficult to justify keeping the position out of the union if the case managers do not perform any of the functions typically considered as management functions, such as hiring/firing and evaluation of other staff.

Service Line Versus Unit-Based

The case managers can be assigned to specific product/service lines or clinical areas or be unit-based. They may also be assigned to physician groups or geographical areas, depending on whether your department is in the hospital or in the community. This decision will ultimately drive your staffing patterns and needs. Decisions must be made carefully because of their impact on performance, productivity, and the possibility of ending up with unnecessary unproductive time such as travel time between units, departments, or different locations.

Reporting Structure

A strong infrastructure is important to the success of a case management department. Be sure that the case managers have a clear line of authority and are well supported as they perform their functions.

Staffing Patterns/Case Loads

A typical mistake made when designing case management departments is to not provide the proper staffing patterns to support the role functions selected. Be sure that the caseloads are not so great that the case managers cannot perform their functions effectively or efficiently. This will surely be a formula for failure. Staffing patterns should also depend on whether you go with service line case managers or unit-based case managers, patient acuity levels, and length of stay.

Hours of Operation

Select hours of operation that best meet the operational needs of the department and the patients. Increase the number of staff at busier times, and decrease the number of staff at quieter times. Consider evening, weekend, and holiday needs. Hours of operation should be adjusted to the needs of different care settings and patient populations.

Clinical Practice Guidelines

The format for the organization's clinical practice guidelines should be determined before startup of the department. In this way the case management staff can begin developing the guidelines as soon as the department is implemented.

Variances/Delays

A variance identification system should be developed before implementation. Categories of variances such as patient, system, and practitioner should be selected, as well as a methodology for collecting, coding, aggregating, analyzing, and reporting of variances.

Documentation

Frequency of case management documentation and expected content should be determined and included as a policy and procedure for the case managers. Each organization needs to determine its own specific expectations for documentation while considering JCAHO, National Committee on Quality Assurance (NCQA), Commission on Accreditation and Rehabilitation Facilities (CARF), **Utilization Review Accreditation Commission (URAC),** and other regulatory requirements for documentation.

Orientation

Curricula for orientation of case management staff, other departments, physicians, and administrative staff should be developed, and education should take place before implementation. This will ensure greater organizational support because the reason for the changes will be understood by all involved.

Goals and Objectives

Departmental goals and objectives should be identified before implementation and included in the educational programs. The goals and objectives selected should be consistent with the vision and mission of the organization. These may include measures of cost such as cost per day/cost per case and measures of quality patient outcomes. All should be prospectively identified and should drive the evaluation of the program.

 KEY POINTS

1. There are four basic types of case management, using RNs, physicians, or social workers as case managers.
2. Hospital-based models generally use the RN as case manager, but the RN can be a primary nurse, CNS or nurse practitioner, or utilization review nurse. In some cases the case manager may be a social worker.
3. In some hospital-based models, the RN case manager performs the function of utilization management.
4. In RN/social work dyad models, the two disciplines work as an integrated team.
5. Outpatient case management models can be applied in home care, the community, or along the continuum.
6. Some models focus on management of the chronically ill.
7. Long-term case management can take place in the subacute setting, rehabilitation facility, or chronic nursing home setting.
8. Managed care models use the case manager as either a utilization manager or clinical manager acting on behalf of the MCO.
9. Telephonic and independent/private case management are considered "external" case management services.
10. All case management models must be designed to promote quality care in a fiscally responsible manner.

REFERENCES

Aliotta S, Andre J: Case management and home health care: an integrated model, *Home Healthc Manage Pract* 9(2):1-12, 1997.

American Nurses Association: *Nursing case management,* Kansas City, Mo, 1988, The Association.

Barger S, Rosenfeld P: Models in community health care: findings from a national study of community nursing centers, *Nurs Health Care* 14(8):426-431, 1993.

Blanchfield K, Schwarzentraub P, Reisinger P: Development of telephone nursing practice standards, *Nurs Econ* 15(5):265-267, 1997.

Brueckner G, Glover T: Case management and the continuum of care. In Donovan MR, Matson TA, editors: *Outpatient case management,* Chicago, 1993, American Hospital Association.

Clark KA: Alternate case management models. In Flarey DL, Blancett SS, editors: *Handbook of nursing case management,* Gaithersburg, Md, 1996, Aspen.

Davis V: Staff development for nurse case management. In Cohen E, editor: *Nurse case management in the 21st century,* St Louis, 1996, Mosby.

Deckard GJ, Hicks LL, Rountree BH: Long-term care nursing: how satisfying is it? *Nurs Econ* 4(4):194-200, 1986.

DiBenedetto D: The role of occupational health nursing in disability management, *Case Manager* 8(3):45-47, 1998.

DiBenedetto D: Back to work, *Adv Providers Post Acute Care* 2(5): 28-29, 1999.

DiBenedetto D: *Role of the rehabilitation professional: navigating the rehabilitation maze of return to work,* Case Management Systems Course Handout, Case Management Graduate Program, New York, 1999, Pace University, Leinhard School of Nursing.

DiBenedetto D: Navigating workers' compensation, *Continuing Care* 20(6):12, 14, 2001.

Diers D: Advanced practice, *Health Manage Q* 15(2):16-20, 1993.

Evashwick J: Definition of the continuum of care. In Evashwick J, Weiss L, editors: *Managing the continuum of care,* Gaithersburg, Md, 1987, Aspen.

Feldman C, Olberding L, Shortridge L, et al: Decision making in case management of home healthcare clients, *J Nurs Adm* 23(1):33-38, 1993.

Goodwin DR: Nursing case management activities: how they differ between employment settings, *J Nurs Adm* 24(2):29-34, 1994.

Hamric A: Creating our future: challenges and opportunities for the clinical nurse specialist, *Oncol Nurs Forum* 19(suppl 1):11-15, 1992.

Hicks LL, Stallmeyer JM, Coleman JR: *Role of the nurse in managed care,* Washington, DC, 1993, American Nurses Publishing.

Hosack K: The value of case management in catastrophic injury rehabilitation and long-term management, *J Care Manag* 4(3): 58-67, 1998.

Knollmueller RN: Case management: what's in a name? *Nurs Manage* 20(10):38-42, 1989.

Koerner J: Building on shared governance: the Sioux Valley Hospital experience. In Goertzen IE, editor: *Differentiating nursing practice into the twenty-first century,* Kansas City, Mo, 1991, American Academy of Nursing.

Lynn-McHale DJ, Fitzpatrick ER, Shaffer RB: Case management: development of a model, *Clin Nurs Spec* 7(6):299-307, 1993.

Mullahy CM: *The case manager's handbook,* Gaithersburg, Md, 1995, Aspen.

Mullahy CM: *The case manager's handbook,* ed 2, Gaithersburg, Md, 1998, Aspen.

Norris MK, Hill C: The clinical nurse specialist: developing the case manager role, *Dimens Crit Care Nurs* 10(6):346-353, 1991.

Pacala JT, Boult C, Hepburn KW, et al: Case management of older adults in health maintenance organizations, *J Am Geriatr Soc* 43(5):538-542, 1995.

Powell S: *Case management: a practical guide to success in managed care,* ed 2, Philadelphia, 2000, Lippincott Williams & Wilkins.

Powell S, Ignatavicius D: *Core curriculum for case management,* Philadelphia, 2001, Lippincott Williams & Wilkins.

Rantz MJ, Bopp KD: Issues of design and implementation from acute care, long-term, and community-based settings. In Cohen E, editor: *Nurse case management in the 21st century,* St Louis, 1996, Mosby.

Rutenberg C: Telephone triage, *Am J Nurs* 100(3):77-81, 2000.

Sampson EM: The emergence of case management models. In Donovan MR, Matson TA, editors: *Outpatient case management,* Chicago, 1994, American Hospital Association.

Schroer K: Case management: clinical nurse specialist and nurse practitioner, converging roles, *Clin Nurs Spec* 5(4):189-194, 1991.

Siefker J, Garret M, Van Genderen A, et al: *Fundamentals of case management: guidelines for practicing case managers,* St Louis, 1998, Mosby.

Smith J: Changing traditional nursing home roles to nursing case management, *J Gerontol Nurs* 17(5):32-39, 1991.

Stahl DA: Case management in subacute care, *Nurs Manage* 27(8): 20-22, 1996.

Trella B: Integrating services across the continuum: the challenge of chronic care. In Cohen E, editor: *Nurse case management in the 21st century,* St Louis, 1996, Mosby.

Trella RS: A multidisciplinary approach to case management of frail, hospitalized older adults, *J Nurs Adm* 23(2):20-26, 1993.

Van Dinter M: Telephone triage: the rules are changing, *Am J Matern Child Nurs* 25(4):187-191, 2000.

Vierling L: Return to work: a transition process, *Case Manager* 8(3): 55-57, 1999.

Wells N, Erickson S, Spinella J: Role transition: from clinical nurse specialist to clinical nurse specialist/case manager, *J Nurs Adm* 26(11):23-28, 1996.

Zawadski RT, Eng C: Case management in capitated long-term care, *Health Care Financ Rev* Spec No:75-81, 1988.

4 Role of the Case Manager

The advent of the case manager's role has improved healthcare delivery. It changed the provision of care from a multidisciplinary to an interdisciplinary one. The old days of *"parallel play"* in providing healthcare, in which the different disciplines involved in patient care worked in isolation, are outdated. Today's customers demand high-quality care that can be best achieved through *"interactive play,"* where ongoing interaction and cooperation among members of the various disciplines is key. With the creation of the case manager's role as the focal point of the interdisciplinary approach to care, the age of isolation, territoriality, fragmentation, redundancy, duplication, lack of communication, and the use of unnecessary tests/procedures is gone. The new age of patient care is characterized by collaboration, integration, coordination, continuity, consistency, interaction, and open communication. Today's healthcare customer is happier and more satisfied with the care received. Case managers play an integral role in this accomplishment.

The role of the **case manager** is designed to maximize these efforts. The role has been implemented in almost all care settings in the majority of healthcare organizations. Currently, case managers can be found working in insurance companies and managed care organizations (MCOs); acute, intensive, and ambulatory care settings (including emergency departments, nursing centers, and outpatient clinics); long-term care facilities, nursing and group homes; hospices; senior citizen centers; and home care. Their job description may vary from one setting to another, but the roles, functions, responsibilities, and skills required for success in the role are very similar. This chapter describes the **case management** process through which the various roles and responsibilities assumed by case managers are discussed.

The extent of responsibilities provided for case managers is dictated by the job description defined by each healthcare organization. Description of the role is affected by the operations of the organization, placement of the case manager in the table of organization, power embedded in the role, cost incurred, goals of the case management model, and organizational and specific nursing goals. In addition, the focus of the role of the case manager is determined by the area of practice or the care setting in which it is implemented. Although the common theme is patient care management, there still exist some differences that are reflected by the type of services needed in relation to the care setting.

CASE MANAGEMENT PROCESS

The case management process is a set of steps and activities applied by case managers in their approach to patient care management. It delineates the roles and responsibilities of case managers toward patient care from the time of admission until discharge and in some instances after discharge. The case management process is a modified version of the nursing process (Table 4-1). Both the case management and nursing processes are similar in that they identify the plan of care of patients by assessing needs, diagnosing the problem(s), planning and implementing the care, and evaluating **outcomes.** The nursing process is applied to the care of every patient by all nurses in any care setting regardless of the patient care delivery model followed by the organization. However, the case management process is used by case managers in an environment in which case management is the patient care delivery model, and in some organizations it is applied only to a select group of patients who meet specific predetermined criteria.

TABLE 4-1 Comparison of the Nursing and the Case Management Processes

Nursing Process	Case Management Process
Assessment	Case finding/screening and intake
	Assessing needs
Diagnosis	Identifying actual/potential problems
Planning	Interdisciplinary case conferencing
	Establishing goals of treatment and expected outcomes of care
	Developing/individualizing the case management plan
Implementation	Implementing the case management plan/interdisciplinary plan of care
	Facilitating/coordinating patient care activities
Evaluation	Monitoring the delivery of patient care services
	Evaluating outcomes of care/patient responses to treatment
	Discharge/disposition
	Repeating the case management process

The case management process is a systematic approach to patient care delivery and management (Figure 4-1). It identifies what the case manager should do at what time during the patient's hospitalization or course of care. The process provides the framework for the role of the case manager. It also helps organize and simplify his or her work. Each step in the process requires the case manager to be astute and to exhibit specific skills. The combination of these skills is the token for success in the role.

The case management process is discussed in this chapter in a linear fashion; however, this process is not linear. The case manager may go back and forth or skip some of the steps depending on the situation being handled and the needs of the patient. Similar to the role of the case manager, the case management process focuses on three major functions: clinical care management, **utilization management,** and transitional/discharge planning. For the purpose of clarification, these functions are presented as separate processes in Table 4-2. However, in real patient care situations, case managers approach the delivery of case management services in an integrated way.

Case managers are active members of interdisciplinary teams of various healthcare providers working toward a common goal (i.e., provision and management of cost-effective, efficient, and high-quality patient care). Membership of the interdisciplinary team varies based on the patient's problems and the plan of care. Some members are always represented, such as the case manager, physician, housestaff, nurse practitioners, physician assistants, registered nurses (RNs), and patients and their families. Other members are called upon in consultation, such as the social worker, physical therapist, occupational therapist, respiratory therapist, and nutritionist.

Case Finding/Screening and Intake

The initial step in case management is case finding (i.e., identifying the patients who require case management services). The purposes of case finding/screening are to identify the patient problems and determine the needs for case management services and the patient's eligibility for these services (Bower, 1992). Case managers may identify such patients in four different ways. They may (1) screen all admissions to select those who are in need of case management services, (2) screen only those patients who are referred for services by other healthcare providers, (3) not screen any patients but consider them all in need of some sort of case management services, or (4) respond to a referral or request made by the patients or families themselves.

It is important, however, for each organization to define the method of patient referrals/identification for such services. **Guidelines** or policies must be established at the same time that case management systems are implemented and case manager roles are defined and established. The clearer the system for case finding, the easier the role of the case manager becomes and the faster the patients are referred or identified for case management services. The efficiency of the system impacts on the cost and increases the effectiveness of the case management model. To expedite case finding, interdisciplinary healthcare team members are encouraged to make referrals to case managers within 24 hours of patients' admission to a hospital, **subacute care facility,** or long-term care facility. In other care settings such as clinics or emergency departments, patients should be referred as soon as their needs for case management services are identified. In home care settings, patients are referred for case management services in the home while still on the premises of a healthcare facility, or within a few days of discharge from a hospital setting.

Private physicians, housestaff, primary nurses, social workers, utilization managers/reviewers, discharge planners, nurse practitioners, physician assistants, physical therapists, and nutritionists can refer patients to the case manager. Generally each case manager is made responsible for identifying patients in his or her service or area of responsibility. Healthcare organizations may need to prospectively define the patient selection criteria to make this responsibility easier. It is important to

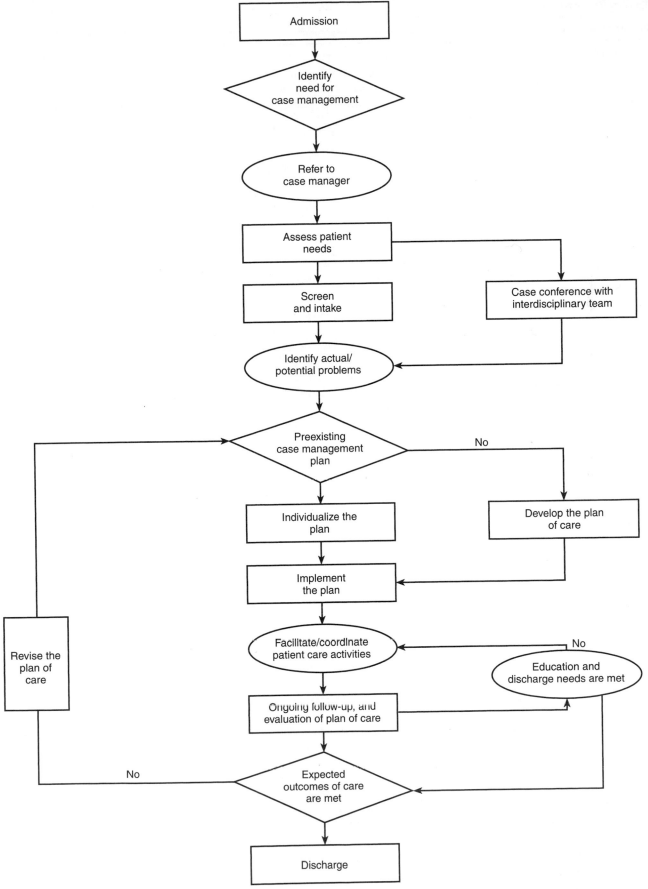

Figure 4-1 Flow diagram: the case management process.

TABLE 4-2 The Relationship Between the Case Management, Utilization Management, and Transitional/Discharge Planning Processes

Case Management Process	Utilization Management Process	Transitional/Discharge Planning Process
1. Case finding/screening and intake	1. Patient's admission/encounter • Evaluate appropriateness for care and level of care using predetermined guidelines	1. Patient's admission/encounter • Screen patient for postdischarge needs • Identify need for discharge services
2. Assessment of needs	2. Assessment of resources • Assess patient's needs for healthcare resources based on medical condition • Assess patient's financial status and insurance benefits	2. Assessment of discharge/transitional planning needs • Agree on needs with patient, family, healthcare team • Assess available resources and type of resources
3. Identification of actual and potential problems	3. Development of resource management plan • Identify patient's problems and need for resource management • Identify areas that require authorizations/certifications • Identify criteria for discharge (i.e., discharge outcomes) • Identify postdischarge needs that require payer's approval	3. Developmet of transitional/discharge plan • Design action plan for meeting patient's discharge needs • Agree on goals of plan and expected outcomes
4. Interdisciplinary care planning	4. Implementing resource management plan • Conduct concurrent review with MCO • Obtain authorizations for services • Discuss need for extended length of stay as needed • Transition patient to next level of care	4. Implementation of plan • Put plan into action • Coordinate necessary activities • Broker services with community agencies, etc. • Educate patient and family regarding healthcare needs
5. Implementation of interdisciplinary plan of care	5. Evaluation of resource management plan • Identify potential denial areas and implement action • Monitor outcomes and appropriateness of plan • Determine patient's readiness for transfer to next level of care • Confer with healthcare team, patient and family, and payer	5. Evaluation of transitional plan • Monitor appropriateness of plan • Examine outcomes of plan • Exchange information with postdischarge agencies as needed
6. Evaluation of patient care outcomes	6. Discharging patient • Identify patient's readiness for discharge based on discharge outcomes determined earlier in process • Confirm discharge with patient and family and healthcare team • Obtain authorizations for postdischarge services from the payer	6. Preparing patient for discharge • Confirm patient's discharge • Confirm postdischarge services

TABLE 4-2 The Relationship Between the Case Management, Utilization Management, and Transitional/Discharge Planning Processes—cont'd

Case Management Process	Utilization Management Process	Transitional/Discharge Planning Process
7. Patient's discharge and disposition	7. Repeating the process • Reexamine resource management process and revise based on patient's needs, conditions, and treatment plan	7. Patient's discharge • Complete actual patient's discharge • Transfer patient to another facility
8. Repeating the process		8. Repeating the process • Reapply transitional planning process based on changes in patient's condition

establish patient referral criteria, especially if the case management model followed identifies patient referrals as the major source for selection of patients for case management services rather than waiting for case managers to screen every admission to the hospital. These criteria eliminate any confusion that may arise when a member of the interdisciplinary team evaluates whether a patient needs to be referred to the case manager.

Box 4-1 presents a list of examples of patient selection criteria for case management services. Some of these criteria are generic; can be applied to any care setting; and are based on issues that may affect the patient in terms of quality of care, length of stay, and/or cost of care. Other criteria are based on the service/setting and are only appropriate to that specific service/setting. The list serves as a guide for case managers to use to establish the criteria specific to their area of responsibility.

Whatever the case finding method is, case managers still have to evaluate the appropriateness of patients for case management services and determine the necessity for "intake." The decision of whether a patient requires case management services (i.e., intake) is made based on screening (initial assessment) of the patient's needs, review of the medical record, and a discussion with the referring personnel. It is then determined whether the patient meets any of the selection criteria for case management. When the intake decision is made, the case manager flags the medical record, identifying that the patient is accepted for case management services, and writes an intake note in the patient's record.

Assessment of Needs of the Patient and Family

Once the case manager has identified patients who meet the predetermined selection criteria, a case management assessment must take place. This assessment is comprehensive and covers a wide range of areas, including the following:

■ The chief complaint that required the patient to seek medical attention

■ The physical, mental, spiritual, and psychosocial status of the patient.

■ The healthcare insurance coverage and, when needed, whether the patient's admission has been approved (i.e., **precertification**) by the MCO

■ The patient's social support system and coping mechanisms

■ Adjustment to illness and hospitalization

■ The health education needs of the patient and family

■ The projected **discharge planning** needs

■ The resources required for caring for the patient and family

The assessment data that case managers collect and analyze fall into two important categories: *subjective* and *objective*. The information told by the patient and family is the subjective data. It is related to the chief complaint and the history of the problem(s) that made the patient seek medical attention in a clinic or an emergency department, or it is the reason for hospitalization. Case managers should be careful when interpreting such data because of its subjectivity. Objective data, however, include the physical examination, laboratory test results, and other diagnostic tests. The objective data are important because they help validate the subjective data and interpret the patient's history more accurately by providing a basis for comparison.

The subjective and objective information case managers collect when interviewing the patient and family, the physical examination, the results of laboratory tests, and the results of the diagnostic procedures make up the assessment **database,** which is necessary for better identification of the patient's actual and potential problems. The goal of the "assessment of needs" step of the case management process is to gather and record information that is most helpful in designing the most appropriate plan of care for the individual patient.

Assessment data collection can be extensive, and some of it may not be necessary at times. Case managers may limit the type of assessment data they collect by answering the following questions: What data should be collected? How should data be collected? How should data be organized for better care planning decisions? What data are most relevant for identifying the necessity for case management services and actions?

Case managers may elect not to perform a physical assessment of the patient. However, they should review the medical record, particularly the admission history and assessment completed by the primary nurse, the physician, and other providers such as social workers and physical therapists and the paperwork from transferring facilities. The assessment of needs requires collecting and synthesizing data from multiple sources across providers and various care settings and/or services, including the patient and family (Strassner,

1996). The initial encounter of the case manager with the patient and family is the beginning of an unwritten contract (Newell, 1996) that dictates the rest of the relationship. It also is essential to the case management process because it helps establish rapport and promote trust in the relationship. This is maximized through the case manager's professional attitude and effective and skillful communication and interviewing techniques. Performing an assessment of needs that is accurate and relevant to the patient's presenting problem(s) requires case managers to possess interviewing and technical skills that are invaluable (Case Manager's Tip 4-1).

Other important aspects of the initial assessment are appropriateness of the patient's admission to that level of care and the postdischarge needs. As the case manager interviews the patient and family and reviews

---

BOX 4-1 Criteria for Case Management Services

This is a list of examples of criteria for referral and/or acceptance of patients for case management services. It is not an exhaustive list. However, healthcare organizations may adopt some of these criteria into their guidelines.

Generic Criteria

1. Physiological instability and complexity
2. Inability to assume self-care as a result of physical dependencies and/or neurological status
3. Mobility impairment/disability
4. Lack of social support from significant other
5. History of nonadherence with medical/surgical regimen (e.g., medications, follow-up)
6. Pain management problems
7. Complexity of diagnosis
8. Fluctuating emotional status
9. Prone to problems/complications
10. Involvement of several disciplines in the care
11. Multiple readmissions in a short period
12. Complex discharge, need for placement in a particular facility
13. Need for intensive healthcare education of patient/family
14. Death and dying/end-of-life issues, hospice care
15. Managed care insurance carrier
16. Medicare or Medicaid managed care carrier
17. Financial risk to the hospital (i.e., inadequate healthcare coverage/financial support)
18. At risk for prolonged length of stay
19. Required treatment in various care settings in one hospitalization (e.g., intensive care unit, telemetry, regular unit)
20. Preexisting problems accessing healthcare

21. Need for durable medical equipment
22. Guardianship issues
23. Interinstitutional transfer; acute to acute transfer
24. Potential or suspected abuse

Service/Unit-Specific Criteria
Emergency department/clinic

1. Homelessness
2. Lack of primary care physician
3. Inconsistency in medical follow-up
4. Requiring admission into the hospital
5. Multiple visits in a short period

Neonate/pediatric

1. Age
2. Chronic illness (e.g., asthma, croup, HIV/AIDS)
3. Prematurity, less than 32 weeks' gestation
4. Vaccination
5. Child abuse
6. Newborn weighing less than 1500 g
7. Requiring individualized instructions such as cardiopulmonary resuscitation (CPR)
8. More than 3 medications on discharge
9. Requiring a home care referral for postdischarge services and follow-up
10. Needing durable medical equipment at home, such as a glucometer

Obstetrics/gynecology

1. First pregnancy
2. First baby, multiple newborns
3. High risk/complicated pregnancy (e.g., gestational diabetes, preeclampsia)
4. No prenatal follow-up

BOX 4-1   Criteria for Case Management Services—cont'd

5. Substance abuse during pregnancy
6. Delivery of a premature baby
7. Teenage pregnancy

Geriatric

1. Elderly, lives alone, with functional impairment and/or exhibiting mental status changes
2. Requiring placement in a nursing home
3. Dementia/Alzheimer's disease
4. Medically complex condition and requiring multiple services
5. Frail elderly
6. No social support system
7. Elder abuse
8. Frequent emergency department visits
9. Extended length of hospital (or other facilities such as subacute care) stay
10. Potential discharge problems such as inadequate financial status, living arrangements, or caregiver support

Intensive care unit(s)

1. Ventilator dependency/weaning
2. Organ transplant
3. Multisystem failure
4. End-of-life issues or withdrawal of treatments
5. Ethical issues
6. Transfer to another acute care facility
7. Need for psychosocial counseling for patient or family

Regular/medical-surgical unit

1. Diagnosis specific (e.g., stroke, heart failure)
2. First-time diagnosis
3. Leaving (or history of leaving) against medical advice
4. Complex discharge plan
5. Medical complications
6. Physiological instability
7. Three or more physicians actively involved in care
8. Requiring multiple services and community services postdischarge

Renal

1. Complications with dialysis access: thrombosed access, infection
2. Newly diagnosed end-stage renal disease
3. Newly put on dialysis treatments
4. Decision making regarding treatment modality
5. Candidate for organ transplantation
6. Educational needs
7. Need to establish diet and exercise regimens
8. No insurance coverage
9. Inadequate home environment
10. Lack of social support
11. Frequent readmissions
12. Need for transportation services
13. End-of-life decision making/termination of treatment

HIV/AIDS

1. Newly diagnosed HIV (6 months or less)
2. Medical complexity, more than one opportunistic disease
3. Repeated hospitalizations
4. Lack of insurance or inadequate coverage
5. No housing
6. Counseling and psychosocial support
7. Termination of treatment
8. Lack of or inadequate social support system

Neuroscience

1. Ischemic stroke or intracranial hemorrhage
2. Brain and spinal cord diseases: brain tumors, traumatic spinal cord injury
3. Tracheostomy
4. Cerebrospinal fluid drainage
5. Deficit requiring intensive postdischarge services and resources
6. Multiple providers/services involved in care provision
7. Complex discharge/transitional plan
8. Transfer to another facility

Psychiatry

1. Complex medication therapy
2. Complex medical condition
3. Compromised behavioral condition requiring one-to-one therapy
4. Legal risk
5. Acute depression and suicide
6. Homicidal behavior
7. Need for extended hospitalization
8. Coordination of postdischarge services and community resources
9. Increased frequency of hospitalizations and recidivism
10. Lack of or inadequate social support system
11. Complex discharge/transitional plan
12. Seclusion

Oncology

1. Metastasis
2. Complex chemotherapy and radiation therapy protocols
3. Terminal stage
4. Withdrawal of treatment
5. Hospice/palliative care
6. Complex discharge/transitional plan
7. Lack of or inadequate social support system
8. Pain management
9. Extended hospital stay
10. Multiple physicians/services involved in care provision

CASE MANAGER'S TIP 4-1

Effective Interviewing of Patients and Families

1. Introduce yourself, indicating your full name, your title and responsibility, and what you prefer to be called.
2. Inform the patient and family of the reasons for your visit.
3. Make them aware of what you can do to help them survive and cope well with the current episode of illness.
4. Review the medical record before you approach the patient.
5. Discuss the reasons for case management services with the person referring the patient before you conduct the interview.
6. Obtain as much information as possible about the patient and family before you interview them.
7. During the interview, ask open-ended questions to obtain an appropriate history of the problem/chief complaint. Also, ask direct questions based on the needs you may have identified during the chart review and the discussion with the person who referred the patient.
8. Maintain privacy and confidentiality during the interview.
9. Obtain information related to the patient's social support system, healthcare insurance coverage, education needs, and needs after discharge. These questions are important in evaluating appropriateness for case management services.
10. Discuss with the patient and family the next step(s) regarding the plan of care and case management.
11. Provide the patient and family, in writing (e.g., on a business card), your name and how you can be reached.

the medical record, he or she evaluates the appropriateness of the level of care the patient is to receive, using certain criteria such as InterQual or Milliman & Robertson (see Chapter 5). If the case manager finds that the admission or the level of care is inappropriate, he or she will initiate some action to correct the situation. This may require the case manager to discuss the situation and negotiate a better plan with the physician and other members of the healthcare team. This is important for ensuring reimbursement for the services provided.

At the same time the case manager assesses the appropriateness of the admission, he or she identifies the patient's and/or family's postdischarge healthcare needs. This assessment acts as the beginning of the transitional/discharge planning process (see Chapter 6). The utilization management and **transitional planning** assessments are important because they affect the follow-up actions and determine the plan of care.

Identification of Actual and Potential Problems

A thorough assessment of the needs of the patient and family provides the basis for identifying the actual and potential problems (e.g., nursing diagnoses). Identifying these problems dictates the types of interventions and treatments necessary to achieve the desired outcomes. Accurate and comprehensive identification of these problems has a significant effect on the quality of care, incurred cost, **reimbursement,** course of care, and **length of stay** or treatment. Case managers are always advised to seek the collaboration of the interdisciplinary team and the patient and family in identifying the actual and potential problems. This strategy improves outcomes and promotes agreement on the plan of care and increases consistency and continuity in the provision of care among the various disciplines involved.

Regardless of the patient's clinical condition, case managers should always identify any needs or problems the patient and family may have related to healthcare teaching, discharge/transitional planning, and social support systems. The earlier such problems are identified, the sooner they are incorporated into the plan of care. This results in better control over the length of stay and ensures that patients' needs are met. It also expedites the process of resolving the problems.

During the time case managers identify the patient's problems, they elect to reassess the patient's needs to validate uncertain or incomplete areas that existed in the previous assessment. It is important for case managers to be certain of the patient's needs before finalizing the problems list or sharing it with members of the interdisciplinary team.

Interdisciplinary Care Planning

Interdisciplinary care planning helps establish a seamless approach to patient care. It requires the involvement of members of the various disciplines that will be caring for the patient. In addition, it is important to involve the patient and family. The first activity in this step of the case management process is case conferencing. The case manager presents the findings of the assessment of patient's needs and the identified actual and potential problems to the interdisciplinary team. The team then prioritizes the patient problems, selects appropriate intervention/treatment modalities to resolve these problems, and establishes the expected outcomes of care. During this discussion the plan of care is developed.

A care plan that is interdisciplinary and well developed helps decrease the risk of incomplete tasks or incorrect/inappropriate care. It also provides a seamless approach to care that supports the standards of care of regulatory agencies such as the Joint Commission on Accreditation of Healthcare Organizations (JCAHO). Such a plan provides direction to all the disciplines involved in the care of the patient, opens the lines of communication among these disciplines and the patient and family, and ensures continuity and consistency of the care provided.

During this step of the case management process, case managers establish the goals of treatment and the projected/desired outcomes of care. They also include goals for utilization management and transitional planning. It is important to establish these goals and desired outcomes in collaboration with members of the interdisciplinary team. An interdisciplinary approach to setting the goals and expected outcomes is the key to cost-effective and quality care.

With their assessment skills, clinical expertise, and holistic approach to patient care, case managers ensure that a comprehensive interdisciplinary plan of care is developed and that it is succinct with the patient's and family's goals. They also verify that it contains the identified patient's actual and potential problems, the mutually determined and agreed-on goals with the interdisciplinary team members and the patient and family, the required patient care activities that reflect all of the involved disciplines (specifically the nursing interventions and medical treatments), and the preventive measures for complications or undesired outcomes. In addition, the plan should always include patient and family teaching and discharge planning components (Tahan, 1993; McNeese-Smith et al, 1996).

The interdisciplinary plan of care developed is the **case management plan (CMP)** (see Chapter 12) to be followed by all disciplines in the care of individual patients. If a CMP (specific to the patient's diagnosis/procedure) already exists, the case manager presents it to the interdisciplinary team during case conferencing for review and individualization to meet the patient's and family's needs. The CMP then becomes the tool used to identify, monitor, and evaluate the treatments and interventions and the care activities and outcomes. It is constantly evaluated and revised to reflect the changing needs of the patient and family.

Planning an appropriate patient's course of care is a skill required by case managers. To be effective in their role, they should be knowledgeable about the available hospital and community resources necessary for the care of patients, the various care settings, management of resources, cost, and reimbursement (Strassner, 1996), and they should be clinically astute.

Implementation of the Interdisciplinary Plan of Care

In this step of the case management process, the interdisciplinary plan of care/CMP is put into action. Each member of the interdisciplinary team ensures that his or her responsibilities, as indicated in the CMP, are met within the projected timeframes. Implementation encompasses all of the interventions (medical, nursing, and others) that are directed toward meeting the preestablished goals, resolving the patient's problems, and meeting the patient's healthcare needs and predetermined care outcomes.

Reassessment skills possessed by case managers are the key to success in this role. When reassessing the patient and the care, case managers usually answer questions such as the following:
- Does the patient have any new needs?
- Does the interdisciplinary plan of care/CMP meet the patient's needs?
- Does the plan need to be revised?
- Are the projected patient care activities indicated in the plan appropriate and timely?
- Will the patient's problems be resolved during this episode of care?
- What is the appropriate timeframe for resolving the identified problems?
- Does the transitional plan meet (or continue to meet) the patient's and family's needs?
- Are **authorizations/certifications** obtained from managed care companies for the treatments instituted or to be implemented?
- Are the patient and family or caregiver aware of and in agreement with the plan of care?

Answers to these questions help case managers to confirm that the planned interventions remain appropriate to the patient's condition and projected/desired outcomes. When case managers identify any problems, they are responsible for bringing them to the attention of the interdisciplinary team, discussing them, recommending necessary changes in the CMP, and ensuring that the plan is revised to meet the patient's latest condition.

Case managers are pivotal in facilitating and coordinating patient care activities. They informally direct the work of the interdisciplinary team members in an effort to promote cost-effective and appropriate care and to ensure that services are provided in a timely manner and patients are well informed and advocated for.

Case managers facilitate and coordinate patient care activities related to required tests, procedures, and treatments; patient and family teaching; and discharge planning and the need for community resources. They are responsible for confirming that tests, procedures, treatments, and interventions coincide with those recommended in the CMP, are preauthorized/certified by the insurance company, and are scheduled and completed in a timely fashion. They also make certain that changes in these activities are dictated by the patient's condition and are not arbitrary.

Case managers act as **gatekeepers** of the interdisciplinary teams they belong to. With their continuous follow-up on the implementation of the patient care activities and evaluation of outcomes and reassessment of the patient's condition and needs, they keep all of the interventions in order and ensure that what is supposed to occur is taking place. They may remind members of the team of any incomplete or inaccurate activities; expedite tests and procedures; eliminate or prevent any fragmentation, duplication, or unnecessary services; and prevent any confusion or misunderstanding. When case managers identify delays, variations, or deviations in the care from the CMP, they immediately act on the issue and attempt to correct it.

Because of their understanding of the total picture of the care of the patient, they are invaluable in coordinating the scheduling of the different tests and procedures required for a patient's workup and treatment. They ensure that these tests or procedures are not scheduled at the same time. Their careful attention to such situations prevents the occurrence of any conflicts, delays, duplication, or fragmentation of care. Case managers are also instrumental in facilitating timely reporting of results of the tests and diagnostic and therapeutic procedures. This function allows the interdisciplinary healthcare team to make timely decisions pertaining to the appropriateness of care, to change interventions and treatments to more effective ones as indicated by the clinical status of patients and supported by objective data (i.e., results of tests and procedures), and to validate that the recommended patient care activities outlined in the CMP or interdisciplinary plan of care are achieved in a timely fashion.

Facilitating and coordinating the patient and family teaching activities are important functions of case managers. They are able to manage these activities efficiently and effectively because of their extensive knowledge of the healthcare system, their clinical experience and skills, and their familiarity with the adult learning theory and the health-belief model. Case managers may

be directly or indirectly involved in patient and family teaching activities. They are more likely to be directly involved in teaching in situations such as the following:

■ *Patients with complex diagnoses that lead to complicated teaching needs* (e.g., patients with multiple problems such as chronic renal failure, diabetes, hypertension, and heart failure). Patients with such conditions require intensive teaching plans. Case managers may elect to develop such plans in collaboration with the interdisciplinary team, including the patient and family and the primary nurse. They may conduct some teaching sessions pertaining to specific topics or needs (e.g., insulin self-injection) or supervise and/or ensure the completion of teaching activities related to other topics (disease process, signs and symptoms, or medications) by the primary nurse or other members of the interdisciplinary healthcare team.

■ *Patients with multiple admissions in a short period of time.* These patients may have problems that are beyond the understanding of the disease process and signs and symptoms. After careful assessment of the patient's and family's teaching needs, case managers may find that the real problems of repeated admissions are inconsistent clinical follow-up, non-adherence to the medical/surgical regimen, or an inappropriate social support system. In such situations, active involvement of the case manager is essential. The case manager then concentrates on the real issue and works closely with the patient and family to prevent readmission to the hospital and improve compliance with the treatment.

The role of patient and family educator can be challenging to most case managers as hospital length of stay decreases and patient acuity increases and the shift to providing healthcare services in the home, subacute care, and ambulatory settings is becoming more popular. This role is important in maximizing patient care outcomes, minimizing cost, and promoting the patient/family independence in care (McNeese-Smith et al, 1996). Case managers can function as role models and experts in patient teaching to primary nurses and other members of the healthcare team. Their responsibility toward patient and family teaching starts at the time of admission in assessing the teaching needs and initiating the teaching plan that helps meet these needs. They also coordinate the teaching activities, based on the plan, to be completed by the different members of the healthcare team, including the primary nurse.

The patient and family education role requires case managers to be astute in assessing patient teaching needs and readiness, identifying any existing barriers and limitations to teaching, and selecting the appropriate methodology. They are also required to be sensitive to the patient condition, culture, values, and belief system. Case managers should demonstrate competency in how to incorporate these factors into the patient and family teaching plan and help members of the interdisciplinary team choose the most effective method and plan for teaching.

Case managers are key players in effective discharge/transitional planning. They play an important role in coordinating and facilitating the patient's discharge. Their role in discharge planning starts with admission of the patient to the hospital, or at the time the patient seeks medical attention, and during the first encounter with the patient and family. They are responsible for assessing the patient's needs for safe and appropriate discharge and coordinating the process of getting these services approved and perhaps instituted before the patient is discharged.

Case managers collaborate with the patient and family, physician, primary nurse, social worker, home care planner, and other members of the healthcare team in establishing the patient's most appropriate discharge plan and work closely with them to achieve this plan. Case managers update and revise the plan as needed based on their ongoing reassessment of the patient's condition and needs. They also discuss and communicate any changes in the discharge plan to the members of the team informally or formally during case-conference meetings.

Facilitation and coordination of discharge planning activities may require case managers to communicate with external services such as medical equipment providers, home care agencies, or representatives from other healthcare facilities. They may also need to contact case managers in MCOs to obtain certification for the postdischarge services or transfers to other facilities as required by patients. These functions demand that case managers be skillful in negotiation techniques and brokerage of services. They also need to possess excellent communication skills and be knowledgeable in managed care contracts, entitlements, federal and **third-party payers,** other reimbursement methods, laws and regulations, policies and procedures, and the variety of available community services and agencies. Seasoned case managers can be found to have established successful business relationships with key people in the different agencies they contact on a regular basis. Such relationships are instrumental in providing case managers with a wide networking circle and expediting the process of approval, certification, and delivery of discharge services.

Evaluation of Patient Care Outcomes

In the evaluation of the patient care outcomes step of the case management process, case managers evaluate the effectiveness of the interdisciplinary plan of care/CMP and the patient care activities and outcomes. They are also responsible, in collaboration with members of the interdisciplinary healthcare team, to continuously monitor the patient's condition, responses to interventions, and progress toward recovery. Ongoing communication with the healthcare team regarding the appropriateness of the plan of care in relation to the patient's changing condition and needs, and whether the plan is realistic, is important for timely revision of the plan and implementation of new interventions and treatments.

When evaluating patient care, case managers should answer the following questions:

- Were the patient care activities accurate and timely?
- Were the goals of the patient and family and the healthcare team accomplished?
- Have the patient and family needs been met?
- Has the patient's condition progressed toward recovery, deteriorated, or remained the same?
- Which interventions or treatments need to be changed or added?
- Should patient care outcomes, activities, and/or goals be reprioritized?
- Is the care being delivered in the appropriate setting or at the right level?
- Is the transitional/discharge plan relevant?
- Have certifications been obtained for services before their delivery as indicated in the managed care contract?
- Are the patient, family, and/or caregiver in agreement with the plan of care?

Answers to these questions by the interdisciplinary team members at case conferences or by case managers when reviewing medical records and evaluating the appropriateness of patient care activities and outcomes help the healthcare team remain focused and make timely revisions to the plan of care. This function of case managers is important in ensuring that high-quality and cost-effective care is delivered at all times.

Case managers are responsible for monitoring and evaluating **variances** of care on a continuing basis. They identify and track deviations from the CMP (i.e., variances of care) as they relate to the following:

- Patient (e.g., refusal of test or procedure, deterioration in condition)
- Practitioner (e.g., medication errors, delay in scheduling or performing a certain test, visiting nurse not showing up, certifications not obtained)
- System (e.g., unable to complete a test because the machine is broken, no physical therapy available on weekends, MCO not certifying/approving home care

services). (See Chapters 9 and 14 for more detailed discussion on variances.)

They also keep members of the interdisciplinary healthcare team well informed of the presence/ occurrence of variances and together attempt to resolve these variances. Early detection and resolution of such variances are essential to prevent **complications** or undesired outcomes, delays in the length of stay, increased cost, and deterioration in patient and family satisfaction.

Case managers are also made accountable for evaluating the fiscal, quality, and clinical outcomes of care (Strassner, 1996). These outcomes are interrelated, and a deficit in one usually affects the others negatively. *Fiscal outcomes* are those related to the organizational goals rather than the patient's health. Examples of fiscal outcomes are cost and revenue of care, resource use, length of stay, inappropriate admissions, and system-related variances. Traditional *quality outcomes* have been those directly related to a patient's health and functioning. Examples of quality outcomes are nosocomial infection rates, independence, health perception, readmissions, inappropriate discharges, complications, and patient and family satisfaction. *Clinical outcomes* are those directly related to patient care activities. These outcomes are identified proactively by members of the interdisciplinary team and included in the CMP, and they are expected to be achieved while caring for the patient and family. Some examples are the intermediate and discharge outcomes (see Chapters 9 and 14). Through timely facilitation and coordination of patient care activities, patient and family teaching, and discharge planning, case managers are able to maintain a delicate balance of these outcomes.

While monitoring and evaluating care; reviewing medical records; or communicating with the patient and family, primary nurses, members of the interdisciplinary team, and ancillary departments, case managers continually collect data related to variances and outcomes of care. They then aggregate the data based on similarities in issues and diagnoses, conduct a trending and analysis review, and finally generate reports to be shared with appropriate personnel (e.g., **quality improvement** department, case management department, interdisciplinary team members, chiefs of services/departments [nursing, medical, and ancillary], and administration). Case managers are instrumental in their feedback related to the critical issues, particularly system problems that require administrative attention and initiation of quality improvement task forces for resolution.

Throughout the evaluation of the patient care outcomes step of the case management process, case managers exhibit certain skills that are essential to

the role. These skills are problem solving, decision making, critical thinking, clinical reasoning, consensus building, quality improvement, leadership abilities, networking, partnership, collaboration, communication and feedback, and negotiation. It is through these effective skills that case managers are able to make a difference in patient care management and to meet the goals of the case management model and the organization.

Patient's Discharge and Disposition

It is important for case managers to bring their relationship with the patient and family to closure. Discontinuation of case management services, whether it is due to the patient's discharge from the hospital/ facility or because case management services are deemed no longer required by the patient, is the last step in the case management process. During this phase case managers hold a "case-closing" conference with the patient and family and the interdisciplinary team, during which the plan of care is evaluated for its completion, particularly the appropriateness of the discharge plan and the effectiveness of patient and family teaching. This is the time when case managers confirm that the transitional plan is appropriate and that all post-discharge services required by the patient are in place and the necessary paperwork is completed. If a problem is identified, it should be resolved before the time of the patient's discharge.

Case managers ensure that all discharge activities are completed effectively before the time of discharge or transfer to another facility for follow-up care such as rehabilitation. They evaluate the patient's readiness by making sure that the **discharge outcomes** are met and that all of the required interdisciplinary activities have been successfully achieved or the receiving facility has already accepted the transfer and arranged for a bed for the patient. It is essential to answer the patient's and family's last questions regarding care after discharge and provide them with emotional support. Sometimes it is helpful for them to have the case manager's phone number; this is a safety or reassurance mechanism for patients and families that reduces their anxiety and fear of discharge. It is also important for case managers to provide them with written instructions pertaining to the care after discharge and the scheduled follow-up appointment(s).

Some institutions require case managers to make follow-up phone calls to the patients after discharge and evaluate their level of functioning and adherence to the medical regimen and follow-up appointments and to answer any questions. This practice may prevent readmissions of patients for the same problems (chief complaint or diagnosis). It also increases the patient's and family's satisfaction and faith in the institution.

Repeating the Case Management Process

Case managers usually repeat the case management process every time they are in contact with the patient and family. This function is not considered a true or direct step in the case management process. Reassessment of patients, ongoing evaluation of patient care activities and outcomes, and constant checking and ensuring that care is delivered as scheduled in a timely fashion are all examples of tasks that require going through every step of the case management process. Case managers are constantly repeating the process.

Repeating the case management process is one way of ensuring that the provision of care is appropriate, the quality is not compromised in the name of cost containment, and the patient is discharged safely. Case managers have the opportunity and obligation to repeat the case management process every time a task is not completed effectively, a delay in any care activity is identified, an expected outcome is not met, or the patient or a family member are in disagreement with the plan. When repeating the process, case managers implement new interventions and activities to resolve the identified problem(s). Repeating the case management process functions as a safety net for ensuring that appropriate care is delivered and as a method for developing an action plan for problem solving.

VARIOUS ROLES PLAYED BY CASE MANAGERS

Case managers are involved in many different situations throughout the day. They may provide a patient and/or a family with care instructions and may teach staff members about new trends in patient care. They may also ensure approval/certification of services by MCOs or negotiate home care services with an agency. The varied scope of roles, functions, and activities they may provide increases their challenge for ensuring that high-quality and cost-effective care has been delivered.

This wide range of responsibilities requires case managers to put more than one role or function into action at the same time. The interrelatedness of these roles is the key to success. Case managers may be found assessing or reassessing patients while monitoring and evaluating outcomes. They may be scheduling a test while trying to resolve delays related to tests or procedures. Their various roles are important for timely patient care delivery and outcomes. The various responsibilities and roles of case managers and their ongoing planning and prioritization of the tasks to be completed require them to be

CASE MANAGER'S TIP 4-2

Time Wasters Case Managers Should Avoid
1. Lack of ongoing prioritization and planning
2. Unrealistic goals and time estimates
3. Overambition and desire to impress superiors
4. Inattentiveness and insufficient communication and feedback
5. Tendency to be perfectionists
6. Confusion with regard to responsibilities, functions, and boundaries
7. Insecurity, fear of failure, and lack of confidence and self-esteem
8. Failure to follow up on incomplete tasks
9. Ego and feeling of overimportance
10. Sense of unnecessary obligation
11. Inability to say *no* when needed
12. Failure to obtain important information when it is required to do so, or collecting unnecessary information
13. Being an "extra pair of hands" to everyone
14. Inability to delegate
15. Treating every problem as a crisis (overreaction)
16. Procrastination
17. Leaving tasks unfinished
18. Being unaware of importance of things
19. Socializing

astute in time management, which is integral to the effectiveness of their role (Case Manager's Tips 4-2 and 4-3).

Clinical Expert

Case managers are chosen for their role because of extensive clinical experience and knowledge of patient care. They bring excellence in clinical practice to the role (Case Manager's Tip 4-4). They act as role models and resources to nursing, medical, and other staff members. They exhibit clinical competence in assessing patient and family needs; establishing the actual and potential health problems, goals for treatment, and desired outcomes; applying the nursing process; planning, implementing, evaluating, and coordinating the care activities to meet the patient and family goals and expected outcomes; using advanced treatment modalities and technologies; and dealing with patients as biopsychosocial systems with the treatment plan directed toward the system as a whole rather than just the disease.

Consultant

Because of their clinical experience and knowledge of the institutional operations/systems, policies and procedures, and standards of care and practice, case

CASE MANAGER'S TIP 4-3

Strategies for Effective Time Management

1. Set objectives, goals, priorities, and deadlines.
2. Use "to do" lists for the day. List activities in order of priorities/importance based on the number of tasks to be completed. Update your list continually. Keep your priority list current.
3. Distinguish the urgent from the truly important.
4. Delegate the activities and tasks that can be delegated.
5. Avoid being a perfectionist. Lower your standards to what is reasonable and acceptable.
6. Communicate effectively.
7. Collect appropriate data and necessary information only. Determine what is needed for planning activities, making decisions, and providing feedback.
8. Clarify your job responsibilities, power, and boundaries with your supervisor.
9. Constantly check progress and follow up on unfinished tasks.
10. Refuse to spread yourself too thin. Say no, give reasons, and provide alternatives. You may say, "Sorry, I cannot. I do not have the time, but I have a suggestion..." or "Thanks for the compliment, but I am afraid I have to decline."
11. Make no assumptions, and avoid being critical.
12. Recognize that things may take longer to complete than planned. Accept this fact. Impose realistic deadlines on tasks.
13. Seek the help and guidance of your superior as needed. Avoid struggling with uncertainties on your own.
14. Avoid socializing, distractions, or unnecessary interruptions.
15. Respect deadlines. Avoid procrastination.

 CASE MANAGER'S TIP 4-4

Maintaining Clinical Expertise

1. Become a member in professional organizations and/or nursing societies.
2. Subscribe to journals that pertain to clinical practice.
3. Stay abreast of the healthcare literature and the changes in technology.
4. Attend organization-based continuing education sessions.
5. Participate in conferences, particularly those related to case management.
6. Seek the help of other experts when faced with a situation that is uncertain or unfamiliar.
7. Make every effort to learn new skills and gain new knowledge when opportunities arise.
8. Participate in clinical activities such as case study presentation, case conference, or clinical research.
9. Spend some time in the library (at least 1 hour a week) searching for new knowledge.
10. Attend medical staff/student teaching rounds.
11. Seek higher education.

managers can be called on as consultants by physicians, nurses, and other case managers and members of the interdisciplinary team. They are helpful in solving clinical and administrative issues when members of the interdisciplinary team are in doubt.

Case managers, particularly those who work in an ambulatory care setting, may provide telephone consultations to MCOs or other healthcare insurance companies, patients and families, and home care agencies.

Coordinator and Facilitator of Patient Care

Case managers spend a great deal of their time coordinating and facilitating patient care activities and expediting the completion of tests and procedures.

They also ensure that results of the tests and procedures are available within a reasonable turnaround time. This function is important in reducing length of stay and treatment and eliminating delays and variances in patient care activities. In collaboration with members of the healthcare team, they help patients move smoothly and safely through the hospital and healthcare systems.

In this role function, case managers prevent any fragmentation or duplication in the provision of care. Their timely intervention when a patient's condition changes increases the efficiency and **effectiveness of care.** When necessary, they ensure that authorizations for services are obtained before initiation of treatment. In addition, they coordinate the patient's teaching and discharge plans and ensure the completion of all discharge activities in a timely fashion to prevent unnecessary hospital stay. This role is important in controlling the use of resources and containing cost.

Manager of Patient Care

Case managers function as managers of healthcare services through controlling the use of resources to what is required to achieve the desired outcomes. They act as gatekeepers of the interdisciplinary team to ensure that all patient care activities are accomplished by each team member within the projected timeframes.

CASE MANAGER'S TIP 4-5

Strategies for Better Patient Care Management

1. Maintain constant knowledge of the patient's plan of care. Update your information as indicated by changes in the patient's condition.
2. Prevent delays in patient care activities.
3. Ensure that tests and procedures are prescheduled.
4. Obtain timely results of tests and procedures, and adjust the plan of care accordingly.
5. Become knowledgeable about the contracts of managed care companies and federal and third-party reimbursement procedures.
6. Encourage patients' timely discharge.
7. Maximize the use of outpatient testing and same day of admission procedures.
8. Communicate with the interdisciplinary team on an ongoing basis.
9. Ensure the involvement of the members of the interdisciplinary team in patient care–related decisions and problem solving.
10. Maximize the involvement of the patient and family in such decisions.
11. Prevent redundancy, duplication, or fragmentation of patient care activities.
12. Eliminate any unnecessary or inappropriate tests or procedures.
13. Seek administrative support as needed.
14. Seek the guidance of experts when uncertain of a particular situation.

One of their main responsibilities is direct supervision of the process of patient care to ensure quality outcomes. Case Manager's Tip 4-5 lists some strategies for managing patient care.

Educator

The role of educator is twofold. Case managers are involved in patient and family education and staff education. Regarding patient and family, they ensure that all healthcare needs are met within a reasonable timeframe during the hospital stay. They usually incorporate the teaching plan as part of the CMP and transitional plan as early as the time of admission or care encounter. They may provide direct patient teaching activities or supervise their completion by the primary nurses and/or other team members. Case managers may also be involved in developing patient and family teaching materials and planning and conducting patient teaching classes (Case Manager's Tip 4-6).

Regarding nursing and other staff members, case managers are instrumental in mentoring the less

 CASE MANAGER'S TIP 4-6

Strategies for Effective Patient/Family Education

1. Educate patients and families only when they are ready.
2. Identify the barriers or limitations to learning before you conduct a patient's education session.
3. Maximize the family's/caregiver's involvement.
4. Use visual aids such as handouts, drawings, audiotapes, and videotapes.
5. Assess the need for low-level reading materials. At the same time, avoid being "cutesy." Adult learners might feel insulted.
6. Apply the concepts of adult learning theory in your teaching sessions/activities.
7. Encourage the patient's/family's participation in the decision-making process regarding learning needs.
8. Include return demonstrations or verbalization of material taught.
9. Adapt the teaching strategy to the patient's level of understanding, capabilities, or preferences.
10. Involve other professionals (e.g., pharmacists, staff nurses, clinical nurse specialists) in educating patients/families.
11. Limit the material to be taught to what the patient is able to grasp in one session.
12. If possible, schedule the next teaching session with the patient/family.
13. Evaluate the ability of the patient/family to retain the information taught.
14. Be consistent in the information provided, especially if other professionals are involved in teaching or reinforcing patient/family education.
15. Put special emphasis on the care needs of patients after discharge.
16. Conduct small group education sessions when appropriate.
17. Allow for questions and answers.
18. Avoid the use of medical jargon. Speak a language the patient understands.
19. Clearly indicate the patient's teaching plan in the medical record.
20. Use patient and family education materials written in the patient's language.
21. Use **Internet** resources as appropriate, especially with patients who are familiar with how to navigate the Internet.

experienced staff. They participate in inservice sessions related to case management and new trends and advances in patient care. Their staff teaching activities may be done as unit-based sessions or formal classes planned and held in collaboration with staff education departments. Either way, they are actively involved in the dissemination of new patient care knowledge and delivery systems.

Negotiator/Broker

Among the other roles assumed by case managers is the role of negotiator and broker of care and services. They are instrumental in getting necessary tests and procedures completed on time. They also negotiate the best treatment plan possible with the healthcare team, patient and family, and most importantly, the MCO. Case managers also negotiate with healthcare agencies

 CASE MANAGER'S TIP 4-7

Successful Negotiation

The strategies discussed in this section could be applied when the case manager negotiates services with outside agencies, physicians, consultants, and professional and ancillary staff, as well as when attempting to facilitate and coordinate patient care activities and prevent delays in patient care within and outside the boundaries of the institution.

1. Separate people from positions.
2. Negotiate for agreements—not winning or losing.
3. Establish mutual trust and respect.
4. Avoid one-sided or personal gains.
5. Allow time for expressing the interests of each side/party.
6. Listen actively during the process, and acknowledge what is being said.
7. Use data/evidence to strengthen your position.
8. Focus on interests—patient care interests.
9. Always remember that the process is a problem-solving one, and the benefit is for the patient and family.
10. Never forget that patient care is the priority.
11. Avoid using pressure.
12. Be knowledgeable of the institutional policies, procedures, systems, standards, and the law. Apply this knowledge in the process.
13. Try to understand the other side well. Ask questions and seek clarifications when unsure or uncertain.
14. Avoid emotional outbursts. Do not overreact if the other party exhibits such behavior.
15. Avoid premature judgments.
16. Be concrete and flexible when presenting your stand.
17. Use reason and be reasonable.
18. Be fair.

for community services such as home care, needed for patients' support after discharge from the hospital. In addition, they negotiate with managed care companies for approval of the patient's hospitalization, the need for **durable medical equipment,** or the necessary services needed after discharge. Case Manager's Tip 4-7 lists strategies for effective negotiation.

Patient and Family Advocate

One of the important responsibilities of case managers is patient and family **advocacy** (Case Manager's Tip 4-8). Case managers assume a liaison role between the patient and family and the healthcare team. With their relationship with the patient and family at the time of admission, case managers are able to build trust and establish rapport to help facilitate the implementation of the plan of care. They keep the patient and family constantly informed of the plan of care, tests and procedures, and condition, which makes them the best vehicle through which the care is advocated, negotiated, agreed on, facilitated, and coordinated.

Case managers advocate for patients in case conferences and healthcare team meetings held throughout the patient's hospitalization or care encounter, during which they communicate the needs and wishes of the patient and family. They also advocate for the patient when reviewing plans of care with case managers of

 CASE MANAGER'S TIP 4-8

Advocating Effectively for Patients/Families

1. Know the plan of care of your patients well, including the minute details.
2. Spend enough time discussing the care with the patient and family, and understand their concerns.
3. Be familiar with the Patient's Bill of Rights.
4. Be knowledgeable of the law and the standards of regulatory agencies regarding certain patient care issues such as informed consent and do not resuscitate (DNR) orders.
5. Be honest with the patient and family. Admit when you do not know the answers to their questions.
6. Convey patient/family concerns to the appropriate personnel, obtain answers, and report results back to the patient and family.
7. Identify ethical dilemmas and refer them to the ethics committee in a timely fashion.
8. Provide the patient and family with emotional support as needed. Alleviate their anxieties and apprehension.

MCOs for purposes of obtaining authorizations/certifications and when negotiating with agencies for community services or informing them of a patient's care needs after discharge.

Outcomes and Quality Manager

Monitoring and evaluating patient care quality and outcomes are integral to the role of case managers. They are important because they link case management to quality improvement and help determine whether the patient and organizational goals are met. Case managers monitor the occurrence of variances and outcomes of care as they relate to the CMP. The results of this monitoring process provide important data for quality improvement efforts and evaluating the effectiveness and efficiency of the case management model and the use of CMPs. Case managers also investigate the reasons of variances and attempt to resolve them as soon as they are identified.

Case managers communicate variances, delays, and undesired patient care outcomes to members of the interdisciplinary healthcare team so that the team can revise the CMP as necessary. Together as a team they are better able to convince administration of the need for quality improvement task forces to have a closer

 CASE MANAGER'S TIP 4-9

Strategies for Improving Patient Care Quality

1. Focus on the process, not the people.
2. Listen to patient and family concerns.
3. Identify patient care problems (variances and delays) early and attempt to resolve them in a timely fashion.
4. Attend as an interdisciplinary team, rather than individually, to patient problems.
5. Keep lines of communication open at all levels. Discuss the issues as they arise with the patient/family, superiors, subordinates, and whoever is deemed appropriate.
6. Ensure that the desired/projected outcomes of care are met.
7. Ensure patient's safe discharge.
8. Provide care that is patient focused.
9. Attend customer relations classes. Apply strategies learned to practice.
10. Obtain and read the results of patient satisfaction surveys and quality improvement monitors. Change behavior and practice as indicated by the results.
11. Conduct concurrent or retrospective chart reviews on an ongoing basis.

look at certain system issues and non–value adding processes, particularly those that require immediate attention. Case Manager's Tip 4-9 lists actions to help improve patient care quality.

Scientist/Researcher

Research has been made a part of the case manager's role in institutions in which the required educational background of case managers is a master's degree. In this role, case managers are expected to participate as active members of institution-based research committees. They are also expected to write grant and research proposals, collect research data, and evaluate patient care activities. As advanced practice nurses, case managers are excellent at knowledge development and dissemination and utilization of research. Case managers help nursing departments establish a research-based clinical practice, policies, procedures, and standards of care. Case Manager's Tip 4-10 lists some strategies to help in becoming involved in research.

Risk Manager

Because of their proximity to the bedside and involvement in direct patient care activities, case managers are at the forefront of identifying patient care issues that are considered legal **risk.** They are good at ensuring that the care delivered is in compliance with the standards of regulatory agencies, such as the U.S. Department of Health and Human Services and the JCAHO, and the internal/institution's policies, procedures, standards of care, and standards of practice. Their role in assessment and monitoring of the delivery of patient care activities and evaluation of outcomes makes them crucial in identifying **risk management** issues and bringing them to the attention of the legal department in a timely fashion.

Case managers are able to establish a trusting relationship with the patient and family. Because of this relationship, they are able to prevent problems from

 CASE MANAGER'S TIP 4-10

Strategies for Getting Involved in Research

1. Learn the research process. Take courses in research or seek the help of research experts.
2. Apply research outcomes to practice.
3. Conduct research.
4. Obtain funding; write grants.
5. Participate in institutional research efforts: collect data, identify potential subjects, and so on.
6. Become a member of the research committee.
7. Get involved in research utilization and dissemination programs.

escalating and becoming potential legal risk issues (Case Manager's Tip 4-11). Their advocacy of patient care helps them reduce the seriousness of any problems and makes patients view them as "God-sent angels." They are also helpful to members of the healthcare team.

CASE MANAGER'S TIP 4-11

Reducing Legal Risk

1. Always know the law. Seek the help/advice of the legal and risk management department in your institution when uncertain.
2. Familiarize yourself with the standards of care and practice of regulatory agencies.
3. Familiarize yourself with institutional policies and procedures and standards of care and practice.
4. Refer to the experts or the available reference manuals when unsure of a situation or a decision.
5. Attend to problems immediately as they arise. Do not wait for them to escalate.
6. Do anything possible to prevent problems from occurring.
7. Advocate for patients/families as opportunities arise.
8. Know the details of the Patient's Bill of Rights. Ensure that patients are also educated about their rights.
9. Obtain knowledge of the requirements of federal and third-party payers.
10. Understand well the managed care contracts and their impact and relation to patient care.
11. Monitor and observe patients constantly. Make sure you are aware of the latest changes in your patient's condition.
12. Communicate changes in the plan of care to the patient and family in a timely fashion.
13. Apply the scientific method to the development of CMPs.
14. Base CMPs on the latest therapies, research outcomes, expert opinion, and recommendations/standards of professional societies.
15. Use CMPs as standards of care. Develop and apply one CMP for each diagnosis or procedure.
16. Include a disclaimer in the CMP explaining that it is only a recommended treatment plan and needs to be individualized to the patient's needs when applied. For example, a disclaimer might read: *"This case management plan is a suggested interdisciplinary plan of care. It is a guideline that may be changed and individualized according to patient condition and needs."*

They provide them with answers to their clinical dilemmas and act as resource people to the team when faced with administrative problems. Case managers are excellent in this role because of their knowledge of the institution's administrative and clinical policies and procedures.

Change Agent

Case managers are the *champions of change*. They are the most helpful change agents an institution may have while implementing a new case management model (Case Manager's Tip 4-12). Case managers act as

CASE MANAGER'S TIP 4-12

Instituting Effective Change

1. Become familiar with change theories and processes.
2. Recognize and foster the attitude that change is inevitable.
3. Learn the goals and objectives of the change happening at your institution. Communicate them to all those involved.
4. Give special consideration to all the aspects of change: physical, emotional, conceptual, perceptual, individual, and organizational.
5. Acknowledge that an organization cannot change unless all staff buy into the change.
6. Reduce turf battles.
7. Educate all staff about the change, reasons, goals, new processes/systems, mission, and philosophy.
8. As a case manager, act as a change agent, champion, coach, and mentor.
9. Identify and communicate the benefits of change.
10. Avoid surprises. Be as open as possible.
11. Keep lines of communication open. Invite questions and provide answers.
12. Invite participation of all those interested. Encourage and support them in promoting the change.
13. Admit to difficulties.
14. Attend to those resistant to change. Investigate their reasons and concerns. Consider their recommendations for improving the situation.
15. Recognize and reward everybody's efforts regardless of their position in the organization or degree of participation. Every little effort is important.
16. Involve informal leaders and those who are powerful.
17. Maintain ongoing follow-up and reinforcement.
18. Establish/clarify new policies, procedures, and standards.
19. Establish an open forum for communication and dissemination of information.

role models and resource people and experts in case management to all staff during the transition into case management and thereafter. They are knowledgeable in the subject matter, which makes them well versed in case management and able to educate other staff members such as physicians, staff nurses, and ancillary staff.

In their training, case managers are prepared to handle resistance to change and resistant people. Their coaching, mentoring, and teaching approach to staff when facing resistance makes them able to conquer problems. They are well aware that resistance is a normal coping mechanism some people choose to follow when experiencing change. Their professional and mature approach to such situations makes it easier to convince staff to support the change. Case managers are also trained in problem solving, conflict resolution, and negotiation. These skills help improve their outlook and their strategies for preventing resistance. They also help them to build a better response to staff concerns.

Case managers are the main advocates for case management systems an institution is lucky to have. Case managers' commitment to their role and their hard work make them successful and help them to attain excellence in their practice.

Holistic Care Provider

Case managers attend to their patients as whole systems (i.e., biopsychosocial systems). They assess patients and families for any actual or potential health problems regardless of the chief complaint or the disease for which they are being treated (Case Manager's Tip 4-13). They are savvy in their evaluation of the patient's condition; they identify the physical, psychological, financial, and spiritual needs and make sure that these needs are incorporated into the CMP/interdisciplinary plan of care. For example, when a patient is admitted to the hospital for uncontrolled diabetes, case managers not only assess dietary habits, blood glucose levels, and compliance with insulin and follow-up visits, but they also assess the patient for complications of diabetes such as deficiency in vision and foot ulcers. In addition, they assess footwear, skin care, support system, adjustment to the disease, and insurance and benefits.

Case managers ensure that disease prevention and lifestyle changes are addressed with their patients and families. They work with them closely to identify the best strategies to improve compliance with the medical/surgical regimen and disease risk reduction. For example, they may counsel a cardiac patient on strategies for quitting smoking or drinking alcohol or beginning a physical exercise program. They may provide patients and families with important information regarding community services and support groups for the same purpose.

Counselor

Another characteristic in the role of case managers is counseling and support of patients and families (Case Manager's Tip 4-14). Case managers are attentive to the emotional and spiritual needs of patients. They are astute at providing patients with emotional support, and they counsel them regarding adjustment to hospitalization and their coping skills and mechanisms with the disease—particularly if patients are suffering from a chronic disease that requires frequent hospitalization, such as cancer.

 CASE MANAGER'S TIP 4-13

Providing Holistic Patient Care
1. Deal with the patient as a biopsychosocial being.
2. Develop an action plan that meets all of the patient's symptoms and needs rather than just the disease.
3. Attend not only to the patient's actual needs but also to the potential ones.
4. Educate the patient about health promotion activities and strategies for disease risk reduction.
5. Promote a healthy lifestyle.
6. When dealing with the patient, do not forget about the family or the caregiver.
7. Evaluate the impact of the patient's illness on the patient-family system and relationship, not just the patient.
8. Encourage a healthy adjustment to illness (patient and family related).
9. Include health promotion activities in the CMP.

 CASE MANAGER'S TIP 4-14

Effective Counseling
1. Evaluate the patient's and family's ability to cope with and respond and adjust to illness.
2. Alleviate anxieties and apprehension.
3. Address the patient's and family's spiritual, emotional, and psychological needs.
4. Conduct therapy sessions.
5. Communicate therapeutically.
6. Allow for questions and provide answers.
7. Attend to patient and family concerns.
8. Alleviate the patient's fears and concerns regarding care after discharge.

Case managers may also work closely with victims of domestic violence and sexual and physical abuse. Their counseling skills and emotional support to these groups of patients are highly appreciated. They also ensure that these patients are well educated regarding availability of crisis teams and how they can be accessed, and they direct them to local agencies or support groups for further follow-up and support after discharge from the hospital or emergency department.

Utilization Manager

Utilization management (see Chapter 5) is an integral component of case management. It helps contain cost and ensures the provision of appropriate care at the right level and in the appropriate setting. It is a technique used by case managers to ensure that the patient meets predefined criteria to support the level of care being delivered. These criteria are national guidelines applied particularly by MCOs and agreed on with the providers and payers during managed care contract negotiations. Examples of these guidelines are InterQual (InterQual, 1998), which is mostly used for **Medicare** and **Medicaid** populations, and Milliman & Robertson (Schibanoff, 1999), which is mostly used for patients with managed care health insurance. By applying the criteria present in these guidelines, the case manager ensures reimbursement for services provided.

Utilization management is a predominant function in hospital-based case management models. Case managers usually collaborate with members of the interdisciplinary team in transitioning the patient to the appropriate level of care to prevent reimbursement **denials.** Case managers also communicate with other case managers in the MCOs either daily or periodically regarding the services being rendered. This communication is called **concurrent review,** and its purpose is to obtain certifications/authorizations for the plan of care before delivering the necessary services. This process is important because it reviews, monitors, evaluates, and certifies the allocation of healthcare resources and services. Case managers apply the utilization management process for the following purposes:

- Examining the patient's **severity of illness**
- Identifying the **intensity of services**
- Precertification of services
- Authorizations for continued/extended length of stay
- Transitional planning and approval of postdischarge services
- Transitioning patients from one level of care to another of lesser intensity
- Transferring patients from one healthcare facility to another

- Timely delivery of services
- Reimbursement

Case managers in MCOs get involved in utilization management mainly because of their role in telephone triage. In this role, they direct patients to access healthcare services at the appropriate setting; that is, they act as gatekeepers. They also certify the delivery of services requested by other case managers who work for the provider. They do this during the patient care review process, before or during the delivery of care.

Transitional Planner

Transitional planning (see Chapter 6), also known as *discharge planning,* is another predominant function of case managers in the hospital-based setting. It focuses on brokering postdischarge services for patients and their families or caregivers. These services apply to the varied settings across the **continuum of care.** Transitional planning also involves a team approach to care planning, delivery, monitoring, and evaluation. Similar to utilization management, it is integrated with the case management process. Case managers design the transitional plan in collaboration with the interdisciplinary healthcare team and based on the patient's:

- Treatment plan
- Clinical condition
- Financial status and insurance plan
- Support system
- Ability for self-care management
- Postdischarge medical regimen
- Need for rehabilitative services
- Discharge location

Case managers engage in ongoing assessment and reassessment of the patient's condition and needs. They identify any changes and incorporate them in the transitional plan as necessary. They make these efforts to ensure timely, safe, cost-effective, and quality discharge. As they exercise this function of their role, case managers apply the laws and regulations (federal and state) and the standards of accreditation agencies and ensure adherence to these expectations. If they identify any issues, concerns, or problems, they address them accordingly. Sometimes they conduct case conferences with the patient and family and the team for this purpose.

Pursuant to transitional planning, case managers refer patients for evaluation by specialist providers such as physical therapy, nutrition, home care, and social services. These referrals are essential for the development of an appropriate and safe discharge plan and to maintain compliance with the regulations. However, the case manager remains responsible for ensuring that referrals and evaluations are completed in a timely manner and that recommendations from the specialist providers are discussed by the healthcare team and incorporated in the transitional/discharge plan as deemed necessary.

Ethicist

Case managers have long defined themselves as patient advocates. In this role they constantly face ethical dilemmas and challenges. Today's managed care environment has brought about new ethical problems such as inaccessibility to care and denials of services. As coordinators and managers of patient care, case managers are obliged to address and resolve these issues. However, they are not expected to resolve them alone; they do consult with ethics specialists for this purpose. Case managers usually bring ethical dilemmas to the attention of the healthcare team and facilitate their resolution by looking out and advocating for patients and their families and by assisting the team in making decisions that are in the best interest of the patient. Because these deliberations are usually challenging, case managers rely on the guidance of ethicists.

In dealing with ethical dilemmas, case managers apply the principles of **autonomy, beneficence, justice, veracity,** and **nonmaleficence.** They also apply the code of ethics of their profession (e.g., nursing, social work) and that of the Case Management Society of America. These codes guide the case managers in the process of ethical decision making and problem solving (see Chapter 18).

ROLES OF THE CASE MANAGER IN VARIED SETTINGS

Case management models have been implemented in every setting along the continuum of care. This makes the case manager's role available in all settings as well. Although the care settings are different, the basic functions and responsibilities of case managers are essentially the same. The case management process discussed previously acts as a generic process for all settings and shares the important elements of case management that can be slightly modified and individualized to the specific care setting. The main focus of case management services differs between settings. These differences explain the variations of the role. Case managers apply different iterations of the case management process depending on the setting they are employed in and the focus of the case management model. For example:

- Acute care focuses on **utilization review** and transitional planning.
- Admitting department focuses on appropriateness and patients' eligibility for admission to the hospital.
- Emergency department focuses on gatekeeping and appropriateness of patients' admission to the hospital.

- Perioperative care focuses on patients' readiness and eligibility for surgery.
- Community-based care focuses on primary care, wellness, prevention, and health maintenance.
- Home care focuses on chronic care management and self-care management.
- Subacute care focuses on restoration and rehabilitation of function.
- Long-term care focuses on chronic and supportive care management.
- Disease management focuses on population risk stratification and reduction and chronic care management.
- Managed care focuses on utilization management, **demand management,** and gatekeeping.
- **Telephonic case management** focuses on giving advice, triage, and gatekeeping.
- Independent/private case management focuses on disability and rehabilitation care management.
- **Workers' compensation** focuses on rehabilitation services and return-to-work planning.

Case management activities in all of these settings include aspects of clinical care management, utilization management, and transitional planning. However, the main focus may differ depending on the setting. For example, in MCOs, the main aspect of the case manager's role is utilization management. Table 4-3 presents examples of these functions as they relate to the specific setting. The list is not exhaustive, and further descriptions of the varied models can be found in Chapter 3.

THE SOCIAL WORKER AS CASE MANAGER

As in most clinical arenas, the role of the social work case manager varies greatly from one care delivery setting to the next. Nevertheless, certain elements are considered fundamental to the differentiation of social work case management from that performed by other professionals.

Social work case management has been defined as a method of providing services whereby a professional social worker assesses the needs of the client and the client's family when appropriate. The social worker in this environment arranges, coordinates, monitors, evaluates, and advocates for a package of multiple services to meet the specific complex needs of clients (Case Management Standards Work Group, 1992).

Social work case managers distinguish themselves from other case management professionals by addressing the client's biopsychosocial status and the state of the social system in which case management operates. Social work case managers develop therapeutic

TABLE 4-3 Examples of Case Manager Roles in Varied Settings

Care Setting	Examples of Case Management Roles and Activities	Care Setting	Examples of Case Management Roles and Activities
Acute care	Obtain authorizations for services Develop and implement plan of care and transitional plan Conduct concurrent utilization reviews with MCOs Facilitate interdisciplinary plan of care and communication Educate patient and family regarding care and needs Transition patients across necessary levels of care Expedite diagnostic and therapeutic procedures Conduct case conferences and patient/ family counseling	Home care	Provide postacute care services such as wound care, dressing changes, administration of IV antibiotics Prevent the need for readmission to hospital or emergency department Promote self-care management skills Provide patient and family education regarding healthcare needs and services Coordinate care from home setting with physician and other specialty providers such as physical therapist Monitor treatments rendered by other providers such as infusion therapy, home health aide, social worker Evaluate safety of home environment Coordinate use of durable medical equipment Communicate with MCOs
Admitting department	Assess patients for eligibility of admission Obtain authorization for services Develop preliminary transitional plan Suggest use of alternate level of care	Subacute	Provide services such as weaning from respirators, IV antibiotic therapy, extensive wound management Provide restorative and rehabilitative services Coordinate care and services with physician and other providers/interdisciplinary team Obtain authorizations for services Establish and implement transitional plan Handle end-of-life issues and decisions
Emergency department	Provide timely care and services Arrange for community resources Provide counseling for patients and families Plan patient's admission or discharge Suggest use of alternate level of care Expedite tests and procedures	Long-term	Provide skilled care Provide supportive care and services Communicate and follow up with physicians and other providers on ongoing basis, considering that primary care provider may not examine patient on daily basis Counsel patients and families as needed
Perioperative	Complete preadmission tests Evaluate postdischarge needs and establish transitional plan Discuss discharge options with patient, family, and team Provide psychosocial counseling to patient and family Obtain authorization for services Ensure patient's readiness for surgery: tests, medical clearance, insurance approval, consent Adjust operating room schedule Address delays and cancellations	Disease management	Ensure safety in delivery of care and environment Conduct risk stratification surveys for population served Stratify patients into risk categories Provide case management services based on needs of each risk group Provide telephone support services Educate patients and families regarding medical regimen, self-care management, risk reduction strategies Manage populations with chronic diseases such as asthma, renal failure, HIV/AIDS, heart failure, premature babies Transition patients across continuum of care as needed Coordinate care in collaboration with interdisciplinary healthcare team Facilitate and expedite care and services
Community	Support patient and family to achieve optimal state of wellness and functioning Provide primary care and primary prevention services Conduct patient and family education sessions Coordinate use of community-based resources Prevent need for acute care and services Stratify patients/population into risk groups and provide case management services accordingly Focus on strategies for health risk reduction Promote healthy lifestyle and behavior		

HIV/AIDS, Human immunodeficiency virus/acquired immunodeficiency syndrome; *IV,* intravenous.

TABLE 4-3   Examples of Case Manager Roles in Varied Settings—cont'd

Care Setting	Examples of Case Management Roles and Activities	Care Setting	Examples of Case Management Roles and Activities
Managed care	Coordinate demand management services Conduct health surveys Provide preventive screening services such as mammography, hypertension, cholesterol Distribute patient and family education newsletter and materials Provide gatekeeping services Authorize/certify services Engage in managed care contract preparation and negotiation	Independent/ private—cont'd	Advocate for patient and family Coordinate rehabilitative and restorative services Transition patient along continuum of care Facilitate return-to-work plan Represent patient, provider, or payer, depending on contractual agreement Facilitate communication among different providers Implement complex plan of care and services
Telephonic	Triage patients according to need Facilitate access to healthcare services Act as gatekeeper Provide advice over the telephone Assess patient's condition and needs and coordinate care accordingly Communicate patient's needs to physician and other providers Use algorithms to help in decision making Provide psychosocial counseling services	Workers' compensation	Manage care of on-the-job injured patients Collaborate with occupational health department, risk management, human resources, and lawyers Establish and implement plan of care and transitional plan Coordinate complex plan of care and services and return-to-work plan Obtain authorizations for services Expedite diagnostic and therapeutic procedures Manage patient's benefits Facilitate provision of disability and rehabilitation services Provide psychosocial counseling to patient and family
Independent/ private	Provide case management services to MCOs and providers of healthcare facilities Manage patient's plan of care and clinical and financial services Obtain authorizations for services		

relationships with their clients and may link them to other services that they may require.

Perhaps the most fundamental difference between the social worker as case manager and the nurse as case manager is the deeper focus on the patient's entire social system. An example in Table 4-4 clarifies this difference. The other steps in the case management process are consistent to both groups. In addition, social workers have certain values unique to their profession. These include the primacy of the client's interests, respect for diversity, confidentiality, client self-determination, and respect (Ballew and Mink, 1996).

Social work defines the stages of case management in the following way:

■ Disengaging—building effective relationships
■ Coordinating—organizing services
■ Accessing resources—connecting client and resources
■ Planning—identifying goals
■ Assessing—finding the client's strengths

■ Engaging—negotiating expectation, building trust (Ballew and Mink, 1996)

These stages mirror fundamental components of social work and meld with the goals of case management.

THE ADVANCED PRACTICE NURSE AS CASE MANAGER

Advanced practice nurses assuming the role of the case manager are both clinical nurse specialists (CNSs) and nurse practitioners (NPs). Because of their educational backgrounds and training, each brings a different set of skills to the role and enhances it in specific ways. For example, NPs as case managers are more autonomous and independent compared with CNSs because of their prescriptive privileges and role in primary care. Both professionals bring special aspects of their preparation into the case manager's role as follows:

■ **CNS:** expert clinician, educator, consultant, and researcher, with a main focus in acute care

TABLE 4-4 Guidelines for Referrals: Case Managers and Social Workers, Emergency Department

RN Case Manager	Shared Responsibilities: RN Case Manager/Social Worker	Social Worker
Admission utilization review: Intake assessment of admitted patients	Coordinate/facilitate plans of care for discharged patients	Patient/family having difficulty understanding/accepting and/or following through on medical plans of care and continuing care options
Utilization/insurance calls	Transportation	Interventions regarding issues impacting the ability to access the continuum of care (e.g., immigration problem, primary caregiver or disabled person)
Coordinate/facilitate plans of care for admitted patients	Patient education (e.g., reinforcement regarding follow-up with medical appointments, medical regimen)	
Screening/assessments of patients for psychosocial needs in conjunction with plan of care	Crisis intervention needed for patient/family having difficulty coping with illness, family dysfunction, trauma, death, accidents, injuries, substance abuse	Advocacy and counseling around entitlements or other essential services (e.g., Medicaid, food stamps, housing, medications)
Discharge planning, including equipment, home care, infusion treatment	Referrals for nursing homes, adult homes, shelters	Suspicion or evidence of domestic violence, elder abuse or neglect, child abuse or neglect, sexual assault
Initiate inpatient discharge planning		Ethical or legal concerns (e.g., patient, family, team conflicts related to medical plan of care, guardianship or APS cases, end-of-life issues around Advance Directives)
Participates in the development of ED guidelines for care		
Track data (e.g., variances in patient care standards, systems standards)		Referrals for home supports for psychosocially complex patients
Clinical resource for staff		Referrals needed for marital, individual, or family treatment
Facilitates patients' progress through the ED to disposition		Assistance needed in locating families of unidentified, seriously ill patients
Oversees/facilitates transfers from institution to institution		Tracking of difficult to locate patients for follow-up medical care

APS, Adult Protective Services; *ED,* emergency department.

RN Case Managers and Social Workers, Maternal Child Inpatient Units

RN Case Manager	Social Worker
Performs admission and concurrent utilization management, including insurance calls	Patient/family difficulty coping with diagnosis, lifestyle changes; difficulty understanding/accepting decision making with long-term discharge planning and/or continuing care options
Coordinates/facilitates plans of care	
Facilitates daily rounds and team meetings	
Assesses all patients for psychosocial needs	Psychiatric, cognitive, or behavioral factors that may impede delivery of care and discharge planning process
Discharge planning, including equipment, home care, rehabilitation, and long-term care facilities	Inadequate supports that may impact on compliance with continuing care needs (social workers can offer information to case managers regarding entitlements for patients/families)
Orders transportation	
Discharge planning forms	
Oversight of clinical guidelines	Ethical or legal concerns (e.g., patient, family, team conflicts related to medical plan of care, guardianship cases, or end-of-life issues around Advance Directives such as DNR)
Tracks data (e.g., variances in patient care and systems standards)	
Provides alternate level of care notification	Suspicion or evidence of domestic violence, abuse or neglect, rape, sexual assault
	History of poor medical compliance (e.g., lack of prenatal care, late registration, late immunizations)
	Advocacy around entitlements and community social services

DNR, Do not resuscitate.

TABLE 4-4   RN Case Managers and Social Workers, Maternal Child Inpatient Units—cont'd

RN Case Manager	Social Worker
	Drug or alcohol abuse
	Cannot afford medications and no plan for access in near future
	Bereavement (e.g., terminally ill child, fetal demise)
	Homelessness or unable to return to prior living situation
	Questionable parenting skills or interactions among family members
	Community referrals

■ **NP:** expert clinician, health promotion and disease prevention, referrals to other services, reimbursement for care, and prescribing treatments, with main focus on primary care in inpatient and outpatient settings (Schroer, 1991)

With their advanced education (i.e., master's degree), NPs and CNSs can effectively implement managed care and case management strategies for cost control and the provision of safe and quality care. They can also function as change agents and care decision-makers. The success of the case management model relies heavily on the person who assumes the pivotal role of case manager. The CNS or NP as case manager ensures that the critical link between the patient, the payer, and the provider in the context of complex healthcare systems is kept as simple as possible and at a manageable level. Because of their advanced degree, they are better able to tolerate the challenges of patient care management presented to them as case managers compared with those with a bachelor's degree. Their graduate education allows them to be more confident, knowledgeable, and skillful. Moreover, they demonstrate better skills than those prepared at the undergraduate educational level in problem solving, delegation, critical thinking, clinical judgment, negotiation, interdisciplinary collaboration, and outcomes evaluation.

The case manager role assumed by CNSs and NPs is not any different from the role discussed in this chapter. However, one challenge of the use of advanced practice nurses in the role of the case manager is the area of financial management. Educational programs of both NPs and CNSs lack courses in financial management, cost accounting, and cost-benefit analysis. Because of this limitation, cost control as an aspect of the case manager's role presents some challenges. Therefore healthcare organizations using CNSs or NPs as case managers must prepare them in this area. Suggested focus is training in cost of care, charges, expenses, revenue and loss analysis, and reimbursement methods. Although case managers may spend 5% to 10% of their time in financial management, this aspect makes their role more powerful.

In their various roles, functions, and responsibilities, it is highly important for case managers to be able to work efficiently and effectively with the interdisciplinary team members. Teamwork is essential at all times and in all situations. In addition, case managers are expected to be skilled in time management, organization and prioritization of work and responsibilities, and follow-up on issues continuously until closure or resolution. Their role is a challenging one, particularly because their priorities change throughout the day as a result of changes in patients' conditions, priorities of the interdisciplinary team, or priorities of the healthcare organization.

Box 4-2 provides an example of a day in the life of a hospital-based case manager. This example is a concise version of what needs to be accomplished daily by case managers. It can be used especially by those who are struggling with how to survive their busy day, as a structure for prioritizing what needs to be done on a certain day and as a tool for time management and improving productivity. When electing to apply this example in their daily activities, case managers are advised to adjust the example to meet the constantly changing needs of their patients. In addition, they are urged to reprioritize their task lists to meet the changing demands of their patients.

The role of the case manager is essential to the success of the case management system. It is the key to ensuring that cost-effective and high-quality patient care is provided. This role is designed to maximize collaboration among all members of the healthcare team; integration of the services required for the care of each patient; coordination and facilitation of tests, procedures, and other patient care activities; continuity and consistency in the provision of care across care settings and services; and most importantly, the openness of lines of communication among all disciplines and on all levels. In addition, it is important for integrating

BOX 4-2 A Day in the Life of a Case Manager

To be able to provide efficient and effective case management services for an entire group of patients, case managers may elect to follow the daily routine presented here.

This routine is only one example of how a case manager may spend his or her day to ensure that the important tasks for the day are completed. When adopting this schedule of activities, one should be careful not to be rigid about the timeframes suggested. One should be able to adjust this schedule to the specific organization, area of practice, specialty, and responsibilities of the role as delineated in the case manager's job description of the individual institution.

An important function of the case manager is priority setting. This function is essential for time management, organization of activities and responsibilities, and completing the most important tasks first. Case managers adopting this schedule of activities should factor in the need to constantly revise their "to do" lists based on the significant changes in the conditions of their patients and the constantly changing priorities. They ought to understand that the key here is flexibility and fluidity.

07:30–08:30

1. Obtain informal report from night staff regarding significant changes in patients' condition, new admissions, and new referrals.
2. Review medical records of new admissions and screen potential patients requiring case management services.
3. Identify/make a list of patients to be seen before discharge.

08:30–09:30

1. Participate in interdisciplinary rounds.
2. Check on all patients scheduled for discharge and ensure that all discharge planning activities have been met (e.g., patient teaching, home care services, follow-up appointment).
3. Conduct case conferencing with the interdisciplinary team and communicate patients' needs.

09:30–11:00

1. Complete the assessments of those patients who meet the criteria for case management services.
2. Confirm, finalize, and follow up on or update the plans of care/CMPs of those patients who are a part of the caseload.
3. Facilitate and coordinate patient care activities (e.g., call ancillary departments and expedite scheduling of tests and procedures, obtain results), investigate and attempt to resolve delays in the provision of care, and initiate appropriate consults and referrals—particularly those necessary for timely discharge planning.

11:00–12:00

1. Communicate with managed care insurance companies regarding appropriateness of and necessity for patients' continued hospitalization.
2. Follow up on the patients scheduled for discharge and verify that discharge has occurred.
3. Start documenting in patients' medical records.

12:00–13:00

Lunch break.

13:00–15:00

1. Perform/reinforce appropriate patient/family teaching (e.g., preoperative and postoperative teaching, discharge teaching).
2. Meet with patients and families to discuss the plan of care, answer questions, and provide emotional support.
3. Complete necessary paperwork for patients' discharge. Continue documenting in patients' medical records.
4. Attend to any consultations called for by primary nurses or other case managers.

15:00–16:00

1. Review scheduled discharges for next day and ensure patients are ready.
2. Follow up on tests that are not completed. Ensure tests/procedures that were discussed in morning rounds are scheduled appropriately.
3. Continue documenting in patients' medical records.

In addition, case managers conduct patient care rounds informally with the attending physicians when they visit their patients, and they discuss the plans of care. They attend to emergency situations as they arise. They also collect/track patient care variances and follow up on resolutions of problems identified. Case managers are also expected to collaborate with other disciplines (e.g., utilization review, social work, nutrition, physical therapy) as needed. They may also attend certain meetings (e.g., patient/family teaching committee, CMP development teams) and conduct staff inservice education regarding case management.

the patient's, provider's, and payer's perspectives and interests in healthcare delivery and management.

The case manager's role is successful only when full support and commitment of hospital and nursing administrators are evidenced and their belief in case management becomes part of the culture and values of the institution. The description of the role presented in this chapter is extensive and could seem to be overwhelming in terms of the amount of responsibility that goes with the case manager's role. However, it is important to keep in mind when studying this role description that it is a thorough approach to the functions and responsibilities of case managers. Healthcare administrators are urged to evaluate this description and only adapt to their institution what seems to be appropriate to their needs based on their systems, procedures, policies, standards, operations, financial status, care settings, and, most importantly, the goals of their case management system/model and what they are attempting to achieve through this role.

 KEY POINTS

1. Case managers function as an integral part of the interdisciplinary healthcare team.
2. Case managers usually manage, coordinate, and facilitate patient care. They ensure timely patient and family teaching and discharge planning.
3. Case managers perform their role functions in virtually all healthcare settings across the continuum.
4. Case managers have many different roles and responsibilities, which are defined differently in each institution. Sometimes their responsibilities cross the boundaries of a particular care setting.

5. Social workers, in collaboration with case managers, play an important role in case managing the biopsychosocial needs of patients.
6. Advanced practice nurses are emerging as case managers in a variety of care delivery settings.
7. Today, case managers work in all patient care settings. They are found to be effective in reducing length of stay and healthcare cost and improving quality and patient and family satisfaction.
8. Case managers should be clinically competent and astute in time management, problem solving, negotiation, and teamwork.

REFERENCES

Ballew JR, Mink G: *Case management in social work,* Springfield, Ill, 1996, Charles C Thomas.

Bower KA: *Case management by nurses,* ed 2, Kansas City, Mo, 1992, American Nurses Association.

Case Management Standards Work Group: *NASW standards for social work case management,* 1992. Available online at http://www.social workers.org/practices/standards/casemgmt.htm.

InterQual, Inc: *System administrator's guide,* Marlborough, Mass, 1998, InterQual.

McNeese-Smith D, Anderson G, Misseldine C, et al: Roles of the professional registered nurse in case management and program director. In Flarey DL, Smith-Blancett S, editors: *Handbook of case management,* Gaithersburg, Md, 1996, Aspen.

Newell M: *Using case management to improving health outcomes,* Gaithersburg, Md, 1996, Aspen.

Schibanoff JM, editor: *Health care management guidelines,* New York, 1999, Milliman & Robertson.

Schroer K: Case management: clinical nurse specialist and nurse practitioner, converging roles, *Clin Nurse Spec* 5(4):189-194, 1991.

Strassner LF: The ABCs of case management: a review of the basics, *Nurs Case Manag* 1(1):22-30, 1996.

Tahan HA: The case manager in acute care setting: job description and functions, *J Nurs Adm* 23(10):53-61, 1993.

5

Utilization Management

RELATIONSHIP BETWEEN UTILIZATION MANAGEMENT AND CASE MANAGEMENT

Utilization management is a technique used by **case managers** to ensure that the patient meets preestablished criteria to support the level of care being delivered. Criteria that guide the process of determining the appropriate level of care and setting have been established for acute, subacute, and home care and virtually all levels of service across the continuum. A match between the patient's clinical picture and needed care interventions and the level of service being provided will greatly increase the likelihood that the provider will be reimbursed for the services rendered. When a match cannot be achieved, the case manager is responsible for working with the interdisciplinary team to transition the patient to the appropriate level. This may mean that the patient will either need a higher level or a lower level of service. For example, the patient may be receiving care in the acute care setting, but after intervention and stabilization, the patient may be appropriate for transition to a subacute setting. Conversely, a patient in a nursing home may become acutely ill and require a transfer to an acute care setting to receive acute care services.

Before the introduction of **case management** in acute care settings, utilization management was a discrete function generally performed by registered nurses (RNs). More commonly known as **utilization review** (UR), it was introduced as a function in the 1960s for matching patient needs to necessary care interventions with the goal of reducing waste and overutilization of resources. At the time, UR was limited to acute care settings. The UR nurse was responsible for reviewing the patients' medical records and for communicating with physicians when there were delays in care delivery or when a patient did not meet the criteria for the level of service being provided.

Although the terms *utilization management* and *utilization review* are used somewhat interchangeably, they are not the same. Table 5-1 summarizes the differences between these two terms. Both UR and utilization management describe activities or programs used by healthcare providers, review agencies, and managed care organizations (MCOs) to ensure medical necessity, appropriateness, efficiency, and cost-effectiveness of the healthcare services being provided. The process also includes a review of services to ensure that they are being provided in the most appropriate setting.

Utilization management is the term used to describe programs that focus on planning, organizing, directing, and controlling healthcare resources and services in an effort to ensure the provision of cost-effective, appropriate, and high-quality care. UR, however, describes the process, technique, or method by which a healthcare organization reviews, monitors, and evaluates its use and allocation of resources and services. UR is subsumed under the umbrella of utilization management. It enhances an organization's ability to meet the standards of regulatory and **accreditation** agencies and the policies and procedures of MCOs.

For example, a UR nurse might try to intervene when it is noted in the medical record that the patient had been waiting for an extended period for a computed axial tomography (CAT) scan or other diagnostic tests. In this case, the UR nurse might contact the department responsible for performing the test and facilitate its completion. The UR nurse also might communicate with the discharge planner when there are perceived delays in discharging the patient from the hospital.

There were inherent problems with this type of review process, which became more obvious after the inception of the acute care **prospective payment system** in the mid-1980s. The UR nurse performed chart reviews and seldom actually interviewed, assessed, or

TABLE 5-1 The Differences Between Utilization Review and Utilization Management

Category	Utilization Review	Utilization Management
Medical record review	Yes	Yes
Process	Retrospective	Prospective/concurrent
Use of criteria	Yes	Yes
Patient contact	No	Yes
Monitoring of resources	Allocation	Necessity/appropriateness
Authorization of services	No	Yes
Scope of responsibility/service	Limited	Wide
Providers contact	Indirect	Direct
Cost	Containment	Effectiveness
Setting	Acute care	Across the continuum of care
Focus on transitional planning or level of care	Minimal	Maximal
Interaction with MCOs	No	Yes
Contribution to the plan of care	No	Yes
Case conferencing with providers	No	Yes
Case conferencing with patient/family	No	Yes
Reimbursement appeals function	Minor	Major

MCOs, Managed care organizations.

met with a patient. In some organizations, the UR nurse was not allowed to speak directly to a patient. It was believed that such interactions would prohibit the UR nurse from being completely objective in her analysis of whether the patient was meeting the criteria for the level of service being provided. The lack of direct patient contact limited the UR nurse's review and analysis to only what was documented in the medical record. If certain assessments, interventions, or outcomes were not documented, the UR nurse would have no way of knowing that they existed or had occurred.

After the inception of prospective payment, the need for better management of these UR processes became increasingly evident. Reimbursement was limited to the **diagnosis-related group (DRG)** payment, and excessive use of resources would mean that the total case rate **reimbursement** would be chipped away at by the excessive or redundant use of resources. In addition, it was clear that the UR nurse was, by design, disconnected from the patient, the healthcare team, and the other care processes. This was particularly problematic as it related to the discharge planning process. In some instances the UR and discharge planning functions overlapped and the practitioners found themselves "bumping into" each other. In other instances, lack of communication might mean that issues "fell through the cracks" and were either addressed late or not at all. This led to system inefficiencies, higher cost, and poorer quality of care.

As the 1980s waned, higher and higher managed care penetration in various parts of the country heightened the need for more efficient utilization management. Most MCOs required "reviews," meaning that communication of clinical and service delivery interventions be given to the company on a regular basis while the patient was in the hospital or under the care of a healthcare provider in another setting. It became evident that the clinician providing this information needed to have a working knowledge of the factors related to that patient's hospital stay. If the UR nurse had to rely on others to continuously obtain that information, the process was delayed and was clearly less efficient. If he or she referred the MCO to another clinician, this made it more challenging for the MCO to navigate the hospital system and added to the inefficiencies.

In the early 1990s these "passing of the baton" models of care no longer met the needs of a changing healthcare delivery system. These models required some drastic modifications to be more relevant to the changing marketplace. Many acute care hospitals realized that economies of scale would need to be designed to respond to the changing needs of the environment and to make their organizations more productive and efficient.

The Move Toward Case Management

In an effort to improve efficiency and optimize dwindling resources, many acute care settings began to integrate some functions that previously had been disconnected in hospital settings. Many of the early case management models in acute care settings were designed to integrate the functions of clinical coordination/facilitation, **discharge planning,** and utilization management. The new care providers to take on these integrated functions were titled case managers (Case Manager's Tip 5-1).

Some argued that integrating the utilization management function with the other case management functions would switch the focus of the role to a solely financial one. However, forward-thinking organizations recognized the benefits to such an approach.

 CASE MANAGER'S TIP 5-1

Utilization management is one of the typical role functions of a hospital-based case manager.

CASE MANAGER'S TIP 5-2

Added Responsibilities to the Case Manager's Role as a Result of Utilization Management

- Review the medical record for appropriateness of documentation that reflects intensity of service and severity of illness (i.e., necessity for care provision in the specific care setting).
- Obtain authorizations/certifications for services before providing care regardless of setting (e.g., operative procedures, home care).
- Conduct ongoing medical record reviews and communicate results to appropriate members of the healthcare team, staff of MCOs, or other third-party payers.
- Ensure timely discharge from acute care settings, efficient transfer/transition to a different level of care, or termination of treatments/services.
- Ensure the provision of cost-effective services as reflective of the patient's healthcare benefits package or health plan.
- Appeal reimbursement denials or denied services based on necessity and appropriateness and within specific timeframes.
- Collect quality assurance data related to resource utilization and reimbursement for services rendered.
- Collaborate with medical director or physician advisor as needed (e.g., when reviewing or addressing challenging situations/cases).
- Report on outcomes of reviews and identify opportunities for improvement.

By integrating these previously disconnected functions, the case manager would manage all functions indirectly related to patient care. This concept of "one stop shopping" enabled the case manager to coordinate all aspects of care from clinical coordination and facilitation to resource management, to ensuring reimbursement, to transitioning the patient to the next care setting when appropriate. By having this "big picture" focus, the new acute care case manager could successfully assist the hospital in becoming more streamlined, efficient, and consumer-focused. Adding the utilization management function to the case manager's role resulted in added responsibilities. These additional responsibilities are outlined in Case Manager's Tip 5-2.

THE REVIEW AND CERTIFICATION PROCESS

The majority of today's **third-party payers** require that the hospital provide information from which a decision to approve reimbursement for the stay, or a portion of the stay, is made. This review includes three processes: **precertification, continued stay,** and discharge planning.

Precertification (Also Known as Prior Authorization)

Patients whose care is being reimbursed by an MCO are required, as per their contract, to obtain precertification before rendering any nonemergent care. Therefore a patient being admitted for elective surgery (or in the case of a planned medical admission) will require that the MCO be notified and a "precert" number be obtained. For elective surgical patients, this process is generally completed by the physician's office staff. The hospital may need to verify the precertification number with the third-party payer. In some situations the third-party may request additional clinical information. The actual process of precertifying a patient is strictly a clerical function and does not require an RN or other clinician to perform it. When MCOs request additional clinical information, a clinical person should be identified to provide this information. This may be a case manager, the physician, or his or her designee. It is clearly a waste of resources to have an RN case manager obtain all precerts. Generally this function should remain with either the admitting department or the finance department. Under any circumstance, it is important to remember that failure to obtain precertification before the service is rendered can result in partial or full denial/lack of payment (Case Manager's Tip 5-3).

First-Level Reviews

First-level reviews are conducted while the patient is in the hospital. Care is reviewed for its appropriateness and may include the following:

- **Medical necessity on admission:** to determine that the hospital admission is appropriate, clinically necessary, justified, and reimbursable.
- **Continued stay:** to determine that each day of the hospital stay is necessary and that care is being

 CASE MANAGER'S TIP 5-3

The Sharing of Utilization Management Functions
Not all utilization management functions need to be performed by a registered nurse. Functions such as precertification can be delegated to clerical support staff. Controversial situations that may result in reimbursement denials must be handled by clinicians such as case managers.

rendered at the appropriate level. Examples include acute care, critical care, and subacute care.

- **Overutilization and underutilization of resources:** Using a clinical practice guideline, clinical pathway, or other established criteria as a guide, determination is made as to whether the patient is receiving all appropriate services, or that those services are redundant or overused.
- **Appropriateness of setting:** to determine if the care needed is being delivered in the most appropriate and cost-effective setting possible.
- **Delay in service:** to identify delays in the delivery of needed services and to facilitate and expedite such services when necessary.
- **Levels of service:** to identify and verify, based on the patient's condition and the needed level of service, that the patient is receiving care at the appropriate level.
- **Quality monitoring:** to ensure that care is being delivered at or above acceptable quality standards and as identified by the organization or national guidelines.

The Process

The insurance company requesting or receiving information regarding the patient's condition and the delivery of services will do so either by telephone, by fax, or electronically, depending on the specific system in the hospital. The turnaround time for responding to a request for a review will depend on the organization's contracts with the MCO. Generally the information will need to be provided by the end of the business day and usually by a specific predetermined time of day. The case manager must provide the MCO representative (e.g., case manager) with the clinical evidence that supports the level of service being provided. The case manager must provide supportive evidence that the patient's plan of care is reflective of the clinical condition and that the interventions/treatments support the level of service. Preestablished and nationally acceptable criteria are usually used for this purpose. Examples are InterQual and Milliman & Robertson.

CRITERIA USED FOR UTILIZATION REVIEW

One of the more commonly used sets of criteria, particularly for the Medicare and Medicaid populations, are the InterQual criteria (InterQual, 1998). The InterQual criteria were developed in 1978 by a physician and an RN to assist in identifying and supporting the level of care and services provided to patients to ensure reimbursement. Consistent with the healthcare environment of the time, the criteria were strictly hospital-based.

 CASE MANAGER'S TIP 5-4

Criteria for Utilization Review

As a case manager performing utilization review functions, you have a right to know what criteria the third-party payer uses for certification purposes. These criteria should be made accessible and you must apply them to the reviews you conduct.

 CASE MANAGER'S TIP 5-5

Logic for Combining Coordination/Facilitation with Utilization Management Functions

Through the process of clinical coordination and facilitation, case managers can familiarize themselves with the intensity of service and severity of illness criteria. By combining the functions of coordination/facilitation and utilization management, the processes become more streamlined and efficient.

The criteria help to support the **intensity of service** (IS) and **severity of illness** (SI) of the patient; they also identify discharge criteria. They have been updated over the years and now address the **continuum of care** and include observation, critical care, telemetry, acute care, subacute care, rehabilitation, and home care. The criteria are used as a tool to facilitate appropriate admissions, transfers, and discharges. The case manager should know which criteria the third-party payer is using (Case Manager's Tip 5-4) and should apply the criteria by asking the following questions:

- Is the patient a candidate for the requested level of care?
- How sick is the patient? (SI)
- What treatments/services is the patient receiving? (SI)
- What resources does the patient require? (IS)
- Is the patient stable and ready for discharge?

As discussed in Case Manager's Tip 5-5, the functions of coordination/facilitation and utilization management are interrelated. Combining them is efficient and effective.

CRITERIA USED FOR UTILIZATION REVIEW—INTERQUAL
Severity of Illness

Determining the patient's SI is completed through the use of objective indicators reflective of the patient's illness. The SI criteria include clinical, imaging, electrocardiogram (ECG), and laboratory findings. Time definitions are also included as part of the criteria for each category of findings. For example, acute onset would be within the past 24 hours, recent onset would be within the past week, and newly discovered would be at the present episode of illness.

Clinical findings are composed of chief complaints, vital signs, and working diagnoses as identified by the physical examination and patient interview.

Findings related to imaging include the results of diagnostic radiology procedures such as x-ray, ultrasound, magnetic resonance imaging (MRI) or positron emission tomography (PET) scanning, echocardiography, and nuclear medicine studies.

Laboratory findings include blood gases, pulse oximetry, and arterial blood gas measurements; hematology, which are tests related to blood and blood-forming organs; chemistry, which includes chemical analysis of blood, tissue, secretions, and excretions; microbiology, which includes analysis of blood, tissue, secretions, and excretions for identification of microorganisms; and cerebrospinal fluid analysis.

The criteria include clinical parameters for each of the findings. The parameters are based on abnormal states/values indicating the need for care. For example:
Blood Gases
Arterial $PO_2 \leq 59$ mmHg (7.9 kPa)
Arterial $Pco_2 \geq 51$ mmHg (6.8 kPa)
Arterial pH ≥ 7.50

Intensity of Service

IS criteria are diagnostic and therapeutic services generally provided at a specific level of care (i.e., intensive care, telemetry, and so on). The IS component contains one element, treatments/medications, which includes those modalities of medical and other professional care provided at a designated level. Within the treatment/medications category, there are two types of IS criteria:
1. Nonasterisked (IS)
2. Asterisked (*IS)

Nonasterisked criteria (IS) signify those treatments/medications that generally cannot be provided at a less intensive level of care. For example, intravenous (IV) nitroglycerin can only be provided at the critical level of care.

Asterisked criteria (*IS) reflect treatments/medications that could be safely rendered at a less intensive (and usually less costly) level of care. These criteria are important case management flags and allow the case manager to consider the need for an **alternate level of care** for the patient, such as rehabilitation, subacute, or home care. The general time requirement for IS assessment is "at least daily"; for example, once in 24 hours. Some IS criteria specify a frequency such as

"IV antiinfectives $\geq 3\times/24h$." This refers to the services being rendered greater than or equal to 3 times over a 24-hour period and overrides the "at least daily" requirement.

The acute-body system criteria subsets include an IS criterion for postsurgery/procedure care. This criterion has a time limit assigned depending on the body system. For example, in the cardiovascular section, the time limit for postsurgery/procedure care is $\leq 24h$, whereas the time limit in musculoskeletal/spine is ≤ 3 days. Day 1 begins the day the surgery/procedure is performed.

Discharge Screens

The InterQual criteria also include discharge screens (DS) that identify the parameters of patient stability indicating discharge readiness from a specified level of care. The DS component contains one element only, discharge indicators. These indicators are the parameters of a patient's clinical stability and relative safety the case manager uses to assess the patients' readiness for discharge or transfer to another level of care.

For example, the discharge indicators for the acute-cardiovascular criteria subset include the following:
- Vital signs stable last 8 hours
- Syncope: cardiac etiology ruled out
- Pericardial effusion resolving

The case manager must refer to the "rules" as outlined in the InterQual criteria for each level of service. For example, the rule for SI critical-noncardiac stipulates that this level of care would be appropriate if the patient required intensive care after surgery and/or a procedure (e.g., after a craniotomy, or if one SI criterion contained in that subset was met).

The IS rule indicates which criteria must be met for each clinical system. The rules differ for critical, acute-body system, and acute-other. Case managers must become familiar with the rules for the clinical areas most covered by them.

The rule driving the application of the DS address two critical elements in the evaluation of discharge readiness from a level of care: clinical stability and necessity for continuing care. The first element to consider is clinical stability. This refers directly to the causative factors (SI) for this episode of illness. However, individuals with comorbidities or chronic illnesses may never reach optimal stability. Therefore the degree of clinical stability required is that which allows safe transfer to the next level of care.

Applying the Criteria

Selection of the patient's level of care and the criteria subset is based on the patient's clinical findings and actual treatments/medications. For example, available clinical information indicates that the patient is scheduled for cardiac surgery and requires cardiac monitoring postoperatively. The case manager would select and apply the critical-cardiac subset.

SI, IS/*IS, and DS must all be selected from the same criteria subset. For example, a case manager must not apply criteria related to the musculoskeletal system when working with a cardiology patient. A new criteria subset may be selected during the hospital stay to reflect clinical findings associated with either a change in the SI or a new episode of illness.

An admission review is conducted when there is a change in the SI and a subsequent transfer to a critical care (cardiac, noncardiac, or telemetry) level from any other level is necessary, or when a patient moves to or from a specialized acute care (other) level.

Types of Reviews

The types of reviews are as follows:
- Preadmission review
- Admission (initial) review
- Subsequent (continued services) review
- Discharge review

Preadmission review takes place for any elective inpatient (scheduled) surgery/invasive procedure. The procedure must be scheduled to be performed on the same day as the planned admission and must appear on the designated inpatient hospital list. InterQual's *Guidelines for Surgery and Procedures in the Inpatient Setting* can be found in the *Intensity of service/Severity of illness/Discharge* (ISD) Master Appendix.

The admission review is a review done within 4 hours of the decision to admit the patient to the critical care or acute level. An SI criterion and all corresponding elements of the IS criteria subset must be met on admission to the critical or acute care level.

Subsequent reviews are performed daily to ensure that the patient requires continued care in the particular setting. An IS criterion also must be met daily. If one IS criterion cannot be met, then three *IS criteria are required to justify the level of care. If only *IS criteria is met, the case manager should review the discharge criteria and explore other level of care options. If at least three *IS criteria are met and the DS are not met, the case manager should approve the level of care.

Once the case manager knows the reason for admission, it is logical to expect to find documented SI criteria in the medical record. If the patient is sick enough to require services, then the physician's orders for treatment should validate the need for providing care at the level to which the patient is admitted.

Example

A 55-year-old male with a history of angina has been treated with nitroglycerin for approximately 3 months. He arrives at the emergency department (ED) via ambulance after a 2-day history of shortness of breath. On physical examination, he has rales one-third up bilaterally, his chest film reveals pulmonary edema, and his ECG shows uncontrolled atrial fibrillation. Based on this information, the case manager should set an expectation of care and search the record for such therapies as IV inotropics, continuous cardiac monitoring, continuous oxygen therapy, serial ECGs, pulse oximetry, and intravenous/sublingual (IV/SL) nitroglycerin.

As seen in this example, the clinical indicators for hospitalization (SI) are demonstrated by the patient's signs, symptoms, and clinical findings. The expected treatment plan (IS) is found in the patient's medical record. The information gathered during the admission review is used by the case manager to validate that the criteria of the level of care are met. This is accomplished by approaching the medical record both systematically and expectantly: The record of emergency services documents the patient's vital signs, clinical findings, chief complaint, and laboratory and x-ray findings; the physician's admitting note provides the reason for admission, the pertinent history, the physical findings, and the plan of treatment.

THE CONTINUUM OF CARE

The case manager must always be cognizant of the continuum of care and be sure to apply the appropriate criteria to the patient's current setting or review the criteria to determine the appropriateness of transitioning the patient to another setting (Case Manager's Tip 5-6).

Subacute Care

To qualify for subacute level of service, there must be an expectation for continued recovery. The patient must be

 CASE MANAGER'S TIP 5-6

Criteria Must be Applied to the Appropriate Setting

Criteria are available for all levels of service along the continuum of care and must be applied by the case manager appropriately. Criteria designed for a particular care setting (e.g., acute care) must be applied to that setting only. However, case managers need to be familiar with and knowledgeable about the criteria for all levels of service so that they can effectively and efficiently transfer patients to other levels of care as their medical conditions warrant transfer.

cleared medically for less than acute care. Finally, there must be a need for more IS than a skilled nursing facility or home care would provide. Examples would include concomitant conditions, post-major acute conditions, and medical **complications.** Patients who are end stage and who need complex care, comfort, and dignity would also qualify for this level of service.

Rehabilitation Care

Rehabilitation care is defined as coordinated, goal-oriented, multidisciplinary programs for individuals who have had an illness/injury or exacerbation of known disease with resulting functional deficits and whose expectation for improvement is reasonable. Rehabilitation programs are designed to meet the patient's physical, social, psychological, and environmental needs. They require that the patient actively participate in rehabilitation activities/exercises and that there is an expectation of functional improvement. Patients are often medically frail and on-site physician presence is expected. This is in contrast to subacute care, in which treatments are provided for the patient but there is not necessarily an expectation that a level of patient's participation be present. Physician presence may be more sporadic as well.

Home Care

Home care is considered a comprehensive approach to healthcare services for individuals who have experienced an episode of acute illness, injury, or exacerbation of a disease process and where the potential for complications and/or deterioration exists. Both professional and paraprofessional services are provided in this level of care.

The case manager should always consider that home care is a cost-effective alternative to inpatient care when the patient's clinical needs can be appropriately met in the home setting.

APPLYING ISD CRITERIA

Case managers should follow these steps when applying the criteria:

1. Apply body system first, then generic criteria.
2. Generic criteria are considered part of each category.
3. SI criteria from one category must be matched by IS criteria in the same category.
4. DS must be from the same category as the SI and IS.
5. Review at a maximum of 3-day intervals.

Admission Review

1. Either one SI or the specified number of IS must be met on admission.
2. Both an SI and the specified number of IS criteria from the same category must be met within 24 hours.

Exceptions

1. An aggregate of marginal findings may meet the SI requirement.
2. Elective admissions generally do not meet SI criteria.
3. ED admissions must meet both SI and the specified number of IS criteria at the time of admission.

Special Unit Admission

1. The specific criteria for each unit must be met.
2. The patient must meet both SI and IS criteria at the time of admission to the unit.

   Exception: Patient scheduled for special unit admission postoperatively after an elective major surgical procedure generally does not meet SI criteria but *must* meet IS criteria.

Continued Stay Review

1. IS criteria must be met every day.
2. If the IS met under treatments/medications is IS criteria, SI criteria must also be met.

Discharge Review

1. In case the IS criteria are no longer met and the clinical/functional DS are met, the patient should be scheduled for discharge. The only exception to this would be patients with severe, chronic abnormalities who may never meet clinical/functional DS because they do not have the potential to return to physiological normalcy.
2. When IS criteria are met and SI criteria are not met but clinical/functional DS are met, an alternate level of care should be explored.

As case managers complete the reviews, they identify deficient areas and opportunities for improvement. They also address/correct the issues as they arise. Examples are documentation reflective of SI and IS, necessity for continued care provision in the same level of care, appropriateness of transfer to another level of care, avoidable days or services in case of patients not meeting predetermined criteria, complete plan of care and transitional plan. Success of the case manager in this role relies on certain conditions such as those presented in Box 5-1.

MILLIMAN & ROBERTSON

In addition to the InterQual criteria, another set of commonly used criteria are the Milliman & Robertson Health Care Management Guidelines (Schibanoff, 1999). These guidelines, commonly known as the *M & R Guidelines,* are most typically used by managed care companies for UR purposes. The guidelines have been designed based on a commercial population and to the exclusion of the Medicare and Medicaid populations.

BOX 5-1   Success Factors in the Case Manager's Utilization Review/Management Role

- Use of established criteria such as Milliman & Robertson and InterQual
- Clearly defined job description and responsibilities
- Clearly defined and well-communicated process for utilization review and utilization management
- Availability of a medical director or physician advisor for consultation and help when needed
- Clear identification of scope of responsibilities, role boundaries, and collaboration with other departments (e.g., admitting office, finance, patient accounts, medical records, managed care contracts, information technology, and management)
- Appropriate caseload and staffing patterns
- Automation and electronic communication and exchange of information including financial and quality performance/productivity reports
- Formal denials and appeals process in place with clear delineation of responsibilities of personnel

---

Therefore it is important for the case manager to remember that the M & R Guidelines may not strictly apply to these populations. They are intended to be applied as the most efficient practices for "ideal" patients supported by an "ideal" infrastructure. Unfortunately, many insurance companies do not adhere to this application but instead follow the guidelines to the letter of the law, even when a guideline clearly is not a good match with either the patient or the healthcare delivery system.

The M & R Guidelines are also called *Optimal Recovery Guidelines (ORG)* and follow a specific format and apply to specific diseases and surgical procedures. The elements of each ORG are as follows:

- ORG description, International Classification of Diseases, Ninth Revision, Clinical Modification **(ICD-9-CM),** and/or **Current Procedural Terminology (CPT)** code
- Case management actions
- Adequate reasons for admission
- Inadequate reasons for admission
- Alternatives to admission
- Day 1 (expected patient progress in best practice)
- Day 2
- Day 3
- Goal length of stay in days

The M & R Guidelines can be matched to the patient's specific diagnosis, while the InterQual criteria are applied using body system criteria.

There are certain assumptions made concerning the application of the guidelines. The case manager must have an understanding of these assumptions to work

with the insurance company and to optimize reimbursement for the provider. The first assumption is that the patient has an uncomplicated course of treatment. The patient does as well clinically as the physician hoped he or she would. The second assumption is that all necessary continuum of care infrastructures are in place and available. The third and final assumption pertains to an expectation that there exists the cooperation of the patient, the family, and any other caregivers.

M & R research indicates that 80% of commercial **health maintenance organization (HMO)** members and 50% of Medicare HMO members fit the definition of uncomplicated patients (Schibanoff, 1999).

The structural requirements needed to fulfill the M & R requirements are as follows:

- A rapid treatment site (and/or observation)
- Ambulatory surgery access
- Ancillary services 24 hrs a day/7 days a week
- Discharges 7 days a week
- Home infusion and healthcare
- Skilled nursing facility and rehabilitation availability

Because the M & R Guidelines are based on clinical diagnoses and/or surgical procedures, it may become more difficult to apply a single guideline that will single-handedly manage the length of stay and clinical outcomes. Case managers must use their best clinical judgment when selecting and applying a guideline and must work with the third-party payer to ensure that the patient's other clinical needs are addressed as well. In general, the guideline most closely matching the primary reason for hospitalization should be used as the best guide for that hospital stay.

In addition to adequate reasons, inadequate reasons for hospitalization are also outlined in the guidelines. This data can be a powerful tool used by the ED and admitting department's case managers to assist in the identification of other treatment modalities when hospitalization may not be the most appropriate option. Like InterQual, M & R provides the case manager with care interventions for other care delivery sites across the continuum, such as home care, skilled care, and subacute care. As in the case of acute care, the guidelines provide clinical interventions and outcomes appropriate to those settings.

Proper Use of the M & R Guidelines

The guidelines are based on clinical outcomes that are expected to be achieved during a predetermined timeframe; for example, daily in acute care settings. The acute care case manager should be well skilled in the use of these designated timeframes. For example, day 3 of the Community Acquired Pneumonia Guideline calls for the patient to have a declining temperature, to be breathing comfortably at rest, to have microbiology culture reports completed, and to be discharged. Although it may indeed be day 3 of the hospital stay, the patient may not have achieved all of these outcomes and therefore discharge would be clinically inappropriate. Perhaps the patient's temperature has not declined significantly. The acute care case manager should discuss this clinical outcome with the case manager at the MCO/health plan the patient is enrolled in. Negotiations should be made for an additional day of hospital reimbursement because the patient was not clinically ready to move to the next phase of care. In this case, the acute care case manager should indicate to the insurance-based case manager that day 3 will be repeated until the patient has met the expected clinical outcomes and is then ready for discharge. This extension of the hospital stay is appropriate and should be approved for reimbursement. The acute care case manager should think of the expected outcomes in terms of "phases" of care rather than as true days, as some patients may not achieve these outcomes in perfect 24-hour intervals. If the managed care case manager (i.e., the acute care case manager) you are providing the review to does not understand this, then you should ask to speak to that individual's supervisor or to the medical director (Case Manager's Tip 5-7).

The acute care case manager should also use this logic when reviewing the criteria for discharge. Once again, if the patient cannot meet the clinical outcomes necessary for a safe and appropriate discharge as per the guidelines, the discharge should be held until they are met.

As an acute care case manager, be sure that you have access to copies of any criteria you are being asked to use by any third-party payer. You cannot adequately do your job without having access to the same criteria being looked at by the third party. The third-party payer should tell you which criteria they are using so that you are able to make the review as efficient and complete as possible. You have a right to know which standards you are being held to and you should expect to be told which criteria are in use and to have copies of these criteria.

 CASE MANAGER'S TIP 5-7

Strategies for Using the M & R Guidelines

When following the M & R Guidelines, the case manager may need to request a continued stay authorization when the outcomes for that day have not been met. Each set of outcomes can be considered in terms of phases rather than days.

DENIALS AND APPEALS

During the concurrent review process, the third-party payer's case manager will either approve or deny payment for the hospital stay or a portion of the hospital stay. You will most likely be informed of this information during the review, or by an "end of day" report. You may also be informed at a later point in time by a letter. Once a **denial** of payment has occurred, an **appeal** should take place. As per the hospital's contracts, as well as the insurance and public health laws (Table 5-2), there will be time limits to this process. You will generally have between 30 and 60 days to appeal a denial of payment. The insurance company must respond to your appeal within similar parameters. An appeal may result in the entire denial being upheld, a portion of the stay being denied, or a complete reversal of the denial. As an acute care case manager, you may or may not be directly involved in the written formulation of an appeal. This function may be performed by the admitting physician or by designated nurses in the case management department who take responsibility for writing letters of appeal.

Writing Letters of Appeal

Whenever possible, the individual writing the appeal should be the attending physician of record (Case Manager's Tip 5-8). If this is not possible or realistic in your organization, the case should, at a minimum, be reviewed with the physician of record before the appeal letter is written and submitted. The physician of record is in the best position to argue for why he or she cared for the patient in the manner that he or she did and why the hospital should be reimbursed for the services provided. Regardless of who is writing the appeal, the appeal should use the criteria of the third-party payer as the basis for its argument. Information as to which criteria are used is usually found in the managed care contractual agreement. If the third-party payer follows M & R, the person writing the appeal should refer to the appropriate M & R guideline for the case and match the criteria and outcomes in the guideline against the patient's care interventions and achieved outcomes. This puts the hospital in the best position to reverse the denial and increases the chances of reversal.

Reasons for Denial

Each organization may categorize its denials in various ways (Box 5-2). Broadly speaking, though, the categories will fall into either clinical or nonclinical groupings. Clinical denials are related to the patient's condition and decided on based on appropriateness and necessity of the clinical care delivered. An example is denying reimbursement for a diagnostic or therapeutic

TABLE 5-2   Utilization Review and Payment Provisions, Timeframes, and Accompanying Sections of Law

Law	Major Provisions	Section(s) of Law
Prompt Payment	Insurers must make payment to healthcare providers within 45 days of receipt of claims for services rendered.	§ 3224-a (a) Insurance Law
	Insurers must abide by the 45-day rule except in instances when their obligation to pay it is not reasonably clear.	§ 3224-a (a) Insurance Law
	In instances when the obligation of the insurer is not reasonably clear due to a good faith dispute, the insurer shall pay any undisputed portion of the claim and notify the healthcare provider within 30 days of receipt of the claim that:	§ 3224-a (a) Insurance Law
	It is not obligated to make payment, stating the specific reasons why it is not liable, *or*	§ 3224-a (b) (1) Insurance Law
	To request all additional information needed to determine liability to pay the claim	§ 3224-a (b) (2) Insurance Law
	Each claim in violation of this section of Law constitutes a separate violation, and insurers are obligated to pay the full settlement of the claim, plus interest.	§ 3224-a (c) Insurance Law
Utilization Review Determinations	UR agents must make a UR determination involving healthcare services that require preauthorization and provide notice of a determination to the healthcare provider by telephone and in writing within 3 business days of receipt of the necessary information.	§ 4903 (b) Insurance Law and § 4903 (2) Public Health Law
	UR agents must make a determination involving continued or extended healthcare services or additional services in connection with a course of continued treatment and provide notice of such determination by telephone and in writing within 1 business day of receipt of the necessary information.	§ 4903 (c) Insurance Law and §4903 (3) Public Health Law
	A UR agent must make a UR determination involving healthcare services that have been delivered within 30 days of receipt of the necessary information.	§ 4903 (d) Insurance Law and § 4903 (4) Public Health Law
Internal Appeals of Adverse Determinations	Expedited appeals must be determined within 2 business days of receipt of necessary information to conduct such an appeal.	§ 4904 Insurance Law (b) and § 4904 (2) (b) Public Health Law
	A UR agent must establish a period of no less than 45 days after receipt of notification by the insured of the initial UR determination and receipt of all information to file the appeal from said determination. The UR agent must provide written acknowledgement of the filing of the appeal to the appealing party within 15 days of such filing and make a determination with regard to the appeal within 60 days of the receipt of necessary information to conduct the appeal.	§ 4904 (c) Insurance Law and § 4904 (3) Public Health Law
	Failure by the UR agent to make a determination within the applicable time periods shall be deemed to be a reversal of the UR agent's adverse determination.	§ 4904 (e) Insurance Law and § 4904 (5) Public Health Law
External Appeals	Healthcare providers acting in connection with retrospective adverse determinations have the right to request an external appeal when services were denied on the basis of medical necessity or services were denied on the basis that they were experimental in nature.	§ 4910 (b) Insurance Law and § 4910 (2) Public Health Law
	Providers have 45 days to initiate an appeal after a final adverse determination is issued.	§ 4914 (b) (1) Insurance Law and § 4914 (2) (a) Public Health Law

UR, Utilization review.

Continued

TABLE 5-2 Utilization Review and Payment Provisions, Timeframes, and Accompanying Sections of Law—cont'd

Law	Major Provisions	Section(s) of Law
External Appeals—cont'd	The external appeal agent must make a determination on a standard appeal within 30 days of receipt of the insured's request. The external appeals agent has the opportunity to request additional information within the 30-day period, in which case the agent has up to 5 days to if necessary to make such determination.	§ 4914 (b) (2) Insurance Law and § 4914 (2) (b) Public Health Law
	The external appeal agent must make a determination on an expedited appeal within 3 days of the request.	§ 4914 (b) (3) Insurance Law and § 4914 (2) (c) Public Health Law

 CASE MANAGER'S TIP 5-8

The Physician of Record

Whenever possible, the attending physician of record should participate in writing the letter of appeal because the physician is in the best position to make a case for why reimbursement for the care provided is appropriate.

procedure such as endoscopy that is not justified or pre-certified as an inpatient procedure. The nonclinical reasons for denials refer to those that have nothing to do with the patient's clinical situation or need for care. They usually indicate factors in the organization's contracts that were not met such as delays in submitting claims.

Appealing Nonclinical Denials

Nonclinical denials tend to be much more difficult to appeal. Because the reason for the denial is generally based on the contract with that insurance company, the basis of an appeal may be rather limited. Your own department must decide whether it will or will not take the time to appeal such denials. One must weigh the odds of winning such an appeal against the cost of generating the appeal in the first place. It is very difficult and rare to win nonclinical appeals.

Appealing Clinical Denials

The case manager, or whoever is writing the appeal, should review the case against the established review criteria in use. Whenever possible, the criteria should frame the argument for the appeal. In writing the appeal, it should refer directly to how the patient did meet the criteria if this is indeed true. These criteria will form the greatest likelihood of a reversal of the denial. If the criteria are truly not met, the appeal may be much more difficult to win. Other arguments may need to be introduced, such as the unavailability of subacute care beds or home care services. These sorts of arguments do not generally win an appeal. The case manager in the acute care setting needs to know the "philosophy"

BOX 5-2   Denial Reasons

Nonclinical (Administrative) Reasons for Denial

1. *Technical*—Medical record not produced by requested deadline.
2. *Appropriateness of setting*—Procedures that should be performed in outpatient setting (e.g., ambulatory surgery, ED). These cases can be billed to these settings.
3. *Delay in service/treatment*—Primarily on weekend days when patients are waiting for tests.
4. *Initial noncovered services*—Services usually not covered by payer (e.g., cosmetic surgery, dental care for Medicare FFS patients).
5. *Precertification*—No prior authorization from third-party payer. Emergency admissions require notification to payer within 24 hours.
6. *DRG*—Payment for a different DRG than originally billed.
7. *Untimely billing*—Bill submitted greater than 60 days after discharge.
8. *HINN issued incorrectly*—HINN letter given to Medicare patients when services are no longer covered by Medicare (e.g., custodial care or awaiting home care). PRO decides if patient is still covered by Medicare.
9. *Preop/preprocedure days*—All elective cases should be admitted on the day of surgery/procedure.
10. *Pass day*—When a patient is discharged and later readmitted for treatment of the same medical condition within 60 days, hospitals are to bill the two admissions as one (e.g., the patient was either admitted with or develops an infection that must be resolved before surgery).
11. *Payment inconsistent with service*—Payment is determined contractually (i.e., case rate, human immunodeficiency virus [HIV] or psychiatric per diem rate, when such contractual billing agreements are not followed).

Clinical Reasons for Denial

1. *Continued stay*—Patient should have been discharged—no longer meeting acute care criteria.
2. *Medical necessity on admission*—Admissions and treatments that do not meet inpatient care criteria.

BOX 5-2 Denial Reasons—cont'd

3. *Necessity of procedure*—No documentation to support need for surgical procedure.
4. *Premature discharge*—Patient readmitted within 31 days—PRO denies second admission—if they decide patient discharged prematurely on first admission.
5. *Alternate level of care*—Patient no longer meets acute care criteria but could not be discharged without continued services (e.g., nursing home, home care).
6. *Level of care reduction*—Payer decreases payment to subacute rate for inability to meet acute care criteria.

 CASE MANAGER'S TIP 5-9

Templates Make Writing Appeals More Efficient

By creating a template for letters of appeal, the process can be greatly streamlined. Whenever possible, the criteria (M & R or InterQual) should be referred to in the letter.

of the organization to know whether there is an expectation that such appeals will be written. Once again, the likelihood of winning such an appeal must be weighed against the cost of the labor spent on writing it when those resources might be better spent on writing an appeal with a greater likelihood of being won.

See Box 5-3 for a template of a sample appeal letter that includes all of the information necessary to include when writing an appeal. As mentioned in Case Manager's Tip 5-9, using a template can streamline and expedite the appeal writing process.

PEER REVIEW ORGANIZATIONS

Your hospital will most likely have contracts with one or more **peer review organizations (PROs).** These PROs are contracted with to perform a number of functions; among these may be the review of selected medical records for the purpose of UR. This function is most commonly performed for **Medicare** and **Medicaid.** As with any denial and appeal process, the case manager needs to know which criteria the PRO is using and to frame the appeal against those criteria. Once your PRO has requested some medical records for review, it will also review the record for quality issues and anything else it deems necessary. Because the hospital's exposure is greatly increased during an appeal process, some consideration should be taken as to whether the organization wants to conduct the appeal. If other issues are obvious in the record, it may be more prudent for the

hospital to skip that particular appeal rather than open the organization up to an audit.

Hospital Issued Notice of Noncoverage for Medicare—Fee for Service

Hospital-issued notices of noncoverage (HINNs) are issued when Medicare no longer maintains the financial responsibility for a hospital admission and financial responsibility is being transferred to the patient. Preadmission reviews may reveal that the inpatient setting is not the appropriate setting for the particular level of service that the patient requires, or the hospital may determine that the level of care is custodial. A HINN may also be issued when the patient is at a skilled level of care and the patient or representative has refused the first available bed in a nursing home. The hospital may also issue a HINN when the medical record clearly documents a discharge plan and the patient/representative is not compliant with the hospital's attempts to execute the discharge plan in a timely manner.

Before issuing a HINN, the case manager should be sure that the medical record contains the following:
- Discharge planning process, clearly documented
- Documentation of all conversations with the patient/representative regarding the discharge planning process
- Evidence of repeated noncompliance by patient/representative, clearly documented
- Evidence that at least three skilled facilities are contacted at least twice weekly
- If a behavioral health patient, clear documentation that the patient/representative is competent to understand the regulations concerning his or her Medicare benefits
- Clear documentation of all conversations between the hospital and patient concerning the patient's financial liability when the first available nursing home bed is refused
- Finally, a copy of the HINN, signed by the patient, should be placed in the medical record.

HINNs can be issued before or at the time of admission. The attending physician does not have to agree to the issuance. If the HINN is being issued for continued hospital stay, if the admission was appropriate then the attending physician may or may not agree. If the attending physician disagrees, the hospital can issue the HINN once the case has been reviewed by the PRO and it agrees with the issuance.

An admission HINN should be issued before 3:00 PM on the day of admission. Continued stay HINNs issued and appealed to the PRO by the patient or representative before noon on the first working day after receipt of the HINN entitles the patient protection from financial liability until noon of the day after notification of the PRO's determination.

BOX 5-3 Template for Appeal Letter

Organization Name

Address

Address

Patient Name *[Organization Reference Number]*

Date

Dear: *[Name of Third-Party Payer]*

We are writing to appeal your decision to *[concurrently or retrospectively]* deny payment of medical benefits for *[Patient Name]*. Your decision to deny *[level of care]* *[type of service]* from *[start date]* to *[end date]* for reasons described in your denial letter as *[content from denial letter]* is not supported by *[basic evidence]*.

[Describe the particular services rendered]

Below, we present the application of *[state your hospital]* medical necessity criteria* to the services that your organization has denied. We believe that our criteria are consistent with managed care industry standards and that the evidence to substantiate our claim to cover services is compelling.

Medically necessary means a service or supply that the physician has determined to be:

_____

*an adequate and essential therapeutic response provided for evaluation or treatment consistent with the symptoms. Proper diagnosis and treatment appropriate for the patient's illness, disease, or condition as defined by standard diagnostic nomenclature.

{Following this, state why your service provided fit this criteria.}

_____

OR

†reasonably expected to improve the patient's illness, condition

{Following this, state why your service provided fit this criteria.}

_____

OR

‡safe and effective according to nationally accepted standards as recognized by professionals or publications

{Following this, state why your service provided fit this criteria.}

_____

OR

§the appropriate and cost-effective level of care that can safely be provided for the patient's diagnosed condition

{Following this, state why your service provided fit this criteria.}

We will appreciate your careful consideration of this information and prompt reversal of your earlier determination. Should this not be your conclusion, we will expect you to communicate to us the reasoning behind your decision at a level of detail that substantiates the application of your specific criteria to this specific case.

If you have any questions, please call *[name]* at *[number]*.

Sincerely,

WHAT CASE MANAGERS NEED TO KNOW ABOUT MANAGED CARE CONTRACTS

Organizations contracting as providers for a specific MCO usually negotiate contracts that include elements such as rates and types of reimbursement per case and UR activities and functions (may also be referred to as case management). Once the specific contract has been signed by both the provider and payer, the provider becomes responsible for following all of the agreed on elements in the contract. If not followed precisely, the MCO has the right to deny payment for services rendered, even if those services were medically necessary and appropriate. For example, if a patient is admitted for cardiac surgery but the admission was not precertified as per the contract, it is possible that payment will be denied for part or all of the admission (Case Manager's Tip 5-10).

The functions of utilization or case management are fundamental to any contract. Whenever possible, a case management representative from the provider organization should be present during contract negotiations. When this is not possible, the contract, once written, should be reviewed by the UR or case management department. This process will ensure that the agreed-on elements are realistic and achievable. For example, the contract may call for reviews to be performed 7 days a week. The case management department may not be staffed 7 days a week and therefore would not be able to meet the requirements of the contract, thus resulting in denials of payment for services rendered, especially those provided on days when the department is closed.

A case manager working in a hospital setting needs to know the reimbursement elements of the contract. For example, the case manager should know whether a particular case type is being reimbursed as discounted billed charges, a per diem rate, a case or DRG rate, or a capitated rate. Some contracts may include certain case types that may be reimbursed under any of these methods. Therefore a single contract may include per diem and case rates within it. The risks assumed by the organization change as the reimbursement changes.

A discounted **fee-for-service (FFS)** structure is least risky to the provider. Because reimbursement may be between 20% and 50% below the nondiscounted rates, the case manager will need to ensure that all provided services are reasonable and necessary so that resources are not overutilized.

Per diem rates are daily reimbursement amounts that are agreed to as part of the contract. Once again, the case manager will need to know that a per diem rate is in effect. In a per diem rate methodology, the MCO may deploy continued stay denials when it believes that the patient is no longer meeting acute care criteria and should be downgraded to a lower level of service. This method creates higher financial risk to the provider.

Case rates or DRG rates may apply to particular types of patients as identified in the contract. When a case rate is applied, the provider should not receive continued stay denials or denials for delays in service because the financial burden of a length of stay extension becomes that of the provider.

Finally, the contract may call for capitated rates. In capitated arrangements the entire financial burden falls on the provider. In these circumstances the provider is incentivized to reduce the inappropriate use of resources and to aggressively manage the length of stay.

Other elements of the contract that should be communicated to case management would include clinical review criteria. These criteria should include the frequency and type of reviews, as well as the expected turnaround time. Finally, case management should be aware of all precertification and authorization processes.

WORKING WITH PATIENT ACCOUNTS

The patient accounts or billing department is the department that submits the hospital's bills for reimbursement. The patient accounts department must work closely with case management or the denial/appeals staff if they are separate from the case management staff. Patient accounts receives third-party payments and should be electronically interfaced with the case management department.

The case management department should keep a **database** of all denial and appeal activities. This database should be supported by the actual dollar amounts denied or reimbursed by third-party payers. In this way case management can keep accurate statistics as to days and dollars denied, appealed, won on appeal,

 CASE MANAGER'S TIP 5-10

Case Managers and Managed Care Contracts

A case management representative should be given an opportunity to review the utilization management portion of any managed care contract before it is signed. The review should focus on the appropriateness of the demands made by the MCO and the likelihood that the provider/agency (i.e., hospital) is able to comply with the contract and deliver the agreed-on services within the agreed-on timeframe.

	Dollars*	Percent
Denials	11,767,300	—
Recoveries	3,231,665	27.50
Denials net recoveries	8,535,635	72.50

*Dollars shown are for demonstration purposes only
and do not represent the actual performance of any organization

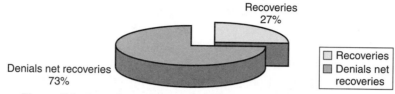

Figure 5-1   Denial summary 2000-2002 (as of December 31, 2002).

or lost on appeal. When it is time for the organization to renegotiate its contracts, the performance of the MCO in terms of its denial rate relative to other payers should be considered. Patterns and types of denials should also be tracked and trended by payer. For example, does one payer routinely deny for precertification at a higher rate than another, and on appeal is it often determined that the precertification number had indeed been obtained? Does another MCO deny for continued stay at a higher rate than the others?

The case manager should stay informed and up-to-date on the organization's contract status and the expectations of both organizations as it relates to case management and utilization management functions. When possible, the case managers should have timely access to this information and be kept informed as specific elements change.

REPORTING UTILIZATION MANAGEMENT DATA

Utilization management data can be reported in a variety of ways, depending on the focus and needs of the organization. Regardless of the data reported, it should be tracked and trended over time and used for quality improvement opportunities when the data shows a downward trend. The case management department should be able to show a relationship between the data and the department's interventions to improve the processes that the data represents. For example, if it is noted that continued stay denials have consistently increased for two quarters of a given year, case management will need to show that a process improvement plan was initiated to identify the reasons for the negative trend and the processes put into place to correct it.

Figure 5-1 demonstrates one way of reporting aggregated denial and appeal data for discreet periods. The figure shows denial and appeal activity including a pie chart of the data for a 3-year period. In this example, the organization received a total of $11,767,300 in denials of payment between 1998 and 2000. Of those initial denials received, the organization recovered $3,231,665 or 27.5% after appealing the denials. Another 72.5%, or $8,535,635 is pending appeal or has been lost following the appeal process. This number represents monies currently outstanding or not available to the organization.

Figure 5-2 reports a subset of the previously mentioned data for 1 specific year. It also reports the cases recovered (43.2%) and the cases lost on final appeal (56.8%).

Another way to reference the data might be by reason for the denial. This data can be reported in days denied or in dollars denied. It can also be reported based on the date the denial is received. Figure 5-3 represents denials received regardless of when the patient was admitted to the hospital.

	Dollars	Percent
Cases closed	3,889,000	—
Recoveries	1,680,000	43.20
Final denials	2,209,000	56.80

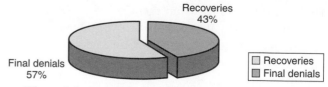

Figure 5-2   Recovery rate for cases closed year 2002.

	1Q02	2Q02	3Q02	4Q02	2002 Total	Total (percent)
Continued stay	466	414	390	459	1,729	31.7
Precertification	245	370	235	272	1,122	20.6
Med necessity	256	230	298	242	1,026	18.8
Care level reduction	98	148	106	174	526	9.6
Other	159	290	345	254	1,048	19.2
TOTAL	1,224	1,452	1,374	1,401	5,451	100.0

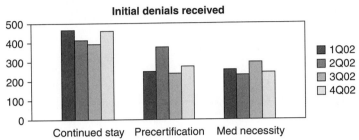

Figure 5-3   Denials based on reason—reported in total days denied.

	2001	2002	Variance
Initial denial days	4,687	3,500	(1,187)
Patient days	163,438	165,536	2,098
Percent of patient days	2.87	2.11	−0.76

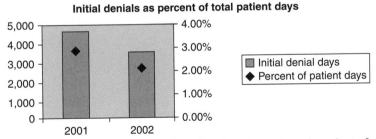

Figure 5-4   Initial denials as percentage of total patient days—based on date of service.

Denial can also be reported based on when the patient was in the hospital. This data indicates the performance of the organization at a particular point in time. In the case of Medicare or Medicaid denials, the denial may be received months or even years after the patient was in the hospital. This data can be reported as a percentage of patient days because it correlates to all of the patients who were in the hospital at that point in time. Figure 5-4 demonstrates how an organization might report this type of data. Organizations will want to keep their denials as a percentage of total patient days as low as possible because this statistic directly relates to the organization's financial performance at that point in time.

KEY POINTS

1. Effective utilization management techniques, as performed by the case manager, can increase the percentage of reimbursed services for a healthcare provider.
2. Case managers must be very familiar with the criteria used by the third-party payers they interact with.
3. Commonly used criteria include the InterQual criteria and the Milliman & Robertson Health Care Management Guidelines.
4. The criteria used should always match the patient's location along the continuum of care.
5. Denials can be cataloged as either nonclinical (administrative) or clinical.

6. Case managers should be familiar with the managed care contracts negotiated in their organization.

7. Utilization management data should be collected, tracked, and trended on a regular basis and reported through the organization's internal structure.

REFERENCES

InterQual, Inc: *System administrator's guide,* Marlborough, Mass, 1998, InterQual.

Schibanoff JM, editor: *Health care management guidelines,* New York, 1999, Milliman & Robertson.

6

Transitional Planning and Case Management

In these times of fixed payments, whether they are due to prospective payment or managed care reimbursement systems, healthcare organizations no longer can afford to keep patients at one level of care for an extended period of time. Without ongoing assessment for timely transfer to a more appropriate level of care, these organizations risk either no reimbursement for services rendered or denial of payments for all or a portion of these services. **Transitional planning,** traditionally known as **discharge planning,** is the process case managers apply daily, in conjunction with **utilization management.** It ensures that appropriate services are provided and that these services are provided in the most appropriate setting (i.e., level of care) as delineated in the standards and guidelines of regulatory and **accreditation** agencies (federal and private). This chapter focuses on the transitional planning process and its relationship to case management. Utilization management is discussed in Chapter 5.

Transitional planning places the **case manager** in a pivotal position in the patient care delivery process, especially where decisions are made to ensure quality, safe, efficient, cost-effective, and continuous care and transitional plan. Transitional planning is defined as a dynamic, interactive, collaborative, and interdisciplinary process of assessment and evaluation of the healthcare needs of patients and their families or caregivers during or after a phase/episode of illness. Transitional planning also includes planning and brokering of necessary services identified based on the patient's condition. In addition, it ensures that these services are delivered in the patient's next level of care (i.e., setting) or after discharge from a hospital. This process is systematic and aims to facilitate the transition of patients from one level of care to another more appropriate,

necessary, and reimbursable level without compromising the quality and continuity of care or the services being provided.

Transitional planning involves a team of healthcare providers from within the healthcare organization: the patient, family, case manager, and other relevant providers, such as the managed care case manager, physician, social worker, physical therapist, occupational therapist, speech pathologist/therapist, pharmacist, and financial screener/reviewer. This team may also include other representatives from agencies that are external to the organization, such as home care, skilled nursing facilities, hospice, and transportation. Not every member of this transitional planning team is involved to the same degree. Some members may only be involved based on their specialization and as they relate to the needs of patients. For example, a patient with cardiovascular disease would not routinely require the services of a speech pathologist/therapist, whereas a patient who has had a stroke would. The case manager usually ensures that the appropriate members of the healthcare team are involved in the transitional planning process as the condition of the patient warrants.

TRANSITIONAL PLANNING OR DISCHARGE PLANNING

Transitional planning was not born by happenstance. Over the years and as in any evolutionary process, some sociopolitical factors contributed to the advent of discharge planning and later to its evolution into transitional planning. Discharge planning was not a component of case management until the late 1980s, when healthcare organizations began to view unnecessary use, fragmentation, and duplication of resources as wasteful and cost-ineffective. In addition, certain pressures such as the prospective payment system in acute care settings forced hospitals to reduce the patients' length of stay, which was basically accomplished through discharging patients expeditiously. However, the shift to transitional planning did not occur until legislative changes in reimbursement and care delivery (i.e., the Omnibus Budget Reconciliation Act [OBRA] of 1986 and the Balanced Budget Act of 1997) took place, coupled with the increased incidence of **managed care** in the 1990s. Only then did transitional/discharge planning evolve to a necessary function of every acute care hospital and every case management program.

Rather than *discharge planning,* the term *transitional planning* better demonstrates the essence of this process and its intent. This can be substantiated in three ways. First, transitional planning describes the act of transitioning patients from one level of care into another within or outside the acute care organization (i.e., from intensive care to intermediate step-down, or regular floor, and then discharge), whereas discharge planning basically focuses on discharging patients from acute care settings to another facility or to home, discounting the different levels of care within the acute care setting. Second, transitional planning means the beginning of a new phase of care, whereas discharge planning denotes ending care. The use of the term *discharge planning,* then, is not truly reflective of case management because case management also includes the act of managing patients' transitions across the healthcare continuum and services instead of focusing on the care provided in a single setting or level of care. Third, transitional planning, as a terminology, reflects the way managed care reimbursement functions, that is, reimbursement based on the level of care provided and the transitioning of patients from one level to another, less complex level until the patient is ready for discharge from the service or the setting.

Driving Forces for Transitional Planning

Transitional planning as a function performed by case managers is important for several reasons, some of which follow.

- Existing pressures and limits on hospital length of stay
- Shift in reimbursement methods, with **fee-for-service (FFS)** being the least popular mechanism
- Focus on improved and cost-effective resource management and allocation methods
- Demand on healthcare providers and agencies to justify why the care is provided in a certain setting and at a specific level of care

- Managed care organizations (MCOs) denying reimbursement for a portion of or all services provided
- Ensuring the identification of the patient's and family's potential needs for referrals to specialty healthcare providers and for community resources after hospital discharge
- Availability of varied and numerous options for patients after discharge from an acute care setting such as subacute care, acute rehabilitation, home care, skilled nursing facilities, assisted living facilities, Meals on Wheels, day care centers, and so on
- Physicians are no longer the sole decision-makers as to what types of services a patient may require and in what setting
- Heightened awareness and knowledge of healthcare consumers of their benefits and entitlements and their demand for patient-centered care
- Scrutiny by MCOs and accreditation and regulatory agencies
- The current perception of utilization management and discharge planning as "real" and essential clinical work and not a "nuisance" or external to patient care delivery and management
- Managing patients in an increasingly complex environment characterized by multiple payers, providers, sites, and settings

Mandates of Regulatory Agencies and Professional Societies

Transitional planning has been mandated or advocated for by federal agencies in the form of legislation, by accreditation agencies in the form of accreditation or performance standards, and by professional organizations/associations in the form of policies or practice guidelines (Box 6-1). For example, OBRA mandates that hospitals have a transitional planning program in place to meet the Medicare's conditions of participation or to be eligible for providing services to Medicare patients (OBRA, 1986). The **continuum of care** standard of the Joint Commission on Accreditation of Healthcare Organizations (JCAHO) calls for hospitals to have explicit policies and procedures for discharge planning that ensure early identification of patients' needs for postdischarge services and to have a process in place for the coordination and arrangement of these needs. JCAHO also requires hospitals to establish a process for the assessment of available and appropriate resources for this purpose. This process entails gaining knowledge of the resources available for patients within the internal and external healthcare environments (JCAHO, 2001).

To assist in meeting the requirements of federal and accreditation agencies and to help hospitals develop

BOX 6-1 Examples of Entities That Mandate or Advocate for Transitional Planning

Legislation
The Omnibus Budget Reconciliation Act (OBRA) of 1986
The Social Security Act
Balanced Budget Act of 1997

Accreditation Agencies
Joint Commission on Accreditation of Healthcare Organizations (JCAHO)
Commission on Accreditation of Rehabilitation Facilities (CARF)

Professional Associations
American Hospital Association (AHA)
American Nurses Association (ANA)
Case Management Society of America (CMSA)

BOX 6-2 Case Management Society of America's Standards on Discharge Planning

Although not exactly phrased as discharge planning standards, the Case Management Standards of Practice (CMSA, 1995) identify some roles and responsibilities of the case manager regarding discharge planning. These are as follows:
1. The case management plan identifies immediate, short-term, and ongoing needs, as well as where and how these care needs can be met.
2. The case management plan sets goals and timeframes for achieved goals that are appropriate to the individual or his or her family and agreed to by the client/family and treatment team and ensures that funding and/or community resources are available to implement the plan.
3. Plan with client/family a goal-oriented care process that analyzes and gives direction to a treatment plan that moves the client toward health, wellness, adaptation, and/or rehabilitation.
4. Focus on accountability for quality care and cost or benefit to clients consistent with payer, provider, and consumer expectations.
5. Be knowledgeable and educated with regard to the roles and capabilities of various professionals and research the various resources for determining the type and quality of these resources.
6. Refer, broker, and/or deliver care based on the ongoing healthcare needs of the client and the ability, knowledge, and skill of the health and human services providers.
7. In conjunction with the client/family, link the client/family with the most appropriate institutional or community resources.
8. Procure and coordinate healthcare services.

solid discharge/transitional planning programs, the American Hospital Association (AHA) published its guidelines for discharge planning in 1984. These guidelines apply mainly to the acute care settings. They explain the essential elements of discharge planning: early identification of patients in need for postdischarge services, patient/family education, assessment and counseling, development of the discharge plan, coordination and implementation of the discharge plan, and follow-up after hospital discharge (AHA, 1984).

The American Nurses Association (ANA) in its *Standards of Clinical Nursing Practice* described the role and responsibilities of the nurse in discharge planning and continuity of care (ANA, 1991). According to these standards, the nurse is expected to collaborate and consult with other providers in the provision of safe and quality patient care. This entails the assessment of patients' needs, making referrals to other providers, identifying and securing appropriate services available to address patients' health-related needs, ensuring continuity of care, and educating patients and their families regarding health needs and condition.

The AHA **guidelines** and the ANA standards functioned as resources for healthcare organizations to use in the development, implementation, and enhancement of their discharge planning programs and processes. Today there are specific case management standards and guidelines available that explain the role and responsibilities of case managers in discharge/transitional planning. These are advocated for by the Case Management Society of America (CMSA) (Box 6-2). In addition, certifying bodies for case manager's certification, such as the Commission for Case Manager Certification (CCMC) and the American Nursing Credentialing

Center, include transitional planning as a topic or dimension of the certification examination (Box 6-3). This makes it necessary for case managers to assume the role of transitional planner and be knowledgeable in this function.

With the advent of case management, healthcare organizations, particularly acute care hospitals, reexamined who is best to assume the role of the discharge planner. The traditional method of having either a social worker or a registered nurse (RN) designated solely to this function/aspect of patient care became no longer acceptable. The pressures for efficient, quality, and cost-effective care delivery processes influenced healthcare executives to design models of practice and patient care delivery that eliminated the problems of fragmentation and duplication of services, roles, and responsibilities. Case management programs and delivery models became most popular because of their focus

---

BOX 6-3 Discharge Planning as Evident in Case Manager's Certification Tests

Topics included in the Commission for Case Manager Certification's certification exam (CCMC, 2000) that refer to discharge/transitional planning are as follows:

1. Levels of care
2. Community resources and support programs
3. Rehabilitation service and delivery systems
4. Public benefit programs such as Medicare, Medicaid, and Social Security Income
5. Assistive technologies
6. Healthcare benefits and insurance principles
7. Life care planning

Topics included in the American Nurses Association's certification exam that refer to discharge/transitional planning are as follows:

1. Determining treatment options
2. Designation of appropriate care setting
3. Negotiation and management of financial aspects of care
4. Delineation of appropriate level of care
5. Referrals to other providers for services
6. Coordination of services
7. Continuity of care

---

on addressing these pressures through consolidation of departments such as utilization management; quality improvement and management; clinical care management; social services; and, most importantly, discharge planning. Hence this became the beginning of an integrated case manager's role. Today this role most commonly integrates transitional planning, clinical care management, and utilization management (Case Manager's Tip 6-1). Such integration has demonstrated the best cost, quality, and consumer-related outcomes.

THE CONTINUUM OF CARE

Before we explain the role of the case manager in transitional planning, it is important to review the continuum of care. A focus on the continuum of care is instrumental for success in transitional planning and case management. To simplify the discussion, we decided to divide the continuum of care into three types of services and settings: preacute, acute, and postacute care and services. These are distinct in terms of scope, type, and cost of services (Table 6-1). The services provided in each of these settings are highly regulated and warrant that case managers be knowledgeable of the clinical, reimbursement, and eligibility guidelines for the provision of services in each setting. In addition, they must apply these guidelines when they collaborate with the members of the healthcare team in the

 CASE MANAGER'S TIP 6-1

Integrating Transitional Planning in the Case Manager's Role

When integrating transitional planning into the role of the case manager, you must consider the following:

- The cost incurred since expanding the scope of responsibility of the case manager may require adding more case managers to the department and perhaps limit the number of patients seen by each
- Clearly defined roles and boundaries; of particular interest must be clarifying the difference between the role of the social worker and the case manager
- The impact on the relationship of the case manager with other staff in the organization such as the primary nurse, physician, admitting office staff, emergency department staff, and others
- The impact on the relationships of the case manager with outside agencies such as MCOs, skilled nursing facilities, and home care
- Reassessment of the role of the primary nurse
- Making clerical staff available to assist case managers in clerical/secretarial functions so that case managers can spend the majority of their time in the clinical area and with their patients or the healthcare team
- Assigning case managers to the clinical areas in a way that maximizes productivity and reduces downtime/unproductive time
- Use of automation and technology (e.g., electronic communication)

---

development of the transitional plans for their patients (Case Manager's Tip 6-2). Moreover, case managers must be able to match the patient's condition to the appropriate next level of care with adequate consideration of the patient's health insurance plan and its related benefits (Case Manager's Tips 6-3 and 6-4).

- *Preacute services* are those offered to prevent illness or deterioration/changes in the patient's health condition that may warrant the need for acute care or hospitalization. Examples of these services are health risk screening (e.g., cholesterol and blood pressure/hypertension screening, mammography, prostate screening), patient and family education materials for health promotion and illness prevention, health advice lines, triage services, and counseling. Settings included in this type of services are MCOs, ambulatory/clinics, physician offices or group practices, and community-based health centers.
- *Acute services* are those provided during an acute episode of illness and in a hospital setting. Examples

TABLE 6-1 Characteristics of the Continuum of Care

Settings	Preacute	Acute	Postacute
Cost	Low and in some instances free	High	Moderate to high
Complexity of care	Least complexity	Most complex	Moderate complexity
	Proactive	Reactive	Reactive
	Self-directed care	Total/assisted	Assisted
Type of services	Primary/prevention	Secondary/tertiary	Long term
	Risk assessment	Acute care	Rehabilitative
	Screening for illness	Intensive care	Maintenance
	Fitness	Operative procedures	Restorative
	Health promotion	Emergency care	Custodial
	Self-care management	Specialty care	Skilled
	Counseling		End of life
	Behavior modification		Supportive
			Home care
Institutionalization	Rare (ambulatory)	Always (hospital)	May be necessary depending on type of care (community)
Case management services	Minimal	Intensive	Moderate to intensive
	Telephonic	Comprehensive	Self-care management
	Health appraisal		
	Risk reduction strategies		

 CASE MANAGER'S TIP 6-2

Determining the Level of Care

As a rule of thumb, case managers must deliver care that is patient centered. Focusing on the patient's condition rather than the level of care provides the most desired benefits for both the patient and the healthcare organization. It is the patient's condition that drives the decision as to the level of care that is appropriate. For example, a home care case manager may transfer a patient to an acute care hospital when he or she notices that the patient is experiencing an acute hyperglycemic episode, or a case manager may transfer a patient from an intensive care setting to a regular inpatient unit when the patient's signs, symptoms, and treatments are able to be managed in a lower level of care setting.

 CASE MANAGER'S TIP 6-3

Matching Patients to the Level of Care

It is important for the case manager to understand what constitutes the different levels of care and settings (e.g., skilled nursing facilities, acute rehabilitation, home care) and the different insurance coverage for these settings when matching patients for the next level of care.

 CASE MANAGER'S TIP 6-4

Managed Care and the Level of Care

It is imperative for the case manager to be aware of the rules for coverage as delineated by the MCO/health insurance plan and to obtain authorizations/certifications before rendering the services. The case manager must also be aware of or assess what the patients have already exhausted from their benefits and determine whether what is left is adequate to cover the next needed service.

are emergency and trauma care and operative procedures such as coronary artery bypass graft surgery. Settings included in this type of services are hospitals, acute rehabilitation facilities, postanesthesia and intensive care units, and emergency departments (EDs).

■ *Postacute services* are those provided for patients after an acute episode of care whether in a facility setting or at home. They usually aim at rehabilitation and health maintenance. Examples include subacute care, geriatric rehabilitation services, and visiting nurse services. Settings included in this type of services are long-term

care facilities, skilled nursing facilities, assisted living facilities, hospice, and home care agencies.

Case managers are responsible for matching patients to the next appropriate level of care, which in most instances requires either the discharge or the transfer of a patient to another institution or care site. Tables 6-2, 6-3, and 6-4 provide examples of the types of patients

TABLE 6-2 Types of Services and Patients in Preacute Service Settings

Setting	Types of Services and Patients
Telephonic/triage	Offering advice regarding care, triage services, provision of authorization to pursue access to healthcare services, crisis intervention
Managed care organizations	In addition to telephonic and triage services, offering health risk assessment and screening; counseling; identifying at-risk health behavior; instituting an action plan for behavior modification; patient/family education and counseling using materials, fact sheets, newsletters, electronic communications, and support groups
Ambulatory/clinic/ community health centers	Medical follow-up services, disease management services, routine health appraisals, health behavior counseling such as nutrition counseling, exercise and fitness services, crisis intervention, patient/family education

There is no need for one to be ill to access the services offered in any of these settings. They are provided for both healthy and ill persons and are aimed at maintaining health and functioning.

TABLE 6-3 Types of Services and Patients in Acute Care Settings

Setting	Types of Services and Patients
Acute care	Inpatient/in-hospital care, operative procedures, invasive diagnostic and therapeutic procedures, invasive monitoring and supervision, intensive care
Acute rehabilitation	Acute rehabilitation such as geriatric rehabilitation services (however, patient must be able to tolerate 3 hours of rehabilitation activities per day), recent functional loss, trauma victims, dependence on the assistance of another person, expected significant improvement in condition
Emergency department	Conditions requiring urgent care such as myocardial infarction, new onset stroke, life and death situations, trauma, unclear condition requiring complex and immediate workup
Transitional hospitals	Complex medical conditions that do not require an acute phase of care and are too complex to be in a skilled nursing facility, mechanical ventilation dependency or requiring weaning, use of total parenteral nutrition, extensive wound management, coma recovery, complex intravenous medication management

and services that are cared for in the different preacute, acute, and postacute settings, respectively. As case managers assess the conditions of their patients to make decisions pertaining to transitional planning, they apply the criteria of admission and discharge to and from the various care settings. In the case of **Medicare**- and **Medicaid**-participating organizations, these criteria are usually driven by federal reimbursement regulations (i.e., InterQual guidelines). For example, to transition a patient into an acute rehabilitation facility, the patient must be able to tolerate and participate in therapy for a minimum of 3 hours per day.

Case managers also apply the criteria used by managed care agencies (i.e., Milliman & Robertson) when indicated by the patients' insurance or health plans. In a practical or operational sense the InterQual and Milliman & Robertson criteria are usually referred to as either of the following:

1. **Intermediate outcomes;** that is, outcome indicators when met by the patient's condition indicate the need to transition the patient to the next level of care. For example, a cardiology patient in an intensive care setting is transferred to the telemetry unit when the patient's condition no longer requires invasive hemodynamic monitoring.

2. **Discharge criteria;** that is, outcome indicators when met by the patient's condition indicate the discharge of the patient completely from the healthcare organization/setting. Usually these criteria are applied for discharging a patient from a hospital/acute care setting. For example, a pediatric patient admitted for acute exacerbation of asthma is discharged home when he or she is breathing comfortably and shows adequate oxygenation or improvement in peak expiratory flow.

The JCAHO has greatly influenced the healthcare organizations' view of and focus on the continuum of care and services in its accreditation standards. According to the JCAHO (2001), case management services must aim at coordinating care and services across the continuum of care. This is necessary especially because patients may need to receive a range of services in multiple settings and from multiple healthcare providers. This makes it essential for hospitals to view the care they provide to patients as part of an integrated system of

TABLE 6-4   Types of Services and Patients in Postacute Care Settings

Setting	Types of Services and Patients
Subacute care	Skilled nursing, physical therapy, occupational therapy, speech therapy, respiratory therapy, restorative care, social services and activities *Examples of patient types:* Requiring intravenous therapy and antibiotics, daily injections, tube feedings and tube care, ventilator monitoring and weaning, wound care and more frequent dressing change, peritoneal dialysis, maximum assistance in ADLs, building self-care activities, skilled therapies, total bladder and bowel incontinence
Home care	Skilled nursing, physical therapy, occupational therapy, home health aide, companion, hospice, social services and activities, respiratory therapy, durable medical equipment, intravenous infusion therapy, and chemotherapy *Examples of patient types:* Homebound, requiring assistance with ADLs, intermittent and skilled care, wound care, ostomy care, Foley catheter, tube feeding, patient teaching for self-care management, phlebotomy, vital signs monitoring, medication supervision, death and dying support
Long-term care	Custodial care, oxygen therapy/administration, tube feedings, skilled nursing, social services and activities, hospice care, respite care *Examples of patient types:* Requiring skilled nursing, complex or chronic medical conditions, severe mental retardation, lives alone and cannot care for self, cognitive or functional impairment, lack of social support, unsafe home environment, chronic illness and deteriorating, 24-hour supervision, long-term/unweanable ventilator
Respite care	Custodial care, social services and activities *Examples of patient types:* Patients are appropriate for long-term care facilities but wish to stay at home or with family members, caregivers needing a rest
Residential facilities/ custodial	Assisted living, assistance with ADLs, medications supervision, social interactions and activities, transient/intermittent episodes of confusion or impaired judgment *Examples of patient types:* Requiring skilled nursing, 24-hour supervision, stand-by assistance in ADLs, bowel and bladder incontinence, assistance with grocery shopping and cooking

ADLs, Activities of daily living.

settings, services, healthcare providers, and care levels. These characteristics make up the continuum of care. Therefore it is in the best interest of hospitals to ensure that they have a process in place that addresses compliance with the continuum of care standard described by the JCAHO. This process is the transitional planning process and must be applied for all patients and at every encounter. It is best ensured if case managers assume the responsibility for transitional planning, especially because they are better prepared for this function compared with other providers (Case Manager's Tip 6-5).

The JCAHO defines the continuum of care, focusing on the role acute care organizations (i.e., hospitals) play in transitional planning. Case management programs and delivery models enhance compliance with the continuum of care standard because of their natural focus on the care coordination activities JCAHO delineates in this standard in terms of the process of patients' admission and discharge from a hospital (Box 6-4). Not surprisingly, these activities

 CASE MANAGER'S TIP 6-5

Success of Case Managers

The success of case managers in providing care across the continuum is dependent on their knowledge, skills, and ability to do the following:

- Provide the *right care*
- At the *right time*
- In the *right place/setting*
- Reinforcing that it is provided by the *right provider*
- In consideration with the *right cost* and insurance benefits
- Aiming for the *right outcomes*
- Ensuring the *right quality*

are essential components of the transitional planning process.

In addition to the care coordination activities, JCAHO identifies six standards with which hospitals must

---

BOX 6-4 The Sequence of Activities for Care Coordination as per the JCAHO Continuum of Care Standard (JCAHO, 2001)

1. *Before admission:* The hospital must identify and use available information sources about the patient's needs and communicate with other care settings for this purpose.
2. *During admission:* The hospital provides services that are consistent with its mission and the population it serves. It must make arrangements with other facilities to facilitate patients' admission or transfer as indicated by their needs and based on intensity, risk, and staffing levels. In addition, it must refer patients to clinical consultants and providers of contractual agencies as appropriate.
3. *While in the hospital:* Continuity of services must be maintained through the phases of assessment, treatment, and reassessment of patients, and the care provided must be coordinated among all providers.
4. *Before discharge:* The patient's postdischarge needs must be evaluated and arrangements made to meet these needs, including patient/family teaching regarding such care.
5. *At time of discharge:* The patient must be referred to other providers or agencies to provide the postdischarge services needed. Such arrangements must also be reassessed and confirmed before discharge. The hospital is required to communicate relevant information to the agency that will assume responsibility for continuing care after the patient's discharge.

---

maintain compliance to meet the requirements of the continuum of care function. These standards are as follows:

1. The hospital must have a process in place to ensure that patients access the appropriate level of care and services they require based on their assessed needs.
2. The hospital must accept patients to an appropriate level of care and services based on a completed assessment of needs. This assessment must be completed based on predefined criteria with regard to the patient information necessary to make appropriate decisions regarding the level of care, service, and setting.
3. The hospital must have a process in place to ensure continuity and coordination of care and services over time.
4. The hospital assesses the patient's needs and readiness for discharge, referral, or transfer to another level of care, setting, or provider. Such a decision must be made based on the hospital's and other facility's ability to meet the patient's needs. The hospital is obligated to inform the patient in a timely manner of the plan of discharge or transfer.

5. The hospital must exchange appropriate and necessary information with other facilities and providers when transferring patients. This information is usually related to the services required for a patient's care.
6. The hospital must have a clearly defined procedure for resolving denial of care conflicts. Such procedure must take into account the needs of patients as they are (re)assessed on an ongoing basis.

These standards are relevant to case management and transitional planning. It is natural then to design a case manager's role that incorporates these functions. For example, standards 1 and 2 can be incorporated in the screening and case identification function of case managers, standard 2 can be addressed in the planning care function, standard 3 relates to the care coordination and facilitation function, standards 4 and 5 are appropriate components of the discharge/transitional planning function, and standard 6 can be incorporated in the utilization management function.

The Centers for Medicare and Medicaid Services (CMS), formerly known as the Health Care Financing Administration (HCFA), is the federal agency that defines the standards of discharge planning in the form of Medicare's Conditions of Participation. These standards are available online in the *State Operations Manual, Interpretive Guidelines for Hospitals,* Tag Numbers A330 through A344, Medicare Conditions of Participation §482.43 (HCFA, 2001). Similar to the JCAHO's continuum of care standard, they focus on the process of transitional planning. A summary of these standards follows. More detailed information is available in Table 6-5. According to these regulations, hospitals are expected to do the following:

- Have a discharge planning process applicable to all patients, and the related policies and procedures must be made available in writing.
- Identify the patients in need of discharge planning and postdischarge services at an early stage of hospitalization.
- Provide a timely discharge planning evaluation for patients who require it and those who request it regardless of need.
- Have a licensed professional, such as an RN or social worker, develop or supervise the development of the discharge planning evaluation.
- Include an evaluation of the patient's need for posthospital services and the availability of the services.
- Evaluate the patient's capacity for self-care or the possibility of returning to the prehospital environment.
- Share the discharge plan with the patient or designee for approval and counseling.
- Assess the patient's discharge needs on an ongoing basis while hospitalized, revise the plan when necessary, and prevent a delay in the patient's discharge.

TABLE 6-5   Centers for Medicare and Medicaid Services' Regulations and Interpretive Guidelines for Hospitals: Transitional Planning

Tag Number	Regulations	Interpretive Guidelines
A330	§482.43 Discharge Planning The hospital must have in effect a discharge planning process that applies to all patients.	The written discharge planning process must reveal a thorough, clear, comprehensive process that is understood by the hospital staff.
A331	The hospital must identify at an early stage of hospitalization all patients who are likely to suffer adverse health consequences upon discharge if there is no adequate discharge planning.	The hospital must set the criteria for identifying patients who are likely to suffer adverse health consequences upon discharge without adequate discharge planning. The following factors are of importance: functional status, cognitive abilities, and family support. The hospital must identify patients at risk for posthospital services through a screening process that must be done as early as possible.
A332	The hospital must provide a discharge planning evaluation to the patients identified in need of postdischarge services and to other patients upon their request or the request of the person acting on their behalf, or the request of the physician.	The postdischarge needs assessment can be formal or informal and generally includes an assessment of factors that impact on an individual's needs for care after discharge from acute care setting. These may include assessment of biopsychosocial needs, the patient's and caregiver's understanding of discharge needs, and identification of postdischarge care services.
A333	A registered nurse, social worker, or other appropriately qualified personnel must develop or supervise the development of the evaluation.	Responsibility for discharge planning is often multidisciplinary and includes disciplines with specific expertise. The hospital has the flexibility in designating the responsibilities of discharge planning to the registered nurse, social worker, or other qualified personnel. The responsible person should have experience in discharge planning, knowledge of social and physical factors that affect functional status at discharge, and knowledge of community resources to meet postdischarge needs.
A334	The discharge planning evaluation must include an evaluation of the likelihood of a patient needing posthospital services and the availability of the services.	The hospital is responsible for developing discharge plan that is based on the following: (1) implementation of a needs assessment process with high-risk criteria identified; (2) complete, timely, and accurate assessment; (3) maintenance of a complete and accurate file on community-based services and facilities including long-term care, subacute care, home care, or other appropriate levels of care to which patients can be referred; and (4) coordination of the plan among various disciplines responsible for patient care.
A335	The discharge planning evaluation must include an evaluation of the likelihood of a patient's capacity for self-care or of the possibility of the patient being cared for in the environment from which he or she entered the hospital.	The capacity for self-care includes the ability and willingness for such care. The choice of a continuing care provider depends on self-care components, as well as availability, willingness, and ability of family/caregivers and the availability of resources. The hospital must inform the patient/family of their freedom to choose among providers of posthospital care. Patient preferences should also be considered. Patients should be evaluated for their return to the prehospital environment. Hospital staff should incorporate the information given by the patient/family or caregiver to implement the discharge plan.

Continued

TABLE 6-5   Centers for Medicare and Medicaid Services' Regulations and Interpretive Guidelines for Hospitals: Transitional Planning—cont'd

Tag Number	Regulations	Interpretive Guidelines
A336	The hospital personnel must complete the evaluation on a timely basis so that appropriate arrangements for posthospital care are made before discharge and to avoid unnecessary delays in discharge.	The timing of the discharge planning evaluation should be relative to the patient's clinical condition and anticipated length of stay. Assessment should start as soon after admission as possible and be updated periodically during the episode of care. Some information is best collected on admission such as age and sex and medical diagnosis; however, other information is best collected close to discharge such as functional ability, indicating more accurately the patient's continuing care requirements.
A337	The hospital must include the discharge planning evaluation in the patient's medical record for use in establishing an appropriate discharge plan and must discuss the results with the patient or individual acting on his or her behalf.	The hospital must demonstrate its development of discharge plans for patients in need and the initial implementation of the plan. Documentation of these activities is expected. The hospital is expected to document its decision about the need for a discharge plan and the existence of the plan when needed and indicate what steps are taken to implement the plan. Evidence of an ongoing evaluation of the discharge plan is also expected to be an important factor in documentation. The hospital must have documented evidence that the discharge plan is discussed with the patient/ family, other interested persons, and the next caregiver.
A338	A registered nurse, social worker, or other qualified personnel must develop or supervise the development of the discharge plan if the discharge planning evaluation indicates the need for a discharge plan.	It is a management function of the hospital to ensure proper supervision of its employees. Existing training and licensing requirements of a registered nurse and social worker in discharge planning are sufficient; other appropriately qualified personnel may include a physician. The hospital should determine who has the requisite knowledge and skills to do the job. However, because posthospital services and ultimately the patient's recovery and quality of life can be affected by the discharge plan, the plan should be supervised by qualified personnel to ensure professional accountability.
A339	In the absence of a finding by the hospital that a patient needs a discharge plan, the patient's physician may request a discharge plan. In such a case, the hospital must develop a discharge plan for the patient.	The physician can make the final decision as to whether a discharge plan is necessary. The hospital must develop a plan if a physician requests one even if the interdisciplinary team determined one to be unnecessary.
A340	The hospital must arrange for the initial implementation of the patient's discharge plan.	The hospital is required to arrange for the initial implementation of the discharge plan. This includes arranging for necessary posthospital services and care and educating the patient, family, or caregiver.
A341	The hospital must assess the patient's discharge plan if there are factors that may affect continuing care needs or the appropriateness of the discharge plan.	The discharge planning evaluation should be initiated as soon as possible after admission and updated as changes in the patient's condition and needs occur and as close as possible to the patient's actual discharge.
A342	As needed, the patient and family members or interested persons must be counseled to prepare them for posthospital care.	Evidence should exist that the patient and/or family and/or caregiver is/are provided information and instructions in preparation for posthospital care and kept informed of the progress. The use of family/caregivers in posthospital care should occur only if they are willing and able to do so. It is appropriate to use community resources with or without family support whenever necessary.

TABLE 6-5 Centers for Medicare and Medicaid Services' Regulations and Interpretive Guidelines for Hospitals: Transitional Planning—cont'd

Tag Number	Regulations	Interpretive Guidelines
A343	The hospital must transfer or refer patients, along with necessary medical information, to appropriate facilities, agencies, and outpatient services as needed for follow-up or ancillary care.	The hospital must ensure that patients receive proper posthospital care within the constraints of a hospital's authority under state law and within the limits of a patient's right to refuse the discharge planning services. Documentation of the refusal of the discharge plan/services is recommended. Medical information may be released only to authorized individuals or those involved in the discharge plan and its coordination. Examples of necessary information include functional capacity of the patient, requirements for healthcare services, discharge summary, and referral forms.
A344	The hospital must reassess its discharge planning process on an ongoing basis. The reassessment must include a review of discharge plans to ensure that they are responsive to discharge needs.	The hospital must have a mechanism in place for ongoing reassessment of its discharge planning process. Although specific parameters or measures that would be included in a reassessment are not required, the hospital should ensure the following factors in the reassessment process: (1) the effectiveness of the criteria to identify patients needing discharge; (2) the quality and timeliness for discharge planning evaluations and discharge plans; (3) that the hospital discharge planning personnel maintain complete and accurate information to advise patients and their representatives of appropriate options; and (4) that the hospital has a coordinated discharge planning process that integrates discharge planning with other functional departments, including quality assurance and utilization review activities of the institution, and involves various disciplines.

■ Refer or transfer the patient to other facilities and providers as needed for follow-up care and share the necessary information for that purpose.

It is evident in these regulations that hospitals must focus on the continuum of care in the provision of healthcare services. Similar to the JCAHO's standards, each of these requirements can be fit in one or more step of the transitional/discharge planning process. Therefore case management models and programs in acute care and other settings enhance compliance with Medicare's Conditions of Participation and JCAHO's standards of accreditation. Moreover, case managers, who are licensed professionals as stipulated in the regulations, are best suited to assume the responsibility for these functions. They can apply the transitional planning process for this purpose.

THE CASE MANAGER'S ROLE IN TRANSITIONAL PLANNING

Case managers are responsible and accountable for transitional planning in virtually every institution that employs case management delivery services. This section discusses the role of the case manager in transitional planning through the application of a systematic process (Figure 6-1) especially designed for that purpose. The goals of the transitional planning process are, but are not limited to, the following:

1. Facilitating high-quality, cost-effective, and patient/family-centered care
2. Providing linkages among the varied providers within and outside the healthcare organization
3. Providing linkages between healthcare providers and organizations and MCOs/payers
4. Influencing a multidisciplinary healthcare team approach that includes patients and their families or caregiver for the planning of care and service delivery
5. Ensuring optimal services and continuity of care for patients and families, especially after discharge from acute care settings
6. Brokering community services/resources for patients and their families as deemed appropriate
7. Ensuring adherence to guidelines and standards of regulatory and accrediting agencies and MCOs
8. Examining the outcomes of the discharge plans and services provided in preparation for or after discharge

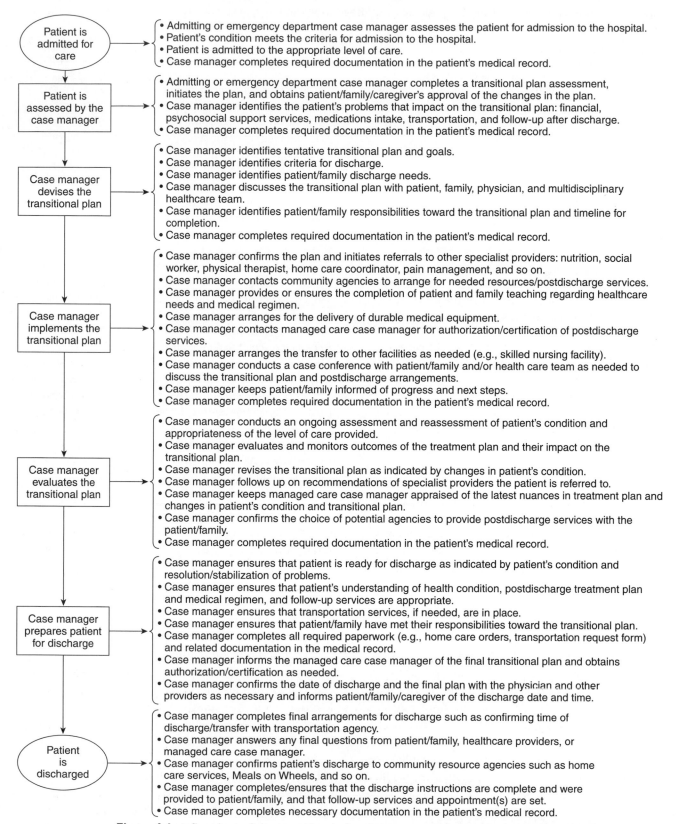

Figure 6-1 A flowchart of the transitional planning process and the case manager's roles.

As noted in the previous section, a particular focus of the continuum of care is coordination of care or services provided by a healthcare organization to meet the ongoing identified needs of individuals. This includes referrals to appropriate community resources and liaison with others, such as the individual patient's physician; other healthcare organizations; and community services involved in care or services. The transitional planning process assists healthcare organizations in the implementation of the plan of care and prevents the use of unnecessary duplication of services. It consists of six steps or phases in the care of the patient. As noted in Figure 6-1, these are as follows:

1. Assessment of the patient's condition, risks, and needs
2. Development of the transitional plan, including the goals of treatment and discharge
3. Implementation of the plan
4. Evaluation and ongoing monitoring of the plan
5. Confirmation of and final preparation for the patient's discharge
6. Discharge of the patient to another level of care or to home

The steps in this process, although listed in a linear fashion, are not necessarily linear. They also are not limited to an acute care setting focus, even though the patient may be receiving care while in the hospital at this point (Case Manager's Tip 6-6). Case managers usually shift back and forth between the steps while engaged in functions such as assessing/reassessing the patient's condition and discharge planning needs, accounting for the latest changes in the patient's condition when revising the plan of care, attempting to confirm the transitional plan with MCOs, and making the final arrangements for transferring a patient to another facility.

Step 1: Assessment of the Patient's Condition, Risks, and Needs

On admission to the hospital and as early as possible, case managers usually screen patients to determine what their needs are and whether these needs may require case management services. As they complete this assessment, they pay special attention to identifying the discharge planning needs and the conditions that will necessitate the transition of patients from one level of care to another. In this assessment, case managers apply criteria for admission to the hospital as indicated, for example, in the Milliman & Robertson or InterQual criteria. To illustrate this point, let us assume that a patient is seen in the ED with a possible stroke and is admitted to the hospital if he or she meets any of the following criteria (these are select examples):

1. InterQual: inability to move limb(s), unconsciousness, aphasia, need for surgery, uncontrolled seizure activity

 CASE MANAGER'S TIP 6-6

The Continuum of Care
Case managers must always remember that the continuum of care is virtual in perspective and is not limited to a particular setting. It is a state of mind and not a physical place. Case managers are expected to focus their efforts on coordinating the care of their patients across the various settings and not just the location in which they work. This aspect of care coordination is essential to the success of the transitional plan and usually ensures the safety of the patient's discharge and the continuity of care/services.

2. Milliman & Robertson: intracranial hemorrhage, hemiparesis, need for physical therapy and/or speech therapy evaluation as a result of the disease, requiring anticoagulation therapy

Case managers can see in this example that the criteria from InterQual and Milliman & Robertson are essentially the same. In this example, case managers evaluate the appropriateness of the admission to the acute care setting/hospital, which means the transfer of the patient from the ED level of care to the inpatient level of care. Based on the complexity of the patient's condition, that is, the severity of the presenting illness and the intensity of the required resources, the patient may be transferred to either an intensive care unit or a regular inpatient unit as needed. The case manager initiating the preliminary assessment of this patient can also identify the patient's potential postdischarge/hospital needs and include these needs in the transitional plan for follow-up and ongoing evaluation.

Institutions may have an ED or an admitting office-based case manager complete such assessment and develop an initial transitional/discharge plan. ED case managers can apply the InterQual or Milliman & Robertson criteria to determine the need and appropriateness to transition a patient from the ED to an inpatient level of care/setting.

After admission to the inpatient unit/level of care, inpatient case managers can then follow up on the plan already developed in the ED. They first reassess the patient's condition and needs, then revise the plan of care, including the transitional plan. Next they begin the interdisciplinary process for service delivery planning, facilitation, and coordination. Before developing the transitional/discharge plan, the case manager should complete a thorough assessment and evaluation of the patient's:

■ Current treatment plan
■ Financial status or health insurance benefits

- Psychosocial status and support system
- Medication intake and management
- Medical history and previous services
- Need for rehabilitative services
- Need for transportation services at the time of discharge
- Need for community-based postdischarge services
- Potential discharge location (i.e., transfer to another facility)

Step 2: Development of the Transitional Plan, Including the Goals of Treatment and Discharge

After completing the initial assessment based on the previous list, case managers can develop the transitional plan in conjunction with the interdisciplinary plan of care. The transitional plan must focus on the identified patient problems or areas of deficit and concern. For example, these may be related to the following:

- Assisting the patient in applying for Medicaid because of lack of insurance and the possibility that the patient meets the Medicaid eligibility criteria
- Lack of social support and inability to care for self after discharge
- Complex medication regimen that may require visiting nurse services
- Limited functional ability or mobility that may require home care rehabilitation services or the transfer to an acute or subacute care facility
- Eligibility for transportation services to and from the dialysis center
- Arranging for community services such as Meals on Wheels, support groups, senior citizen's social activities, and the like

As case managers identify and confirm these needs, they establish the goals of the transitional plan that are reflective of the problems identified. Therefore the transitional plan focuses on the issues case managers intend to resolve in conjunction with the patient and family/caregiver and the healthcare team. Before they initiate their action plans, case managers confer with the patient and family and the appropriate members of the healthcare team such as the physicians to approve and finalize the plan. During this step, case managers communicate their expectations of the patient and family and explain their responsibilities to them. For example, case managers may request certain documents that are in the possession of the patient/family and necessary for the Medicaid application. Therefore they may establish a timeline with the patient and family for completing the Medicaid application and follow up with them if they do not meet the timeline.

In addition to the transitional plan, case managers focus on the medical plan of care and its impact on

CASE MANAGER'S TIP 6-7

Use of Criteria When Transitioning Patients
When considering transferring a patient from one level of care to another, case managers must apply the criteria (usually level of care-based) that guide the transitional planning process.
1. The InterQual criteria: intensity of service and severity of illness
2. Milliman & Robertson Guidelines: intermediate outcomes

However, when planning the patient's discharge, case managers must evaluate the patient's condition for discharge readiness. This decision is made based on the discharge criteria that are available for each diagnosis and is in the form of:
1. Discharge screens in InterQual criteria
2. Discharge outcomes in Milliman & Robertson Guidelines

transitioning patients from one level of care to another. They usually evaluate the patient's condition and the treatments being provided for their appropriateness to the level of care/setting the patient is in (Case Manager's Tip 6-7). This is important because of their role in transitioning the patient to the next level in a timely fashion. This function results in preventing reimbursement denials or an unnecessary hospital stay. In addition, this evaluation facilitates the implementation of the discharge/transitional plan. These activities bring to life the act of integrating utilization management and transitional planning for a seamless approach to case management care delivery. For example, when a patient admitted to the coronary care unit because of acute myocardial infarction undergoes uncomplicated angioplasty or a coronary stent placement, the case manager may ensure the patient's transfer to a telemetry or cardiac unit after the procedure. This is indicated because the patient's stable condition no longer meets the criteria for an intensive care setting/level of care. In this case, the case manager not only is expediting the transition of the patient toward discharge but is preventing inappropriate/unnecessary utilization of a higher level of care that may jeopardize reimbursement.

Step 3: Implementation of the Plan

Before the case managers implement the patient's transitional plan, they may arrange for a case conference(s) with the patient and family or the healthcare team. They may elect to conduct the conference either with all parties combined or with the patient and family separate from the team. Such a decision is made based on the complexity of the issues and treatment plan and the concerns to be discussed or by a request from the patient and family, the physician, or the team. Regardless of how the case conference is held, the purpose remains to reach consensus on the plan of care, including the transitional plan, and to answer any challenging questions regarding the care. Some examples of the reasons for holding a case conference are discussing end-of-life issues and decisions about continuing or discontinuing treatment, do not resuscitate (DNR) order, disagreement among

family members regarding the plan of care, managed care denial of continuing services, or merely a patient and family education and counseling session.

To implement the transitional plan, case managers may need to request the involvement of specialists in the care of the patient such as physical therapy, speech therapy, occupational therapy, pharmacy, home care, pain management, social services, and nutrition. Following predetermined referral criteria facilitates this process and enhances consistency in the delivery of quality care. Examples of these criteria are available in Box 6-5.

BOX 6-5 Sample Criteria for Referral to Other Specialty Healthcare Providers

Sample Referral Criteria to Nutritionist
1. History of unintentional weight loss or gain greater than or equal to 10% in 1 month
2. Inadequate nutrition due to poor oral intake (e.g., less than 25% of meal for 3 days or longer)
3. Nausea, vomiting, or diarrhea for 3 days or longer
4. Difficulty chewing or swallowing
5. Total parenteral nutrition/hyperalimentation
6. Newly initiated enteral feedings
7. Albumin level less than 2.5 g/dl
8. Stage III or IV pressure ulcer
9. Nonhealing wound
10. Malabsorption
11. Substance abuse: alcohol or drugs
12. New diagnoses such as diabetes, heart failure, pre- or post-organ transplantation, end-stage renal disease/dialysis, hypertension, lipidemia, inflammatory bowel disease

Sample Referral Criteria to Social Work/Services
1. Assistance with coping with illness, hospitalizations
2. Patient lacks appropriate decision-making skills regarding care
3. Suspicion of patient abuse or neglect
4. Current substance abuse: alcohol and drugs
5. Patient with mental/behavioral health illness
6. Need for placement in a skilled nursing facility, long-term care, hospice, foster care
7. Homeless patient
8. Elderly patient who lives alone and cannot care for self independently
9. New functional deficit
10. Uninsured patient
11. Recent confusion, disorientation, cognitive impairment
12. Absent psychosocial/family support system
13. Need for transportation arrangements

Sample Referral Criteria to Physical Therapy/Rehabilitation
1. New functional deficit requiring occupational or physical therapy such as retraining in activities of

daily living (ADLs): grooming, bathing, dressing, feeding, toileting
2. Need for training on the use of a prosthetic device such as artificial leg
3. Need for training on the use of durable medical equipment such as a wheelchair, bedside commode, crutches, or other prostheses
4. Need for building an exercise regimen after surgery
5. Need for training in transfers from/to bed or chair
6. Need for chest physiotherapy or pulmonary toileting
7. Training in weight bearing or non-weight bearing movements

Sample Referral Criteria to Home Care Services
1. New or problematic wounds, drains, ostomies, and catheters
2. Multiple and complex medication regimen (polypharmacy)
3. Intravenous fluid therapy and medication therapy
4. Pain management and control
5. Peritoneal dialysis
6. Home oxygen therapy including mechanical ventilation
7. Home respiratory therapy
8. Skilled care at home such as physical therapy and exercise, psychosocial counseling, assessment and monitoring of vital signs
9. New diagnoses such as diabetes, heart failure, pre- or post-organ transplantation, end-stage renal disease/dialysis, hypertension, lipidemia inflammatory bowel disease

Sample Referral Criteria to Pain Management Services
1. Patients with chronic pain
2. Oncological conditions
3. Palliative care situations
4. Unrelieved pain regardless of multiple attempts with different types of pain medications
5. Patient's request
6. Need for alternative therapies for pain management

Consultations with specialist providers is necessary, especially when a confusing situation arises that requires their intervention and input or because of the need to adhere to the regulations that govern the practice of that particular discipline. For example, a patient may not receive home care services unless assessed by the home care staff first and deemed eligible for home care services after discharge. Another example is the requirement of a rehabilitation evaluation by a physiatrist before establishing a physical therapy plan of care for rehabilitation purposes. Using a list of criteria to clarify the need for referrals is essential for providing better quality of care, eliminating confusion as to when a patient may need the care of a specialist provider, and expediting the implementation of the transitional plan.

Other important case management functions in this step of the transitional planning process are patient and family education, managed care authorizations for discharge services, and brokerage of services from community agencies. Case managers may not always be involved in patient and family education; however, they make sure that other providers such as primary nurses provide this service (Case Manager's Tip 6-8). In some instances it behooves case managers to educate their patients and families or caregivers themselves. Examples of these situations are confusion about aspects of the care such as managed care health plans and how they operate, insurance benefits and entitlements, the authorization and certification process, transitioning the patient to another less complex or more complex level of care, and the need to transfer a patient to a long-term care facility. Sometimes case managers are involved in

 CASE MANAGER'S TIP 6-8

Education Is Integral to the Transitional Planning Process

In preparation for discharge, the staff nurse is responsible for educating patients and their families/caregivers about medication administration and management; wound care and dressing changes; tube care such as a Foley catheter, feeding tube, or any other drainage tubes; and use of equipment such as a glucometer. Other providers may educate patients about specialty needs such as activity and exercise by a physical therapist, healthy eating or special renal diet by a nutritionist, and oxygen therapy at home by a respiratory therapist. The case manager is responsible for making sure that these educational interventions are completed before the patient's discharge and to prevent delays in these educational efforts.

educating the patient and family about complex care situations or treatment regimens that are unusual to other nursing staff members.

As for discharging patients to another care facility such as a nursing home or subacute care, case managers coordinate such a transitional plan with the rest of the healthcare team, the patient and family, and appropriate representatives from the external facility. Depending on the type of the patient's insurance plan, they may also contact the case manager of the MCO for **authorization** of this type of transition. In the case of a Medicare or Medicaid patient, they apply the eligibility criteria for such transfer available from HCFA or the CMS. If the case managers assuming this role are not social workers, they may consult with social workers for collaboration on such transfers. This aspect of the transitional plan highlights the need for case managers to apply utilization management knowledge and skills while making these plans and the integration of utilization management and transitional planning into a seamless process of care coordination.

Patients' transitional plans may sometimes require the coordination of postdischarge services available in the community. These community services are either volunteer and free or reimbursable by the patient's insurance carrier. Examples include the following:

- Medical supplies
- **Durable medical equipment**
- Transportation
- Lifelines
- Pastoral care
- Meals on Wheels
- Support groups
- Social clubs for senior citizens
- Volunteer agencies/services
- Shelters
- Foster care
- Respite care

If case managers arrange for any reimbursable services, they are required to follow the rules and benefits indicated in the patient's insurance/health plan. For example, in the case of Medicare and Medicaid the eligibility criteria must be consulted when arranging for durable medical equipment. In the case of managed care health plans, case managers must contact the managed care case managers for certification of durable medical equipment before it is arranged for, otherwise reimbursement for such service may be denied.

Step 4: Evaluation and Ongoing Monitoring of the Plan

Evaluation and ongoing monitoring of the transitional plan is important because this aspect of the case manager's role keeps the care provision process in check. Evaluating the transitional plan is essential because it helps case managers determine the plan's continued appropriateness for the patient and ensures that the patient's needs are addressed. However, one cannot evaluate the transitional plan without ongoing reassessment of the patient's medical condition and plan of care. In addition, it is as important to keep abreast of the nuances of care by seeking daily feedback from the patient, family, healthcare team, specialist providers involved in the patient's care, and the representative of any outside agency the patient is referred to for postdischarge services. Based on the new information, case managers usually revise the transitional plan to reflect the changes in patient's condition or wishes regarding discharge services and place.

Case managers also evaluate the appropriateness of the level of care being provided based on the patient's latest condition. Again, in this function case managers apply the InterQual or Milliman & Robertson criteria for this purpose. If the patient's condition is found to meet the next level of care and the patient is not yet transitioned, then the case manager facilitates such transfer. He or she may need to meet with the healthcare team and the patient and family to discuss the transfer or to ensure that it is carried out. Other evaluation and monitoring aspects of the case manager's role in this step of transitional planning are as follows:

■ Completeness of the necessary patient and family education efforts
■ Authorizations from MCOs for services to be rendered
■ Recommendations of specialist providers are implemented or incorporated in the transitional plan
■ Patients and their families/caregivers are in agreement with the plan
■ Community services are arranged for
■ Transportation services needed upon discharge are arranged for

Based on the outcomes of these evaluations, the transitional plan is adjusted as needed. To eliminate conflicts or fragmentation in care, sometimes case managers may resort to a case conference so that agreements are reached and concerns of any member of the healthcare team or patient/family are discussed and resolved. Decisions made during the conference are then implemented in the transitional plan or the medical plan of care as necessary.

Step 5: Confirmation of the Plan and Final Preparation for Patient's Discharge

This step of the transitional planning process focuses on the patient's readiness for the next level of care or discharge. Confirmation of the plan is done while the case manager is evaluating the plan. The decision to transition the patient to the next level of care or discharge is made based on the patient's medical condition and resolution of the problems the patient presented with at the time of admission to the hospital. Other factors that influence this decision are the patient's agreement with the transitional plan, the decision regarding disposition and the date and time of discharge, the position of the MCO/insurance carrier regarding the plan and postdischarge services, readiness of the facility to assume responsibility for the patient's care postdischarge to accept the patient's transfer, and views of the healthcare team, particularly the physician, about the plan and the patient's readiness for it (Case Manager's Tip 6-9).

To determine the appropriateness of the time and condition of a patient's discharge, case managers apply the InterQual or Milliman & Robertson discharge criteria. An example is presented in Box 6-6. Other criteria are as follows:

■ Afebrile during the last 24 hours without antipyretics
■ Fluid and food intake meets nutritional needs
■ Switching from intravenous to oral medications
■ Passing of flatus or bowel movement after abdominal surgery
■ Voiding appropriate amount of urine
■ Serum medication levels (e.g., digoxin) within therapeutic range
■ Patient or caregiver able to care for patient after discharge
■ Refusal of continued inpatient treatment
■ Availability of postdischarge services

To determine the most appropriate disposition for a patient, case managers should consider the discharge possibilities based on regulations and admission criteria that may be different for the different facilities or options. Case managers are encouraged to

 CASE MANAGER'S TIP 6-9

Use of Criteria to Assist in Resolving Transitional Planning Conflicts

Sometimes conflicts may arise between the case manager and the physician related to the timing of discharge or the patient's readiness for discharge or transfer to the next level of care. In these situations, the case manager is advised to use the Milliman & Robertson or InterQual criteria in addressing the conflict. The case manager must focus on the length of stay, reimbursement denials, and position of the managed care case manager when resolving such conflicts.

BOX 6-6   Sample Discharge Screens

InterQual's Cardiovascular-Related Discharge Criteria
- Last prothrombin time (PT) within therapeutic range with anticoagulants
- Potassium between 3.5 and 5.5 in the last 12 hours
- Controlled anginal pain
- Controlled dysrhythmias
- Controlled dyspnea, edema
- No significant ECG changes

Milliman & Robertson's Discharge Criteria for Unstable Angina
- Pain-free
- No significant ECG changes
- Creatine kinase (CK) negative for myocardial injury
- No need for immediate invasive therapy in the next 24 hours
- No parenteral medication therapy such as heparin or nitroglycerine

---

be knowledgeable about these regulations or consult with those who are at their institutions so that appropriate decisions are made and safe, quality, and cost-effective discharge is ensured. Some of the discharge options are as follows:
- Skilled nursing facilities
- **Subacute care facilities** or units
- Rehabilitation facilities or units
- Intermediate care facilities
- Home care
- Hospice care
- Outpatient care
- Residential care

In this step, case managers also revisit the patients' and families' responsibilities toward the transitional plan as agreed on initially after the patient's admission to the hospital and while the plan was being finalized. They examine whether the patient or family made the arrangements they were expected to make, and if not, a decision is made about the next expected step and who is responsible for handling the situation. In addition, case managers are expected to provide the patient, family, or caregiver with a written discharge notice confirming the discharge. This notice acts as a formal and documented notification for discharge, a copy of which usually is kept in the patient's medical record. As discussed in Chapter 5, if the patient and/or family disagree with the discharge, they are entitled to appeal the decision by notifying the **peer review organization (PRO).** If they appeal, the discharge is then held until a

decision by the PRO is reached and the patient and the organization providing the care are informed.

A final function of the case managers in this step is confirming the following:
- The final transitional/discharge plan with the physician, patient, and family; the facility the patient is to be transferred to (only in such cases); and the case manager of the managed care company
- The date of transfer or discharge
- That any required paperwork is completed, such as transportation request form, home care orders, and interinstitutional transfer notes
- Date and time of delivery of durable medical equipment
- Follow-up appointments if indicated

Step 6: Discharge/Transferring of the Patient to Another Level of Care

On the day of discharge, the case managers may not be involved in any major activities other than confirming that the discharge takes place as planned. Any change in the patient's condition that may require continued hospitalization is addressed, and the case manager, in consultation with the healthcare team, determines if the discharge should be cancelled. If the discharge is cancelled, then the case manager reapplies the transitional planning process, revises the plan, or develops a new transitional plan reflective of the patient's condition and needs.

In this step of the transitional plan, the case manager may answer any final questions the patient/family or the MCO may have. The case manager also provides the facility to be responsible for the postdischarge care (whether a skilled nursing facility, a long-term care facility, or a home care agency) with the appropriate information regarding the patient's condition and the required care. This information is important because it ensures continuity of care.

As part of every step of the transitional planning process, case managers are responsible for documenting their plans, interventions, outcomes of coordinating the postdischarge services, and next action steps.

It is evident that the transitional planning process is an integral component of case management, and it cannot be completed without consideration of utilization management. Although the discussion presented in this chapter focused mostly on transitional planning, case managers are advised to be careful in their interpretation of this discussion and to consider the steps presented here within the larger context of case management and their roles and responsibilities. At any time and in any given situation, case managers are always applying the concepts of transitional planning,

TABLE 6-6   The Relationship Between the Case Management and Transitional/Discharge Planning Processes

Case Management Process	Transitional/Discharge Planning Process
1. Case finding/screening and intake	1. Patient's admission Screening patient for postdischarge needs Identifying need for discharge services
2. Assessment of needs	2. Assessment of discharge/transitional planning needs Agreeing on needs with patient, family, healthcare team Assessing available resources and type of resources
3. Identification of actual and potential problems	3. Development of transitional/discharge plan Designing action plan for meeting patient's discharge needs Agreeing on goals of plan and expected outcomes
4. Interdisciplinary care planning	4. Implementation of the plan Putting plan into action Coordinating necessary activities Brokering of services with community agencies Educating patient and family regarding healthcare needs
5. Implementation of interdisciplinary plan of care	5. Evaluation of transitional plan Monitoring appropriateness of plan Examining outcomes of plan Exchanging information with postdischarge agencies as needed
6. Evaluation of patient care outcomes	6. Preparing patient for discharge Confirming patient's discharge Confirming postdischarge services
7. Patient's discharge and disposition	7. Patient's discharge Actual discharge to home Transferring patient to another facility
8. Repeating the process	8. Repeating the process Reapplying transitional planning process based on changes in patient's condition

clinical care management, and utilization management into their action plans and the decisions they make to resolve problems. Table 6-6 summarizes the relationship or correlation between the processes of case management and transitional/discharge planning.

TRANSFERRING PATIENTS TO OTHER FACILITIES

Not every patient is discharged to the home setting after a hospitalization. Some patients may need to be transferred to another facility such as a skilled nursing facility, whereas others may need to be transferred back to the facility they came from before hospitalization. Case managers play an important role in the process of transferring patients from one hospital or level of care to another. They ensure that the transfer packet contains the complete information that is necessary for continuity of care and decision making in the receiving hospital. The transfer information must include the following:

■ Copy of the medical record that contains the patient's radiographic reports, blood work, medical history and physical examination, ECG reports, assess-

ments from specialist providers, and social services assessment
■ Copy of any DNR order, **healthcare proxy**, or **living will**
■ Patient's consent for the transfer
■ Physician transfer orders
■ Treatment plan and postdischarge care expected to be continued in the new facility
■ Accepting physician's name and medical service

It is important to arrange for these documents to prevent patients from being returned to the transferring facility. Sometimes, and in some states, it is required that a pretransfer evaluation be completed and that this evaluation document the appropriateness of the transfer and that the accepting facility approves the transfer before the patient's transfer. Case managers can confirm that such regulations are followed and that such an evaluation is completed before a patient's transfer.

In 1998 the CMS passed a regulation regarding transferring Medicare patients that fall in 10 **diagnosis-related group (DRG)** categories. These DRGs are listed in Table 6-7. This regulation was passed to curtail the

TABLE 6-7 The 10 Transfer Diagnosis-Related Groups

DRG	MDC	Title	GMLOS (Days)
14	M	Specific cerebrovascular disorders except TIAs; examples are subarachnoid hemorrhage, subdural hemorrhage, cerebral aneurysm, nonruptured cerebral aneurysm, CVA	4.9
113	S	Amputations for circulatory system disorders except upper limb and toe; examples are lower limb amputation, below knee amputation, above knee amputation, disarticulation of hip	4.8
209	S	Major joint and limb reattachment procedures of lower extremity; examples are total hip replacement, total knee replacement, limb reattachment	4.9
210	S	Hip and femur procedures except for major joint; examples are open reduction of fracture of the head of femur with various hardware	6.1
211	S	Hip and femur procedures except major joint without complications or comorbidities	4.7
236	M	Fractures of hip and pelvis; examples are fracture of pelvis such as acetabulum and pelvis, femoral neck fracture such as subtrochanteric or intratrochanteric fractures	4.1
263	S	Skin graft and/or debridement for skin ulcer with complications and comorbidity; examples are skin graft for cellulitis (any site), decubitus ulcer, chronic skin ulcer	8.8
264	S	Skin graft and/or debridement for skin ulcer or cellulitis without complications or comorbidity; examples are skin graft for cellulitis (any site), decubitus ulcer, chronic skin ulcer	5.4
429	M	Organic disturbances and mental retardation; example is organic brain syndrome	5.2
483	S	Tracheostomy except for face, mouth, and neck diagnosis	34.0

CVA, Cerebral vascular accident; *DRG*, diagnosis-related group; *GMLOS*, geometric mean length of stay; *M*, medical; *MDC*, Major diagnostic category; *S*, surgical; *TIA*, transient ischemic attack.

increased number of transfers of patients to subacute care facilities, especially those who are transferred within a few days of an acute care hospital stay. At the time, subacute care was fairly new and not yet under the **prospective payment system** structure. Acute care institutions found it a rewarding opportunity to transfer patients such as those with strokes, pneumonia, and orthopedic problems early on during their treatment plan for rehabilitation in subacute care settings. Such transfers left acute care hospitals with more desirable lengths of stay and better fiscal states, considering the pressures of the acute care prospective payment system.

As stated in the regulation, patients in any of these 10 DRGs are considered transfers if (1) they were to receive care in a skilled nursing facility or home care after discharge from the hospital, (2) the services are related to the patient's condition during the hospitalization, and (3) these services are provided within 3 days of hospitalization. The condition of 3 days can be translated into a rule of not transferring any patient in any of the 10 DRGs before the acute care length of stay reaches the geometric mean length of stay identified in the DRG system. If this happens, the acute care facility will be penalized.

Case managers can prevent this penalty from happening and can enhance compliance with this regulation through their role in the transitional/discharge planning process. They can incorporate such a regulation

 CASE MANAGER'S TIP 6-10

Transferring Patients to Other Facilities

The case manager must consider the following three scenarios when transferring patients to other facilities:

1. If a Medicare or Medicaid patient is transferred from one hospital to another, the receiving hospital receives the full DRG payment. The transferring hospital, however, receives a per diem payment for each day of the patient's stay based on the DRG rate applicable. The case manager should examine all cases that are transferred before transfer for appropriateness in an effort to prevent financial loss and maximize reimbursement.

2. If a patient is transferred from one level of care to another within the same hospital (e.g., from an intensive care unit to a medical unit), the hospital receives one payment. The case manager should evaluate patients as necessary for a timely transfer from one level of care to another less intensive or complex to ensure the delivery of cost-effective and appropriate level of care.

3. If a patient is transferred from one unit in a Medicare- or Medicaid-participating hospital to another hospital or unit that is exempt, the patient is dealt with as a discharge. However, the case manager is responsible for ensuring that the transfer is appropriate so that reimbursement is not jeopardized.

as a criterion of transfer when they evaluate their patients' readiness for discharge or transfer to another facility. They can also educate the rest of the healthcare team about this regulation to improve compliance and prevent the hospital from being penalized by the CMS in case of lack of compliance. Another strategy to increase compliance is for case managers to apply this criterion when they are coordinating post-discharge services for their patients with subacute care facilities or home care agencies. Also refer to tips presented in Case Manager's Tip 6-10 for more information about patient transfers.

KEY POINTS

1. Case managers play a pivotal role in ensuring that the transitional plan is safe, timely, and meets clinical criteria such as InterQual or Milliman & Robertson.
2. The continuum of care can be aggregated into preacute, acute, and postacute care and services.
3. Matching the patient to the clinically appropriate level of service will result in increased reimbursement to the provider organization.

4. The case manager should use the steps of assessing, planning, implementing, evaluating, confirming, and transitioning the patient through the continuum of care.
5. Transitional planning is highly regulated. Case managers should stay up-to-date on all relevant regulations, both at the state and federal levels.

REFERENCES

American Hospital Association: *Guidelines: discharge planning,* Chicago, Ill, 1984, The Association.
American Nurses Association: *Standards of clinical nursing practice,* Kansas City, Mo, 1991, The Association.
Case Management Society of America: *Standards of practice for case management,* Little Rock, Ark, 1995, The Society.
Commission for Case Manager Certification: *CCM certification guide,* Rolling Meadows, Ill, 2000, The Commission.
Health Care Financing Administration: *State operations manual: interpretive guidelines for hospitals,* Baltimore, Md, 2001, HCFA. Available online at http//:www.hcfa.gov/pub...5Fsom/somap%5Fa%5F109 %5Fto%5F123.html (accessed on 11/23/01).
Joint Commission on Accreditation of Healthcare Organizations: Continuum of care. In: *Accreditation manual for hospitals,* Oakbrook Terrace, Ill, 2001, JCAHO. Available online at http//:www.jcaho.org/ CAMH/cc2.html (accessed on 11/23/01).
Omnibus Budget Reconciliation Act of 1986: *Conference report to accompany H.R. 5300,* Section 9305, Washington, DC.

Disease Management

Gerri S. Lamb, PhD, RN, FAAN, Paul S. Shelton, EdD, and Donna Zazworsky, MS, RN, CCM, FAAN

Disease management (DM) is a comprehensive and evidence-based approach to caring for populations with chronic healthcare conditions. The concept of DM emerged over the past decade in response to growing concern about the quality and costs of healthcare for groups of individuals with common and expensive health problems such as diabetes or heart disease. Proponents of early DM programs believed that a more systematic and evidence-based approach to caring for populations of individuals with chronic conditions would not only improve clinical outcomes but would save significant dollars for healthcare plans, consumers, and providers. The recent growth and popularity of research-based practice **guidelines** has supported and propelled DM in many new directions (Box 7-1).

DM programs seek to create better systems of healthcare targeted for patients with chronic conditions. Based on current scientific knowledge about prevention and treatment of common health problems and their **complications,** these programs focus on improving processes of care to ensure that patients receive appropriate interventions at the appropriate time. For example, a diabetes DM program would include strategies for identifying patients at risk for developing diabetes and tools to increase the likelihood that patients with an established diagnosis of diabetes receive foot and eye examinations within recommended timeframes. A comprehensive diabetes DM program also would establish criteria for referring high-risk patients for **case management** services and would provide an infrastructure for the role of the case manager (Case Manager's Tip 7-1).

BOX 7-1 Factors Contributing to the Growth of Disease Management

- Growing concerns over the cost and quality of healthcare
- The need for systematic processes to manage individuals with chronic illnesses
- The growth and popularity of research-based practice guidelines
- Consumer focus on outcomes of care, safety, and error-free healthcare

---

 CASE MANAGER'S TIP 7-1

Disease Management and the Case Manager
DM provides a structure for case managers to manage high-risk and vulnerable patient populations.

For case managers, DM programs can offer an effective structure and state-of-the-art tools for practice with high-risk patients. This chapter provides an overview of the evolution of current DM programs and their impact on the quality and costs of care. Current approaches to DM are described, including key strategies for success. The chapter concludes with a detailed example/case study of a DM program implemented in a clinic setting.

EVOLUTION OF CURRENT DISEASE MANAGEMENT PROGRAMS

During the 1990s the U.S. healthcare system experienced increased levels of financial risk for patient medical management. At the same time it was being held more accountable for providing appropriate, cost-effective, quality care (Rosenstein, 1999). These pressures mounted in an atmosphere characterized by a lack of skilled staff, increased consumer dissatisfaction with **managed care,** and constant turnover in clinical and administrative personnel. It was within this rapidly changing environment that DM programs came of age, emerging from **outcomes** research—a discipline that attempts to improve clinical practice and control costs through well-designed effectiveness studies.

DM programs have been implemented in **managed care organizations** (i.e., **health maintenance organizations [HMOs]**) and hospital and physician group practices. DM programs were initially developed and promoted by pharmacy benefits management organizations to address the inadequacies of the healthcare system. They focused on the small number of patients who consumed a large portion of resources, were complex cases to manage, or were patients with specific chronic conditions. The rationale for developing DM programs was that short-term costs in one specific disease arena would be offset by longer-term savings (Harris, 1996). Commercial companies were the first to develop DM programs and to sell them to HMOs, employer groups, and healthcare organizations. They provided mechanisms for identifying patients with chronic diseases and patient education materials and classes aimed at lifestyle modification and self-management skills, such as help with quitting smoking, nutrition/exercise for cholesterol reduction, and stress management. They also offered assistance with medication management through the tracking of pharmacy **claims.**

However, not all DM services were provided by commercial DM companies. At the same time these programs were growing, a number of leading healthcare organizations developed their own "in-house" programs (Wagner et al, 1999). These newer programs attempted to overcome some of the deficiencies of earlier programs by focusing on individuals with multiple chronic illnesses and integrating physicians into the process (Leider, 1999; Fernandez et al, 2001). They developed interventions that relied on multidisciplinary teams and care providers of varied specialties. They emphasized population-based care and included formalized treatment plans to assist patients in navigating the complexities of healthcare systems, self-management education, and continual follow-up (Wagner, 2000).

In the future, demographic trends can be expected to drive continued growth of team-based DM programs for chronically ill individuals. It is estimated that over 100 million Americans suffer from multiple chronic illnesses today (Hoffman, Rice, and Sung, 1996). With the aging

 CASE MANAGER'S TIP *7-2*

Future Drivers for Disease Management Programs
- An aging population
- Increased growth of chronically ill individuals
- Increased demands to reduce variation in the management of chronic disease processes
- Increased need to implement best/research-based practices
- Increased consumer demand for innovative and effective programs to manage chronic illnesses

of the population and the large baby boom generation, in particular, these numbers will continue to increase, as will the customers' expectations for improved systems of care (Bodenheimer, 1999). There will be increased demand to reduce wide variations in patterns of care for the same disease(s) and to implement and monitor best practices of care (Coye, 2002). Increased access to information via the **Internet** and growing familiarity with the various managed care structures also will propel consumer demand for innovative and effective programs for chronic illness management (Bazzoli et al, 2002; Coye, 2002). Case Manager's Tip 7-2 describes the issues that will drive future DM programs.

DISEASE MANAGEMENT AND CASE MANAGEMENT

Although current models of DM emerged after the rapid growth of case management in the 1980s and 1990s, they provide an important context for effective application of case management. Generally, DM programs address the full **continuum of care** for patients with targeted chronic and complex health conditions. They are concerned with health promotion and prevention of illness, as well as treatment of advanced complications of diseases. They consider the needs of patients at all levels of risk for adverse outcomes to ensure that patient needs are matched to an appropriate level of intervention.

Case managers fulfill an essential component of DM programs. Working at the high-risk end of the DM spectrum, case managers focus on the care of individuals and populations who are most likely to have complications and adverse health outcomes. In many practice settings, it is likely that it will be these high-risk patients who trigger the interest of healthcare providers in starting a DM program. Examination of service use patterns or expenses may reveal a population that is hospitalized more than expected or costs more than the norm. Once this pattern is discovered, it leads to discussions of

CASE MANAGER'S TIP *7-3*

A Process for Disease Management

In DM programs, case managers apply the process of assessment, planning, monitoring, coordinating, and evaluating patients at highest risk. This is consistent with the case management process.

---

how care for this population may be managed more effectively and efficiently. The case manager is in a pivotal position to help the team understand the usual trajectory of illness and care for high-risk members of the populations and to guide them in looking at strategies to prevent patients from becoming high risk or to reduce the risk once it occurs.

DM can provide a useful framework for case managers to explain their interventions and justify their value to the organization. If DM is described as the overarching approach to working with populations with one or more chronic conditions, it is relatively easy to show how and where case management fits into a DM process. That is, case managers are most concerned with assessment, planning, monitoring, coordination of care, and evaluation for patients at the high-risk end of the population (Case Manager's Tip 7-3). From there, case managers can further emphasize their importance in the DM process by highlighting the complexity and costs associated with providing healthcare for this group.

Not surprisingly, however, case managers have been in the forefront of developing DM programs. Armed with their perspective and experience with highly vulnerable and expensive populations, case managers have led the way in designing better systems of care for patients who are not yet at risk and can potentially avoid future complications and threats to their quality of life.

IMPACT OF DISEASE MANAGEMENT ON QUALITY AND COST

DM programs focus on the care and management of populations with a greater volume of high-cost, chronic health conditions. As outlined in Box 7-2, expected outcomes of these programs include a decrease in overall healthcare costs for the population, reductions in avoidable hospitalizations and emergency care, improvements in disease-specific clinical outcomes and patient satisfaction with care, as well as increased adherence to national treatment guidelines.

Numerous clinical trials testing diverse interventions have documented improvements in a number of selected outcomes for specific chronic illnesses, including patients with asthma (Homer, 1997), diabetes

---

BOX 7-2 Expected Outcomes of Disease Management Programs

Decrease in	Improvements in
Overall healthcare costs	Disease-specific clinical outcomes
Hospitalizations/acute care	Patient satisfaction
Emergency department visits	Adherence to national treatment guidelines
Reactive approach to care	Proactive approach to care

(Berger and Muhlhauser, 1999; Clark et al, 2001), and heart failure (McAlister et al, 2001; Rich, 2001). The literature describing DM programs' impact on outcomes and cost savings is less compelling. Initially, most of the reported benefits of DM programs were anecdotal and based on cursory evaluation of changes in outcomes before and after the program was implemented (Hunter and Fairfield, 1997; Todd and Ladon, 1998; Bodenheimer, 2000).

Typically, DM programs have been able to demonstrate reductions in acute care hospitalizations and/or emergency department visits in the short run, usually 6 to 12 months, and an increase in patient satisfaction. Despite their potential, they have not consistently documented overall cost savings, improved clinical outcomes, or quality of care indicators.

Recently, Mathematica Policy Research, Inc. (MPR), conducted a comprehensive review of best practices in chronic illness care coordination (Chen et al, 2000). Participants in their study were identified through an extensive process that included literature review, word-of-mouth recommendations, and invitations to share detailed program descriptions. Over 150 programs that met specified eligibility criteria volunteered information. To participate, programs needed to have (1) published evidence of reductions in hospital admissions or total medical costs and (2) services in place to coordinate care for adults with chronic conditions. Two types of coordinated care programs emerged: (1) DM programs that served patients with a specific disease or condition; and (2) case management programs that served patients with multiple **comorbidities.**

The principal finding from this review showed no single potentially effective way of coordinating care. Characteristics of the successful programs included interventions that targeted specific disease(s), worked most effectively in integrated healthcare organizational structures, had staff resources and capabilities to conduct rigorous program evaluations, and willingness to share the stories of the programs with others.

BOX 7-3   Common Features of Disease Management Programs

- Utilization of nursing case management as core component.
- Case managers are either baccalaureate- or master's-prepared nurses.
- Case managers collaborate with primary care physician to develop a written plan of care.
- Case managers establish an ongoing relationship with patients and families.
- Case managers deliver and coordinate aspects of the care plan.
- Case managers continually monitor interventions and reassess the plan as needed.

 CASE MANAGER'S TIP *7-4*

A Challenge for Disease Management Programs

A challenge that any DM program faces is designing an evaluation strategy that includes meaningful comparisons between the DM program and usual care or alternative interventions.

Although each DM program was different, they had a number of common features that are outlined in Box 7-3. The DM interventions took a proactive outlook and viewed case management and care coordination as preventive activities (i.e., providing services to patients in the present to prevent adverse health outcomes and limiting hospitalizations in the future). For those readers who are interested in a more in-depth review of the programs MPR evaluated, refer to the report by Chen et al (2000). The report is accessible via the Internet.

One of the primary reasons DM programs have not demonstrated success is that many healthcare organizations do not have adequate internal resources necessary to evaluate program outcomes. As a result, the effectiveness of DM has either not been tested or has been shown to be minimally effective. Future programs will need to address this deficit (Case Manager's Tip 7-4).

Although DM programs might not have all of the resources necessary to conduct vigorous scientific research, there are some "rules of thumb" that should be considered.

Rule of Thumb #1

First, as noted previously, the "gold standard" for any evaluation strategy is to make comparisons between the tested intervention and usual care or alternative interventions.

Ideally, these comparisons include a treatment and control group based on patient randomization into each group. When randomization is not possible or feasible, program outcomes should be compared with some other type of group—a defined group of patients who resemble the treatment group but do not necessarily receive all aspects of the DM intervention. Another evaluation strategy can be the use of the same group; data can be collected before and after the DM intervention is implemented.

Rule of Thumb #2

It is important to build in a data collection strategy early in the process of designing a DM program.

Having credible data is essential to program sustainability. At a minimum, try to include data that describe the patients served in the DM program and a few key measures of outcomes. Descriptive information about the patients being served might include age, gender, race, marital status, education, and insurance, as well as living conditions (e.g., live with spouse, live alone, live with a relative, live in a retirement community), presence or absence of a caregiver, existing chronic health condition(s), functional status/limitations (e.g., activities of daily living [ADLs] and instrumental activities of daily living [IADLs] for establishing disability levels), and perceptions of overall health.

Rule of Thumb #3

Selection of outcome measures must be tied to the goals of the DM program.

Measurement of DM outcomes might include patient and provider satisfaction; targeted clinical outcomes; and service use patterns such as the number of hospitalizations, hospital bed days, emergency department visits, ambulatory care visits, and physician visits. This is discussed in greater detail in a later section of this chapter.

Rule of Thumb #4

Although it may not be feasible or practical to randomize patients or even have a comparison group, it is usually possible to collect the same information on all patients at different points in time.

Data can be collected on all patients when they enter the program (baseline measure) and then again at predetermined intervals (e.g., 6, 9, or 12 months) to evaluate changes in patient outcomes over time.

DESIGNING DISEASE MANAGEMENT PROGRAMS

The majority of DM programs include a number of common features. Increasingly, evidence-based practice guidelines and protocols are used as a framework

CASE MANAGER'S TIP 7-5

Steps in Setting up the Disease Management Program

1. Defining the target population
2. Establishing goals and outcome indicators
3. Identifying key stakeholders in the care of the target population
4. Defining core interventions for the targeted population, such as the following:
   - Prevention/health promotion
   - Health education
   - Monitoring
   - Coordination
   - Case management
5. Facilitating the implementation of key processes required to achieve objectives, such as the following:
   - Patient selection criteria and risk screening
   - Use of practice guidelines
   - Coordination and communication
   - Data management
   - Evaluation
6. Overseeing the evaluation of the program and process improvement activities

for core program interventions. Interventions are selected to match the illness and care trajectory of the population and may include a unique mix of self-care education, prevention, medical management, and care coordination and case management components. DM programs rely on information systems capable of identifying potential program patients and providing detailed reports to track and monitor clinical, utilization, and cost outcomes. **Continuous quality improvement (CQI)** tools and processes are typically integrated into all aspects of the DM programs.

A systematic process may be used to design, implement, and evaluate programs that incorporate each of these core features of DM. Most commonly an interdisciplinary team is brought together to select the target population and to oversee the development of the program. The team works through a number of steps in setting up the program. Case Manager's Tip 7-5 outlines the key steps in the process, which are reviewed in detail.

Step 1: Defining the Target Population

The first step in designing a DM program is to define the target population. Typically this is done based on an analysis of the frequency and costs associated with various medical diagnoses in a practice or health

plan. Initial programs usually focus on common diagnoses associated with high expenses, increased hospitalizations or emergency department use, and/or a high incidence of adverse outcomes. The diagnoses tend to include diseases that are chronic and complex.

Selecting diagnoses that are associated with well-developed evidence-based guidelines facilitates the start-up process. Guidelines provide an important benchmark for gauging the effectiveness of changes in clinical practice that are part of DM programs. Some of the more common diagnoses chosen for DM are diabetes, asthma, and heart failure, each of which is common and associated with high service use, complications, and costs.

Increasingly, DM programs are designed to address comorbid conditions and health problems that tend to go along with major chronic illnesses. Examples of such conditions are hypercholesteremia, hypertension, and renal failure/insufficiency. Decisions about the scope of the program should be made during the initial planning phase.

Step 2: Establishing Goals and Outcome Indicators

The analysis of common diagnoses, practice patterns, and costs used to select the target group also should be used to establish the expected goals or outcomes for the program. Depending on the type of organization and its **incentives, credentialing,** and regulatory guidelines, expected outcomes will include a combination of clinical, service use, cost, and provider and patient satisfaction indicators. Reductions in cost per patient, emergency department visits, and hospitalizations are commonly tracked over time. Most settings also desire to achieve improvements in disease-specific clinical indicators targeted in current practice guidelines, such as blood glucose or blood pressure levels.

Selection of specific outcomes may be based on a combination of current outcomes and a plan for incrementally improving the outcomes to a target or benchmark level. For instance, a hospital-based clinical or **quality improvement** team identifies that one third of patients admitted with heart failure are readmitted within 30 days for the same problem. Review of current literature on heart failure indicates effective interventions that can diminish exacerbation of the disease and reduce the 30-day readmission rates. The team may set an initial goal of cutting readmissions by half during the first 6 months and then establish a plan for continuing to lower the readmission rate incrementally over the following year. At the same time, the team may identify other positive outcomes for this population that they want to track at the same time, such as the percentage of discharged patients on angiotensin-converting enzyme (ACE) inhibitor medications or the percentage of patients who can correctly identify when to contact their primary care provider.

Step 3: Identifying Key Stakeholders

At the same time that the target population and goals are being discussed, it is important to identify each of the key groups that are major participants in the care of the population and likely to influence reaching the desired goals. Common stakeholder groups include patients and their families, members of the health-care team, agency administrators, and health plan representatives. Although each of these groups may share common goals for a DM program, such as high patient satisfaction, there may be some differences in priorities based on individual or organizational view-points and financial incentives. As specific targets for each outcome are agreed upon, the perspectives of each group of stakeholders should be considered. Representatives of key stakeholder groups should be invited to participate in the design of the program and/or asked to review program plans as they emerge. The initial plan for developing the DM program needs to identify how and when the perspectives of each group will be incorporated in the design and outcomes of the program.

For example, a health plan considering the development of a comprehensive DM program for its members with diabetes identifies several influential groups involved in diabetes care. These include patients with diagnosed diabetes and their families, members in their plan who represent populations at high risk for developing diabetes, primary care providers, endocrinologists, diabetes educators, case managers, and community organizations focused on diabetes education and care. Initial discussions should consider the goals and priorities of each of these groups for diabetes management and how they will affect support for various program outcomes. The administrators of the health plan might be expected to emphasize member satisfaction and a reasonable return on investment. In addition to satisfaction and costs, primary care providers and diabetes educators can be expected to focus on improving clinical indicators linked to reducing severe complications of diabetes such as foot ulcers and diabetic neuropathy and retinopathy.

In contrast, a hospital-based team thinking about developing a program for community-acquired pneumonia might identify a different set of stakeholders. Key players for this condition might include pulmonologists, respiratory therapists, staff nurses, pharmacists, dieticians, and infection control staff. Regardless of group composition, a major challenge in designing DM programs is to keep stakeholder priorities and incentives in balance with the program goals and resources.

Step 4: Defining Core Interventions

Characteristics of the target population and desired outcomes will guide the selection of interventions and the scope of the DM program. Programs seeking to prevent the development of the condition or detect it in an early stage will, by necessity, be more comprehensive than programs focused on reducing complications and **adverse events** in already diagnosed populations. Expected timeframes and resources for achieving program outcomes will shape the priority placed on different services and interventions.

Today, most DM programs are concerned with chronic illnesses that commonly span several years between prevention, detection, treatment, complications, and death. Many of the triggers to these conditions may be found in early lifestyle choices, such as smoking and diet, or environmental factors. Once disease is detected and diagnosed, it may be several more years before complications are evident. Some of the most challenging decisions in designing DM programs are determining when and where the program will interact with the usual illness trajectory and how resources will be allocated to the various stages of disease development and its related care. Although it may be considered highly desirable to have interventions targeted to each stage, from prevention to life-threatening illness, realistic concerns about time and available reimbursement are likely to affect program design. For instance, health plans with high turnover rates may not be willing to invest heavily in prevention programs that can take several years to show an impact on cost savings. Low reimbursement for prevention and education activities may require creative problem-solving strategies to ensure that these activities are incorporated in ways that are not cost-prohibitive.

One practical way to craft DM programs is to begin by drawing out the disease trajectory for the targeted illness. Review of current and evidence-based literature will help to identify essential and state-of-the-art interventions for each stage of illness from prevention to managing life-threatening complications. Next, factor in the goals of the key stakeholders. What are the key outcomes that major groups will use to determine the success and cost-effectiveness of the program? Where in the illness trajectory are the interventions most likely to achieve the expected outcomes in the expected timeframe? Answers to these questions will help determine where energy and resources may best be targeted, especially for the initial stages of program implementation. In general, prevention activities take longer to demonstrate significant cost savings than interventions targeted at reducing expensive outcomes (e.g., hospitalizations and emergency department use) in populations already found to be at high risk for these outcomes.

Clearly, there is no "one-size fits all" DM program for all organizations and stakeholders. Although the availability and standardization of evidence-based guidelines has improved the content and targeted interventions, there is considerable room for flexibility and creativity about how much, where, and when different interventions are applied. The program must be tailor-fit for the organization, the population to be served, the stakeholders, the timeframes, and the resources available. The growth in common processes and tools for DM make it much easier for program customization.

In sum, the initial stages of designing DM programs require considerable analysis and discussion. Key stakeholders must come to some agreement on the target group, goals, and primary services to be offered. Decisions need to be made about the scope of the program and the components of the illness trajectory that will take priority.

At this point, a planning team might summarize: *"After considerable study, our program will focus on the population of people with heart failure in our system. Our goals are to (1) reduce hospitalizations and emergency department visits for this population by 50%, (2) increase the percentage of patients on ACE inhibitors by 25%, and (3) reach 90% satisfaction rate of patients who receive services in the program. Our initial focus will be on patients at high risk for hospital admission and emergency department visits."*

Another planning team might conclude *"Our program is aimed at improving outcomes for all patients in our system who have diabetes or are at-risk of developing diabetes. Our goals are to (1) screen 100% of the patients in our clinic for their risk of developing diabetes, (2) increase by 50% the percentage of patients who have a hemoglobin A_{1c} of less than or equal to 7%, and (3) reduce by 25% the percentage of patients with high low-density lipoprotein (LDL) cholesterol."*

Each of these examples requires interventions of different focus and scope. The first example emphasizes working with high-risk patients and is likely to incorporate case management as a key intervention. The second example encompasses early detection and screening, as well as treatment, and will likely include a range of interventions to assist patients in reaching clinical outcome targets.

Step 5: Implementing Disease Management: Tools and Strategies

After there is initial agreement on program focus and goals, attention then turns to plans for program implementation. Fortunately there are many resources available to assist with this, from descriptions of setting up programs to written tools and instruments to help stay on track.

Most DM programs are based on a common set of core processes that begin with identifying the target population and proceed through matching patients to appropriate interventions and evaluating the impact on outcomes. Underlying most of the descriptions of current DM programs are a sequence of steps that include risk screening, systematic application of evidence-based practice guidelines, mechanisms for communication and coordination of patient progress, evaluation, and process improvement.

One framework uses the acronym *FAST* to alert clinicians to essential steps in the DM process (Lamb and Zazworsky, 2000). FAST stands for **F**ind, **A**ssess, **S**tratify, **T**reat, **T**rain, and **T**rack. Once the target population for the program is determined, a variety of information sources are used to *"Find"* patients who meet the criteria for participating in the program once privacy regulations are met. Patients with various diagnoses or clinical experiences (e.g., readmission to the hospital, emergency department use, high expenses) may be identified by diagnostic codes, service use files, or financial information. Patients fitting the program criteria are then *"Assessed"* for their level of risk using standardized risk assessment tools. Risk assessment tools are available to identify the risk for hospitalization and the likelihood of experiencing clinical complications and other adverse events. Examples of risk tools are described in a later section of this chapter. Using the results of the risk assessments, patients are *"Stratified"* into low-, moderate-, or high-risk groups. Each group has a specific plan to *"Treat," "Train"* (educate), and *"Track"* (communication, coordination, evaluation) their progress based on their level of risk, complexity, and intensity of need.

There are a variety of tools that have been developed to support the core elements of the DM process. Risk assessment tools provide a standardized way of measuring a person's level of risk for experiencing adverse outcomes or further progression of the disease. CareMaps are used to track patient progress in achieving outcomes and reasons why there may be a difference between the expected and actual outcomes.

Risk Assessment Tools

The most extensively used screening tool to identify patients at risk for adverse outcomes is the Probability of Repeat Admissions (PRA) questionnaire (Boult et al, 1993). This eight-question survey has been found to be a valid and reliable indicator of future adverse health events in a variety of community-dwelling elderly populations (Pacala, Boult, and Boult, 1995; Pacala et al, 1997). The PRA was specifically designed to measure the probability of being hospitalized in the next 4 years.

A defined risk score identifies a patient as "high risk." A risk score of 0.50 or higher, based on the instrument's scoring algorithm, places the patient in the high-risk category. However, this "cut point" is somewhat arbitrary, and there are other ways to interpret the scores for classification purposes. A useful way of analyzing the risk scores is to examine their distribution from lowest to highest and then select those patients whose scores fall in certain percentiles. As an example, all patients whose scores are in the 70th percentile (70% to 100%) or 80th percentile (80% to 100%) could be identified as potential high-risk candidates. Those with scores in the 50th percentile (50% to 70%) could be of moderate risk, and those with scores that fall below the 50th percentile could be identified as low risk.

Another example of a screening tool is The Community Assessment Risk Screen (CARS) (Shelton, Sager, and Schraeder, 2000). The CARS is intended to identify elderly patients who are at increased risk of a hospitalization or emergency department visit in the next 12 months. The CARS consists of three questions that identify preexisting chronic illnesses (heart disease, diabetes, myocardial infarction, stroke, chronic obstructive pulmonary disease [COPD], or cancer), the number of prescription medications (five or more), and hospitalization or emergency department use in the preceding 6 to 12 months. Based on answers to these questions, patients are classified into either high- or low-risk groups.

Both the PRA and CARS were designed to be short, easily administered risk screening tools. They were developed to identify elderly (age 65 and older) populations at risk for future hospitalizations and increased healthcare costs. Data used to construct the instruments were collected from self-report mailed questionnaires. Mailed surveys used to collect health-related information should be used with caution. First, the response rate to mailed surveys generally achieves response rates of only 50% to 60%, and nonrespondents tend to be older and sicker than respondents. Second, low socioeconomic status and literacy rates can lead to even lower response rates. Third, administration and data entry for mailed surveys can be expensive, and these costs must be considered with any DM program (Vojta et al, 2001). Finally, all individuals who are categorized "at risk" by any screening tool or mechanism should undergo further evaluation and in-depth clinical assessment to reduce the incidence of false positives (i.e., identifying those patients who are identified as "at risk" but by clinical evaluation are not).

There are many other instruments that can be used to screen potential patients for DM programs. For a review of many of these instruments the reader should refer to the article by Ware (1994).

Use of Case Management Plans

Treatment recommendations usually find their way into DM programs in a variety of forms, including practice guidelines, clinical pathways or **multidisciplinary action plans (MAPs),** and specific practice **protocols.** Although providers may initially resist the use of these case management tools, guidelines, pathways, and protocols offer a template or framework to organize interventions and maximize the likelihood that patients receive effective treatment in a timely way.

Evidence-based guidelines are recommendations for desired elements of practice and outcomes for a specific population based on a compilation of research findings. Support for each recommendation is provided, including an analysis of the scientific merit of the studies underlying each recommendation. In recent years, federal healthcare agencies and professional associations have put considerable effort into developing consensus around outcomes and performance measurement for several chronic conditions, such as hypertension and diabetes.

Step 6: Overseeing the Evaluation and Process Improvement Activities

DM programs rely on systematic data collection and tracking to monitor and refine expected outcomes. Although program goals are identified early in the process of designing DM programs, it often requires considerable time and effort to develop and maintain reliable and valid systems of outcome measurement. Tracking outcomes may require complex linkages between financial, clinical, and service use data. Access to credible and timely data is the key to demonstrating program value and thus to the survival and sustainability of DM programs.

All team members must be committed to collecting complete and accurate information and making sure it is documented or entered into a computer **database** and in a timely way. Information systems personnel must be relied on to create user-friendly processes to track data and generate reports.

PUTTING IT ALL TOGETHER: THE DISEASE MANAGEMENT TEMPLATE

Planning and implementing DM programs requires that all of the steps come together in a coordinated and seamless process. Patients who meet the criteria for the program must be identified and matched to the right interventions and right quantity at the right time. Entry and exit of key stakeholders need to be closely orchestrated. Plans for outcome evaluation must be built into the earliest stages of program design and then implemented using reliable and valid tools.

The DM template provides a blueprint for action. It defines and operationalizes each of the components of

 CASE MANAGER'S TIP 7-6

Standardizing the Disease Management Plan

A DM template is useful in assisting team members to organize the steps of the process, establish timelines, and clarify responsibility for each activity.

the DM program (Case Manager's Tip 7-6). It specifies expected timelines and individual and team responsibilities. Some of the usual elements in a DM template are shown in Figure 7-1. Common issues and questions that drive template development are discussed as follows.

Risk Assessment

Each of the steps involved in selecting, implementing, and evaluating a risk assessment tool can be incorporated into the template. These steps might include the following:

1. Defining the type of **risk** that will be tracked (e.g., risk for hospitalization or high costs)
2. Reviewing the literature for standardized tools to measure this risk
3. Selecting a risk tool(s)

	Date	Person
1. Risk assessments		
2. Patient education		
3. Staff education		
4. Reporting structures (see specific reports)		
5. Information systems support		
6. Physician coordination		
7. Care coordination		
8. Communication plan		
9. Community referrals		
10. Patient and caregiver support		
11. Pharmacy		

Figure 7-1 Disease management template.

4. Pilot testing the risk tool with a small sample of target population
5. Developing a protocol(s) for collecting and interpreting risk data, and so on

Each of the decision steps should be reflected, including the following: Will the DM teams use a standardized tool, or will they design their own? Will the risk information be collected by chart review, patient interview, or both? Who will be responsible for designing and implementing the risk assessment process?

Patient Education

The team will evaluate the patient education materials necessary and their appropriateness for age, reading level, and culture. In addition, the method of delivery must be specified. For example, will the patients receive individual or group education in the hospital or community setting?

Staff Education

Preparation of staff for implementation of DM programs requires careful consideration and planning. Not only is it necessary to assess the level of knowledge about the disease being addressed, the staff must have a basic understanding of patient behavioral change processes and influencing factors, such as age, sensory deficits, and cultural beliefs. In addition, it is essential to provide staff members with an overview of the DM process and each of its components.

Evaluation and Reporting Structures

Identifying the clinical, quality, and financial outcomes will be the first goal in the evaluation plan. Next, a plan for the generation and distribution of reports may be outlined in this section. Decisions about the type and frequency of reports to various stakeholders should be included. In other words, what information does the executive team, medical staff, and/or DM administrative and practice team need to have and how often? As noted earlier, each stakeholder group may have different needs and priorities for information.

Information System Support

Demands for data tracking and management in DM require early involvement of information system (IS)

 CASE MANAGER'S TIP 7-7

Role of Physicians in Disease Management Programs
The presence of a physician champion can be integral to the success of the program.

experts. This section of the template should define the process and timeframes for development and testing of automated data collection tools and reports.

Physician Coordination

One of the earliest criticisms of DM programs was the lack of physician involvement. Ideally, one or more physicians are members of the development team. The physician coordination component of the template identifies how and where physician participation will be needed in the DM process. For example, in hospital-based DM programs there may be a need for standing orders guided by evidence-based protocols. In the outpatient setting it is common to see interdisciplinary practice guidelines for common chronic illnesses. Physician education on the DM process and tools also may be specified here (Case Manager's Tip 7-7).

Care Coordination

DM programs typically address the needs of patients who require integration of services across multiple settings and care providers. Plans for referrals and coordination across providers and settings are addressed in this component of the template. Team members integral to ensuring continuity and consistency of care are identified, and plans are put in place to ensure smooth transitions. This may involve case managers, social workers, staff nurses, utilization managers, and admitting personnel, as well as community resources and health plan representatives.

Communication Plan

Support of the public relations and marketing department may be enlisted to facilitate internal and external communication about the progress and outcomes of the DM program. Keeping major stakeholders informed is essential for program support and sustainability. The template should address how and when each stakeholder group will be contacted.

Community Referrals

This section of the template describes how community referrals will be documented, communicated, and tracked. Often, referrals are initiated, but very little is incorporated into the DM program to determine if the patient seeks and/or receives the intended services. Clear feedback loops and accountability for tracking and communicating of referrals should be delineated.

Patient and Caregiver Support

New support systems may be required for patients to achieve desired outcomes. In this component of the DM template, members of the team identify essential supports and resources for the target population. Strategies for overcoming barriers to care, such as lack of transportation or funds for medications, are included.

Pharmacy/Equipment

This element considers the medication and equipment needs specific to the targeted chronic conditions. In some cases it may address pharmacy protocols and how they will be managed across service settings. Equipment needs for various populations are included here. For example, in a congestive heart failure (CHF) program, plans typically are made to provide all participants with a scale for weighing themselves. Issues related to ordering and distributing scales may be included in this part of the template.

The DM template is best used as a working tool and blueprint for rolling out the DM program. Completing each component of the template ensures that both patient and programmatic needs will be identified and addressed. Potential gaps in key DM processes or available resources may be anticipated and prevented. An example of how to use the template is included in Case Study 7-1.

ST. ELIZABETH OF HUNGARY CLINIC'S DISEASE MANAGEMENT PROGRAM
Step 1: Defining the Target Population

In 1999 St. Elizabeth of Hungary Clinic (SEHC) brought together a multidisciplinary committee, the Clinical Care Support Committee, to oversee the process of identifying patient needs and improving patient care practices and outcomes. The committee established several objectives. To identify priorities for action, committee members decided as one of their first steps to conduct a comprehensive needs assessment, including surveys of both professionals and patients and a review of SEHC's database.

The results of the clinic needs assessment indicated that the most common health conditions of SEHC's patients were hypertension, acute infection, and pregnancy. For many of the visits associated with these conditions, diabetes was identified as a primary comorbidity. A random chart audit indicated that out of 5,000 patient records reviewed approximately 600 patients (12%) were diagnosed with and being treated for diabetes (adult onset or gestational). Limited information was available in the medical records on diabetes management, suggesting a significant opportunity for improvement.

As a result of the analysis of the clinic needs assessment, members of the Clinical Care Support Committee decided to target the population of individuals at SEHC at risk of developing diabetes and those already with a diagnosis of diabetes. Their broad objective was to identify at-risk individuals as early as possible and immediately implement core interventions to prevent the onset of diabetes. Another objective was to implement necessary interventions to reduce the incidence of complications for those who were already diagnosed with diabetes.

Step 2: Establishing Goals and Outcome Indicators

The objectives of the diabetes DM program were twofold: (1) to improve diabetes clinical care and outcomes and (2) to enhance patient and provider satisfaction. Although there were a number of process objectives defined, these two goals reflect the ultimate outcomes that were important to the clinic.

Specific goals were to do the following:

- Screen 90% of the patients registering for services at SEHC for risk for diabetes
- Complete a diabetes flow sheet on at least 80% of patients who have a diagnosis of diabetes
- Achieve an HbA_{1c} level of less than or equal to 7% for 50% of moderate- to high-risk patients with a diagnosis of diabetes

Step 3: Identifying Key Stakeholders

For SEHC, the key stakeholders of the diabetes DM program initially included patients and their families and the clinic administrative staff consisting of the medical director (MD), nursing director (ND), clinic administrator (CA), home health director (HH), registration supervisor (REG), and business manager (BM). The administrative staff brought in a certified diabetes educator (CDE) and an evaluation consultant from the University of Arizona College of Nursing to work with them.

For the implementation stage a new set of stakeholders was added. SEHC clinic staff, including nurses and medical assistants, became primary stakeholders, as did the clinic's primary care providers.

Step 4: Defining Core Interventions

SEHC goals for the diabetes DM program required a comprehensive approach that included prevention, early detection, systematic treatment, and a range of interventions to minimize the development and progression of complications. Given the desired scope of the program, the menu of interventions that was envisioned included screening and risk assessment, primary care using evidence-based guidelines, patient education, and case management services.

Once the goals and scope of the diabetes DM program were established, members of the team began to work on the DM template (Figure 7-3). Each of the steps required for program implementation was identified. Expected timeframes and individuals accountable for leading each step were also specified.

CASE STUDY 7-1 ■ Disease Management in a Clinic Setting

Since 1961, St. Elizabeth of Hungary Clinic's (SEHC) mission has been to provide healthcare and social services to underserved and uninsured individuals and families in southern Arizona. In 2000 SEHC had more than 18,000 active clients and more than 46,000 visits for SEHC services. The vast majority of individuals seen at SEHC are Hispanic. SEHC provides services for individuals of all ages and races.

Operating with a staff of two full-time physicians and three nurse practitioners, SEHC has more than 150 volunteer physicians and dentists who deliver primary and specialty care at the clinic or in their private offices. SEHC also has a home health and outreach service that provides home visiting and community case management. For the past 3 years, SEHC's home health and outreach services have used state funding to create and coordinate a volunteer health professional program that delivers health education programs to vulnerable groups in the community, such as senior centers, assisted living centers, homeless shelters, and foster care homes.

SEHC has established community partnerships with numerous agencies that support its mission. For example, the local Catholic Social Services offers a variety of bilingual social support and case management services. It also provides counseling for multicultural patients who have behavioral health issues such as anxiety, depression, domestic violence, parenting problems, as well as other services. The

Portable, Practical Education Program (PPEP) is another large community agency that offers behavioral health services with a primary focus on domestic violence and substance and chemical abuse. The local YWCA offers a very experienced Promotora (Community Health Advisor) Outreach Program that provides lay health workers who deliver health education and social service referrals that focus on chronic illness management and women's health issues in multicultural communities. The community-wide network of programs and services targeting similar populations provides an excellent infrastructure for integrated DM across service settings.

SEHC's delivery model is illustrated in Figure 7-2. The model is adapted from Lamb and Zazworsky's Chronic Illness Model (Lamb and Zazworsky, 2002). It emphasizes an integrated approach to primary prevention, DM, and acute care episode management through a continuum of low-cost or volunteer care and community partnerships.

SEHC operationalizes this model through two standing committees. The multidisciplinary Clinical Care Support Committee tracks and analyzes monthly referrals and oversees process improvements related to patient barriers and system/practitioner issues. The Quality Improvement Committee follows AmbuQual II Guidelines for ambulatory care and addresses issues related to access, satisfaction, and clinical practice.

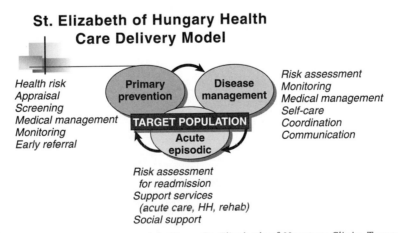

St. Elizabeth of Hungary Health Care Delivery Model

Health risk
Appraisal
Screening
Medical management
Monitoring
Early referral

Primary prevention

Disease management

TARGET POPULATION

Acute episodic

Risk assessment
Monitoring
Medical management
Self-care
Coordination
Communication

Risk assessment
for readmission
Support services
(acute care, HH, rehab)
Social support

Figure 7-2 Disease management model. (From St. Elizabeth of Hungary Clinic, Tucson, Arizona.)

Step 5: Implementing Disease Management: Tools and Strategies

The Diabetes DM program at SEHC adapted the FAST approach to DM (Lamb and Zazworsky, 2000). The model was operationalized as follows:

■ **F**ind: Identify the patients at the time of enrollment (proactive) or through database query (retrospective).

■ **A**ssess: All patients are assessed through a standardized risk assessment tool.

■ **S**tratify: Patients are stratified into low-, moderate-, and high-risk categories to receive appropriate interventions.

■ **T**reat, **T**rain, and **T**rack: All patients receive medical treatment and self-care education based on their level of risk and treatment guidelines. In addition,

	Date	Person
1. Risk assessments		
a. Establish risk assessment tool for current patients wih diabetes.	June	HH, MD, ND
b. Identify risk assessment process for new/potential patients with diabetes upon registration.	June	HH, MD, ND
c. Train appropriate staff on risk assessment processes.	August	HH, CDE
d. Perform risk assessment on current patients with diabetes.	Sept-Oct	
e. Implement risk assessment for new/potential patients with diabetes	November and ongoing	
2. Patient education		
a. Develop interventions for low, moderate, and high-risk patients with diabetes.	July	CDE, MD, HH, ND
b. Develop interventions for patients who are at low and high potential risk for developing diabetes	July	CDE, MD, HH, ND
c. Develop patient education into provider guidelines	July	CDE, HH
3. Staff education (physicians, nurses, MAs, dieticians, registration, etc.)		
a. Educate staff guidelines for patient education and case management inteventions.	August	CDE, HH
b. Educate staff on provider clinical protocol flow sheet	November	CDE, MD, HH
c. Educate staff on outcome measures	August	CDE, MD, HH
4. Evaluation and reporting structures (attach specific reports)		
a. Develop financial tracking with business office of grant expenditures.	July	HH, CA, BM
b. Develop clinical care support quarterly report of participants referred to nutrition counseling and nurse case management	July	HH
c. Develop evaluation plan for outcome measurements: • Clinical (HbA$_{1c}$) • Satisfaction (patient, provider, staff)	July	MD, ND, HH, CDE
5. Information systems support		
a. Establish codes in patient data base for nutrition visits, diabetes education visits, and nurse case management visits	June/July	CA, BM, HH
b. Establish risk assessment clinic codes	June/July	HH
c. Establish quarterly query of ICD-9 diabetes codes	June/July	CA
6. Physician coordination		
a. Establish provider clinical provider flow sheet	November	MD, CDE, HH
b. Identify clinical outcomes measures.	June/July	MD
7. Care coordination (specify care coordination efforts in hospital, community, rehab, etc.)		
a. Establish referral process with clinical care support system: • Diabetes patient education • Nurse case management/home health • Nutrition counseling	July	HH, ND
8. Communication plan		
a. Develop and disseminate patient communication materials	September	HH, ND, CA
b. Develop provider referral forms	September	HH, MD
c. Include in clinic brochures for patients and volunteers	September	HH, CA
d. Develop poster for community and clinic displays	September	HH, CA
e. Write regular articles in clinic newsletter and brochure	Ongoing	HH
9. Community referrals		
a. Identify community partnerships (YWCA, hospital programs, American Diabetic Association, etc.)	August	HH, ND, CDE
b. Develop available services and referral criteria.	August	HH, CA
10. Patient and caregiver support		
a. Identify barriers to care and support needs	July and ongoing	HH, MD, ND, support staff
11. Pharmacy/equipment		
a. Obtain grants and patient assistance programs to support medication needs.	November	HH
b. Obtain grant support for glucometers and strips	November	HH
c. Obtain grant to purchase DCA machines for on-site HbA$_{1c}$	January	HH

Note: Dates and initials are used as examples only.

Figure 7-3 St. Elizabeth of Hungary Clinic Disease Management Template: diabetes. (From St. Elizabeth of Hungary Clinic, Tucson, Arizona.)

patients are tracked in a database to monitor adherence to the DM protocols and the outcomes achieved. This model was implemented in 2001 after the FAST action plan discussed here.

Find:

- Identify all new patients at the time of enrollment to the Main Clinic or Outreach Clinics.
- Identify existing patients through the database by International Classification of Diseases, Ninth Revision, Clinical Modification (**ICD-9-CM**) codes.

Assess:

- During eligibility/enrollment, perform the American Diabetes Association's (ADA's) Diabetes Risk Assessment for potential risk for diabetes.
- Perform chart audits on all existing patients with type 2 diabetes, following the risk assessment tool. The diabetes consultant assisting SEHC in implementing the diabetes DM program developed the chart audit tool.

Stratify:

- Place patients into low-, moderate-, and high-risk categories. These categories are important because they assist the staff in deciding on the core interventions.

Treat:

- Develop and implement treatment guidelines and protocols according to risk categories.
- Develop self-care education guidelines and programs for patients according to risk categories.
- Specify interventions by risk category (Box 7-4).

Train:

- Develop and implement education guidelines and programs for patients.
- Train staff on the use of guidelines and other program materials.

Track:

- Develop systems to track the following outcome indicators:

- Patient outcomes (clinic visits, home visits, nurse case management visits, education visits, adherence to treatment, HbA_{1c})
- Cost outcomes (hospitalizations, complications, service utilization)
- Patient and provider satisfaction
- Generate reports at specified intervals.

Disease Management Tools

Two tools provided a prospective and retrospective risk assessment process for newly enrolled patients (Unknown Risk for Diabetes) and the currently active clinic patients diagnosed with diabetes (Known Persons with Diabetes).

1. *Unknown Risk for Diabetes*: A commercially available automated Diabetes Risk Assessment tool was used. Several similar tools that follow the standard questions from the ADA diabetes risk questionnaire may be used.
2. *Known Persons with Diabetes*: The certified diabetes educator consultant developed this risk assessment tool. The tool uses a Likert-type scale for parameters specified in current diabetes standards of care, including HbA_{1c}, blood pressure, low density lipoprotein (LDL), foot examination, urine protein level, and eye examination for retinopathy.

Integration of Practice Guidelines and Pathways

The Diabetes Quality Indicator (Figure 7-4) was developed as a flow sheet for the SEHC clinical record. The form incorporated the current collaborative evidence-based standards developed by the American Medical Association (AMA), the ADA, and the Joint Commission on the Accreditation of Healthcare Organizations (JCAHO) (http://www.ama-assn.org\ama\pub\category\3798.html). The recommendations cover each of the core areas of diabetes management. The flow sheet integrates management of the comorbidities associated with diabetes, such as hypertension, decline in kidney function, retinopathy, and periperal neuropathy.

For efficiency, several practitioners can be involved in documenting the data on the flow sheet. At SEHC, medical assistants perform and document vital signs on the flow sheet while the physician or nurse practitioner

---

BOX 7-4 Interventions by Risk Category for Diabetes Disease Management Program

Low (Potential Risk)	Moderate (Diabetes Controlled)	High (Diabetes Controlled)
Clinic visits	Clinic visits	Clinic visits
One-to-one education	One-to-one education	One-to-one education
Lobby education	Lobby education	Lobby education
CDE consult	CDE consult	Nurse case management

CDE, Certified diabetes educator.

St. Elizabeth of Hungary Clinic
Diabetes Quality Indicators: Clinical

St.Elizabeth of Hungary Clinic
140 W. Speedway Blvd
Tucson, AZ 85705-7698
(520) 628-7871

Patient: _____ DOB: _____

MR# _____ Provider: _____

		Frequency	Baseline	3 mo	6 mo	9 mo	1 year
	Date/Initials						
Assessment	FS blood glucose R or F	qvisit					
	HbA$_{1c}$	quarterly					
	Blood pressure 130/80	qvisit					
	Urine protein dip	Annual					
	Height	Annual					
	Weight	qvisit					
	Body mass index (BMI)	qvisit					
Lab	Chol/TG <200/200	Annual					
	HDL/LDL >45/<100	Annual					
	Micro Protein (If protein dip negative)	Annual					
	BUN/Creatinine	Annual					
Interventions	Oral agents Y or N	qvisit					
	Insulin Y or N	qvisit					
	ACE inhibitor if hypertensive Y or N	qvisit					
	ACE inhibitor if proteinuric Y or N	qvisit					
	Statin Y or N	qvisit					
	ASA Y or N	qvisit					
	Vaccines Specify (i.e., flu, pneumonia, etc)	Annual					
PE	Full physical exam Y or N	Annual					
	Eye exam Re or C	Annual					
	Foot exam Re or C	qvisit					
Self-care	SMBG and records S or SME	qvisit					
	Meal plan S or SME	qvisit					
	Physical activity S or SME	qvisit					
	Medication instruction S or SME	qvisit					
	Tobacco cessation S or SME	qvisit					

S=Satisfactory   SME=Self-Management Education Referral   R=Random   F=Fasting   Re=Referred   C=Completed

This flow sheet indicates recommended services to be provided in the continuing care of persons with diabetes. The frequency of each service is a recommendation from the American Diabetes Association. Document values where indicated. Any discussions with patients or significant others should be documented in the "notes" section in date order.

Signature	Initials	Signature	Initials

Figure 7-4 St. Elizabeth of Hungary Clinic Diabetes Quality Indicator: clinical. (From St. Elizabeth of Hungary Clinic, Tucson, Arizona.)

documents laboratory results, specific examinations, medications, and self-care management interventions. Charting by exception expedites this type of documentation system. The provider only charts problems (i.e., abnormal findings) in the progress notes. In this scenario, the problem is noted along with interventions and plan of care. This type of framework facilitates the CQI process and outcomes management. Information is readily accessible and easy to audit. The format also can be computerized.

Key recommendations from guidelines also may also be integrated into clinical pathways/case management plans, improvement action plans, and flow sheets to provide more detail to guide decision making and interventions.

Procedure: Diabetes case management	
Date/Time MAP initiated:	
Followed by case manager:	YES [ ] NO [ ]
(If yes) name:	
Social worker (if applicable):	
Goals mutually set with patient and/or family:	

	YES [ ]	
	NO [ ] EXPLAIN:	

Date	Name/Signature	Initials/Title

Figure 7-5 Multidisciplinary action plan. (From St. Elizabeth of Hungary Clinic, Tucson, Arizona.)

Continued

For example, clinical pathways and MAPs are usually organized to track whether goals have been achieved and to determine what alternatives to consider if there are any differences between expected and actual goals.

The Diabetes Case Management MAP (Figure 7-5) is an example of a tool developed by SEHC to mirror the Diabetes **Quality Indicator.** This tool continues to support the recommended evidence-based interventions outlined by the AMA, ADA, and JCAHO. It also incorporates case management interventions that are appropriate for high-risk patients with diabetes.

The Diabetes Case Management MAP is completed for patients at regularly defined intervals, usually once a month for high-risk individuals. This tool follows the same charting by exception process as the Clinical Quality Indicator Flow Sheet. The only time additional notes need to be written are when the patient has a **"variance"** from the desired outcome (i.e., a deviation from the norm). Anytime a variance occurs, the case manager documents in the progress notes the reason for variance and notes the interventions and/or changes needed to be made in the plan of care.

The risk assessment and practice guideline tools were implemented using a systematic process. SEHC implemented a 3-month pilot program in which all registration personnel administered the Diabetes Risk Assessment for all new and reenrolled patients into the clinic. More than 500 patients were assessed for diabetes risk during this period. Of the patients who completed the Diabetes Risk Assessment, 22% rated high risk for diabetes. All current patients with diabetes were followed using the Clinical Quality Indicator Flow Sheet. High-risk patients were assigned to case managers for case management services and interventions.

Step 6: Overseeing the Evaluation and Process Improvement Activities

The results of the pilot demonstrated benefits and opportunities for improvement in the new DM program. Early identification of at-risk patients was a major benefit. However, registration staff were unable to manage this new responsibility at the same time that new state requirements for insurance screening were put into place. Systematic tracking of patients' experiences suggested that certain populations had higher clinic "no-show" rates than others and did not follow up on recommended referrals. Additional staff needs for education also were identified during the pilot program.

St. Elizabeth of Hungary Clinic
Nurse Case Management Assessment
Elements of Care

Physician/NP:
DIAGNOSIS:
DATE:

MAP DOES NOT REPLACE MD ORDERS		NOTES
Tests/ procedures/ treatment	FBG and Random Lipids (Clinic visit) HbA_{1c} (Qtrly clinic visit) Proteinuria (Clinic visit) Annual retinal exam	
Assessments	Height and weight Blood pressure and pulse/heart rate Foot exam	
Medications	1. Diabetic (none, sulf, biguaride, TZD, Megal, Alpha Glu, Insulin-type) 2. Cardiac 3. Antihypertensives 4. Statins 5. Other	
Activities of daily living—functional limitations	Employment Functional status Tolerance of physical activity Recreation Mechanisms of adaptation	
Patient's perceptions of needs	Potential for rehabilitation Relationships with significant others, care givers Roles in life (e.g., mother, teacher, wife, daughter) Hope/s, goal/s for the future Depression	
Patient education	Survival skills: 1. Meal plan 2. Medications 3. Treat low blood sugar 4. When to call 5. Self blood glucose monitoring	
Dietician	Meal plan	
Social work	Family, money, transportation	
Consults/ referrals	Endocrinology Dermatology Cardiology Wound management Ophthalmology Psychology/psychiatry Podiatry Nephrology Infectious disease Clergy Other:	

Figure 7-5—cont'd   Multidisciplinary action plan. (From St. Elizabeth of Hungary Clinic, Tucson, Arizona.)

The SEHC Quality Improvement Committee analyzed these system and patient issues that created barriers to effective program performance. A quality improvement plan was developed and implemented to reduce barriers and improve key processes. For example, SEHC expanded its community partnerships to increase outreach to high-risk populations with high "no-show" rates and poor follow-up on referrals. Training sessions were provided on-site to SEHC's nursing and support staff.

Today, SEHC's diabetes DM program has been in place for over 1 year. Evaluations of targeted outcomes show the following results:

■ 46% of the moderate- to high-risk patients with diabetes have reduced their HbA_{1c} levels

■ 85% of the records have completed Diabetes Quality Indicator flow sheets

New information systems have been implemented that permit tracking of other outcomes of interest. SEHC currently analyzes the number of primary care, dietician, education, and nurse case management visits for each patient. In the future, members of the diabetes DM program will be able to link program interventions and the achievement of targeted outcomes.

DM programs have considerable promise for organizing and improving the care of populations commonly served by case managers. Emerging models of DM emphasize aspects of care that are essential to case

St. Elizabeth of Hungary Clinic
MULTIDISCIPLINARY ACTION PLAN

PATIENT PROBLEM AND NURSING INTERVENTION	EXPECTED PATIENT OUTCOME AND/OR DISCHARGE OUTCOME	ASSESSMENT/ EVALUATION		
Physiological outcomes **Potential for altercation in:**				
1. HbA$_{1c}$ 2. FBG and Random 3. Height and weight (BMI) 4. Blood pressure 5. Heart rate 6. Foot exam	1. 6-7 2. <100 FBG or <140 RBG 3. 26 4. <140/90 5. <100 6. 0 or 1			
Medications outcomes **Potential for nonadherence to medication regimen:**				
1. Provide patient with list of prescribed meds, purpose of each, and times to take. 2. Prioritize meds list for patient to rank order of importance. 3. Review meds list with patient monthly	1. Patient will be able to describe meds taken and carry list of those taken daily. 2. Patient will report perceived side effects and changes in med regimen to NCM. 3. Patient will maintain or modify regimen based on directions by provider.			
Educational outcomes **Potential for knowledge deficit related to:**	**Patient describes/demonstrates:**			
1. Meal plan 2. Treat low blood sugar 3. When to call physician/NP or NCM 4. Adequate self blood glucose monitoring 5. Medication regimen 6. Importance of skin integrity to avoid infection *Review appropriate information for any unmet desired outcome in this category*	1. Good nutrition and diet restrictions 2. S/S of low blood sugar and how to treat. 3. When to call Physician/NP or NCM 4. Consequences of inadequate self blood glucose monitoring 5. Prescribed meds, their purpose, and times taken 6. Adheres to recommended skin checks			
Psychological outcomes **Potential for intolerance of plan of care:**				
1. Involve family in support with adherence to treatment regimen and follow-up appts. 2. Discuss/review consequences of inadequate self-care management. 3. Discuss/review long-term effects of gradual inadequate self-care management.	1. Will be able to describe conditions and their responsibilities in maintaining health status. 2. Will show up for scheduled appts. 3. Will complete all scheduled treatments.			
Psychological outcomes **Potential for depression:**				
1. In the last 4 weeks, how much of the time have you felt downhearted or blue? (a) all (b) most (c) some (d) little (e) none *Discuss with patient and/or refer to appropriate counseling resources*	1. Patient reports some, little, or no feelings of down-heartedness.			

Figure 7-5—cont'd Multidisciplinary action plan. (From St. Elizabeth of Hungary Clinic, Tucson, Arizona.)

management practice, including coordination, continuity, and communication. In addition, these models focus on achieving important quality and cost outcomes based on systematic attention to evidence-based guidelines, case management services, and quality improvement processes.

As DM programs continue to evolve, case managers have a significant opportunity to lead the development of systematic and innovative interventions for individuals at risk. Armed with the principles and tools of DM, case managers can improve health-care for increasingly vulnerable populations.

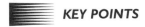 **KEY POINTS**

I. DM programs are designed to create better systems for managing common high-risk chronic conditions.

2. Case managers are key to the DM process because they focus on individuals and populations most likely to have complications or adverse health outcomes.

3. The overall effects of DM programs on cost and quality are still unclear and require additional research.

4. Evidence-based practice guidelines are an important tool and framework for the core program interventions of a DM program.

5. Risk assessment tools are valuable in placing patients into risk categories, which then drive the appropriate type and intensity of case management interventions.

REFERENCES

Bazzoli GJ, Shortell SM, Ciliberto F, et al: Tracking the changing provider landscape: Implications for health policy and practice, *Health Affairs* 20(6):188-196, 2002.

Berger M, Muhlhauser I: Diabetes care and patient-oriented outcomes, *JAMA* 281(18):1676-1678, 1999.

Bodenheimer T: Disease management: promises and pitfalls, *N Engl J Med* 340(15):1202-1205, 1999.

Bodenheimer T: Disease management in the American market, *BMJ* 320(7234):563-566, 2000.

Boult C, Dowd B, McCaffrey D, et al: Screening elders for risk of hospital admission, *J Am Geriatr Soc* 41:811-817, 1993.

Chen A, Brown R, Archibald N, et al: *Best practices in coordinated care, Mathematica Policy Research*, Inc., Reference No. 8534-004, 2000. Available online at http://www.mathematicampr.com/3rdLevel/bestprac.htm/ (accessed April 1, 2001).

Clark CM, Snyder JW, Meek RL, et al: A systematic approach to risk stratification and intervention within a managed care environment improves outcomes and patient satisfaction, *Diabetes Care* 24(6):1079-1086, 2001.

Coye MJ: No Toyotas in health care: why medical care has not evolved to meet patients' needs, *Health Affairs* 20(6):44-56, 2002.

Fernandez A, Grumbach K, Vranizan K, et al: Primary care physicians' experience with disease management programs, *J Gen Intern Med* 16(3):163-167, 2001.

Harris JM: Disease management: new wine in new bottles, *Ann Intern Med* 124(9):838-842, 1996.

Hoffman C, Rice D, Sung HY: Persons with chronic conditions: their prevalence and costs, *JAMA* 276(18):1473-1479, 1996.

Homer CJ: Asthma disease management, *JAMA* 337(20):1461-1463, 1997.

Hunter DJ, Fairfield G: Managed care: disease management, *BMJ* 315(7099):50-53, 1997.

Lamb G, Zazworsky D: Improving outcomes fast, *Advance for Providers of Post-Acute Care* 39(1):28-29, 2000.

Leider HL: Gaining physician buy-in for disease management initiatives, *Dis Manage Health Outcomes* 6(6):327-333, 1999.

McAlister FA, Lawson FME, Teo KT, et al: A systematic review of randomized trials of disease management programs in heart failure, *Am J Med* 110:378-384, 2001.

Pacala JT, Boult C, Boult L: Predictive validity of a questionnaire that identifies older persons at risk for hospital admission, *J Am Geriatr Soc* 45:373-377, 1995.

Pacala JT, Boult C, Reed R, et al: Predictive validity of the Pra instrument among older recipients of managed care, *J Am Geriatr Soc* 45:614-617, 1997.

Rich M: Heart failure disease management programs: efficacy and limitations, *Am J Med* 110(5):410-412, 2001.

Rosenstein AH: Measuring the benefits of clinical decision support: return on investment, *Health Care Manage Rev* 23(2):32-43, 1999.

Shelton P, Sager M, Schraeder C: The Community Assessment Risk Screen (CARS): identifying elderly persons at risk for hospitalization or emergency department visit, *Am J Manag Care* 6(8):925-933, 2000.

Todd WE, Ladon EH: Disease management: maximizing treatment adherence and self-management, *Dis Manage Health Outcomes* 3(1):1-10, 1998.

Vojta CL, Vojta DD, TenHave TR, et al: Risk screening in a Medicare/Medicaid population: administrative data versus self-report, *J Gen Intern Med* 16:525-530, 2001.

Wagner EH: The role of patient care teams in chronic disease management, *BMJ* 320(7234):569-572, 2000.

Wagner EH, Davis C, Schaefer J, et al: A survey of leading chronic disease management programs: are they consistent with the literature? *Manag Care Q* 7(3):56-65, 1999.

Ware JE Jr: The status of health assessment 1994, *Annu Rev Public Health* 16:327-354, 1994.

8

Skills for Successful Case Management

Professional nurses, case managers, and social workers have been key advocates in the provision of quality healthcare. Their broad skills and training allow them to assess patients' needs and to work well with families and other members of the healthcare team. Negotiating, collaborating, communicating, team building, precepting, educating, and consulting are the basis of what a successful case manager brings to the care setting each day.

The application of the nursing and case management processes is concerned with the whole person and the full range of patient needs. This clearly leads to comprehensive and consistent care. Much has been written about the nursing process and its unique qualities. Yura and Walsh (1983) noted the following, which is still applicable today: In contrast to the goals of the other members of the health profession, the nurse is involved with human needs that affect the *total* person rather than one aspect, one problem, or a limited segment of need fulfillment.

Case management is no different in its approach to successful coordination of patient care than that of nursing or those applied by other professionals. The role of the **case manager,** by its definition as outlined in the *Case Management Society of America's Standards of Practice for Case Management* (2002), upholds and expounds on the nursing process. **Case management** is a collaborative process used to assess, plan, implement, coordinate, monitor, and evaluate options and services to meet individuals' health needs through communication and available resources to promote quality, cost-effective **outcomes.**

The case manager's expertise is the vital link between the individual, the provider, the payer, and the community. Successful outcomes cannot be achieved without using all of the specialized skills and knowledge applied through the case management process. It must

be emphasized that the skills necessary to be a successful case manager are not possessed by everyone. Case managers need to be clinically astute and competent in areas of practice. It is important for case managers to be skilled in the application of the case management process and to acquire the assessment skills that make them better able to identify the patient's actual and potential health problems. This allows them to implement the required interventions to successfully resolve these problems and to evaluate the outcomes of care and responses to treatments (Bower, 1992).

Not all nurses acquire the professional credentials, education, and expertise in the application of the nursing process to succeed as a case manager. Case managers are notoriously consummate organizers, paid to be in control of what many would regard as sheer chaos. Does their skill for organization derive from a compulsive personality, years of experience, mastering the nursing process, or a balanced blend of all of these components? One would believe the latter to be true. As long as there is a subtle balance of the dynamics a case manager possesses, there will be a positive effect.

How does this overview translate and apply to the required skills necessary for today's successful case managers? The section that follows categorizes and details each function and skill that becomes a critical element when providing the services of an effective case manager (Box 8-1).

NURSING PROCESS
Assessment

Assessment is an ongoing and continuous process occurring with all patient–case manager interactions. It is during the assessment phase that the case manager seeks a better understanding of the patient, the family

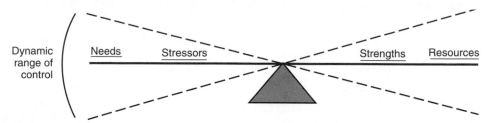

Figure 8-1 The health balance model. (Redrawn from Rorden JW, Taft E: *Discharge planning guide for nurses,* Philadelphia, 1990, WB Saunders.)

BOX 8-1 Functions and Skills for Effective Case Management

Nursing Process
1. Assessment
2. Planning
3. Implementation
4. Coordination
5. Evaluation

Leadership Skills
1. Patient advocate
2. Facilitator
3. Negotiator
4. Quality improvement coordinator
5. Utilization manager
6. Educator
7. Financial analyst/consult
8. Decision maker
9. Critical thinker
10. Data manager and analyst

Communication/Interpersonal Skills
1. Team building
2. Customer relations
3. Public speaking
4. Conflict resolution
5. Delegation
6. Information sharing
7. Systems thinking
8. Emotional intelligence

---

dynamics, and the healthcare beliefs and/or myths. An assessment generally involves three phases, which at times seem inseparable: gathering data, evaluating data, and determining an appropriate nursing diagnosis. Case managers use a multifaceted subgroup of skills (Rorden and Taft, 1990) to assess a patient's needs accurately:

- Interviewing skills that include the ability not only to listen but also to formulate insightful questions
- Interpretation skills that allow the case manager to understand what patients say about their concerns and symptoms and to transmit this information

to other **caregivers** using concise and appropriate terminology
- Nonverbal communication skills that permit the case manager to recognize responses to treatments that reflect the patient's moods, attitudes, and psychosocial needs
- Relationship skills that cut across potential social and cultural barriers to promote trust with patients, family members, and professional colleagues
- Observational skills that allow the case manager to distinguish normal from abnormal functioning and to recognize subtle changes in patients' responses to treatments
- Evaluation skills that permit the case manager to consider the facts about a patient's condition, as well as the interconnection and balance between strengths and weaknesses
- Goal-setting skills that help the case manager see beyond the immediate needs to identify intermediate and long-term goals of care

As an assessor, the case manager must obtain relevant data through skillful investigation. All of the information related to the current plan must be evaluated with a critical eye to objectively identify trends, set and reset realistic goals, and seek viable alternatives as necessary.

Part of being a successful assessor is to find a delicate health balance for each patient. Needs and demands are balanced by strengths and resources. When there is a balance between these factors, there can be positive movement. When a patient is in acute distress, patient needs may be only the obvious; however, if a health balance is to occur or to be restored, the case manager must uncover factors that influence the relationships between needs, strengths, and resources. A representation of this health balance model is shown in Figure 8-1 (Rorden and Taft, 1990). Case Study 8-1 presents an example of the use of the health balance model during the assessment of a patient.

A vital case management skill is the ability to recognize a patient's health problems and formulate diagnoses based on the subjective and objective data collected during the assessment. The diagnoses express

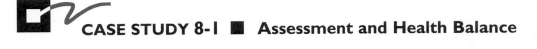

CASE STUDY 8-1 ■ Assessment and Health Balance

Ms. J. Mazure is a 50-year-old professional career woman. She recently noticed excessive vaginal bleeding. A Pap smear revealed a malignancy, leading to the need for a hysterectomy. From this you must begin to assess the health needs of the patient and work toward the balance.

You will use a range of skills to help you identify the changes in this patient's health balance as a result of her hysterectomy.

You must also explore the patient's strengths and resources, such as insurance benefits and employee sick leave, as well as evaluate stresses and demands such as the self-imposed pressure of missing work, work responsibilities piling up in her absence, and familial obligations that she temporarily will not be able to handle. By using the health balance, you can connect the physical and the psychosocial aspects of the patient's care with the patient's strengths and available resources.

---

the case manager's judgment of the patient's clinical condition, functional abilities, responses to treatments, healthcare needs, psychosocial support, financial status, and postdischarge needs.

Planning

Planning is the next step in managing the patient's care. This is accomplished by planning the treatment modalities and interventions necessary for meeting the needs of patients and families. During the planning phase the case manager, in collaboration with the other members of the healthcare team, determines the goals of treatment and the projected **length of stay** and, immediately on admission, initiates the transitional plan of care. The determination of goals is vitally important because it provides a clear timeframe for accomplishing the care activities needed (O'Malley, 1988). Case managers must identify immediate short- and long-term needs, as well as where and how these needs will be met.

Planning is initiated as the patient is admitted or before admission to any healthcare setting. The case manager's clinical expertise is quickly tapped into when establishing whether the treatment plan and interventions are appropriate. Data are assimilated, diagnoses are established, and a multidisciplinary plan of care begins to unfold.

Throughout the acute hospital, subacute, home care, or long-term care stay, the case manager monitors and reevaluates the plan for accuracy as the patient's condition changes. As a planner, the case manager identifies a treatment plan while remaining cognizant of the patient outcomes and minimization of payer liability. The case manager must include the patient and family in decision making and consider the patient's goals as an integral part of the care plan. Alternate plans must always be incorporated in anticipation of sudden shifts in the treatment process or in response to treatments yielding complications. Case Study 8-2 illustrates the principles of successful planning.

Implementation and Coordination

Implementation and *coordination* involve building the plan, determining the goals of patient care, and deciding what needs to be accomplished to make a viable and realistic plan move to completion. The aim of the case manager at this point is to give the patient and family the knowledge, attitudes, and skills necessary for the implementation of the established plan. Through communication, collaboration, and teaching, the case manager works with the multidisciplinary team to motivate the patient to succeed in fulfilling the plan of care determined by all of the participants. Abraham Maslow (1970), in his theory of the hierarchy of needs, suggested that everyone seeks fulfillment of general needs and that these needs motivate behavior. At a time of high stress or ill health, people seek to fulfill more basic needs, such as survival and safety. The higher needs of self and creativity do not seem as much a priority at this time (Maslow, 1970).

The case manager needs to be aware of this theory of motivation when trying to elicit decisions about **discharge planning** or future goals for a patient. The patient and family must first reach a level of awareness that enables them to focus on the goals of the care plan. They must then reach a level of understanding at which they learn in greater depth what the patient's needs and the available options are, the likely consequences of these options, and what aspects of self-care need to be learned. It is at this juncture that motivation will take place and the implementation of the plan will come to fruition.

As the patient nears discharge, the case manager can take three steps to improve the chances of effective implementation of the plan: clarifying the transfer of responsibilities of care, reviewing the plan to ensure that nothing has been overlooked, and making last-minute alterations and arrangements for the immediate discharge period. Following these steps will confirm the plan for continuing care (Case Manager's Tip 8-1). Case Study 8-3 presents an

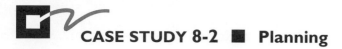

CASE STUDY 8-2 ■ Planning

Mrs. Smith is a 25-year-old married woman with a history of miscarriage and no living children. She is now hospitalized for the second time during her pregnancy. She is admitted with a diagnosis of preterm labor at 30 weeks gestation with a low-lying placenta. Mrs. Smith was home only 2 days after her first hospitalization before cramping and vaginal bleeding began and she was readmitted. She is very anxious about delivering early. She lives in an upstairs apartment and has no family support to help her. You have assessed her needs to include the following:

■ Preterm labor requiring medical intervention
■ Teaching about her preterm labor to reduce her anxiety
■ Motivation to comply with the probable bedrest regimen that is ahead of her

■ Investigation of the need for home care to follow up on her pregnancy and medical regimen while at home

You quickly establish that the patient's apartment is a problematic setting and determine the need to put home care into the plan because visits to the physician's office would need to be minimized and bed rest maximized. You also educate Mrs. Smith's husband about preterm labor and the importance of his wife's maintaining bed rest. The overall plan includes the patient's goal of returning home as soon as possible. You plan clear guidelines for patient compliance and establish community resources to meet the goal of leaving the hospital. By using a step-by-step planning process and going beyond the walls of the acute care setting, you are able to meet the needs of this patient while maintaining quality, safe care.

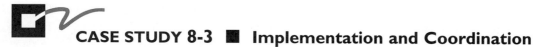

CASE STUDY 8-3 ■ Implementation and Coordination

You recently thought all steps were taken to provide a safe discharge plan for your cardiac patient. The patient's plan included an ambulance to bring the patient home from the hospital because he had no family support or means of transportation. Shortly after his departure from the hospital, the ambulance driver called the medical unit rather displeased with the lack of assessment and planning done for this patient. Apparently the address given for the patient's home did not exist and was a vacant lot.

After investigating the situation further it was discovered that the patient's medical record had an address from a previous hospitalization that was no longer valid. No one had verified where the patient lived or reconfirmed his address during the assessment or planning phase. This situation could have been avoided by following the simple steps to implementation, thus avoiding a distressful and embarrassing situation for the patient, you, and the hospital.

CASE MANAGER'S TIP 8-1

The Importance of Confirming the Plan

Taking the time and making the effort to confirm the plan greatly increase the probability of the plan's effective and efficient implementation. Follow-through will help ensure that the goals are met.

example of what can happen to implementation if a step-by-step approach of assessment, diagnosis, planning, and coordination does not take place.

Evaluation

The final step in the nursing process, *evaluation*, is designed to measure the patient's response to a formulated

plan and at the same time to ensure the appropriateness of the care plan and the quality of the services and products being offered to the patient.

To achieve successful evaluation and outcomes, the case manager must routinely assess and reassess the patient's status and progress toward reaching the goals set forth in the plan of care. If the situation is at a halt or regressing rather than moving forward, the case manager must then make appropriate adjustments and alter the plan accordingly.

The following important questions must be asked as the evaluation proceeds:

■ Were the patient's needs identified early in the hospital stay?
■ Were learning goals identified and teaching documented?
■ Were referrals complete and timely?

CASE MANAGER'S TIP 8-2

Applicability of Skills to Different Settings

Keep in mind that all of the skills delineated in this chapter are applicable to all forms of case management, including acute care, subacute care, home care, and insurance case management.

- Was the patient/family clearly able to verbalize the goals of the plan of care?
- Were the patient's/family's problems resolved?
- Did the patient/family seem satisfied with the plan and the decisions surrounding the plan?
- Did the patient/family comply with medical advice and follow the recommendations of the case manager?
- Were the services provided appropriately authorized by the managed care organization?

These questions will help the case manager to determine if the overall discharge plan for a particular patient was effective and will assist with **quality improvement** efforts for future patients. This information also is valuable when evaluating the facility's total case management program. Throughout the evaluation process, all participants in the interdisciplinary team will identify system, process, clinician, patient, and family **variances** and trend them. These trends will be further analyzed in **continuous quality improvement (CQI)** teams to improve, fine-tune, revamp, and reorganize the processes of care delivery.

The case manager must use many skills and functions of leadership to effectively master the nursing process (Case Manager's Tip 8-2). A more specific and comprehensive breakdown of these skills will add to the role dimensions of the case manager.

LEADERSHIP SKILLS AND FUNCTIONS

Because case managers function as problem solvers, resource people, and members of the multidisciplinary healthcare team, they should be highly skilled in various leadership qualities. Nursing case managers must be adept at negotiating and contracting and capable of making sound decisions and resolving conflicts. To do this successfully, they should acquire critical thinking and problem-solving skills. Because of their managerial responsibilities, case managers must be involved in quality improvement efforts, speak publicly, and write for publication.

Advocacy and Facilitation of Care Activities

The case manager's work as an *advocate* (Case Manager's Tip 8-3) for the patient is one of the most critical

 CASE MANAGER'S TIP 8-3

Advocacy Skills

Case managers can best advocate for patients and their families if they apply the following strategies:

- Keeping the patient's best interest paramount in the process of care delivery
- Recommending, coordinating, and facilitating the most effective plan of care
- Protecting the rights of patients and their self-determination
- Communicating to other providers and documenting the patient's care preferences
- Facilitating the patient's and family's decision-making activities by keeping them well informed of their rights, options, and so on.
- Clarifying the goals of therapy and treatment
- Determining the appropriateness of the postdischarge services and the discharge/transitional plan
- Ensuring that the interventions are consistent with the patient's needs and goals of treatment
- Maintaining the patient's privacy and confidentiality
- Negotiating on behalf of the patient/family with the managed care organization for authorizations of services
- Facilitating resolution of ethical conflicts
- Maintaining current knowledge of the legal and ethical requirements and standards of patient care delivery
- Preventing delays and variances in care delivery

---

elements of the role. The patient–case manager relationship is built on the ability of the case manager to be trusted; to foster mutual respect between himself or herself and the patient; and to establish a rapport that facilitates communication among the family, caregivers, payers, and other healthcare team members. As case managers gain clear understanding of the patient's needs, care desires, and goals, they communicate this understanding effectively to the members of the healthcare team. They also impact the course of treatment to effect an earlier discharge, negotiate better fees for medical supplies or equipment, or arrange for more efficient home care services.

As a *facilitator,* the case manager can be a catalyst for change by empowering the patient or family members to seek solutions throughout the acute care phase and beyond the hospital setting. The case manager is always on the lookout for quality improvement that could result in potential cost savings or possibly prolong the healthcare benefits of an individual.

The patient's best interests are always the focal point for the case manager's advocacy and care facilitation efforts, whether for needed funding, treatment options, appropriate and timely home health services, or reassessment and evaluation of goals. Case managers are concerned with every detail, sifting through the complex array of paths that can easily lead to confusion for any patient. Case managers advocate for their patients/families in three main ways. These are as follows:

1. Defending patients' rights to treatments and options
2. Helping patients to discuss their needs and preferences and to make informed choices that are consistent with their values and beliefs
3. Respecting and honoring patients' values and beliefs and helping them maintain their dignity (Powell and Ignatavicius, 2001)

Clinical Reasoning and Critical Thinking

In the practice of case management, patient, family, and healthcare provider problems continually arise. Therefore it is important that case managers are able to solve these problems. The ability of case managers to provide safe, efficient, and competent case management services depends heavily on their skills in problem solving, clinical reasoning, and critical thinking. These skills have one thing in common: they all entail the generation of possible solutions to problems, issues, or concerns regarding patient care delivery and options. Case managers use their clinical knowledge and expertise and their leadership skills for this purpose. They capitalize on their role as informal leaders of the healthcare team and facilitators of patient care delivery to solve the problems that may arise.

Case managers are constantly making decisions. They decide what observations should be made in encountered situations, derive meaning from the observations made and data collected, and decide on the actions/interventions to be taken to care for the patient or resolve the situation. The overall goal is the delivery of optimal, cost-effective, quality care.

Case managers use a framework for decision making and problem solving (Figure 8-2) that bridges the present and the future. They assess the patient's and family's current state and, based on this assessment, they envision the future state by deciding on the goals and expected outcomes of the treatments. They then implement an action plan to bring the patient and family to the desired future state. This framework enhances an outcomes-based approach to the delivery of case management services. The plan is usually interdisciplinary in nature and implemented only after approval by the healthcare team and consent and agreement by the patient and family. Understanding that the action plan may not always result in a resolution of the patient's and family's problems, issues, and concerns, case managers engage in constant reassessment, monitoring, evaluation, and revising of the plan until the desired outcomes (i.e., the future state) are achieved. Case managers complete these activities using a testing technique applied to examining the appropriateness of the action plan and the relevance of its outcomes.

The case manager's skills in decision making and clinical reasoning and judgment must always help the patient to work through the confusion he or she faces in the complex healthcare environment. Case managers operate by answering questions pertinent to the development of the plan of care, actual delivery of care, and evaluation of the discharge plan, such as those following. These questions are examples of how case managers engage in evaluating the case management action plan using the problem-solving framework shared in Figure 8-2.

- Is the current treatment plan appropriate enough to resolve the patient's problems?
- Will the current case management action plan prevent the patient from needing readmission?
- Are the treatments provided the best possible treatments for the patient and family?
- Are healthcare team members in agreement with the plan?

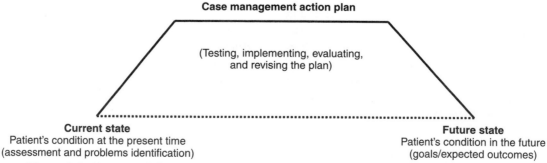

Case management action plan

(Testing, implementing, evaluating, and revising the plan)

Current state
Patient's condition at the present time
(assessment and problems identification)

Future state
Patient's condition in the future
(goals/expected outcomes)

Figure 8-2 Framework for decision making and problem solving in case management.

- Do the patient and family have any issues or disagreements with the plan?
- Should any changes be made to the plan of care or the discharge plan?
- Will the electricity in the home support a mechanical ventilator?
- Does the patient have safe access to a bathroom on the main floor of the house?
- Is it worth the hospital's financial support to fly a patient home to Florida rather than incur the cost of an extended length of stay?
- Is the family capable of learning how to perform tracheal suctioning so that their loved one can go home with them rather than to an extended nursing facility?

Answers to these questions influence the type of care a patient will receive and how it will be accomplished to ensure the best possible outcome for a patient in the most cost-effective manner. Case managers who are able to apply critical thinking and clinical reasoning skills in the decision-making process ensure appropriate, effective, and efficient care delivery. This makes certain that the patient and family will receive the necessary support, potential obstacles to the treatment plan will be avoided, the potential for readmission will decrease, the educational component of care will be reinforced, and a positive outcome and promotion of health will take place.

Negotiation

Negotiation is a skill that is not primarily taught in nursing or social work education programs. To be a successful negotiator, a case manager must be a good time manager. Along with managing their own time, case managers must learn to determine what work others can and should do in assessing a patient's needs when preparing a patient's plan of care. This understanding allows them to negotiate more effectively.

Negotiation in case management is an everyday occurrence. It is a skill used with payers and providers, with vendors for **durable medical equipment,** with the patient and family/caregiver, and even with physicians reluctant to opt for a home care discharge plan or placement in a long-term care facility. The purpose of negotiation is to reach an agreement. Fair negotiation requires trust, rapport, and complete honesty with regard to a patient's care needs. Successful negotiation (Case Manager's Tip 8-4) is achieved by being well prepared to present the facts clearly and succinctly. To know if you have negotiated your case well, you must be a good listener who tunes in to verbal and nonverbal cues; otherwise, windows of opportunity could be missed. On the financial side of the equation, we know

 CASE MANAGER'S TIP 8-4

Negotiation Skills
Strategies for better negotiation in case management
- Always have clear, factual, and pertinent data.
- Do not lose sight of your long-term goal.
- Know the players well, including their values, beliefs, and scope of responsibilities.
- Plan, prepare well, and practice before you start negotiating.
- Always have alternate solutions or options in mind.
- Cultivate an interactive, collaborative relationship rather than an antagonistic relationship.
- Focus on interests and not positions.
- Focus on the exchange of the information.
- Do not give up—persevere.
- Avoid becoming emotional.
- Trust the person you are negotiating with; distrust is destructive.
- Do not miss your chance.
- Focus on negotiation as a process and not an event.
- Ask questions.
- Avoid talking too much.
- Wait for the right moment to make your pitch
- Listen carefully and acknowledge the person you are negotiating with.
- Brainstorm for solutions.
- Be creative.
- Appreciate small wins; they are as important as the larger ones.

Strategies to avoid in negotiation
- Make the other side feel guilty.
- Offer options that are only favorable to you.
- Threaten the other side.
- Use sarcasm, cynicism, or putdown statements.
- Play games or tricks.
- Rush the process.
- Jump at the first offer.
- Give away the store.
- Try to score all the points.
- Distort the facts.
- Be emotional.
- Be aggressive.
- Deal with the other person as an enemy.

all too well that healthcare environments are committed to doing more with less and at a lower cost. Financial prowess on the part of the case manager is a must in these times of cost containment. Case managers must work with financial support personnel and help them keep abreast of a patient's insurance **health benefit** plan, no-fault coverage, or a patient's lack of finances that could lead to **Medicaid** eligibility.

According to Umiker (1996), negotiation may take three forms:

1. *Power play:* Assumes that the stronger party will win. The power play process is a form of combat in which one side makes an unfair offer and expects the other side to counter with an equally unfair demand.
2. *Taking positions:* Assumes a win-lose outcome. This is a form of haggling wherein each side adopts a fixed position and assumes an inflexible stand.
3. *Collaboration:* Assumes a problem-solving approach. This form of negotiation results in a win-win situation wherein each side desires to end up with a good deal while preserving the integrity of the other.

Collaboration is the most desired approach for negotiation by case managers. It is the only of the three forms of negotiation that allows all parties involved to win and to be pleased with the outcome. It also makes the process more efficient, positive, and amicable. The other two forms must be avoided because they tend to be unproductive and divisive and to work against building teams and effective relationships. The power play approach is usually aggressive, intimidating, and condescending; in the taking positions (haggling) approach, rather than solving problems, the process of negotiation becomes a contest of wills (Umiker, 1996).

Utilization Review and Management

Case management plans can be useful tools when determining the allocated resources for a particular diagnosis. Variance analysis or comorbid conditions can help a case manager anticipate extra costs, such as the need for longer hospitalizations, expensive antibiotic treatment, or pain management therapy.

Working alongside the hospital's controller to review the expenses incurred for various diagnoses will serve as a checks-and-balances system of appropriate allocation of funds. The case manager has a key role in being able to communicate the overutilization of laboratory tests or repetitive diagnostics or the underutilization of less-expensive antibiotics. Thus the case manager can have a major positive impact on the ability of an institution to provide the same quality of care that it is accustomed to while being more cost-efficient in the process.

Another way in which case managers affect the financial balance of an acute care setting while monitoring quality is through **utilization review** and management (see Chapter 5). Participation on a hospital length-of-stay committee is one way to monitor **utilization.** The healthcare team can then be alerted to an inappropriate admission, an unusual length of stay for a given patient, a planned premature discharge with no clear discharge plan and with potential readmission risk, or inappropriate use of resources. It is case managers who are charged with monitoring these potential financial drains on the healthcare organization. It is their high-quality efficiency that provides the organization with a safety **gatekeeping** mechanism to avoid potential utilization problems. Knowledge of utilization review and management is also effective in subacute, home care, and insurance arenas to justify or nullify care requested.

In this ever-shrinking resource environment, it becomes more and more prudent for the case manager to be an instrumental participant in payer contract negotiation, on resource management teams and **clinical pathway** development committees, and in any groups designed to promote quality care at less cost but with high efficiency. It is the driving force behind every great case manager to maximize patient outcomes and quality of care while being ever cognizant of the dwindling resources to provide that care.

Patient and Family Education

One of the last but certainly not least leadership skills is that of educator. This is a large responsibility within the case manager's role because it covers a broad scope of functions. Being a facilitator of both the patient and the staff is at times a monumental task that brings with it periods of extreme challenge. A good principle to follow is to begin with the end result in mind. First there is the mental picture of the outcome of your patient's plan of care; then you begin to formulate the blueprints and develop your construction plan to get the patient and family to the projected outcome. This idea can be conveyed through the use of the analogy of constructing a house. The blueprint for the house is meticulously designed before any physical creation of the house is begun. Without a developed blueprint, the physical creation will undoubtedly have expensive changes that could double the cost of the house. The case manager, much like the carpenter, must make sure that the blueprint (i.e., patient's plan of care) includes everything needed and that everything has been thought through (Covey, 1989).

Educating the patient and family is part of the blueprint for success. The clearer the understanding of the disease process and the course of the acute level of care, the better the plan will be. Of utmost importance is that the case manager considers educating the patient and family using language that is understood, with consideration for cultural diversity and healthcare beliefs. In our constant awareness of the pressure to reduce lengths of stay, education is sometimes elected to take a back seat. However, timely education is crucial, especially as patients experience shorter hospital stays. Placing education at the bottom of the priority list can have devastating effects on outcomes. For example, a family decides to take their loved one, who is dependent on a ventilator, home. All plans appear to be in place: the respiratory company has been arranged, the home is prepared, and the nursing visits are on standby. Everything seems to be ready, but a crucial element is missing. No one thought about the necessity to teach the family how to care for their family member at home, including expertise in ventilator function and resuscitative measures. Without this most important step of early education, the discharge plan runs the risk of failure, costly extra days in the hospital, or potential rehospitalization of the patient as a result of lack of knowledge on the part of family members or the inability to handle the patient's care.

Do the patient and family respond better to verbal or nonverbal communication, audio or video, written word or pictures, discussion or demonstration? It is the case manager who can impact the education process by serving as the resource for staff to develop or select supporting educational materials and define the best method of conveying the information (Case Manager's Tip 8-5). The case manager may also serve as a member of the patient teaching committee responsible for patient and family teaching materials or documentation tools such as the one shown in Figure 8-3.

Ensuring compliance with standards of patient and family teaching as outlined by regulatory and accreditation agencies is also a required facet of the case manager's role. Case managers are involved in nursing staff development by enhancing and disseminating new knowledge and skills. They act as mentors and preceptors of less senior staff. The knowledge of case management itself must also be conveyed across professional lines and levels of hierarchy. In addition, the community is in need of hearing and learning more about case management; that way, if a person is hospitalized or offered the option of home care, he or she will have an appropriate expectation of case management and how the case manager will be involved in the plan of care.

 CASE MANAGER'S TIP 8-5

Assessing for Readiness to Learn
The case manager must use every possible means of assessing for readiness to learn or potential barriers to learning. The preferred and most appropriate method of education must be determined.

COMMUNICATION AND OTHER INTERPERSONAL SKILLS

Communication and other interpersonal skills are the lifeline that connects each individual in any walk of life and in any organization. As our technological world moves faster, quality communication becomes essential. Many would claim that communication is the core of leadership and decision making. Without a doubt, thorough communication is a core managerial function. Therefore as managers and leaders, case managers must master effective communication to be successful. Communication is the transfer of information, ideas, understanding, or feelings. Case management is working with and through others. Communication is necessary so that each person knows his or her role in the process of accomplishing goals.

Dash et al (1996) define communication as follows:
- A complex, dynamic interchange of verbal and nonverbal messages and meanings between people, the means by which information is transferred
- The process of imparting knowledge
- A social process
- Something continuous and fluid

We take communication for granted, but in the case of quality job performance—as in the role of a case manager—it should not be treated lightly. A miscommunication or a barrier to effective communication could lead to expensive hardship for a hospital, payer, patient, or family. In fact, it is easier to miscommunicate than to communicate clearly. At any stage in the process of communication something can interfere with its effectiveness, clarity, or accuracy. This interference is called *noise*. Noise can be physical, such as a cardiac monitor beeping in a patient's ear; psychological, such as the fear of or anxiety as a result of being hospitalized; or anything else that keeps the message from getting from sender to receiver.

A communication model has at least four elements (Figure 8-4). The first element is the *sender*, as in the case manager, who transmits the communication message. The second element is the *message*, which includes the verbal (i.e., spoken or written) and nonverbal (i.e., facial expressions and body language). The third component, the *receiver*, is the person to whom the message is sent. If all goes well, the message received will be the intended message sent. The fourth component, the *context*, is the surroundings in which the communication takes place. The environment is identified by such factors as the patient's condition, cultural background, health beliefs, and values (Dash et al, 1996).

The *channel* one chooses is also a key to effective communication and must be individualized to the

MERCY
MEDICAL CENTER
1000 NORTH VILLAGE AVENUE
ROCKVILLE CENTRE, NEW YORK 11570

MOTHER / BABY NURSING EDUCATION
RECORD / DISCHARGE SUMMARY
(PAGE 1)

Interview Date:	Person Involved in Patient Teaching/Relationship:

Lives with Patient: ☐ Yes ☐ No	Primary Language Spoken:

Preferred Learning Method:
☐ Listening   ☐ Demonstration   ☐ Reading Pictures   ☐ Other

ADDRESSOGRAPH

Identified Barriers:
☐ Auditory   ☐ Visual   ☐ Cultural/Religious   ☐ Other

Comments:

OUR NURSING STAFF WISH TO GIVE YOU THE INFORMATION YOU WANT AND NEED MOST DURING YOUR STAY WITH US.
PLEASE LOOK OVER THE FOLLOWING LIST OF EDUCATIONAL TOPICS AND COMPLETE THE FORM BY PUTTING A CHECK IN THE COLUMN THAT MOST APPLIES TO YOU, USING THE FOLLOWING SCALE:
1 = MOST IMPORTANT TO LEARN BEFORE I GO HOME   2 = I WOULD LIKE TO REVIEW   3 = I ALREADY KNOW OR AM COMFORTABLE WITH

SELF ASSESSMENT CHECKLIST	1	2	3	Date Time	Nurse Initial	Mode	Code	Date Time	Nurse Initial	Mode	Code	Nurse Initial	Signature
BABY CARE													
DIAPER CHANGE													
BATH SPONGE / TUB													
TEMPERATURE													
DRESSING													
CORD CARE													
SKIN CARE / RASH													
JAUNDICE													
CIRCUMCISION CARE													
UNCIRCUMCISED BABY CARE													
BULB SYRINGE / CHOKING													
CRYING AS COMMUNICATION													
CAR SEAT													
WHEN TO CALL THE PHYSICIAN													
NOTIFY M.D. FOR SIGNS OF INFECTION													
SLEEP POSITIONS													
OTHER													
BREASTFEEDING													
LATCHING ON													
POSITIONING MOM / BABY													
FREQUENCY & LENGTHS OF FEEDINGS / BURPING													
CARE OF BREASTS / NIPPLES												Comments	
BREAST PUMP / PUMPING STORAGE													
WHEN TO CALL THE PHYSICIAN													
BOTTLE FEEDING													
LATCHING ON													
POSITIONING													
FREQUENCY & LENGTHS OF FEEDINGS / BURPING													
FEEDING WATER													
FORMULA PREPARATION													
WHEN TO CALL THE PHYSICIAN													
MOTHER CARE													
VAGINAL DISCHARGE / BLEEDING													
INCISION CARE / EPISIOTOMY CARE													
BREAST CARE-WHEN NOT BREASTFEEDING													
BLADDER / BOWEL FUNCTIONS													
ACTIVITY / REST													
NUTRITION / DIET													
EMOTIONS													
MEDICATION													
WHEN TO CALL PHYSICIAN													
OTHER													

TEACHING MODES: D = DEMONSTRATION   R = REINFORCEMENT   B = BOOKLET   H = HANDOUT   A = AUDIOVISUAL   MT = MEDICATION TEACHING RECORD
I = ICN / NBN DISCHARGE PLANNING FORM

EVALUATION CODES: 1 = UNABLE TO PERFORM / UNABLE TO UNDERSTAND*   2 = NEEDS REINFORCEMENT AND / OR PRACTICE   3 = PERFORMS / VERBALIZES UNDERSTANDING

MB-100A/95

#22110 MBS 11/96

Figure 8-3   Mother/baby nursing education record/discharge summary. (Courtesy Mercy Medical Center, Rockville Center, New York.)

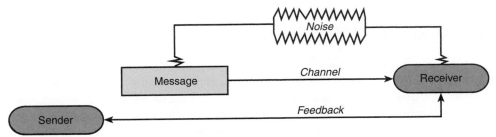

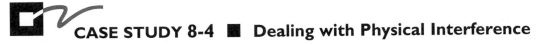

Figure 8-4 Diagram of the communication model. (Redrawn from Rawlins C: *Harper Collins college outline: introduction to management,* New York, 1992, American Book-Works.)

CASE STUDY 8-4 ■ Dealing with Physical Interference

You enter room 410 to speak to Ms. Blondin about her discharge plan. The first thing you notice Is that her television is on, she has two visitors by her bedside, housekeeping personnel are emptying the garbage, and the lunch carts are arriving in the hallway. Obviously, very little effective communication will occur unless the physical barriers are reduced. First, ask the patient's permission to turn off the television; next, invite visitors to participate in the meeting if agreeable to the patient and appropriate to the purpose of your meeting; then explain why you are there and make eye contact. If distractions are still evident, wait until the housekeeper has left the room and the dietary cart has passed in the hallway. Then you can proceed because you have taken control of the physical environment and have reduced the physical interference that would have certainly had a negative effect on your communication effort.

patient's readiness to learn and preferred method of communication (e.g., face-to-face communication, group meeting, or written information). In addition, the listener's receptivity must be established and maintained if quality communication is to take place.

Because barriers to communication are the pitfalls for any case manager to try to avoid, it is helpful to review some examples in depth.

Physical Interference

The first and most important step in improving communication is to make sure that your intended receiver receives the message. The sender (case manager) must take full responsibility for seeing that the physical barriers to communication are reduced. Case Study 8-4 provides an example of such a situation.

Psychological Noise

The root cause of this interference is distraction (thinking about something else). Accuracy is at stake here. Hunger, anger, depression, medication, and fear all have an impact on the way the receiver understands. Asking for feedback, providing feedback, and verifying the accuracy of the message helps identify the existence of a psychological barrier. See Case Study 8-5 for an example.

Information Processing Barriers

Our brains have the miraculous ability to take in enormous amounts of data but can only process consciously one thought at a time. If information is being sent too fast, the brain and therefore the receiver have trouble taking it in (Case Manager's Tip 8-6). *Communication overload* is a classic example of a processing barrier. During communication overload too much information is being sent, and the receiver cannot process it all. The receiver then becomes overwhelmed and shuts down. You have probably seen this occur numerous times. Picture yourself giving a patient instructions on how to test his or her blood sugar. You go on and on reciting the steps of pricking the finger, dabbing a drop of blood on the glucose test strip, and preparing the machinery to accept the strip for reading. When you suddenly try to make eye contact, what you see is a face staring back at you blankly. The patient is overwhelmed by your instruction, is overloaded, and has shut down.

Perceptual Barriers

Each individual brings a unique set of past experiences to communication. These experiences, good or bad, will influence how a person perceives the meaning of your communication. Perception is greatly influenced by our value system. We interpret everything we experience

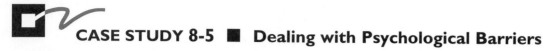

CASE STUDY 8-5 ■ Dealing with Psychological Barriers

You approach Mr. Tumbie, an 80-year-old frail-looking man admitted for dehydration and intractable diarrhea. Your first question, "How are you today, Mr. Tumbie?" gets a nonverbal response of sighs and wringing his hands but a verbal response of feeling fine. Mr. Tumbie's expressions and actions do not match his verbal reply, and you interpret this as anxiety. As you probe further into his apparent anxiety, you learn that he is very tired and is preoccupied with his daughter and son-in-law, who are "after his money."

Your original goal of offering Mr. Tumbie discharge planning options may be too premature in light of the fact that there is a clear psychological barrier that must be tackled first: his relationship with his daughter and son-in-law. It may be his belief that discussing personal or family problems with a nurse is inappropriate; therefore before discussing his personal life you may first need to establish trust with this patient to help him to feel more comfortable. Beginning with a less emotionally charged topic would be advantageous in building rapport and becoming better informed about this patient. You will no doubt be more successful when approaching this sensitive subject with him in the future.

CASE MANAGER'S TIP 8-6

Information Overload and Quality of Communication

Too much information delivered too quickly will result in a poor-quality communication effort.

CASE MANAGER'S TIP 8-7

Limiting the Chain of Communication

The fewer people to whom messages must be relayed, the more effective the communication is.

through mental images, and we tend to assume that the way we see things is the way that they really are and the way everyone else sees them.

Structural Barriers

There are aspects of organizational structure that can affect the quality of communication. These next barriers to communication, as those previously mentioned, can be applied not only to a case manager's patients but also to a case manager's peers, other members of the multidisciplinary team, payers, and upper administrative management.

The more people who are involved in a chain of communication, the greater the likelihood that message interruption can occur (Case Manager's Tip 8-7). You may remember the old game of "telephone" in which a message is whispered into the ear of one person after another. By the time the message reaches the last person it is substantially different from the initial message. Usually the important details such as times, dates, and names become confused.

Defensive Communication

Defensive communication can also be a barrier to the effective transmission of the message. This type of communication occurs when people attempt to protect themselves from a real or perceived threat. The threat could be related to the sender or receiver of the message, or it could be present in the message itself. Defensive communication tends to occur when there is a lack of trust—for example, when the receiver of the message is doubtful or suspicious of the sender's motives. Message-related defensive communication takes place when the message being sent contains challenging content or disregard for the receiver's values, beliefs, worth, or feelings (Lancaster and Lancaster, 1999).

Power

If communication must take place between various levels of authority or power, the differences in *status* can result in poor-quality communication. This is known as *information processing* or *filtering*. Overcoming the communication barrier imposed by status differences is mostly a matter of realizing that it can occur (Case Manager's Tip 8-8). There are generally two types of power:
1. *Directive power,* or power used to affect the behavior of others with the intent of satisfying personal needs
2. *Synergistic power,* or power used to increase the energy and creativity of all participants with the intent of satisfying the needs of all participants
Knowing how and when to enforce power appropriately, along with having the components of a trusting relationship, will result in a shared sense of responsibility and better outcomes. Possessing a solid power base is crucial, and its appropriateness is essential. As an

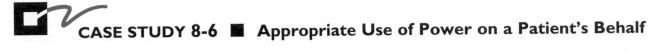

CASE STUDY 8-6 ■ Appropriate Use of Power on a Patient's Behalf

Mrs. Rose is a resident of Florida who came to visit her elderly sister in New York and became ill, requiring hospitalization. The patient has remained hospitalized for 20 days and is now essentially ready for discharge. In the course of the hospitalization, the patient's functional status has deteriorated and the likelihood that she can remain home alone is slim. The patient requires oxygen and a wheelchair. The dilemma becomes how to get the patient discharged when she refuses nursing home placement and wants only to return to Florida where her friends could help her. Many contacts and more hospital days later, it becomes clear to you that it would be less expensive to arrange for medical air transport to Florida than to continue her hospitalization.

The case manager in this scenario has the ability to affect the outcome of this patient's hospitalization by using directive power and educating the hospital's administrative body. It would be soon realized that it is financially more prudent to send this patient back to Florida rather than keep her hospitalized indefinitely. The case manager needs to clearly communicate to the hierarchy holding the purse strings the cost of a few days in the hospital versus the cost of an ambulance and medical air transport.

CASE MANAGER'S TIP 8-8

Power and Communication

Always keep yourself focused on the goals of your communication and do not get intimidated by hierarchical status when quality patient care is at stake. Seeking feedback and verifying the information conveyed will help you maintain power.

---

expert case manager, you must be willing to share expertise, issue directives, follow up on compliance, and attempt to influence as occasions arise (Bass, 1985). Case Study 8-6 provides an example.

Trust

Stress and lack of trust are additional structural barriers to communication. They both interfere with accurate, clear communication, and they both affect the ability to express needs and share information openly and honestly. Building rapport and a trusting relationship usually has the added bonus of reducing stress, thereby increasing the chances of accurate communication.

The following sections outline the four basic qualities a case manager should exhibit to initiate a patient–case manager or case manager–colleague relationship in which trust can be developed.

Warmth

This quality helps others to feel accepted. Nurses who are willing to extend themselves with openness rather than exhibit cold, expressionless, disapproving behavior will gain trust more quickly. Warmth reflects self-respect, self-acceptance, and genuine concern for others, and people respond to this type of behavior favorably.

Respect

Treat others as you would want to be treated; take into consideration personality, culture, opinions, customs, values, and beliefs. To respect another person does not necessarily mean that you must like that person; however, you must accept and value him or her. This becomes important to a case manager when a family's or patient's decisions regarding a discharge plan are not in full agreement with the case manager's recommendation. Keeping patients informed about their care gives them the feeling that they are respected as individuals, not just seen as a bed number or a disease entity.

Empathy

Helping people to feel understood means actively tuning into feelings and thoughts and letting go of stereotypes and prejudices. This is an essential ingredient in trusting relationships. You must really hear, without demanding that someone feel as you think they should in a given situation (Rorden and Taft, 1990).

Genuineness

This final component of verbal communication enhances the trust relationship. This quality allows people to feel that they are interacting with a real person who is interested in their well-being. Consistency is a facet of being genuine. If there is inconsistency between verbal and nonverbal behavior, communication will break down (e.g., the case manager who voices concern about a patient's situation but fails to make eye contact will surely be judged as "put on"). Keep in mind that people who are already stressed by their situation will be more astute to false behavior and inconsistent communication. Armed with the knowledge of the many barriers to communication and the ways in which to avoid or to minimize them, the case manager must now become versed in the communication channels that effectively transmit the message from sender to receiver.

COMMUNICATION PATHS

The path that a communication takes, whether it be formal or informal, has an effect on the communication itself (Rawlins, 1992). Formal communication takes two forms: downward and upward. Downward communication is communication about what to do, how to do it, and when it is to be completed. This communication usually takes place when delegating to subordinates. To delegate effectively, all of the aforementioned barriers should be avoided. An example of upward communication is when a case manager speaks with a chief financial officer (CFO) to request financial approval, as in the previously discussed scenario of flying a patient back to her home rather than incurring the cost of an extended hospital stay. The result is a more accurate managerial process, greater participation, and interactive control of the positive destiny of an organization.

Informal communication usually takes place between smaller groups, such as the case manager and the social worker. Managers in these two areas may get together after a more formal meeting to discuss a policy that may affect both of their departments. This type of communication must be based on mutual trust, or a more formal communication will need to follow.

In addition to becoming aware of typical barriers to effective communication and channels of communication, case managers can take additional steps to improve communication competency. How colleagues work together as a team can determine the success or failure of any work environment. Good relationships are fostered when colleagues respect each others' job duties.

Teams

There is a great difference between an effective team and a group of people who have been thrown together with no clear goals (Haase, 1992). There are generally 10 elements of an effective team. While reviewing these elements, think about the members of your organizational team, whether they be social workers, discharge planners, utilization reviewers, nurse managers, payers, or physicians. Rate the effectiveness of your team effort toward a productive case management program and better patient outcomes. You will begin to see that many if not all of the elements incorporate the communication and interpersonal skills discussed throughout this chapter (Haase, 1992):

1. Team members communicate openly and honestly. They listen with understanding.
2. Team members have common goals and a clear idea of the team's mission.
3. Team members support each other. They have assigned duties and are not engaged in turf wars.
4. Team members take pride in their group's efforts and results.
5. Team members help make decisions on important issues but when necessary are willing to look for guidance for final decisions.
6. Team members feel comfortable expressing ideas, opinions, and disagreements.
7. Team members are encouraged to make the development of new skills a way of life.
8. Team members are encouraged to use their unique skills and talents.
9. Team members realize that conflict is normal and that working out differences can lead to new points of view and creativity.
10. Team members value appropriate humor. Having fun increases openness, enthusiasm, and energy.

These ten elements involve potential attitude adjustment, releasing of power, respect, compromise, and conflict resolution.

Conflict

Administrative pressures for cost control and consumer demands for safe and quality care influence case managers in their daily decision-making activities. Now more than ever it is necessary for case managers to work collaboratively with members of the interdisciplinary team to meet the pressures and demands of healthcare delivery. Case managers must keep in mind that conflict is inevitable and that it is not a negative occurrence as it was once believed to be. Conflict is merely individuals or groups experiencing differences in views, goals, facts, or values that place them at opposite poles. It usually involves areas of differing expertise, practice, or authority.

In most situations conflict falls into one of three categories: *perceived* conflict, the thought that conditions exist between groups that cause the conflict; *felt* conflict, when the conflict evokes feelings of threat, hostility, fear, or mistrust; and *expressed* conflict, which takes the form of debate, assertion, competition, or problem solving. There are five different strategies for resolving conflicts (Box 8-2). However, the most often used tactic to resolve conflict is the collaborative win/win resolution. Groups usually identify solutions that will allow each to maintain their goals and ultimately create a resolution that they can live with (Kirsch, 1988).

The ability to successfully manage conflict is an important skill for the case manager to master. It can help the case manager to increase the total benefits of

---

BOX 8-2   Strategies for Conflict Resolution

1. *Competing:* An assertive strategy in which an individual's concerns are satisfied at the expense of another's. This strategy is useful in a situation in which the solution is urgently needed and time does not allow waiting for a different strategy to be tried first.

2. *Collaborating:* A cooperative strategy in which individuals work together to find mutually satisfying solutions. This strategy is useful when a solution to a particular conflict is complex and requires that all parties involved be satisfied with the outcome.

3. *Compromising:* A strategy in which each of the individuals involved in the conflict must give something up to resolve the conflict. This strategy is useful when the goals of one individual are somewhat important or not important enough compared with the goals of other.

4. *Avoiding:* A passive strategy in which an individual postpones or sidesteps the conflict. This strategy is useful when one party is more powerful than the other and when the risk of confrontation outweighs the benefits or the solution.

5. *Accommodating:* A passive strategy in which an individual focuses on the concerns of others and neglects his or her own concerns. This strategy is useful when one individual has a vested interest in the issue while the issue is unimportant to the other.

From Barton A: Conflict resolution by nurse managers, *Nurs Manage* 22(5):83-85, 1991.

 CASE MANAGER'S TIP 8-9

Positive Effects of Conflict

If conflict is well managed, it can actually increase the effectiveness of an organization.

---

the group efforts by becoming more innovative and creative, with the overall outcome of increasing productivity and achieving goals (Case Manager's Tip 8-9).

One member of the multidisciplinary team, the physician, is a vital communication source. If there are conflicts or obstacles to the case manager–physician communication, then quality patient care will suffer. Professional and up-front communication regarding the case manager's role is a good place to start in building an effective team among the disciplines. Case managers must initiate positive dialogue with physicians and address the stereotypes and stresses of a shifting healthcare system (Mullahy, 1995). Despite sharing the common goal of the patient's well-being, physicians and case managers can easily become adversaries when distrust surrounding the case manager's

intentions is raised. Comments such as "Case managers are the police who work with the insurance payers to deny care" misguide physicians into perceiving case managers as a threat to their medical judgment and their income. As a result of the changing working relationship between case managers and physicians (and others such as nurses, social workers, utilization coordinators, and discharge planners), the transition to a full cooperative and collaborative relationship is at times awkward and frustrating. Being caught up in past traditional roles hinders the establishment of the collaborative alliance necessary to achieve success in the healthcare of the twenty-first century.

We must constantly remind ourselves that we are all here for the patient and must remain focused on that goal. Case managers need to be especially clear on this point—that their interest is in ensuring better quality of care and the best possible outcomes. The physicians (or social workers, utilization coordinators, discharge planners) must be reassured that the case managers are not there to control or dictate practice but are instead there to foster effective, quality communication between members of a multidisciplinary team.

Today's case managers face the challenge of dealing with a diverse customer population. The case manager must be capable of incorporating the communication techniques and skills reviewed in this chapter when communicating with the diversity of groups involved in patient care. For example, a group of growing prominence involved in patient care is the payer source or insurance company. The case manager must listen closely to what the payer is requesting and must clarify any vague communication at the outset. The case manager should not assume that the insurance claims department has all of the necessary knowledge with regard to a patient's discharge plan. The case manager, as educator and advocate, becomes vital to the success of the patient's outcome by sharing his or her medical knowledge of what the patient needs. Case managers must keep in mind that they are the problem solvers and cannot easily accept a simple "No" or "We don't do that." Case managers must be risk takers when communicating with the payer members of the team, or patients could suffer the consequences. The communication with external members of the multidisciplinary team (e.g., payer, community resources, family members) becomes just as important to the success of the patient's outcome as the communication with internal members.

Much of this chapter has been devoted to communication because it is perhaps the most vital skill that case managers must master. Although different communication styles exist (Box 8-3), case managers must use the

---

BOX 8-3 Communication Styles and Their Characteristics

1. Assertive
   - Pushing hard without attacking
   - Expressive and self-enhancing
   - Influencing results/outcomes
2. Aggressive
   - Taking advantage of others
   - Self-enhancing at others' expense
   - Intimidating
3. Nonassertive
   - Inhibited
   - Self-denying
   - Passive

 CASE MANAGER'S TIP 8-10

Improving the Effectiveness of Communication

In addition to improving their basic communication skills of reading, writing, listening, and speaking, case managers can improve their communication effectiveness by withholding judgment, avoiding inconsistencies, and valuing all members of the team, inclusive of the patient and family.

---

assertive style in applying the case management process. However, psychological, physical, and structural barriers can cause turbulence in the information flow. Effective case managers will work fiercely to reduce these barriers. The more rapidly they receive and communicate information, the better the quality of the decisions they make will be (Case Manager's Tip 8-10).

Data Management

The use of data in case management continues to be of great importance. Case managers continually use data for decision-making purposes. They identify, collect, and analyze data when assessing their patients, implementing the required care and monitoring and evaluating the outcomes. This aspect of the case manager's role is important for information management, knowledge development, and enhancing the healthcare delivery system. Therefore case managers must possess appropriate skills in data management to succeed. They also must be able to use certain tools throughout their day for data collection and tracking. Examples of these tools are as follows:

- Variance data collection tools
- **Managed care** review tools

- Documentation tools
- Administrative logs and databases
- Quality assessment, insurance, and improvement tools
- Information systems and electronic medical records

Case managers must also understand the different methods of data collection and management (i.e., retrospective, prospective, and concurrent), their advantages and disadvantages, and when it is appropriate to use each of the methods. In addition, they must be knowledgeable in the types of measures used in data analysis, particularly those that are appropriate for use in case management evaluation, such as the following:

- Numbers: descriptive statistics
- Rates: incidence and occurrence
- Attributes: demographics
- Perceptions: customer and staff satisfaction
- Composites: **case mix index**

With today's reliance on automation in most data management systems and departments, case managers are expected to be able to access databases, run special reports, prepare graphic reports, conduct statistical analyses, and export or download data. Case managers with these skills are the most desirable and successful. When writing reports, they must be able to summarize the important findings, indicate the **outliers** and deviations from the norms or standards, and determine whether there is a need for more detailed or different types of data for better decision making or for more accurate interpretations and conclusions. Furthermore, case managers must be capable of writing concise, readable, and easily understood and interpreted reports.

Big Picture/Systems Thinking

Case management delivery models are grounded in systems theory. The delivery of patient care is dependent on the environment/context in which it is delivered and varies across time and space. For example, intensive care services are not provided in a clinic setting but rather in an acute care setting. Another example is using the emergency department for access to healthcare services at times of emergency and not as a primary care provision setting. Case managers must understand the differences in the types of services provided in the varied settings across the continuum. If they are not systems focused in their thinking and approach to care delivery and management, they will not be successful and effective.

Case managers are expected to interact with their system at three different levels: the individual, the organization, and the environment at large. They manage the care of the individual patients in the context of the care setting or level of care the patient is at. They also coordinate, facilitate, and arrange for the services their patients may require postdischarge or at the next level of care. This requires case managers to interact with other organizations and community agencies or managed care organizations for **authorization** of services; thus they reach out to other organizations and the environment at large. Regardless of the setting they are in, case managers are expected to employ a systems thinking framework and approach to case management care delivery. This framework assures them success and desirable outcomes.

According to Ridge and Bland Jones (in Lancaster, 1999, p. 36), systems thinking is defined as a "powerful problem-solving language that guides the understanding of complex issues within organizations, based on the assumption that organizations are made up of parts with patterns of interaction, rather than discrete structures and components." The complexity of case management models in relation to the scope of services, interdisciplinary approach, and **continuum of care** focus demands a systems approach to care delivery because of its interdependence on the various disciplines involved in care processes. Case managers must be able to pay careful attention to the environment in which they work and to its related inputs, throughputs, and outputs and the degree to which they interact. The inputs, throughputs, and outputs make up the various functions of case management such as resource utilization, strategic plans, care management activities, roles and job descriptions, goals, objectives, performance, productivity, and outcomes.

Senge (1990) views organizations as systems in which staff members interact and function in interdependent teams to accomplish the goals of the organization. This is true for case management systems. Case managers must be able to work collaboratively in teams and to facilitate the achievement of the goals of cost-effectiveness and quality outcomes. Senge (1990) emphasizes systems thinking as the desired approach for achieving such results. He adds that systems thinking is a powerful problem-solving strategy. Case managers must learn how to incorporate this strategy in their daily activities because it focuses on the essential interrelationships of the case management model and helps case managers to see and appreciate the "big picture" and the interconnectedness of the different components of the system or organization. Systems thinking assists case managers in the following ways:

- Managing decision making
- Managing multiple tasks and functions
- Coping with conflict
- Motivating others
- Managing change
- Facilitating negotiation activities

Emotional Intelligence*

During the past decade, **emotional intelligence** has surfaced as a necessary skill for effective industry leaders. It has become even more important for those in healthcare; especially for case managers. Emotional intelligence is defined by Cooper and Sawaf (1996, p. XIII) as the "ability to sense, understand, and effectively apply the power and acumen of emotions as a source of human energy, information, connection, and influence." Goleman (1995, p. 34), however, defined emotional intelligence as the ability to "motivate oneself and persist in the face of frustrations; to control impulse and delay gratification; to regulate one's mood and keep distress from swamping the ability to think; to empathize and hope." Both definitions emphasize the importance of self-awareness of emotions and the need to consider these emotions and feelings in the process of making decisions, instituting actions, or dealing with others.

Feelings and emotions, whether positive, negative, or neutral, serve as a source of vital information used in making decisions, initiating action, or communicating. They cause case managers to act in a certain way. They also influence how case managers may connect with themselves and others and establish relationships. How successful they can be in handling a particular situation or event depends on the following:

- Perception and awareness of one's feelings
- Perception and awareness of the emotions and feelings of others
- The effect of these feelings and emotions on the encountered situation or event

Emotions, if used and managed appropriately by case managers, act as a source of power, motivation, feedback, information, influence, innovation, creativity, success, and freedom. Based on the definitions presented, emotional intelligence enhances case managers' abilities with regard to the following:

- Making influential decisions
- Resolving conflict effectively
- Communicating openly and honestly with others
- Establishing trusting relationships with patients, their families, and members of the interdisciplinary healthcare team
- Building rapport with patients and their families
- Creating an environment of care that is centered on patient and family and is focused on teamwork

---

*This section first appeared in Tahan HA: Emotionally intelligent case managers make a difference, *Lippincott's Case Management* 5(4): 162-167, 2000.

Goleman (1995, 1998) identified five components of emotional intelligence: knowing one's emotions, managing emotions, motivating oneself, recognizing others' emotions, and handling relationships. The first three components are concerned with self-management and regulation skills, whereas the remaining two are associated with building relationships, community, and social skills. These components are described as follows:

1. *Knowing one's emotions* is the state of having a deep understanding of and insight into one's feelings, preferences, internal states, and drives and how they affect self, others, and job performance. Emotionally self-aware case managers are conscious of their capabilities and deficits and have better control over their actions, reactions, and interactions. Their decision-making ability is enhanced and they are more honest and sincere in their practice.

2. *Managing one's emotions* is handling one's feelings, emotions, and internal states appropriately. It is the ability to control one's impulses, delay gratification, and regulate one's moods so that distress is prevented. Case managers who manage their emotions are able to withhold disruptive emotions, reactions, and decision making until relevant information is obtained. In addition, they are able to be flexible in handling change and to be responsible for personal performance. Case managers who manage their emotions are able to self-regulate. They are able to carry on effective internal conversations about feelings, emotions, and experiences so that they feel free of destructive emotions and thoughts and thus are able to channel emotions in useful ways for themselves, others, and the job.

3. *Motivating oneself* is the act of taking the initiative for achieving goals and dreams. It is pursuing solutions to problems without waiting for others to take the lead or provide direction. Self-motivated case managers strive for excellence and align with the goals of the interdisciplinary team and/or the organization. They achieve beyond their own expectations and the expectations of others and what is expected for the job. They are passionate about and take pride in the job they are responsible for. Self-motivated case managers are able to "think outside the box" and to look for nontraditional solutions/approaches to solving problems and improving workflow. Self-motivation enhances their feeling of optimism even after a setback or failure to achieve, or after experiencing frustration.

4. *Recognizing others' emotions* is the ability to recognize the feelings of others and to be more attuned to the subtle signals others send through their behaviors and interactions regarding their needs, wants, and desires. Case managers who have the ability to recognize others' emotions are more aware of others' needs and perspectives. They are able to express their interest in others' concerns and abilities and to work with them on meeting the interdisciplinary team goals. The ability to recognize and acknowledge others' emotions is known as *empathy*. It is essential for understanding and thoughtfully considering the feelings and emotions of others while making decisions or solving problems. Empathy enhances teamwork and unity and helps to bring members of the interdisciplinary healthcare team closer together. It also fosters loyalty to the team and the organization.

5. *Handling relationships* is the ability to manage relationships and others' emotions effectively. Case managers who know how to handle relationships make those around them feel welcome, at ease, and an integral part of the team. They are effective on an interpersonal level and adept at inducing desirable responses in others. The ability to handle relationships well enhances group work and synergy and nurtures influential relationships. It helps to build social skills. This ability allows case managers to foster a sense of community. It is "friendliness with a purpose," moving people in the right direction. Case managers' effectiveness with regard to social skills depends on other components of emotional intelligence; that is, controlling and understanding their own feelings and emotions and empathizing with the feelings and emotions of others.

The desired qualities of case managers are not limited to their technical, clinical, and interpersonal skills, abilities, knowledge, and expertise. These qualities are deemed most effective if they are coupled with the skill and ability to recognize, understand, manage, master, and appropriately respond to one's own emotions and feelings and those expressed by others, such as nurses, social workers, physicians, administrators, patients, and families (Case Manager's Tip 8-11). Case management responsibilities and services demand the presence of case managers who are astute and emotionally intelligent; otherwise these case managers would not be able to provide efficient, effective, safe, cost-effective, ethical, and quality care.

SUCCESSFUL LEADERS

Successful leaders possess quite an extensive list of skills. This is especially true of case managers as leaders. They must be able to incorporate all of the skills

CASE MANAGER'S TIP 8-11

Strategies for Becoming an Emotionally Intelligent Case Manager

1. Knowing one's emotions
   - Identify what information you are using to influence your interpretation of things/events.
   - Identify what influences your mood shifts and the moments you experience them.
   - Know when you are thinking negatively.
   - Know when you are becoming angry or feel frustrated.
   - Know when you are becoming defensive.
   - Recognize when your verbal and nonverbal communications are conflicting.
   - Be aware of what senses you are currently using.
   - Be able to communicate how you feel or what annoys you.

2. Managing emotions
   - Learn to relax when under pressure.
   - Act productively, especially when you are angry, frustrated, or in anxiety-provoking situations.
   - Attempt to calm quickly before you make decisions or respond to unpleasant situations.
   - Be aware of the relationships between your physiological and emotional states.
   - Remain calm when you are the target of anger or criticism from others.
   - Take some time out.
   - Resort to humor.

3. Motivating oneself
   - Regroup quickly after a setback or stressful experience.
   - Change or stop ineffective habits.
   - Develop new patterns of behaviors that are productive and rewarding.
   - Make sure to follow words with actions.
   - Keep the promises you make to yourself and to others.
   - Be persistent.
   - Do not give up.
   - Always attempt to do your best.
   - Complete your responsibilities/duties within the designated timeframes.

4. Recognizing others' emotions
   - Clarify misunderstandings.
   - Ask others how they feel.
   - Validate your perceptions of others.
   - Validate your perceptions of how others think of or feel about you.
   - Recognize when others are feeling distressed, anxious, or distraught.
   - Engage in intimate conversations with others.
   - Manage group emotions appropriately.
   - Help others manage their emotions.
   - Be empathetic.
   - Always provide others with the opportunity to express their feelings honestly.
   - Establish common goals.

5. Handling relationships
   - Work out conflicts.
   - Approach problem resolution as a group.
   - Encourage team-building behaviors.
   - Exhibit effective communication skills.
   - Be honest and sincere.
   - Build trust.
   - Build a sense of community.
   - Influence others and allow others to influence you.
   - Make others feel good and welcome.
   - Seek others for support and advice.
   - Avail yourself to others when they need you.
   - Be approachable.

These are only suggestions and do not reflect an exhaustive list. They are summarized based on Weisinger H: *Emotional intelligence at work*, San Francisco, 1998, Jossey-Bass.

discussed previously into their day-to-day functions with the gracefulness of a gazelle.

As stated earlier, not everyone can be or aspires to be a case manager, even with proper education and development. Successful case managers are likely to demonstrate a special ability to operate in peer relationships, lead others in subordinate relationships, resolve interpersonal and decisional conflicts, communicate with the media, make complex interrelated decisions, allocate resources (including their own time), and innovate (Mintzberg, 1973). Successful case managers must be *leaders*, not *managers*. Leadership skills and abilities are

more desired in case managers than management skills and abilities. Management has a more narrow focus: How can I accomplish certain things? Leadership, on the other hand, deals with the broader picture: What are the things that I need to accomplish? In the words of Peter Drucker and Warren Bennis, management is doing things right, whereas leadership is doing the right things. Management is efficiency in climbing the ladder of success; leadership determines whether the ladder is leaning against the right wall (Covey, 1989).

You can quickly see the important difference between the two if you envision a group of new graduate nurses cutting their way through a jungle. In the front will be the workers cutting through the undergrowth, cleaning it out. The potential managers will be behind them, sharpening their machetes, writing policy and procedure manuals, holding development programs, and setting up work schedules. The potential leader (case manager) is the one who climbs the tallest tree, surveys the entire situation, and yells, "Wrong jungle!" (Covey, 1989).

The metamorphosis taking place in almost every industry, including the healthcare industry, demands professional leadership first and management second. All that has been conveyed in this chapter clearly depicts the leadership qualities needed in today's healthcare environment. Although the title has generally become associated with management, leadership more fully and accurately defines the role of the case manager. Efficient management without effective leadership is "like straightening deck chairs on the Titanic" (Covey, 1989).

Effectiveness does not depend solely on how much effort we expend but whether the effort we expend is in the right place. It is irrelevant if a case manager spends days on a discharge plan, expending much energy, only to find out that as a result of poor leadership vision, the plan was not the right blueprint for the patient.

The pressure for change within our healthcare industry will most definitely intensify rather than diminish in the coming years. This pressure will require nurses to respond with new dynamic transformational leadership to cope with future changes. The transformational leader approaches leadership from an entirely different perspective or level of awareness. The transformational leader, as defined by Bass (1985), is one who does the following:

- Raises levels of consciousness about the importance of certain goals or actions
- Encourages subordinates to transcend self-interests for the good of the team

House (1971), who developed the path-goal theory in the 1970s, depicts the qualities of a transformational leader as someone who does the following:

- Serves as a role model
- Builds an image
- Articulates goals
- Sets high expectations

Although the research of both Bass and House dates back a number of years, perhaps these theorists were ahead of their time. The case manager of the twenty-first century characteristically has all of these qualities, and any organization interested in building a solid case management program should give consideration to them.

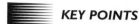

KEY POINTS

1. Utilization of the nursing process—assessment, planning, implementation, coordination, and evaluation—is vital to a successful case manager.
2. Assessment connects the physical and the psychosocial aspects of a patient's care.
3. Planning determines the treatments and interventions necessary for meeting the needs of patients and families.
4. Implementation/coordination builds on the plan and determines the goals of patient care, moving the plan to completion.
5. Evaluation measures the patient's response to the case management plan.
6. Leadership and communication skills such as facilitation, negotiation, utilization management, education, team building, and conflict resolution must be added to the case manager's repertoire and put to use daily.
7. Teamwork is essential to the success of any patient plan. Learn who the members of the team are and develop effective relationships.
8. Acquired skills are applicable to all forms of case management, including acute, subacute, home care, and insurance case management.

REFERENCES

Bass B: Leadership good, better, best, *Organiz Dynam* 13:26-40, 1985.

Bower XA: *Case management by nurses,* ed 2, St Louis, 1992, American Nurses Association.

Case Management Society of America: *Standards of practice for case management,* Little Rock, Ark, 2002, The Society.

Cooper R, Sawaf A: *Executive EQ: emotional intelligence in leadership and organizations,* New York, 1996, Berkley Publishing Group.

Covey S: *The 7 habits of highly effective people,* New York, 1989, Simon & Schuster.

Dash K, Vince-Whitman C, Zarle N, et al: *Discharge planning for the elderly: a guide for nurses,* New York, 1996, Springer.

Goleman D: *Emotional intelligence: why it can matter more than IQ,* New York, 1995, Bantam.

Goleman D: What makes a leader? *Harvard Business Rev* 76(12):93-102, 1998.

Haase J: The 10 elements of an effective team, *Home Care* 38:236, 1992.

House R: A path-goal theory of leadership effectiveness, *Admin Q* 16:321-338, 1971.

Kirsch J: *The middle manager and the nursing organization,* East Norwalk, Conn, 1988, Appleton & Lange.

Lancaster J, Lancaster M: Communicating to manage change. In Lancaster J: *Nursing issues in leading and managing change,* St Louis, 1999, Mosby.

Maslow AH: *Motivation and personality,* ed 2, New York, 1970, Harper & Row.

Mintzberg H: *The nature of managerial work,* New York, 1973, Harper & Row.

Mullahy CM: *The case manager's handbook,* Gaithersburg, 1995, Aspen.

O'Malley J: *Dimensions of the nurse case manager role: case management (Part II),* Gaithersburg, Md, 1988, Aspen.

Powell S, Ignatavicius D: *CMSA core curriculum for case management,* Philadelphia, 2001, Lippincott Williams & Wilkins.

Rawlins C: *Harper Collins college outline: introduction to management,* New York, 1992, American Book-Works.

Ridge R, Bland Jones C: Systems th eory and analysis in health care and nursing. In Lancaster J: *Nursing issues in leading and managing change,* St Louis, 1999, Mosby.

Rorden JW, Taft E: *Discharge planning guide for nurses,* Philadelphia, 1990, WB Saunders.

Senge P: *The fifth discipline: the art and practice of the learning organization,* New York, 1990, Doubleday/Currency.

Umiker W: Negotiating skill for health care professionals, *Health Care Superv* 14(3):27-32, 1996.

Yura H, Walsh M: *The nursing process,* East Norwalk, Conn, 1983, Appleton-Century-Crofts.

9

Case Manager's Documentation

Greater emphasis has been given to the role **case managers** play in the provision of patient care as a result of the redesigning, reengineering, or restructuring of healthcare delivery systems. This change has increased the level of importance of documentation. Documentation has become even more important in institutions that developed and implemented new patient care delivery models such as **case management, care management,** integrated care, and collaborative care. The main reason behind the increased importance of documentation is related to the changes that have occurred in the role of the registered professional nurse and social worker, particularly the introduction of the role of case manager.

The creation of the case manager's role has pressured healthcare providers, nurses, and others to rely more on some of the important functions nurses and social workers play in the delivery of patient care, which have historically been ignored. These functions include but are not limited to the following:

- Coordination of discharge/**transitional planning** activities
- Facilitation and expedition of patient care activities
- **Utilization management** and resource allocation
- Psychosocial assessment of needs of patients and families
- Emphasis not only on actual patient/family problems but also on potential problems
- Evaluation of patient care outcomes and responses to treatment
- Counseling of patient/family regarding knowledge of health needs, preventive measures, and coping
- Service monitoring

These functions have been emphasized greatly in the job descriptions and the roles and responsibilities of

 CASE MANAGER'S TIP 9-1

The Importance of Documentation
The case manager's documentation is crucial because it is the only evidence of the case manager's role in the provision of patient care.

case managers in a variety of institutions and patient care settings.

IMPORTANCE OF DOCUMENTATION

Case managers view documentation as an important aspect of their role (Case Manager's Tip 9-1). Documentation reflects their professional responsibility and accountability toward patient care. In its *Standards of Clinical Nursing Practice,* the American Nurses Association (1991) identifies documentation as an integral part of its six standards of care (Table 9-1). Bower (1992), Cohen and Cesta (1997), and Tahan (1993) also identified documentation as an important role function of case managers. There are several factors that increase the importance of case manager documentation, including the following:

1. Professional responsibility and accountability to patient care
2. Communication of the case manager's judgments and evaluations
3. Evidence of case managers' plans of care, interventions, and outcomes
4. Legal protection; valuable evidence
5. Standards of regulatory agencies (e.g., the U.S. Department of Health and Human Services, the Joint Commission on Accreditation of Healthcare Organizations

TABLE 9-1 Evidence of Documentation in the Standards of Care of the American Nurses Association

Standards	Measurement Criteria
Assessment	Relevant data are documented in a retrievable form
Diagnosis	Diagnoses are documented in a manner that facilitates the determination of expected outcomes and plan of care
Outcome identification	Outcomes are documented as measurable goals
Planning	The plan is documented
Implementation	Interventions are documented
Evaluation	Revisions in diagnoses, outcomes, and the plan of care are documented

Modified from the American Nurses Association: *Standards of clinical nursing practice,* Kansas City, Mo, 1991, The Association.

[JCAHO], the Commission for Accreditation of Rehabilitation Facilities [CARF], National Committee of Quality Assurance [NCQA], and the **Utilization Review Accreditation Commission [URAC]**)

6. Healthcare reimbursement (e.g., the **diagnosis-related group [DRG]** system, managed care organizations, and **third-party payers**)

7. Supportive evidence of quality of patient care

ROLE OF CASE MANAGERS IN DOCUMENTATION

Documentation by case managers is extremely important because it is the only concrete evidence of their role in the provision of patient care. Case managers documentation in the medical record should reflect the case management steps discussed in Chapter 4, the utilization management activities discussed in Chapter 5, and the transitional planning/**discharge planning** functions discussed in Chapter 6. It should include documentation related to the following areas:

1. Method of patient referral for case management services
2. Patient screening for appropriateness for case management services
3. Assessment of needs
4. Identification of the patient's actual and potential problems
5. Establishment and implementation of the plan of care, including the transitional plan
6. Facilitation and coordination of care activities, including the resource/utilization management activities
7. Patient and family teaching
8. Patient discharge and disposition

 CASE MANAGER'S TIP 9-2

Elements to Include in Documentation

The case manager's documentation should include the following items:

1. How the patient was referred for case management services
2. Who made the referral
3. Reasons for the referral
4. Date and time of the referral

9. Evaluation of patient care outcomes
10. **Variances** in patient care

Appendix 9-1 at the end of this chapter presents an example of a case manager's documentation record.

Modes of Patient Referral for Case Management Services

Patient referrals for case management services may take place in three different ways. The first is a direct referral by a healthcare provider such as the primary nurse, private physician, consulting physician, house staff, nurse practitioner, physician assistant, social worker, or physical therapist. Personnel in the emergency department, doctor's office, or the admitting office could also refer a patient for case management services. The second is referral by the patient/family themselves, particularly if they were familiar with the case management process from previous encounters. The third method of patient referral is not a true referral. The case manager may elect to screen all new admissions and identify those who could benefit from case management. In home care settings and insurance companies, case managers may follow all patients regardless of the seriousness of the episode of illness.

In most institutions the case management referral process is preidentified by healthcare administrators and nursing executives in a policy, procedure, or protocol and made clear to all healthcare providers through education and training. Referrals are usually made based on prospectively established criteria similar to those discussed in Chapter 4 (see Box 4-1).

The case manager's documentation (Case Manager's Tip 9-2) should include how the patient has been referred for case management services, who made the referral, the reason(s) for the referral, and the date and time of the referral. If no referral is made and the patient has been identified by the case manager when screening the new admissions, then the case manager's documentation should indicate so.

CASE MANAGER'S TIP 9-3

Elements of Documentation in Telephonic Triage/Case Management

The telephonic triage/case management note must include the following:

1. Date and time of the call
2. Names of the patient and the caller if other than the patient
3. Relationship of the caller to the patient
4. Age and gender of the patient
5. Patient's/caller's telephone number for the purpose of returning the call
6. Name of **primary care provider** (PCP)
7. Whether the patient/caller attempted calling the PCP
8. Summary of problem or chief complaint
9. Type of **protocol** (automated **algorithm**) used
10. Classification of the problem (emergent, urgent, nonurgent)
11. Actions taken such as calling 911, recommending an emergency department visit, calling crisis team, use of Tylenol, ice packs, and so on
12. Whether the patient/caller agrees with the actions taken
13. Whether there is a need for a follow-up call

In some care settings, referrals for case management services by other providers may not exist. Examples are managed care organizations, in which case managers function as **gatekeepers** and demand managers, and **telephonic case management,** in which case managers function as triage nurses. In both settings the patient or family member/caregiver triggers the referral and the case manager completes it by connecting the patient with the appropriate healthcare provider or setting. The interaction between a patient/caller and the case manager in **telephone triage**/case management is limited in time, assessment process, and interventions given. Documentation in these situations is important for reducing legal risk. It should include a summary of the telephone conversation, the assessment made, the actions taken by the case manager, and the outcomes of the telephone call (Case Manager's Tip 9-3).

Patient Screening for Appropriateness for Case Management Services

However the referral is made, the case manager has to conduct a patient/family screening to determine appropriateness for case management activities. A decision regarding the patient's need for case management is

 CASE MANAGER'S TIP 9-4

Elements of the Intake Note

The intake note should focus on the following issues:

1. Reason for patient's hospitalization, need for medical attention, need for postdischarge services such as home care or transportation for follow-up appointment
2. Indications for case management services (i.e., which criteria for selection of patients for case management are met?) (e.g., age, **acuity,** complexity of diagnosis, **noncompliance**)
3. Method of referral (e.g., healthcare provider, patient/family, case manager screening)
4. The date and time patient's screening took place and the time the intake note was written
5. Method of screening (e.g., patient/family interview, discussion with other healthcare providers, review of medical record)
6. **Certification**/approval of current patient's hospitalization or medical services by the managed care organization

---

made based on the "criteria for patient selection into the case management process" discussed in Chapter 4 (see Box 4-1, p. 74). Some of these criteria are patient's acuity, age, complexity of diagnosis and medical condition, teaching needs, discharge/transitional planning, noncompliance with treatment regimen, insurance coverage, social complexity, and financial status.

When patient screening is completed and case management services are deemed appropriate, the case manager then writes an intake note in the patient's record explaining that the patient is accepted into the case management process (Case Manager's Tip 9-4).

Assessment of Needs

Screening of the patient/family for case management services and the initial assessment of needs are usually completed concurrently by the case manager because they are interrelated. The assessment of patient/family needs is made during the case manager's first encounter with the patient/family. Careful assessment and documentation of the patient's/family's needs can enhance the effectiveness of case management. Documentation of the initial assessment of needs by the case manager is a more detailed extension of the intake note (Case Manager's Tip 9-5). Both notes are usually completed consecutively, and in most cases one note is written combining both intake and assessment.

The case manager's documentation should not include a thorough health history or a physical examination. A statement indicating that the medical record,

CASE MANAGER'S TIP 9-5

Elements of the Initial Assessment Note

In addition to the elements of documentation mentioned in the patient's screening section, the initial assessment note should include the following:

1. Chief complaint
2. Risk for injury
3. Discharge planning needs
4. Social support system
5. Health education needs
6. Justification for the need of medical services/ attention, treatment

---

including the patient's history and physical assessment (assessments that are completed and documented by other healthcare professionals, including the primary nurse and the physician), has been reviewed by the case manager is of equal value and importance. However, the initial assessment note should reflect any significant abnormalities and problems identified by the case manager that would dictate the plan of care, the interventions/treatments, and management of the patient's needs.

Identification of the Patient's Actual and Potential Problems

Identification of the patient's actual and potential problems is the starting point for establishing the patient's plan of care. Accurate and comprehensive identification of these problems has a significant effect on patient care **outcomes**. Thoroughly examining the patient's medical record, in addition to interviewing the patient and family or caregiver, makes it easier for the case manager to prioritize the patient's needs that should be stated in the patient's record as actual or potential problems. Regardless of the patient's condition, needs, and chief complaint, the case manager's documentation of the patient's actual and potential problems almost always include problems related to the following:

1. Patient/family teaching
2. Discharge planning and disposition
3. Need for postdischarge services
4. Financial status
5. Social support systems
6. Clinical condition (i.e., signs and symptoms)

The problems identified by case managers with regard to the complexity of patient/family teaching needs, discharge planning, and the absence of a social support system should be clearly and thoroughly documented in the patient's medical record.

For example, an elderly insulin-dependent diabetic patient who is legally blind and unable to self-administer insulin and who is admitted for uncontrolled diabetes cannot be discharged from the hospital before ensuring that he or she has a safe mechanism in place for administration of insulin injections. Another example is a businessman who is newly diagnosed with myocardial infarction and who is going to be started on cardiac medications for the first time. This patient may not be discharged unless patient teaching is completed or visiting nurse services are arranged for postdischarge follow-up and the patient discharge is deemed safe. Case managers are well trained in how to be proactive planners, particularly in how to meet the discharge planning and teaching needs of their patients before discharge.

The documentation of the case manager's assessment of the needs of these two patients on admission should include the potential problems regarding discharge planning and complexity of patient teaching. The plans of care developed should be reflected in the documentation, particularly how the identified needs will be met before the patients' readiness for discharge. Problems similar to the ones discussed in these examples may delay the patient's discharge. Careful documentation of these problems by case managers helps to justify the delay for administrators, insurance companies, and so on. This kind of documentation also justifies the patient's need for services after discharge (i.e., home care). Managed care organizations usually look for such documentation in the medical record, which justifies the need for intensive services, when conducting medical record reviews or making decisions about whether to authorize services.

Establishing and Implementing the Plan of Care

Planning patient care is a key element in the role of case managers. Accurate and careful planning based on the data collected during the initial screening and assessment of patients, as well as the appropriateness of the identified actual and potential problems, enables case managers to provide individualized, efficient, and high-quality care. The plan of care is extremely important because it serves as a communication tool for everyone involved in patient care. Articulating the plan of care in writing and making it clear to all those involved in the provision of care promotes continuity and consistency of care and enhances its efficiency and effectiveness.

Case managers are responsible for making sure that the written plan of care includes the patient's actual and potential problems and/or nursing diagnoses, the

TABLE 9-2   Example of a Patient Problem as Written by a Case Manager in the Plan of Care of a Patient with Fluid Retention Related to Congestive Heart Failure

Patient Problem/Nursing Diagnosis	Expected Outcomes of Care (Patient/Family Goals)	Nursing Interventions
Fluid balance: excess	Stabilized fluid balance	
	Downward trend in patient's weight; no sudden increase	Weigh patient daily before breakfast
	Balanced intake and output	Monitor accurate intake and output
	Adherence to fluid restriction	Restrict fluids intake to 1,000 ml per day
	Electrolytes within normal ranges; no changes in potassium level	Monitor serum electrolytes, notify physician of any abnormal results
	Increased urine output	Give diuretics as ordered and monitor patient's response/urine output
	Reduction in severity of peripheral edema	Assess peripheral edema daily

---

BOX 9-1   Examples of Patient Care Outcomes for a Diabetic Patient with a Nursing Diagnosis of Knowledge Deficit

The patient/family will be able to do the following:
1. Describe the signs and symptoms of hypoglycemia
2. Describe the signs and symptoms of hyperglycemia
3. Demonstrate correct insulin injection technique
4. State the appropriate sites for insulin injections
5. Demonstrate appropriate syringe filling technique
6. Describe the preventive measures of diabetes foot care

 CASE MANAGER'S TIP 9-6

Characteristics of Outcomes
Outcomes should be as follows:
1. Patient- and family-oriented
2. Realistic and practical
3. Clear and concise
4. Measurable and observable
5. Concrete and doable
6. Time- and interval-specific

---

expected/desired outcomes of care, and the interventions/treatments needed to meet the expected outcomes (Table 9-2). It is important for case managers to document in the patient's record the patient/family agreement to the plan of care as discussed on admission and at the time the initial assessment of patient's needs is completed. Documenting that the goals of treatment are collaboratively set with the patient/family, the case manager, the attending physician, and others involved in the care is essential. This improves compliance with the JCAHO standard of patient's rights and **continuum of care** standards.

The case manager should document the goals of care to be met both before and at the time of discharge. These goals are the expected outcomes of care agreed on with the patient and family and the interdisciplinary team. The expected outcomes of care should be documented following a specific format (Box 9-1) and focusing on specific elements (Case Manager's Tip 9-6).

Case managers individualize the treatment plan and nursing interventions based on the signs and symptoms evidenced in the patient's condition. In addition, they include interventions that prevent any undesired

symptoms or untoward outcomes. Case managers formulate interventions that are specific, realistic, individualized, patient/family oriented, and based on the signs and symptoms of the disease or the goals of treatment.

Documentation in the plan of care should reflect the case manager's ongoing evaluation of the patient responses to treatment and the required revisions in the plan of care as necessitated by the patient's responses.

Case managers are also required to reassess the patient and family on a continuing basis, evaluate the patient's condition for any improvements or changes, follow up on the appropriateness of the treatment and nursing interventions, and identify any new problems that may have arisen and ensure their inclusion in the plan of care. When the patient reassessment is completed, the case manager is expected to write a reassessment note in the patient's record (Box 9-2). It is recommended that case managers who work in acute or subacute care settings write a minimum of three reassessment notes for every patient each week of hospitalization. In long-term care settings, one reassessment note every week is considered appropriate. However, in ambulatory care settings such as clinics and

---

BOX 9-2   Issues to be Addressed by Case Managers in the Reassessment Note

1. Assessment of new needs
2. Follow-up on treatments/interventions
3. Patient and family teaching efforts and progress
4. Facilitation and coordination of tests and procedures
5. Patient/family and interdisciplinary team conferences
6. Referrals to and consults with ancillary or specialized services
7. Discharge planning issues and status of discharge plans
8. Evaluation of patient responses/outcomes
9. Necessary revisions in the plan of care
10. Concurrent reviews with managed care organizations and authorizations for services

---

home visits a note is recommended for every encounter with the patient. In telephonic case management, a reassessment note is completed every time the case manager makes a return or follow-up call to the patient or caller. In addition, a reassessment note is suggested as necessitated by the patient's condition.

Facilitation and Coordination of Care Activities

Because case managers are held responsible for coordinating and facilitating the provision of care on a day-to-day basis, their documentation in the patient's record should reflect these functions. Such progress notes include facilitation and coordination of care activities such as the following:

1. Scheduling and expediting of tests and procedures and prevention of any delays
2. Patient care–related conferences with the family and the interdisciplinary team
3. Coordination of complex discharge/transitional plans
4. Preparation of patients and families for operative procedures
5. Transition of patients from acute to subacute or long-term care settings
6. Consultation with other healthcare providers
7. Ongoing communication with managed care organizations
8. Utilization of resources and related authorizations by managed care organizations
9. Referrals made to other providers or care settings

Patient and Family Teaching

Case managers are responsible for supervising the patient and family teaching activities. This role responsibility should be evidenced in their documentation. Case managers make sure that patient/family teaching is included in

 CASE MANAGER'S TIP *9-7*

Documentation of Patient and Family Teaching

The case manager's documentation of patient and family teaching, based on the patient's condition and needs, should include the following:

1. Assessment of healthcare teaching needs
2. Review of the disease process, signs and symptoms, risk factors, possible complications, and preventive measures
3. Review of the medical/surgical regimen, compliance with the treatment, and the importance of continuous medical follow-up
4. Instructions regarding medications intake, dosage, actions, side effects, route, and special observations
5. Preoperative and postoperative teaching
6. Wound care
7. Pain management
8. Instructions regarding the required use of durable medical equipment (e.g., glucometer)
9. Ongoing review of the plan of care and the discharge plan
10. Availability of and the need for support from community resources after discharge
11. The level of understanding of the teachings held, and whether there is a need for further reinforcement of the information shared and discussed

---

the plan of care and appropriately documented in the patient's record. They document all of the patient/family teaching activities they conduct (Case Manager's Tip 9-7).

Patient's Discharge and Disposition

Patient's discharge and disposition are important responsibilities of case managers (Case Manager's Tip 9-8). Assessment of the patient's discharge needs starts at the time of admission and continues throughout the hospitalization until the patient is ready for discharge or transition to another level of care or another facility. Areas of documentation related to the assessment of patient's discharge needs are presented (see Box 9-4).

Documentation of discharge planning to support safe discharge is important because it may be scrutinized by **peer review organizations (PROs)** if the patient is readmitted with the same problem shortly after discharge. Such situations may increase the financial risk of the institution. If the patient is to receive home care services after discharge, the discharge note should then include the reasons for such services and what is expected to take place at home regarding the care of the patient. Because case managers discuss home care

CASE MANAGER'S TIP 9-8

Documentation of Discharge/Transitional Planning

The case manager documents discharge/transitional planning in the following manner:

1. Actual patient's disposition at the time of discharge in the form of discharge note (Box 9-3)
2. Ongoing assessment of discharge needs, because they may change based on changes in the patient's condition
3. Assessment of postdischarge needs in the initial assessment of the patient (i.e., at the time of screening of the patient for case management services) (Box 9-4)

BOX 9-3 Areas of Documentation Related to Patient's Discharge

1. Disposition (e.g., home, nursing home, group home, rehabilitation facility, hospice)
2. Mode of discharge; transportation provided, if any
3. Person who accompanied the patient on discharge
4. Communication with appropriate personnel regarding confirmation of discharge (e.g., home care agency, managed care organization, patient's family)
5. Confirmation of availability of any equipment needed (e.g., wheelchair, crutches, glucometer, walker)
6. Completion of necessary paperwork related to discharge (e.g., medical request for home care, patient review instrument [for patient's placement in a nursing home])
7. Confirmation of services needed by the patient after discharge (e.g., hemodialysis center, special doctor's clinic)
8. Condition of patient at the time of discharge
9. Discharge instructions

---

needs with home care planners or intake coordinators, it is suggested that such discussions and referrals be included in the discharge documentation.

Evaluation of Patient Care Outcomes

Evaluation of the patient's responses to treatments is essential for better decision making regarding the patient's progress and discharge. Progress notes of case managers should reflect documentation of the patient's status in relation to the desired outcomes established at the time of admission and proactively identified in the plan of care. The frequency with which case managers document patients' progress and responses to treatments depends on the institutional policies and procedures regarding documentation, the charting system, the type of treatments and nursing interventions

---

BOX 9-4 Areas of Documentation Related to the Assessment of Discharge Planning Needs of Patients

1. Services used before hospital admission
2. Projected needs of services after discharge (e.g., home care, physical therapy)
3. Availability of adequate social support system
4. Need for referrals to specialized personnel/services (e.g., social work, home care intake coordinator)
5. Patient's condition (e.g., mental stability, functional abilities)
6. Financial status and insurance coverage
7. Necessary paperwork when requesting community services after discharge (e.g., medical request for home care services) or nursing home placement (e.g., patient review instrument)

---

needed by the patient, the standards of care, and **reimbursement** requirements.

Case managers are also required to track variances of care and delays in achieving patient care outcomes (see Chapter 14 for a detailed discussion on variance). They are cautioned not to document any subjective judgments or system and practitioner variances because they increase the institutional liabilities.

Documenting Variances

When documenting the occurrence of a variance, the case manager should describe the event as specifically as possible. The variance should first be categorized at its highest level (e.g., internal system, external system, patient, family, or practitioner) (Box 9-5). Once the highest category has been identified, the case manager should then drill down to the next level. For example, the case manager may have identified that there is a delay in a patient receiving a computed tomography (CT) scan. This would be considered a "system variance," meaning that an issue related to the organization's own internal system processes caused the delay. Once the delay has been identified as "internal system," the case manager should then categorize it as "CT scan delay." Finally, the case manager will want to determine the cause or reason for the delay. This would be the final and most detailed level.

When possible, a prospective list, such as the one in Box 9-5, should be used by all of the case management staff so that staff members who are identifying variances are doing so in a consistent manner. The list should reflect all potential variances and should be as specific as possible. It can be coded and automated in a database. In this way, the case manager need only identify the variance by its code number (Case Manager's Tip 9-9).

By keeping the variances as specific as possible, and by creating the three-tiered system of identification,

BOX 9-5   Sample List of Variances

Internal System Variances

Transfer for procedure that was cancelled

Reasons:
- Cardiac catheterization
- Cardiac surgery
- Clinical complications

Emergency department delay in admission/awaiting bed

Reason:
- Full census

Extended emergency department stay

Reason:
- Observation

Delay in laboratory results

Reasons:
- Equipment failure/malfunction
- Test not available (weekend/holiday)
- Scheduling delay
- Turnaround time (TAT) for reporting >24 hours

Rehabilitation delay

Reasons:
- Weekend/holiday
- Delay in initiating therapy
- Operating room overbooking

Cancellation of an operative procedure, test, or treatment

Reasons:
- Patient condition
- Physician not available
- Overbooking

Unavailable messenger/transport services

Pending infectious disease approval for medication

Nonformulary medications

Unavailable beds on telemetry unit

Delay in transfer to inpatient psychiatric

Delay in catheter laboratory

Reasons:
- Equipment failure/malfunction
- Test not available (weekend/holiday)
- Scheduling delay
- TAT for reporting >24 hours

Delay in computed tomography (CT) scan

Reasons:
- Equipment failure/malfunction
- Test not available (weekend/holiday)
- Scheduling delay
- TAT for reporting >24 hours

Delay in magnetic resonance imaging

Reasons:
- Equipment failure/malfunction
- Test not available (weekend/holiday)
- Scheduling delay
- TAT for reporting >24 hours

Delay in electroencephalogram (EEG)

Reasons:
- Equipment failure/malfunction
- Test not available (weekend/holiday)
- Scheduling delay
- TAT for reporting >24 hours

Delay in electrocardiogram (ECG)

Reasons:
- Equipment failure/malfunction
- Test not available (weekend/holiday)
- Scheduling delay
- TAT for reporting >24 hours

Delay in Haltor monitor

Reasons:
- Equipment failure/malfunction
- Test not available (weekend/holiday)
- Scheduling delay
- TAT for reporting >24 hours

Delay in adenosine/dobutamine stress test

Reasons:
- Equipment failure/malfunction
- Test not available (weekend/holiday)
- Scheduling delay
- TAT for reporting >24 hours

Delay in x-ray

Reasons:
- Equipment failure/malfunction
- Test not available (weekend/holiday)
- Scheduling delay
- TAT for reporting >24 hours

Delay in exercise stress test

Reasons:
- Equipment failure/malfunction
- Test not available (weekend/holiday)
- Scheduling delay
- TAT for reporting >24 hours

Delay in thallium stress test

Reasons:
- Equipment failure/malfunction
- Test not available (weekend/holiday)
- Scheduling delay
- TAT for reporting >24 hours

Delay in Doppler/vascular laboratory

Reasons:
- Equipment failure/malfunction
- Test not available (weekend/holiday)
- Scheduling delay
- TAT for reporting >24 hours

Late discharge

Reasons:
- Physician delay
- Family delay
- Transportation delay
- Patient delay
- Awaiting procedure
- Awaiting laboratory results
- Prescription not written
- Awaiting result of procedure
- Awaiting physical therapy clearance

Continued

BOX 9-5 Sample List of Variances—cont'd

External System Variances

No nursing home bed available

Reasons:
- Weekend
- Patient choice not available
- No beds

Delay in transfer to another institution

Reasons:
- Awaiting physician orders
- Awaiting family
- Awaiting transportation
- Awaiting approval from receiving facility

Delay in ambulette/other transportation

No home care available over the weekend

No rehabilitation bed available

Child protective services late to arrive

Medical equipment delivered late

No subacute bed available

Patient Variances

Unplanned admission from ambulatory surgery

Reasons:
- Patient complication
- Delay in recovery
- More extensive surgery than originally planned
- Unplanned conversion to an open procedure

Unplanned admission from outpatient unit

Reason:
- Patient complication

Readmission within 30 days for surgical wound infection

Readmission within 30 days for surgical complications

Readmission within 30 days for symptoms related to a prior hospital stay

Readmission within 30 days for deep line infection(s)

Readmission within 30 days for exacerbation of chronic illness

Readmission within 30 days planned for staged procedure/chemotherapy

Readmission within 30 days for false labor

Readmission within 30 days for condition unrelated to previous admission

Unplanned return to special care unit

Reason:
- Clinical complication

Medical complication: Aspiration pneumonia

Medical complication: Unexpected cardiac/respiratory distress with intubation

Medical complication: Iatrogenic pneumothorax

Medical complication: Wound dehiscence

Medical complication: Urinary tract infection (UTI) with intravenous antibiotics

Medical complication: Neurologic system

Medical complication: Gastrointestinal system

Medical complication: Cardiovascular system

Reasons:
- New deep venous thrombosis (DVT)
- Other

Medical complication: Genitourinary/renal system

Reason:
- Acute renal failure leading to dialysis

Medical complication: Respiratory system

Reason:
- New acute pulmonary embolism (PE)

Medical complication: Endocrine system

Medical complication: Musculoskeletal system

Medical complication: Multiple systems

Medical complication: Difficulty/inability to wean

Death: Within 48 hours of surgery

Death: Expected death

Death: Nosocomial infection caused or contributed to death

Death: Autopsy performed

Death: Medical examiner case

Death: Certificate of request for anatomical gift present

Death: Unexpected death

Death: Autopsy requested

Postoperative/procedure complication: Difficulty/inability to wean

Postoperative/procedure complication: Wound dehiscence

Postoperative/procedure complication: Wound infection

Postoperative/procedure complication: Neurological system, including any new peripheral neurological deficit within 48 hours of surgery; any new central nervous system deficit with motor weakness within 48 hours of surgery

Postoperative/procedure complication: Gastrointestinal system

Postoperative/procedure complication: Cardiovascular system, including cardiac arrest, new acute myocardial infarction (AMI) with 48 hours of surgery

Postoperative/procedure complication: Genitourinary/renal system

Postoperative/procedure complication: Respiratory system, including new acute PE

Postoperative/procedure complication: Musculoskeletal system

Postoperative/procedure complication: Unexpected excessive bleeding

Postoperative/procedure complication: Hematoma

Postoperative/procedure complication: Unplanned removal/injury of organ

Postoperative/procedure complication: Multiple systems

Postoperative/procedure complication requiring return to operating room, special procedure, or delivery room: Wound dehiscence

BOX 9-5 Sample List of Variances—cont'd

Postoperative/procedure complication requiring return to operating room, special procedure, or delivery room: Wound infection

Postoperative/procedure complication requiring return to operating room, special procedure, or delivery room: Neurologic system

Postoperative/procedure complication requiring return to operating room, special procedure, or delivery room: Gastrointestinal system

Postoperative/procedure complication requiring return to operating room, special procedure, or delivery room: Cardiovascular system

Postoperative/procedure complication requiring return to operating room, special procedure, or delivery room: Genitourinary system

Postoperative/procedure complication requiring return to operating room, special procedure, or delivery room: Respiratory system

Postoperative/procedure complication requiring return to operating room, special procedure, or delivery room: Musculoskeletal system

Postoperative/procedure complication requiring return to operating room, special procedure, or delivery room: Unexpected excessive bleeding

Postoperative/procedure complication requiring return to operating room, special procedure, or delivery room: Hematoma

Postoperative/procedure complication requiring return to operating room, special procedure, or delivery room: Unplanned removal/injury of organ

Postoperative/procedure complication requiring return to operating room, special procedure, or delivery room: Multiple systems

Postoperative/procedure complication requiring return to operating room, special procedure, or delivery room: Difficulty/inability to wean

Preadmission issue: Noncompliance with preadmission procedures

Emergency department issue: Frequent utilization of emergency department services

Treatment of patient: Delay in obtaining therapeutic anticoagulation levels

Patient refuses tests/treatments/procedures

Patient unable to decide on treatment

Patient refuses discharge

Patient noncompliant with medical/surgical regimen, medications, treatment

Unable to wean from respirator (nonsurgical)

Secondary diagnosis with admission

Language barrier

Poor historian

Withholding pertinent information

Signed out against medical advice (AMA)

Refuses discharge due to religious belief, holiday, and/or personal inconvenience

Noncompliant with diet restrictions

Unable to self-administer medications

Unable to learn about disease

Unable to care for self after discharge

No clothes

No keys for home/apartment

Pressure ulcer present on admission

Hospital-acquired pressure ulcer

Cannot afford to buy medical equipment/medication

Procedure cancelled due to patient illness

Physically unable to progress with treatment plan

Psychologically unable to progress with treatment plan

Financial issues
- Awaiting Medicaid
- No insurance
- No healthcare benefits

Elopement

Family-Related Variances

Unable to pick up patient at discharge

Unable to provide support for care after discharge

Language barrier

Late to pick up patient at discharge

Inadequate level of knowledge regarding patient care

Difficulty with compliance

Unable to learn

Want another opinion

Unable to bring patient's clothes until after business hours

Cannot be reached

Cannot afford to buy necessary medical equipment, medication

Delay in bringing needed papers for Medicaid application

Guardianship/conservatorship issues

Practitioner Variances

Preadmission issue: No medical necessity

Preadmission issue: No utilization review approval for preoperative day

Preadmission issue: Documentation and plan of care inconsistent with preadmission statement

Preadmission issue: ≥1 preoperative day

Preadmission issue: Inappropriate transfer from another institution

Preadmission issue: Transfer requiring ≥1 day preoperative with questionable acuity

Preadmission issue: Admission requiring ≥1 day preoperative with questionable acuity

Emergency department issue: Emergency department admission after preadmission denial

Emergency department issue: Emergency department admission for elective procedure

Continued

BOX 9-5   Sample List of Variances—cont'd

Emergency department issue: Emergency department admission from physician office for test/procedure

Emergency department issue: Social admission

Emergency department issue: Incomplete documentation of emergency department findings/treatments

Emergency department issue: Emergency department clerical error

Emergency department issue: Delay in initiating treatment plan

Delay in communicating plan of care

Physician not communicating to patient

Physician not communicating to the family

Wrong test, treatment, procedure ordered

Incomplete admission assessment, hospitalization (hx)

Omission of an order

Delayed request for a consult

No consent for treatment

Delay in processing forms

Delay in initiating treatment/plan of care

Lack of coordination among interdisciplinary team about discharge plan

Patient teaching not done/completed

Inappropriate/early discharge

Physician did not prepare/inform patient of discharge

Delay in medication administration

Delay or omission in transcribing physician orders

Abnormal test results or physical findings not addressed by physician

Plan of care not acute

Incomplete plan of care

TAT to answer consult >24 hours

Weekend or coverage issues delaying changes in treatment

Delay in implementing guideline/multidisciplinary action plan

Repeated unnecessary tests on transfer

Delay in responding to attending physician recommendations

Delay in initiating consult

Reasons:

- Rehabilitation
- Psychiatry
- Medicine
- Surgery
- Other

Delay in switching from intravenous to oral medication

Delay in ordering medication

Delay in ordering test/treatment/procedure

Order exceeds guideline recommendation: Excessive resource utilization

Plan of care inconsistent with guideline

Delay in discontinuing medication

Delay in discontinuing test/treatment/procedure

Delay in implementing guideline/multidisciplinary action plan

Appropriate guideline/multidisciplinary action plan not applied

---

 CASE MANAGER'S TIP 9-9

Specific Documentation of Variances

Variances should always be documented as specifically as possible so that they can be used for quality improvement projects and process redesign.

---

reports can be generated that will reflect any level of detail required. For example, a particular clinical department may want to know first how many total "patient-related" variances it may have had during a specific period. Then that department may want to know how many of each type. Finally, it may decide to focus on specific patient-related variances and will want to know the reasons for these variances. Automating the standard list and tracking of variances makes these reports less time consuming and easier to generate.

During documentation of the variances, the case manager should remember that the "system" and "practitioner" variances SHOULD NEVER be documented in the medical record. These categories of variances are legally protected by being part of the "quality management" initiatives of the organization and considered confidential and privileged information. Conversely, patient and family variances should be documented in the medical record as they relate to clinical and/or psychosocial issues that will need to be clearly communicated. The case manager should always follow the policies and procedures of the organization as they relate to documenting variances in the medical record. If the variances are warehoused in a database, this too will be protected under the quality umbrella.

A variance should be documented as soon as it is identified. If the variances are being entered into a database, the database will be current and the information in it will reflect "real time" issues. If the variances require immediate intervention, the case manager should document the actions taken to correct the situation in the appropriate location as per their policies and procedures. For example, if the patient had a clinical complication such as an infection, the case manager should document this variance in the database and in the medical record. The medical record documentation should reflect the change in the plan of care (medical and transitional plan) that was made in response to the infection, as well as the expected increase in length of stay, if appropriate.

CHARTING BY EXCEPTION

Charting by exception is a system for documenting against a predetermined, standardized set of expected outcomes. The system uses a number of tools, including standardized clinical/case management plans of care such as clinical paths or clinical practice guidelines. Fundamental to the process of charting by exception is the need to have predetermined outcomes against which the practitioner documents. The prospectively identified outcomes are evaluated at predetermined time intervals. The time intervals are specified in the case management plans or pathways. The practitioner assesses the patient and evaluates whether the outcome has been achieved. If the outcome has been achieved, then the practitioner needs only to time and initial the outcome. This indicates that the outcome has been met.

For a charting by exception system to be effective, the following assumptions must be made:

- The clinical practice **guideline** in use is appropriate to the patient.
- Outcomes are evaluated against the patient's progress at clinically appropriate intervals.
- The interdisciplinary team has agreed to the prospectively identified outcomes and their associated timeframes.
- The outcome signed against indicates that the outcome has been positively met.
- If an outcome is not met, a note in the medical record is required indicating the action plan/intervention.

When charting by exception, the expected outcome to be achieved is evaluated based on an (re)assessment of the patient. The assessment may include either a review of the patient's laboratory values, a physical assessment, an evaluation of educational outcomes, or direct reporting from the patient, all depending on the specific outcomes in review. If the patient has met the outcome as stated in the clinical practice guideline, the case manager initials the outcome indicating that it has been positively met and no further action is needed.

When Outcomes Are Not Met

Charting by exception systems require additional documentation only when an outcome has *not* been met. Therefore if an outcome is not met as per the patient assessment and evaluation, additional documentation

is required. The unmet outcome is considered a variance. The variance is the actual outcome that was achieved by the patient. The actual outcome (variance) is then documented in the designated "variance" column in the **case management plan** or **clinical pathway**. Additional documentation of variance in the medical record must include a description of the variance and the action plan executed to correct the situation. Sometimes variances require a complete revision of the plan of care depending on the changes in the patient's medical condition, such as intubation and use of mechanical ventilation because of respiratory arrest.

Every time case managers identify a variance, they must return to their variance documentation system (e.g., automated variance list) to log in the variance and the reason it occurred. This documentation is important because such data are essential for enhancing the case management model and the system or processes of patient care delivery.

Charting by Exception Sample When Outcome Has Been Met

Clinical practice guideline for thoracic laminectomy

Operative day

Intervention	Expected outcome	Assessment/ evaluation
Assess abdomen every 8 hours	Abdomen soft	9/1/03
Check for bowel sounds, distension	Bowel sounds positive No distension	10 AM, AB

AB has placed her initials in the "Assessment/Evaluation" section of the guideline. Her initials indicate that the patient has met the outcome of "abdomen soft, no distension, bowel sounds positive." In this example, no further documentation is necessary.

Charting by Exception Sample When Outcome Has Not Been Met

Clinical practice guideline for thoracic laminectomy

Operative day

Intervention	Expected outcome	Assessment/ evaluation
Assess abdomen every 8 hours	Abdomen soft	9/1/03
Check for bowel sounds, distension	Bowel sounds positive No distension	10 AM Abdomen distended, bowel sounds positive. Patient experiencing some discomfort. MD notified. AB

In this example, the expected outcome of "no distension" was not met on the operative day. Because the outcome was not met, the case manager needed to document what the actual outcome was and what his or her intervention was regarding it. If the unmet outcome resulted in an extension in the length of stay and/or a quality issue, the unmet outcome must also be documented as a variance.

DOCUMENTING PATIENT EDUCATION

The case manager's role in patient education may be one of educator and/or coordinator. In some models the case manager may develop an educational plan of care, perform the educational interventions, and monitor the educational outcomes. In other models the case manager may be coordinating the educational plan and outcomes but may not be directly involved in the actual educational process with the patient.

In any case, the best way to plan, evaluate, and monitor patient education and the outcomes of a patient education plan is through a charting by exception system. As the patient's educational plan is created, expected outcomes should be developed that correlate with each educational intervention. In this way, the case manager can monitor against the achievement of the expected outcomes and update the plan or intervene as necessary.

Educational Outcomes Must Be Measurable

Similar to other types of patient care outcomes, all identified educational outcomes should be measurable. For example, was the patient able to "return demonstration" of what he or she was taught? Or, was the patient able to verbally repeat back the given instruction? These expected outcomes should be prospectively included in the plan, and the case manager or patient educator should chart against them. Whenever a patient is unable to meet an expected outcome, the case manager must revise the plan to reflect new interventions that address the patient's inability to meet the expected outcome and strategies to meet the outcomes at a later time. Also included should be "why" the patient was unable to meet the outcome, and the plan should reflect a change in response to the unmet outcome. In some instances it may be appropriate to refer to a family member or significant other when planning and providing patient education.

Patient Education and Continuum of Care

The case manager should always consider the continuum of care in any educational plan. If the patient is in the acute care setting, the case manager must ensure that the educational plan safely transitions the patient to home or to another level of care or setting. Whenever

possible, the educational outcomes that have been achieved, as well as those that have not been achieved, should be communicated to the providers in the setting to which the patient is transitioning.

Charting by Exception Sample of Patient Education When Outcome Has Been Met
Clinical practice guideline for asthma
Day 1

Intervention	Expected outcome	Assessment/ evaluation
Instruct patient in use of metered dose inhaler (MDI) and spacer	Patient is able to return demonstration of proper use of MDI and spacer	9/10/03 2 PM, RM

RM has placed her initials in the "Assessment/Evaluation" section of the guideline. Her initials indicate that the patient has met the outcome of "able to return demonstration of proper use of MDI [metered dose inhaler] and spacer." In this example, no further documentation is necessary.

Charting by Exception Sample Patient Education When Outcome Has Not Been Met
Clinical practice guideline for asthma
Day 1

Intervention	Expected outcome	Assessment/ evaluation
Instruct patient in use of MDI and spacer	Patient is able to return demonstration of proper use of MDI and spacer	9/10/03 2 PM Unable to return demonstration of proper use of spacer. Will reinstruct later today. Patient properly using MDI after repeated instruction. RM

In this example, the expected outcome of "able to return demonstration of proper use of MDI and spacer" was not met when RM evaluated the outcome at 2 PM of Day 1. Because the outcome was not met, the case manager needed to document what the actual outcome was and what her intervention was regarding it. If the unmet outcome resulted in an extension in the length of stay and/or a quality issue resulted, the unmet outcome would also need to be documented as a variance. Unmet educational outcomes may trigger a need for postdischarge services that may not have been evident at the time of the patient's admission to the hospital. Timely evaluation and documentation of educational outcomes is important because it provides evidence that justifies the need for follow-up services, ensures certification for these services, and ensures that the patient's plan of care remains appropriate throughout the care episode.

CASE PRESENTATION

Documentation by case managers is essential to patient care because it eliminates confusion and uncertainty from the plan of care and promotes its understanding by all of the healthcare providers involved in the provision of care of the particular patient. Documentation reflects the professional responsibility and accountability of case managers toward patient care and provides concrete evidence of their role in the provision of care. To help the reader better understand the case manager's role in documentation, the rest of this chapter is a discussion around a case presentation of an elderly patient with exacerbation of heart failure who needed acute care (Case Study 9-1). Although this case presentation focuses on acute care, the concepts and skills discussed may be applied in any care setting.

Documenting the patient's care in the medical record is an important means of communication between healthcare professionals. It eliminates misunderstanding and improves awareness of the patient's condition, plan of care, and responses to treatments. Case managers' documentation is necessary to the understanding of their role in patient care. The case study and excerpts on documentation shared in this chapter are only examples of case managers' documentation. Case managers are advised to review the policies and procedures related to documentation that are available in the institutions where they work and make every effort to comply with those policies and procedures.

 KEY POINTS

1. Documentation by case managers is important because it is the only concrete evidence of their role in the provision of patient care.

CASE STUDY 9-1 ■ Elderly Patient with Exacerbation of Heart Failure

In this case study, an 86-year-old male was admitted to the coronary care unit (CCU) of a major academic medical center through the emergency department (ED). Mr. D. lives by himself in an apartment building on the fourth floor. He has been admitted to the hospital four times in the past 2 months. Each time he spent 3 to 4 days in the hospital, of which 2 days were in the CCU. This time, he came to the ED with chest pain and shortness of breath even when resting. On physical examination, he was found to have bilateral audible crackles and 3+ edema in the lower extremities, which was worse around the ankles (pedal). No new changes were identified on the electrocardiogram when compared to the ones taken on the previous hospitalizations. According to the results of his blood tests, he was found to have a potassium serum level of 3.3 mEq, a creatinine level of 2.8 mg/dL, and a blood urea nitrogen level of 22 mg/dL.

When Mr. D. was asked about the home care services arranged before discharge during his last hospitalization, he claimed he did not get along well with the visiting nurse and the home health aide, so he asked them not to visit him again. Mr. D. also informed his case manager that he has no relatives or friends, no money, no insurance, and that he has not been taking his medications (diuretics, digoxin, potassium, and angiotensin-converting enzyme [ACE] inhibitor). He has not been compliant with his restrictive

diet and has been eating whatever he could find. Mr. D. was referred to the heart failure case manager by the ED physician and later on by the primary nurse in the CCU.

The heart failure case manager, after meeting with Mr. D. and reviewing his medical history and record, wrote a screening/intake note. She assessed Mr. D. for appropriateness for case management services and wrote an acceptance note while the patient is still in the ED. The following is an excerpt from the heart failure case manager's note.

Case Management Screening and Intake Note
Tuesday, August 13, 1996, 10:00 AM
Called to see patient by Dr. Jones from the ED. An 86-year-old male with frequent hospitalizations (four times in 2 months) with same complaints of exacerbation of heart failure and noncompliance with medical regimen (medications, activity, diet, and community services). Mr. D. has no insurance coverage and no primary physician. Patient is accepted into the case management services program. Will follow up for full assessment and establishment of the plan of care in the CCU.

Jane Doe, MSN, RN, Heart Failure Case Manager

The screening and intake note written by the heart failure case manager is concise and to the point. It includes the source of referral, the reasons for acceptance for case

Continued

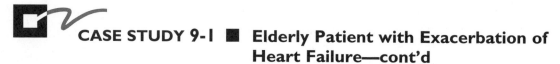

CASE STUDY 9-1 ■ Elderly Patient with Exacerbation of Heart Failure—cont'd

management services, and the necessary follow-up to be made. On arrival of Mr. D. to the CCU, the case manager conducted a thorough assessment of the patient, reviewed the medical record (current and previous hospitalizations), and contacted the cardiologist/heart failure team taking care of Mr. D. to discuss the plan of care. The heart failure case manager then explained to Mr. D. the reason(s) for his hospitalization, the goals of his treatment, and his plan of care (as discussed with the heart failure team). The case manager also involved Mr. D.'s primary nurse in the discussion and in the decisions made regarding his care. The heart failure case manager then proceeded to write an assessment and plan of care note in Mr. D.'s medical record. The note reads as follows:

Case Management Services Follow-Up Note
Tuesday, August 13, 1996, 12:00 PM
A thorough assessment and interview of Mr. D. regarding his past medical history and hospitalizations, medications intake, compliance with medical regimen, insurance coverage, and community services before hospitalization were completed. Medical record was reviewed, and case was discussed with the heart failure team and Mr. D.'s primary nurse.

Assessment of Needs
Mr. D.'s complex condition is related to his noncompliance with the medical regimen and the prescribed community services. His needs are summarized as the following:
1. Healthcare insurance coverage and accessibility to a primary care provider
2. Teaching regarding medical regimen and importance of compliance with the regimen
3. Discharge from the hospital into a safe environment in the community

Plan
1. Verify Mr. D.'s health insurance coverage, and contact outpatient heart failure service for follow-up on Mr. D. after discharge.
2. Teach/ensure patient teaching is done regarding medical regimen and self-care expectations after discharge.
3. Refer patient to home care services. Contact the home care intake coordinator (HCIC). Also refer patient to the nutritionist for dietary counseling.

Jane Doe, MSN, RN, Heart Failure Case Manager

During Mr. D.'s hospitalization, the heart failure case manager continued to work with him, the heart failure team, the primary nurse, and the HCIC to facilitate Mr. D.'s care and expedite his discharge back into the community. She worked on meeting the goals of his hospitalization and the needs that were identified on admission. Every time she was able to confirm the successful completion of Mr. D.'s required care activities, she wrote a note in his medical record. The following are some examples of follow-up notes written by the heart failure case manager during Mr. D.'s stay at the hospital.

Case Management Services Follow-Up Note
Wednesday, August 14, 1996, 9:00 AM
Contacted noninvasive cardiology laboratory to expedite Mr. D.'s echocardiogram. Was able to successfully schedule the echo for today, to be done at 1:00 PM.
12:00 PM
Discussed discharge planning with Mr. D. Reinforced his need for visiting nurse services and home health aide. He states, "I have been very dissatisfied with the agency, the nurse does not answer all my questions…always in a rush"…"the home health aide does not spend the 4 hours with me every day, she frequently tells me that she likes to leave early, because she's got something to do. Could you do something about this?" Reassured Mr. D. of the follow-up.
2:00 PM
Called for results of echo. Preliminary report to be sent to the CCU. Discussed the report with the heart failure team. No significant changes from previous echo that was done 9 months ago. Patient is stable enough to be transferred to a telemetry bed. Arranged for telemetry bed, and primary nurse will transfer Mr. D. out of the CCU by 3:00 PM. Discussed the plan with Mr. D.; he understands the plan and is in agreement. Reassured him of case management follow-up while in the telemetry unit.

Jane Doe, MSN, RN, Heart Failure Case Manager

Case Management Services Follow-Up Note
Thursday, August 15, 1996, 10:00 AM
Home care agency was called; discussed Mr. D.'s concerns, and negotiated a change in the assignment of home care services. The agency agreed to send a different nurse and home health aide. Informed Mr. D. of the change in services; he was pleased. Also discussed the importance of compliance with the medical regimen and the home care services. Mr. D.

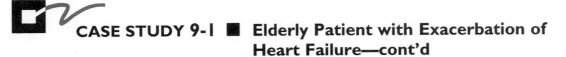

CASE STUDY 9-1 ■ Elderly Patient with Exacerbation of Heart Failure—cont'd

promised to try his best. Contacted the social security and welfare offices and checked on Mr. D.'s insurance. Found out that he has Medicare and Medicaid coverage. Reactivated his coverage and requested new cards, because Mr. D. could not locate the originals. Called the outpatient heart failure services and scheduled Mr. D.'s follow-up appointments for the next 3 months. Arranged for an ambulette for transportation to the hospital for each follow-up appointment.

Jane Doe, MSN, RN, Heart Failure Case Manager

As all case managers do, the heart failure case manager reviewed Mr. D.'s medical record, particularly regarding patient teaching activities, to ensure positive patient care outcomes and to identify any variances in the care of Mr. D. that might require the case manager's interventions. It was noted that Mr. D. has good understanding of his disease process, diet restrictions, and the dosages and actions of his cardiac medications. However, he seemed to experience some problems understanding the importance of fluid restrictions, the side effects of medications, and the necessity of monitoring his weight. The heart failure case manager interviewed Mr. D. regarding teaching and reinforced the areas that still required continued teaching. The case manager then wrote the following note in the medical record.

Case Management Services Follow-Up Note
Thursday, August 15, 1996, 2:00 PM
Mr. D.'s medical record was reviewed. Mr. D. seems to still be experiencing some problems understanding the significance of fluid restrictions and daily weights, as well as the side effects of his medications.

Action
1. Provided Mr. D. with written instructions regarding his medications; reviewed with him the importance of his medications, dosage, schedule, and side effects. Assessed what he was familiar with and reinforced the areas lacking. Reinforced information regarding side effects, particularly the importance and reasons of the need for potassium supplements while on diuretics. Mr. D. was still unable to verbalize complete understanding of the side effects of medications. He was reassured that this issue will be shared with the visiting nurse for further follow-up at home after discharge.

2. Fluid restriction was also discussed with Mr. D. and corrected his impression that restrictions are related to water only. He was provided with instructions on how to control his fluid intake. He was able to verbalize the instructions successfully.

3. When discussed further, it was identified that Mr. D. had no problem understanding the importance of monitoring his weight. The real issue was that he did not have a scale at home. A scale was ordered for him, to be delivered to his house on discharge. He was provided with a daily log to record his weights and instructed to bring it with him every time he is back for a follow-up visit with the outpatient heart failure service.

Jane Doe, MSN, RN, Heart Failure Case Manager

It is as important for the case manager to write a discharge/disposition note in the medical record as it is to write a screening and intake note on admission. Disposition notes usually summarize the patient's progress toward recovery and whether the goals of treatment, identified on admission, are met at the time of discharge. The heart failure case manager summarized Mr. D.'s discharge as follows.

Case Management Services Discharge/Disposition Note
Friday, August 16, 1996, 3:00 PM
Mr. D. is scheduled for discharge on August 17, 1996. The needs identified on admission have been met. His clinical status has improved significantly: no shortness of breath while at rest; able to ambulate around the unit comfortably and without oxygen. He lost 15 pounds with the diuretics. Home care services have been reinstated with new personnel. He has better understanding of his disease and medical regimen. Mr. D.'s healthcare insurance cards will be mailed to him by social services. A scale and oxygen for emergency use at home will be delivered to his house by Saturday morning. Ambulette has been arranged for transportation back and forth on the day of his follow-up appointment. Ambulette service has also been arranged for discharge by 11:00 AM tomorrow. Telephone numbers of the heart failure case manager and outpatient services were provided.

Jane Doe, MSN, RN, Heart Failure Case Manager

2. Documentation acts as a means of communication among healthcare professionals.

3. Documentation improves awareness of the patient's condition, plan of care, and responses to treatments.

4. Documentation by case managers should follow the case management process. For each step in the process, a note is expected.

5. Case managers are responsible for supervising patient education. As part of this responsibility, they should ensure that the educational needs of the patient are planned and documented.

6. Documentation of the discharge planning process is essential to the role of the case manager.

7. The case manager may be responsible for documenting variances or for designing a process for documentation.

8. Charting by exception is a system for documenting against a predetermined set of expected outcomes.

REFERENCES

American Nurses Association: *Standards of clinical nursing practice*, Kansas City, Mo, 1991, The Association.

Bower KA: *Case management by nurses*, ed 2, Kansas City, Mo, 1992, American Nurses Association.

Cohen EL, Cesta TG: *Case management: from concept to evaluation*, ed 2, St Louis, 1997, Mosby.

Tahan HA: The case manager in acute care settings: job description and function, *J Nurs Adm* 23(10):53-61, 1993.

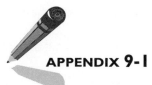

APPENDIX 9-1

CASE MANAGER'S DOCUMENTATION RECORD

This appendix presents an example of a case manager's documentation record. The use of a standardized record streamlines and improves documentation. The record acts as a trigger for better documentation. It also reduces the amount of time required for thorough documentation. Such records can be made flexible to fit the needs of case managers in any patient care setting.

Important Aspects of Documentation

Effective documentation provides a written record of the following items:

- Patient and family needs
- Actual and potential problems
- Patient and family interview on admission
- Goals of treatment
- Case conference
- Assessment and reassessment
- Monitoring and evaluation of outcomes
- **Authorizations** for services
- Patient and family teaching
- Discharge/transitional planning
- Referrals to other services (e.g., home care)
- Managed care reviews/authorizations
- Completion of patient care–related paperwork (e.g., applying for nursing home placement)
- Facilitation and coordination of patient care activities
- Ongoing involvement in patient care activities
- Resolving variances and delays in care activities
- Discharge summary and instructions

EXAMPLE OF A CASE MANAGER'S DOCUMENTATION RECORD

Patient's Name:_____ Date of Admission/Encounter: ____/____/_____

Initial Assessment:

Date: _____/_____/_____ Interviewed: ____Patient ____Family/Caregiver

Review of Medical Record Completed _____Yes _____No

Discussion with _____Physician _____Nurse _____Other: _____

Brief Medical History and Medications Intake:

_____

_____

_____

_____

Diagnosis and Chief Complaint:

_____

_____

_____

_____

Brief Description of Problems (Physiological, Social, Psychological, Emotional, Financial):

_____

_____

_____

_____

Goals of Care (Review of the Plan of Care/Case Management Plan):

_____

_____

_____

_____

Authorization/Certification of Plan of Care and Treatment by Insurer:

Insurer: _____ Contact Person/Case Manager: _____

Authorization #: _____ Telephone #: _____

Type of Needs as Identified by the Case Manager/Focus of Case Management Services:

_____ Medical/Surgical Condition _____

_____ Treatments _____

_____ Acceptance of Illness _____

_____ Emotional Support _____

_____ Grieving Process _____

_____ Support System/Social _____

_____ Nutrition/Diet _____

_____ Activity/Exercise _____

_____ Psychiatry _____

_____ Parenting/Bonding _____

_____ New Parent _____

_____ Health Knowledge _____

_____ Financial _____

_____ Other _____

Consultations (Include Date, Time, and Reason):

_____ Physical Therapy _____

_____ Occupational Therapy _____

_____ Psychiatry _____

_____ Nutrition _____

_____ Social Services _____

_____ Other _____

_____

Meetings/Conferences/Rounds (Include Type, Date, and Time):

_____

_____

_____

Outcomes of Meetings/Conferences/Rounds:

_____

_____

_____

_____

Facilitation/Coordination of Care Activities and Treatments (Include Type, Date, Time):

_____

_____

_____

_____

_____

_____

_____

_____

Patient/Family/Caregiver Education Needs and Activities:
(Use the following key for outcomes of teachings: U, Verbalized Understanding; D, Return Demonstration; R, Needs Reinforcement.)

_____ Signs and Symptoms of Disease _____

_____ Potential Complications _____

_____ Disease Process _____

_____ Tests/Treatments/Procedures _____

_____ Equipment _____

_____ Wound Care _____

_____ Medications _____

_____ Self Care _____

_____ Other _____

_____

_____

Discharge/Transitional Planning:

Level of Care Review: _____ Appropriate Based on Preestablished Criteria (If No, Explain):

_____

_____

Certification for Continued Stay: _____ Yes _____ No Date: _____/_____/_____

_____

_____

Anticipated Discharge Needs:

_____ Equipment _____

_____ Supplies _____

_____ Home Care Evaluation _____

_____ Long-Term Care Facility Placement _____

_____ Short-Term Residence _____

_____ Shelter _____

_____ Rehabilitation _____

_____ Hospice Care _____

_____ Transportation _____

_____ Home, No Needs _____

_____ Home with Home Health _____ Aide _____ Attendant _____ Homemaker

_____ Special Services, Explain: _____

_____

Required Paperwork for Discharge Planning (Include Completion Date):

_____ Personal Review Instrument _____

_____ Visiting Nurse Services _____

_____ Managed Care Authorization/Certification _____

_____ Other _____

Name: _____ **Signature:** _____ **CM**

10 Hiring Case Managers: Role of the Candidate and the Interviewer*

Interviewing or being interviewed for a job is something nearly everyone has to do at one time or another during one's career. It is probably the most important, intimidating, and demanding task one will ever be involved in. The reward of interviewing well is getting hired for the job. Candidates for the **case manager** role face a challenging task. They need to prove to their prospective employers, on paper and in person, that they are the *best candidate* for the role.

The number of experienced candidates for the case manager's role has been increasing because restructuring and redesigning of patient care delivery have resulted in **case management** systems being identified as key delivery models in most institutions. Given this demand, many schools are now including training and education for case management both at the graduate and undergraduate levels. This change has increased competition as recruiters and potential employers select the best candidate for the case manager's role. This chapter discusses the interview process of case managers and the roles of the candidate and the interviewer. In addition, it provides some tips for success in both roles.

CANDIDATE

Employers select their candidates for the case manager's role based on the applicant's clinical and leadership skills and knowledge in case management. The criteria considered in the potential candidate include resourcefulness, flexibility, adaptability, tolerance to stress and hard work, teamwork, dependability, truthfulness, reliability, effectiveness, perseverance, and ability to manage change and conquer challenge. Other criteria relate to clinical expertise in an area of practice (e.g., cardiology or long-term care), specialty certification, and case management certification.

To be hired for the case manager's position, potential candidates should prepare themselves to be "The Candidate." They must go beyond preparing an "attractive" resume. They need not only be able to intelligently market themselves on paper but also to sell themselves even more carefully during the job interview process. This task can be quite intimidating and requires high-level written and verbal skills.

Preparing the Resume and Curriculum Vitae

Today's advertisements (ads) no longer include the telephone numbers of the recruiter or recruitment office; instead a mailing address (electronic or regular), and/or a fax number are provided. This change in advertising makes the resume and curriculum vitae (CV) extremely important. Resumes and CVs are personal marketing and sales tools and should contain accurate information reflective of the candidate's past and current experiences, skills, accomplishments, and honors. They become the only compelling source of information available to prospective employers for targeting candidates for interviews. Resumes and CVs should summarize the candidate's best attributes, including the following:

■ Career objective(s)
■ Employment history, highlighting the most recent experience
■ Education
■ Licensure, certifications, awards, and honors
■ Scholarship activities: previous research, public speaking activities, and citations of published materials

*This material first appeared in Tahan HA: Hiring case managers: the role of the candidate and the interviewer, *Nurs Case Manag* 2(2):85-92, 1997.

- Professional organizations or societies
- Volunteer work or community services
- Other skills (e.g., languages spoken, computer skills)
- Available references

Resumes and CVs require a special type of writing that may not conform to the rules of grammar or punctuation, which makes them easier to write. When preparing their resume/CV, candidates for the case manager role may face some challenges in articulating their previous experiences or conveying the extent of the skills they possess. To overcome this challenge, they may seek the help of professional agencies that specialize in writing resumes, or they may refer to books on business writing (i.e., how to write resumes and cover letters). Such books can be found in public and private libraries and in the business section of bookstores. Today, similar information can be found online (i.e., the Internet). However candidates may seek help for writing the resume, it is important that they make sure the final product provides the potential employer with a comprehensive profile of oneself, stressing what contributions the candidate offers the institution.

Resumes and CVs are different but also somewhat similar. They vary based on length and degree of detail. The length of the resume usually does not exceed two to three pages. However, CVs are generally longer than resumes (they may be longer than 10 pages) and include more details. Although not a standard rule, resumes tend to start with work experience first, while CVs begin with the educational background. This is why CVs are thought of as more academic than resumes. The work history and experience consume most of the length (Case Manager's Tip 10-1). In both resumes and CVs, candidates may highlight their work experience and skills following either a reverse chronological format or a grouping of tasks and skills. The formats are equally appropriate. In the reverse chronological history, the work history is listed starting with the latest job held. In contrast, the grouping of tasks and skills format requires a synthesis of the categories of these tasks and skills based on all previous jobs held. The advantage of the latter format is that the candidate has the flexibility of highlighting the skills, tasks, and qualities most appropriate to the case manager's role regardless of the time they were acquired, performed, or applied. Candidates for the case manager's role who do not have case management experience are advised to prepare their resume following the grouping of tasks and skills format. This format will clearly show the qualities that make them the best candidate for the job.

Box 10-1 presents an excerpt from an ad for a case manager position that one might come across in a newspaper, professional nursing journal, or recruitment

 CASE MANAGER'S TIP 10-1

Suggestions for Writing Resumes or Curriculum Vitae

- Describe your work experience using factual and detailed information.
- Be specific with your educational background, credentials, licensure, and certifications.
- Include the time period of each of your past work experiences and educational background. Be accurate with dates and include the months and years.
- Organize your past experiences and educational background information in the same chronologic order; reverse chronological is preferred.
- Do not include the number(s) of your license(s).
- List your accomplishments; include those that relate to your work and volunteer associations.
- Add a statement about your job objectives and/or goals.
- Make your resume/CV reader-friendly: use a consistent format throughout, font size 12, bulleted lists, and recognizable sections.
- Be concise and to the point in your descriptions: "less is more."
- Include a list of selected publications and presentations.
- Highlight any honors or awards you may have received.

newsletter. Potential applicants should study the ad carefully and be able to identify the qualities, skills, and qualifications the organization is looking for in the candidate (i.e., the bolded areas in Box 10-1). These qualities and skills may not be clearly stated in the ad. It is the responsibility of the candidate applying for the job to synthesize the desired qualifications. The resume or CV should then be written in a way that addresses the identified characteristics of the job. Candidates must not arbitrarily submit a resume or a CV; they must stick to what is specified in the ad.

Cover Letter

A cover letter explaining the candidate's intent to apply for the job is important to have attached to the resume or CV before mailing or faxing the application. In the letter, the candidate should indicate the specific ad he or she is responding to (i.e., specify the job title and the source of the ad). The letter should also include the career objective(s) of the candidate and highlight the acquired qualities and skills that meet the job requirements. For example, if you are responding to the

BOX 10-1 Excerpt from an Ad for a Case Manager's Job

In this position as a case manager you will be responsible for **working with an interdisciplinary team** of healthcare providers and **managing the care** of a select group of patients with complex diagnoses and needs. You are expected to achieve **high-quality care outcomes** in a **cost-effective** manner. You will act as a **patient and family advocate** and a **consultant** for members of the healthcare team within the institution and for **managed care organizations** and **community resource agencies** externally. The ideal candidate will possess a minimum of **4 years' clinical experience** and a current license as a registered professional nurse or certification as a social worker. A bachelor's degree is also required. Excellent **verbal and written communication skills,** case management experience, and certification are a plus.

ad presented in Box 10-1, it is important that you describe your skills in communication, teamwork, negotiation, brokering, facilitation and coordination of patient care activities, and evaluation of care outcomes. It is important to highlight your knowledge of healthcare reimbursement systems, managed care organizations, and patient and family satisfaction issues. It is also beneficial to identify your clinical and leadership skills as they relate to the advertised job.

Because there will be no personal contact with the recruiter or prospective employer to discuss the job, you should put special effort into writing the best resume/CV and cover letter possible to increase your chances for an interview. The resume/CV and cover letter are your selling tools. They reflect your marketability, and they should "paint a picture" of your potential for success in the job. Review them carefully for any typographical or spelling errors, long or run-on sentences, and appropriateness of the adjectives used to describe yourself. Always remember to be concise, clear, and direct.

In the letter, candidates should indicate how their skills and previous experiences can be used in the prospective job or for the benefit of the institution. The style applied in the cover letter should appeal to the recruiter or the prospective employer. Avoid being overly clever or too wordy. Try to be honest, warm, and sincere. Use phrases that will increase interest in you, and emphasize those aspects of yourself that you think will meet the case manager's role and make you look attractive. The cover letter should not be too long or boring to read. It should urge the prospective employer to review the resume/CV and call you for an interview.

Looking Your Best

The interview is the opportunity to prove yourself. It is an act of validating that a potential candidate is the best fit for the job. The interview process should validate for the interviewer that your description of your qualifications and skills, evidenced in the resume/CV and cover letter, is accurate. Your responses to the interview questions should strongly support what you have written in the resume/CV. You should be at your best and look your best.

One way of improving your chances of being hired for the job is by familiarizing yourself with the role or position you are interviewing for. It is important for any case manager candidate to keep abreast of the latest changes occurring in the healthcare industry. A little over a decade ago, case management models were strange to hospitals and healthcare organizations. Training of case managers was held in the healthcare organization itself as part of the orientation to the new work environment and the role. However, because of reengineering and redesign of patient care delivery systems, today these models and roles are more popular, and training in case management has become available in schools of nursing as certificate and degree programs. This shift into case management has increased the competition among the candidates for the case manager's role and helped prospective employers in selecting the best-prepared candidate for the job.

The healthcare-related literature contains a substantial amount of information on case management models and roles. It is important for potential candidates to become knowledgeable in this field before applying for the role, especially if they have not had any prior training or experience in case management.

The case manager's role varies from one institution to another. One's experience as a case manager in one institution might not be transferable. Therefore it is important for a candidate to evaluate his or her previous experience in relation to the skills and qualifications required for the job being interviewed for and to proactively determine how to maximize the benefit of this experience for the interview.

It is important for candidates to obtain the job description of the advertised role and the mission and philosophy statements of the institution before the interview and to study them carefully. This information is invaluable for candidates who are preparing for the interview and is instrumental in familiarizing them with the potential work environment; expectations of the role; and the institution's culture, values, and beliefs. Candidates may ask for this information in advance through a personal letter or a fax addressed to the recruiter at the address/fax number available in the ad.

They also may ask for this information in the cover letter attached to the resume/CV, either at the time it is sent to the recruiter or the prospective employer or when the candidate is contacted to set up a date for the interview. Either way, it is important for candidates to obtain and review this information before the interview.

Candidates must provide evidence to the interviewer that they possess the qualities, skills, and attributes necessary for the position. Sometimes it is helpful to maximize the use of real examples related to previous experiences to convince the interviewer that you are "The Candidate."

Potential case managers should be able to convince their prospective employer that they are the *right* candidates for the job and the organization. One way to accomplish this is by conveying a sense of professionalism. You should clearly articulate your strengths and weaknesses as they relate to the job. You should also explain your willingness to learn and improve in the areas in which you lack experience. The interviewer expects a candidate to be lacking knowledge or experience in some aspects of the job, and candidates who recognize or address this issue demonstrate a clear understanding of the job requirements and willingness to learn. It is also important that you make the interviewers aware of your potential. Explain to them what it is that you are able to bring with you that is considered beneficial to the institution. Concentrate on meeting the organization's mission statement and philosophy. Make an effort to discuss your transferable skills (i.e., the skills you can carry with you to any job or organization).

The outer appearance of potential candidates for the case manager's role is important. It is the first impression you leave with the interviewer/prospective employer. The way you are dressed should create a positive and professional image. This image plays a crucial role in setting the tone for the rest of the interview. You should make an effort to look professional even if you know that the prospective employer has a relaxed dress code. You should *dress for success* (Case Manager's Tip 10-2).

During the interview, candidates should be extra careful in how they respond to the interviewer's questions. They should not appear to be rigid, indifferent, or inflexible. Candidates should avoid using statements that begin with "I never ...," "I don't like ...," or "It is impossible to ..." The following examples illustrate this point.

Do not say: "In my previous job I never attempted to call the private physicians myself because it made them angry. Instead, I always asked the nurse manager to do that." *It is better to say:* "In my previous job I was not expected to contact the private physicians myself, but I

CASE MANAGER'S TIP 10-2

Dress for Success
- What you wear reflects who and what you are.
- Dressing in business attire is preferred.
- Play it safe and stick to conservative colors such as navy blue, black, or gray.
- Keep jewelry and accessories to a minimum; be tasteful in your choices.
- Avoid strong cologne or perfume.
- Stand and sit erect during the interview.

understand the importance of discussing a particular situation with them directly. I am willing and have no problem doing that in this position." *Do not say:* "In the past I found it impossible to discuss the plan of care of each patient with the various healthcare providers." *It is better to say:* "It is a great challenge to discuss the plan of care of each patient with the various healthcare providers, and I understand its importance in improving the quality of care. I will do the best that I can in this area." *Do not say:* "Why should I keep pushing for rescheduling a procedure that is cancelled. It is not my responsibility to do it. It is the responsibility of the department canceling the procedure." *It is better to say:* "I understand how difficult it can be to ensure that a procedure is completed as scheduled. It is important to not delay the completion of a procedure. Otherwise, the patient and the institution suffer (or the cost and quality of care are compromised)."

In their answers to interviewers' questions, candidates are encouraged to use statements that convey an understanding of the case manager's role, flexibility in their opinions and attitudes, openness to change and trying new methods of doing things, and willingness to learn and expand knowledge. Candidates should avoid stating what they have always done in their previous jobs. However, they can use their previous experiences in subtle ways to support their flexibility as practitioners and confirm to the interviewers that they possess the skills and qualities the interviewers seek in the potential case managers.

Questions That May Be Asked by Candidates

It is appropriate for candidates to ask questions during the interview process. However, questions should be asked when opportunities exist. For example, interviewers may ask candidates at some point during the interview process if they have any questions. If this does not happen, then candidates may ask their questions toward the end of the interview. Questions that are considered appropriate include the following:

- Patient population(s)
- Area of responsibility (e.g., inpatient unit, outpatient clinic, both areas)
- Expectations regarding performance
- Expected hours of work (e.g., days, evenings, weekends, rotation)
- Reporting mechanism (i.e., the case manager's position in the table of organization)
- Current status in relation to case management and institutional goals
- Support systems
- Orientation process to the work environment and the role

The salary should not be discussed during the interview unless it is brought up by the interviewer. It is always better to negotiate the salary at the time the job is offered.

Candidates may also ask the interviewer about the timeframe for filling the job or how long it will be before they are notified if they are accepted. Candidates may contact the recruiter and inquire if a decision has been made if the indicated timeframe has passed. It is acceptable to ask about the reasons for not being hired. Interviewing is a demanding skill, and one cannot improve unless if made aware of deficient areas.

CHARACTERISTICS LOOKED FOR IN POTENTIAL CANDIDATES FOR THE CASE MANAGER'S ROLE

The role of the case manager is integral to the success of the case management model. During the interview process candidates for this job should reflect potential for success in the role. There are several significant skills case management leaders look for in candidates for the case manager's role (Box 10-2). These skills are based on the job description of the case manager and are affected by the environment of work and scope of responsibilities (i.e., the operations/systems of the organization, policies, procedures, standards of care and practice, and status and power embedded in the job as compared with other healthcare professionals). The most important skills are those that make the potential candidate able to collaborate effectively with other healthcare providers within and outside the organization.

A person in the case manager position is expected to work with minimum direction and supervision. Because the case manager is an integral member of an interdisciplinary team, he or she is expected to demonstrate excellent decision-making and problem-solving skills. In addition, the case manager should exhibit a willingness

---

BOX 10-2   Case Manager's Skills
1. Clinical
2. Leadership
3. Teamwork
4. Time management
5. Decision making/problem solving
6. Critical thinking
7. Organization
8. Delegation
9. Communication/open-mindedness/assertiveness
10. Diplomacy/politics
11. Tolerance
12. Commitment
13. Education/teaching
14. Role modeling
15. Change agent
16. Conflict resolution
17. Power
18. Cultural sensitivity
19. Information management and reporting
20. Computer literacy

to work with others (i.e., teamwork). Because of the varied responsibilities of this position, the case manager should have superior organizational and time-management skills. This is important for increased productivity and efficiency in the role. Case managers work daily with physicians, nurses, patients and families, and other healthcare providers to ensure that high-quality and cost-effective care and **outcomes** are achieved. These expectations make assertiveness, the ability to communicate well verbally and in writing, diplomacy, and open-mindedness among the many skills required for success in the role.

Case managers spend much of their time facilitating and coordinating patient care activities, advocating for their patients/families, and resolving **variances.** In this role function, they are expected to demonstrate skills in leadership, clinical care activities, tolerance, communication, delegation, and negotiation. When they hold patient and family teaching sessions, they apply the adult learning theory into their practice and follow the strategies derived from the health-belief model, which means that they should be knowledgeable about the available theories on patient and family teaching. In addition, when they are asked for help by a member of the healthcare team, they are looked at as role models and resource people. They are expected to be able to find solutions to challenging situations.

INTERVIEWER'S ROLE

During the interview process, interviewers should evaluate whether potential candidates possess the skills required for the role. If candidates are found to be lacking in any of the skills or functions, interviewers should evaluate them for potential success in learning these skills and functions. The questions to be asked in an interview should cover the affective, cognitive, and behavioral aspects of the role.

The best questions to be asked are open-ended ones (Table 10-1). Potential candidates should also be asked to provide practical examples that support their abilities and help demonstrate competence in their skills. Examples are particularly important because they provide concrete evidence related to a candidate's performance in real work situations. Examples usually validate a candidate's answers because they add an objective flavor to subjective answers. When candidates are found to be struggling with giving examples, the interviewer may use hypothetical situations to help them express their opinion.

The interviewer must be careful not to ask questions that are considered against the law, as determined by the Americans with Disabilities Act, Equal Employment Opportunity Act, and Age Discrimination in

TABLE 10-1 Sample Questions That May Be Asked in the Case Manager's Interview

Questions	Behaviors/Skills Evaluated	Questions	Behaviors/Skills Evaluated
Tell me about yourself.	Personality type Energy Optimism Ego	Tell me about a time when you were able to influence the behavior of others in a positive way.	Encouragement of others Teamwork/team player Ability to provide feedback Interpersonal skills Creativity and paradigm shift Willingness to try new ideas
Give me an example of when you had too many things to do at once, and tell me how you went about accomplishing the tasks.	Time management Organizational skills Prioritization Creating a plan Getting tasks accomplished	Describe a situation when you were able to impact the cost of patient care/resource utilization.	Awareness of healthcare costs Cost-containment strategies Allocation/management of resources
Tell me about a problem you have faced in the past with a patient/family member, co-worker, physician, or superior. How did you handle the situation?	Conflict resolution Problem solving Dealing with stress Affect/temperament Teamwork/independence Effectiveness Assertiveness Comfort level with confrontation	Tell me about a time when you were faced with a problem and needed to collect some information for solving the problem. Describe to me how you analyzed the information to come to your decision.	Problem solving Critical thinking Use of data and evidence Response to stressful situations/affect Willingness to complete a project/task Commitment
Explain to me what makes you the best candidate for the job.	Motivation Self-confidence Self-esteem Ability to discuss strengths and weaknesses Experience Assertiveness	Describe to me a situation when you had to work with little or no supervision. What did you do?	Independence Motivation Commitment Productivity Leadership
From your past experience, tell me about a time when you had to promote change. How were you able to do it? What role did you play in it?	Perseverance Change agent Adaptability and flexibility Openness to change and new ideas Creativity Ability to influence others Assertiveness Risk taking	What is it that you can bring to this role/institution that will make a difference?	Previous experience Ability to identify one's strengths Confidence/self-esteem Visionary
		Tell me about your career goals.	Goal orientation Having a vision Future planning Ability to be focused
In your opinion, what does a case manager do?	Knowledge and understanding Potentials Keeping up-to-date with changes in healthcare	Discuss the biggest mistake you ever made.	Self-confidence Truthfulness Learning Admitting to mistakes

Employment Act. Interviewers should avoid questions such as the following:

- How old are you?
- How many children do you have?
- How old are your children?
- Are you married?
- What religious holidays do you observe?
- What language do you speak when not at work?
- What is your ethnic background?
- What are your political beliefs?

Interviewers should take their time when conducting the interview. They should avoid making candidates feel rushed. A reasonable interview is one that lasts an average of 1 hour. Similar to the candidates, interviewers are required to be poised, clear, direct, articulate, and skillful in the interview process. It is imperative for interviewers not to bore candidates by talking too much about the institution and the job. They should avoid unnecessary rambling.

Interviewers should prepare the interview questions in advance. As much as possible, they should use the same set of questions for interviewing all potential candidates. This pattern makes it easier to compare candidates and select the best one for the job. Most institutions have a standardized interviewing process in place and a predetermined set of questions that can be adapted to each specific job. If this is not the case in your institution, it is helpful to prepare interview questions beforehand.

At the end of the interview, interviewers may summarize the interview by explaining the next step(s) to candidates. This may include whether follow-up interviews are necessary and, if so, with whom, when, and where. It is also important that candidates be informed of the timeframe for filling the position and the method of notifying the selected candidate. This eliminates any confusion candidates may face while waiting to hear from the interviewer/potential employer.

FOLLOW-UP INTERVIEWS

Candidates for the case manager's role are usually interviewed more than once. They are interviewed by the recruiter and the administrator of the case management program. Some institutions also require them to be interviewed by a panel (i.e., representatives from the interdisciplinary team such as physicians, other case managers, directors of nursing, nurse managers, social workers, physical therapists, quality management staff, and home care coordinators). Depending on the job description and roles and responsibilities, potential candidates may be required to interview with chief physicians or chairmen of departments. Candidates should prepare themselves

well for impressive and successful interviews throughout the interview process an institution may have in place.

When interviewed by physicians or chairmen of departments, it is important for a candidate to convey a message of openness, collegiality, collaboration and partnership, and clinical knowledge. It is also important that he or she convey excellence in teamwork, negotiation, leadership, mentorship, problem solving, conflict resolution, and coaching skills.

Candidates are first interviewed by a recruiter, who screens them and selects those who express strong potential for success in the case manager's role. Next they are interviewed by the administrator of the case management program. Those who are found to be impressive and show strong potential are then called for

 CASE MANAGER'S TIP 10-3

Suggestions for the Interviewer

1. Ask open-ended questions: background, behavioral, situational, conversational/nondirective, and directive.
2. Establish rapport at the beginning of the interview.
3. Begin with "ice-breaking" questions (e.g., It is a lovely day today; how was your trip coming here?).
4. Allow silence; the candidate may need to collect his or her thoughts before answering the question.
5. Ask behavioral questions.
6. Control the interview; you may need to redirect the conversation if the candidate starts to ramble around.
7. If you want to take notes, explain why.
8. Prepare the questions in advance. Questions should be based on the related job description and/or the candidate's resume/CV.
9. Ask questions that are based on the candidate's past job experiences. This allows for envisioning the future and investigating the candidate's potential.
10. Ask for contrary evidence, especially when identifying an undesired or a negative skill. Contrary evidence prevents the interviewer from creating a one-sided/subjective picture.
11. Validate responses using reflective statements as needed.
12. Avoid judgment, and be objective. Do not allow intuition or "gut feelings" to interfere in your decision.
13. Familiarize yourself with the skills required for the job (e.g., performance, organizational, interactional).
14. Apply a businesslike approach to the interview process.

CASE MANAGER'S TIP 10-4

Suggestions for the Candidate

1. Ask for the job description and the organization's mission and philosophy statements in advance. Study them well.
2. Research the prospective employer and organization.
3. Arrive for the interview on time.
4. Dress for success.
5. Bring your portfolio to the interview. Be prepared to share concrete evidence of your accomplishments when appropriate.
6. Watch your body language/nonverbal communication. It is a part of the interview too. Sit straight and erect with your head up. Do not fidget.
7. Maintain eye contact at all times.
8. Do not interrupt the interviewer.
9. Avoid rambling around in your answers. Be poised, concise, clear, and direct.
10. Support your answers with evidence (i.e., examples from previous experiences).
11. Be prepared to discuss what it is that you can provide to the organization.
12. Convey your self-confidence, professionalism, and self-esteem through your answers.
13. Do not hesitate to explain your silence at times. The interviewer is aware that you may need a moment of silence to collect your thoughts before answering a question.
14. Avoid speaking fast or stuttering. Be articulate.
15. Be clear in your career goals.
16. Rehearse your interview if that helps you to be better prepared.
17. Apply a businesslike approach to the interview process.
18. Do not downplay your achievements.
19. Avoid criticizing your present employer or supervisor. You do not want to be perceived as a complainer.
20. Be careful and guard against displaying nervous habits.

follow-up interviews. The follow-up interviews, depending on the institution, may include an interview with a physician or the chairman of the department in which the case manager will be working and another with a panel of interviewers, including representatives from the interdisciplinary healthcare team and fellow case managers.

It is important to limit the follow-up interviews to only the candidates who express promising success in the role. The recruiter and the administrator of the case management program may collaborate in selecting these candidates, which usually are limited to two or three in number. Unnecessary interviews waste time and cost money. Candidates should be informed by the interviewer of the next steps, whether follow-up interviews will be conducted, and when they will be informed of such decisions.

Candidates should not forget about the interviewer after the interview is over. It is advisable to send a note or a card thanking the interviewer for the opportunity and the consideration. It is also appropriate for candidates to indicate in the note their continued interest in the job.

Conducting interviews and being interviewed are great challenges. One should learn how to meet these challenges. It is beneficial to read about the interview process or attend seminars to polish your interviewing skills. Sometimes it is necessary to practice role playing before your interview. This practice may help you get the job you desire. Case Manager's Tips 10-3 and 10-4 present some tips for the interviewer and the candidate. These tips should help both the interviewer to be better prepared for evaluating and screening the appropriate candidates for the job and the potential candidates to overcome their fear of being interviewed. The skills necessary for interviewing well are important for everyone to master because one never knows when they may be necessary. You should always remember that the written words (i.e., the resume/CV and cover letter) are the candidate's ambassador to the interviewer. They should be thought of as a glorified list of one's qualities, which when read leaves a lasting impression.

KEY POINTS

1. The interview process is not easy. It requires careful and thorough preparation by the candidate and the interviewer. Practice, role play, or rehearsal before the interview could be helpful.
2. Candidates for the case manager's job should always send a resume/CV with a cover letter to potential employers explaining their intent for applying for an advertised job and summarizing their qualifications for the job.
3. The resume/CV is a compelling source of information for the prospective employer. An impressive resume/CV is one that summarizes the candidate's knowledge, experiences, attributes, and skills.
4. The cover letter should delineate the candidate's acquired qualities and skills that are anticipated to meet the requirements of the job applied for.

5. Avoid being rigid, indifferent, or inflexible during an interview (this is applicable for both the candidate and the interviewer).
6. If interviewing several candidates for a job, use a standardized set of questions that could be prepared based on the job description and should reflect the skills and qualities demanded by the job. It also is helpful to apply a scoring/rating system in the process. This makes it easier to differentiate among the applicants and to select the best candidate for the job.

11 Curricula and Certification in Case Management

Case management has become the most desired approach to patient care delivery. Originally it was a nursing care delivery model. Today, however, most healthcare institutions have adopted case management as their patient care delivery system. Nurses who assumed the case manager's role in the 1980s were basically prepared for the role in healthcare organizations (i.e., hospitals). Training sessions for these nurses were conducted on the premises of the institution itself, particularly at the patient's bedside. Since the early 1990s, however, **case managers** have had opportunities for training in a variety of settings. In addition to the institution-based case management training programs, today there are several programs that are college- or university-based.

Case management is defined by the Commission for Case Manager Certification (CCMC) (2001, p. IV) as "a collaborative process which assesses, plans, implements, coordinates, monitors, and evaluates the options and services required to meet an individual's health needs, using communication and available resources to promote quality, cost-effective outcomes." Case management programs are designed to train case managers in the case management and patient care management processes. The content of these programs is an in-depth review of the CCMC's definition of case management.

BACKGROUND OF CASE MANAGEMENT EDUCATIONAL PROGRAMS

Changes in the structure and processes of patient care delivery have resulted in the development of new educational programs and specializations or the revision of already existing ones. Case management today is considered a basic component of graduate and undergraduate nursing and allied health curricula. In some schools it is provided as an area of specialization as either a postbaccalaureate certificate or a master's degree program (Simmons, 1992; Haw, 1995; Spenceley, 1995; Wells, Erickson, and Spinella, 1996). This is evident in a survey conducted by Haw (1996) of schools of nursing regarding the inclusion of case management content in their nursing programs. The survey was conducted with 108 graduate and 98 undergraduate programs. The results of this survey showed the following:

- 8 (7%) of the schools had a dedicated major in case management at the graduate level but none at the undergraduate level.
- 11 (10%) of the graduate and 1 (1%) of the undergraduate programs had one or more required case management courses.
- 9 (8%) of the graduate and 3 (3%) of the undergraduate programs had one or more elective case management courses.
- 96 (89%) of the graduate and 93 (95%) of the undergraduate programs had some case management–related content in required courses.
- 26 (24%) of the graduate and 12 (12%) of the undergraduate programs required clinical experience.
- 41 (38%) of the graduate and 22 (22%) of the undergraduate programs included optional clinical experience.

Although the results of this survey were limited to the participating schools of nursing, findings do suggest that preparation for the case management role in academia is occurring at the graduate level, and to a limited extent at the undergraduate level. A follow-up article reported an increase in the number of schools offering a graduate degree in case management to approximately 15 programs that offer a combination of theoretical and clinical courses (Toran, 1998).

In 1997 Falter et al (1999) conducted a survey in New York, New Jersey, and Connecticut to assess the need for developing a school-based nursing case management educational program. A sample of 69 hospitals, home care agencies, managed care organizations, and long-term care facilities was surveyed. The results of this survey showed the following:

■ 58 (84%) facilities employed case managers, constituting 85%, 77%, and 57% of the facilities in New Jersey, New York, and Connecticut, respectively.

■ Home care facilities were found to be in the lead of employing nurses as case managers. Next were managed care organizations, then hospitals, then long-term care. No actual frequencies or percentages were provided.

■ 65% of the facilities responded positively to hiring case managers over the next 5 years, 31% responded negatively, and 9% were uncertain.

■ Clinical, home care, and **utilization review** experiences were the top three determining factors for hiring potential case managers.

■ Other factors reported include (in descending order) case management experience, interpersonal skills, management experience, **discharge planning** knowledge, insurance knowledge, **managed care, certification** in case management, **clinical pathways** knowledge, organizational skills, and advanced degree.

■ A master's degree was required by only five (8.6%) facilities, 45 (77.6%) facilities required a Bachelor of Science degree in nursing, and three (5.1%) hired case managers with an associate's degree.

■ 31 (53.4%) facilities agreed that there was a need to educate nurse case managers at the master's level, 25 (43.1%) disagreed, and two (3.4%) were uncertain.

■ 50 (86.2%) were willing to provide financial support for a case manager to attend graduate case management education.

This survey guided the authors in designing a graduate level degree and a post-master's certificate program in case management that were started in the fall of 1998 at Pace University in New York City.

When they were first implemented in the mid-1980s, case management systems were bound to healthcare practice organizations (e.g., hospitals). Education of case managers in these organizations in preparation for these emerging new roles was occurring in the practice setting as part of continuing education. Training sessions were held on the premises of the healthcare organization, both in a classroom and at the patient's bedside.

During the 1990s case management entered the area of nursing education in the form of either lectures on case management or a 3-credit stand-alone course in a graduate and/or undergraduate nursing program. Case

---

BOX 11-1 Content Outline of Case Management Educational Programs

- Overview of case management
- Case management models
- Historic perspectives of case management
- Healthcare delivery systems and organizations
- Roles of the case manager
- The case management, utilization management, and discharge/transitional planning processes
- Managed care and health insurance benefits
- Healthcare reimbursement systems and methods
- Financial management and cost–benefit analysis
- Community resources
- Legal and ethical issues in case management practice
- Interdisciplinary collaboration
- Quality management, performance improvement, and outcomes management
- Clinical pathways
- Case management research
- Clinical practice

---

management programs that exist today are of three types and are classified based on the length of the program and/or the location where they are offered. These are as follows:

■ Certificate programs such as those offered by the New England Healthcare Assembly in Massachusetts and Seton Hall University in New Jersey

■ Noncertificate programs such as those offered through conferences as continuing education units (CEUs) or those offered by healthcare organizations to their own nursing staff

■ Degree programs such as the master's degree program at Villanova University in Pennsylvania

Regardless of the type of program provided, the case management content taught is similar to the content, context, processes, aims, and outcomes of case management discussed in this book. However, the depth and length of the programs vary. The content of case management educational programs has been described by Falter et al (1999), Haw (1995, 1996), Sowel (1997), and Toran (1998). They report the lack of clinical case management courses in schools where no degree in case management was offered but case management content was incorporated into other degree programs. A list of topics addressed in case management educational programs is presented in Box 11-1.

CASE MANAGEMENT CERTIFICATE PROGRAMS

Case management certificate programs are of two types. One is provided by an independent agency or a healthcare institution in the form of a multiday conference. The other is provided by a college or university in the form of multiple credits, usually 12 credits. Enrollment in the independent agency program is open to all nurses and allied health professionals regardless of educational background or specialty. However, the college-based certificate program is limited to those who hold a college degree. Some colleges offer a post-baccalaureate certificate program. Others offer a post-master's program. Both types of programs include theory and clinical courses. Participants in either type of program are provided with a *Certificate in Case Management* after they have successfully completed all of the requirements. New England Healthcare Assembly's certificate program is an example of a non–college-based program, whereas Seton Hall University's program is an example of a college/university-based program.

New England Healthcare Assembly's Case Management Certificate Program

The New England Healthcare Assembly's Case Management Certificate Program (New England Healthcare Assembly, 1996) is designed as an integrated program of three modules. Each module is a stand-alone seminar. However, each is an integral part of the overall program and the scope of case management. Each module is given separately over 3 days of coursework. The whole program requires 9 days of coursework for completion. A participant could complete the coursework within 4 months if registering for the three modules consecutively. A comprehensive examination is required after completing the three modules, after which a certificate of completion can be provided.

The program is offered to clinicians, administrators, and support staff who are involved in designing, implementing, and evaluating case management systems. Healthcare professionals such as nurses, social workers, discharge planners, utilization reviewers, and quality and risk management professionals are eligible for enrollment in this program.

This certificate program includes discussions regarding case management systems in various healthcare settings and managed care organizations. Organizational development, healthcare **reimbursement** systems, and financial analysis processes are also discussed. The skills learned in this program include strategies for successful design, implementation, and evaluation of case management systems and **case management plans;** management of **variances;** and integration of interdepartmental processes for **continuous quality improvement (CQI)** efforts.

The first module includes the following topics:
1. Assessment of the external healthcare environment
2. Managed care and its financial underpinnings

3. Key elements of case management
4. Role of the case manager across the healthcare continuum
5. Management information systems
6. Utilization review and case management

The key concepts discussed in this module include healthcare policy, integration of patient care delivery, managed care, **capitation,** reimbursement systems, cost/benefit analysis, case management models, case management plans, roles of case managers in various models and care settings, critical functions of case managers, variance data collection and analysis, financial and administrative information systems, automation in case management, and utilization review procedures and protocols.

The second module includes the following topics:
1. Patient care across the healthcare continuum
2. Financial reimbursement systems
3. Patient care quality
4. Patient care **outcomes**
5. Evaluation indicators for case management systems

Participants in this module will learn how to coordinate patient care outside the hospital walls. They become astute in identifying and coordinating community resources and in collaborating with patients and their families, primary care physicians, managed care organizations, and community-based case managers. They also learn how to ensure and monitor the quality of patient care in the community. Reimbursement issues are discussed pertaining to **Medicare, Medicaid,** managed care organizations, and other **third-party payers.** How to evaluate a case management model is the last topic learned in this module. Patient care quality, outcome measures and indicators, patient satisfaction, CQI and participation in improvement teams, **length of stay,** and cost containment are among the subjects discussed in this module.

The third and last module provided in this certificate program includes the following topics:
1. Role of case managers
2. Interdisciplinary teams
3. Customer relations
4. Competency of case managers
5. Organizational change

Case managers are given the opportunity in this module to learn the skills required to be an active and efficient participant in an interdisciplinary team. They learn how to effect positive change; manage conflict; and promote case management as an integral part of the organizational culture, values, and philosophy. They also learn the ins and outs of their role and responsibilities, priority setting, and how to respond effectively to multiple needs.

Seton Hall University's Certificate Program

The Seton Hall University Certificate Program (Seton Hall University, 1996) was established in 1996. It is a 12-credit postbaccalaureate program in **nursing case management** that is offered only to nurses. This program combines theory and practice and may fit into any organizational setting. Admission to this program is restricted to those nurses who meet the following criteria:

1. Baccalaureate degree in nursing from a National League for Nursing (NLN)-accredited program
2. Cumulative B average
3. B average in nursing courses
4. Current licensure as a registered professional nurse
5. Minimum of 1 year of clinical nursing experience

Preference for participation in this program is given to applicants who are certified in a clinical nursing specialty and those who are working in the capacity of case managers. The program consists of 6 credits in nurse case management theory, 3 credits of clinical experience/practicum, and 3 credits in nursing resource management.

The Nurse Case Management Theory Course I is designed to teach participants about the role of case managers in a managed care environment and across various healthcare settings. The exploration of community resources for client support and the concepts of healthcare insurance (e.g., Medicare, Medicaid, managed care organizations, and other third-party payers), **utilization management,** legal and ethical issues, discharge planning, and total **quality management** are the selected topics of discussion.

The Nurse Case Management Theory Course II is an extension of Course I. It examines the case management process. Participants are developed in patient screening and selection for case management services, assessment of patient and family needs, development of the treatment plan (i.e., the case management plan), ongoing case management, evaluation of patient responses to treatment, patient and family teaching, and care of the patient after discharge. Healthcare marketing strategies; financial management and healthcare cost accounting, particularly reimbursement systems; standards of care and practice; and public policy legislation are discussed. In addition, research as a vehicle for advancing the role of the case manager is also examined.

The Nurse Case Management Practicum Course provides students with the opportunity to explore, test, and expand the nurse case management theory(ies) in the organizational setting. During this course, enrollees are expected to rotate through clinical areas and be exposed to firsthand experience with case management. They are precepted by seasoned case managers. Socialization with experienced case managers permits the students the opportunity to analyze, synthesize, integrate their learning, and evaluate their effectiveness as potential/future case managers. Students are given control over their clinical experience through designing their own objectives and planning, controlling, and evaluating their learning experiences to achieve these objectives.

The Nursing Resource Management Course emphasizes healthcare organizations as "corporate entities." The business perspective of managing nursing services is a major part of this course. Complex management issues are shared and explored as they relate to managing single departments, as well as the healthcare organization as a whole.

The Seton Hall University's certificate program is a four-semester program in which one or two courses may be taken in each semester. At the successful completion of the program, students are provided with a certificate of completion in nurse case management.

CASE MANAGEMENT NONCERTIFICATE PROGRAMS

Case management noncertificate programs are those offered by healthcare institutions as part of training, orientation, and education of nursing and nonnursing personnel in preparation for the implementation of case management systems. These programs are usually designed by individual institutions based on their policies and procedures and description, roles, and responsibilities of case managers. The design of these programs is affected by who will assume the case manager's role. In addition, the length of these programs varies from one institution to another—2 to 4 weeks depending on the intensity of the program. Some institutions have been able to obtain approval for offering CEUs to the participants in these programs. This is a result of successfully completing an application for CEUs submitted to nursing continuing education credentialing boards such as the American Nurses Association's Board of Continuing Education or to the boards of other allied health professional societies such as the National Association of Social Workers and the Case Management Society of America.

Healthcare institution–based noncertificate programs are generally taught by the nursing continuing education department or the institution's training and development department/office of organizational learning. The staff members of these departments are the instructors of the program, in collaboration with the administrator of the case management service/department. Sometimes these programs are taught by a

CASE MANAGER'S TIP 11-1

Strategies for Developing a Solid Case Management Orientation Program

1. Involve a case management expert or consultant.
2. Develop a program that is reflective of the case manager's job description.
3. Include subject matter experts from your institution on the planning team.
4. Have the subject matter experts teach in the program.
5. Refer to what has been published in this area; limit the topics to what case managers will be involved in.
6. Hold classes and on-the-job training.
7. Make sure that topics taught include finance, reimbursement, leadership skills, conflict resolution, problem solving, communication and teamwork, and negotiation skills.
8. Include teaching strategies such as role play, case studies, and problem-based learning and discussions.
9. Maximize the use of mentoring.

consultant or consulting agency that is charged with overseeing the implementation of case management systems. Topics discussed are similar to those addressed in the certificate programs. The difference, however, is that the noncertificate, institution-based program is individualized to fit the institution's policies, procedures, operations, standards of care, standards of practice, and the job description and extent of responsibilities of those to assume the case manager roles (see Case Manager's Tip 11-1 for strategies for developing a solid case management orientation program).

Other noncertificate case management programs are those offered in schools of nursing as one or two courses, earning 3 to 6 credits, in baccalaureate or master's degree programs. The topical outline of these courses varies from one school to another. However, the basics of case management and managed care, financial reimbursement systems, roles of case managers, case management plans, variance data collection and analysis, **outcomes management,** and performance and quality improvement are common to all schools and programs. The content of these courses is usually approved by the state education department and/or accrediting agencies such as the NLN. Most schools that include case management courses in their programs offer such course(s) as a mandatory part of the curriculum rather than as elective courses.

Students who are enrolled in the school-based programs and nurses who attend the healthcare institution-based programs are eligible to take the certified case manager examination (see p. 209). After completion of these training programs, nurses are deemed knowledgeable in case management systems and ready for practice.

CASE MANAGEMENT DEGREE PROGRAMS

Case management degree programs are full graduate-level programs offered in a college or university setting. They generally are a combination of traditional master's level and newly developed case management systems–related courses. At the successful completion of these programs, students earn a master's degree. The case management curriculum established by the graduate program at the College of Nursing at Villanova University, Villanova, Pennsylvania, is a good example of such programs. Enrollment in this program is limited to students with a baccalaureate degree in nursing from an NLN-accredited school of nursing, a 3.0 grade point average, a minimum of 1 year of clinical experience, and satisfactory performance on the Miller Analogies Test (MAT) or the verbal portion of the Graduate Record Examination (GRE).

In July of 1993 the College of Nursing at Villanova University received a 3-year grant from the Division of Nursing of the U.S. Public Health Service to develop a graduate degree program in clinical case management. It is a 45-credit program designed to prepare case managers for acute care settings, community-based organizations, insurance and disability management companies, and other managed care systems. In addition, it prepares case managers in the provision, management, and coordination of the total care of groups of clients. At the completion of this program, graduates are able to apply the theory and advanced knowledge of case management systems in clinical practice (Villanova University, 1996).

Students in the clinical case manager program take courses in budgeting, organizational systems, case management models, case manager role development, community resources, clinical outcomes, and marketing. In addition, they are required to take some core courses in healthcare delivery systems, nursing science, and nursing research, as well as a theory course and a practicum in a particular clinical specialty. The core courses add up to 15 credits. In addition, there are two elective courses.

Description of the Clinical Case Management Courses

The following description of the courses in the Clinical Case Manager Program at Villanova University is based on the information presented in the 1996-1997 catalog of the university's College of Nursing Graduate Program.

In the *Health Care Organizations and Nursing Care Systems* course, clinical case managers learn about the dynamics, culture, and politics of healthcare organizations and particularly nursing care systems. They analyze the impact of internal and external forces affecting such delivery systems, with a closer look at the impact of these forces on nursing care delivery. In this course, students are exposed to some of the skills required for success in the clinical case manager role, such as negotiation, conflict resolution, change, and motivation.

Budgeting Concepts for Clinical Case Managers is another required course. It prepares case managers in the budgetary process, types of budgets, and budget development and analysis. This course is important because it provides future case managers with a better understanding of healthcare budgeting and the need for cost-containment strategies.

The *Role of the Clinical Case Manager* course prepares case managers for a thorough understanding of their roles and responsibilities with regard to the organization, patient and family, physicians, social workers, physical therapists, and so forth. It puts the various roles assumed by case managers into perspective. This course also analyzes the impact of organizational structures and reference groups on the role of clinical case managers.

Another required course is *Marketing in Health Care,* which includes an analysis of concepts related to creating competitive market planning strategies. Assessment and analysis of the marketplace, demographics, and healthcare needs are also addressed.

Examination of the various models of case management, the impact of legislation and healthcare financing on such models, grant writing, funding sources, and ethical considerations in healthcare are all discussed in the *Models for Case Management* course. In this course, students learn about case management models across the healthcare continuum and their logistics, similarities, and differences.

Community resources and strategies for accessing federal, state, and voluntary agencies, as well as regional resources, are the focus of the *Community Resources* course. This course is important to case managers because of the role they play in discharge planning and patient care coordination. It provides them with an understanding of the regulations regarding community resources and the different entitlements of patients in relation to their healthcare insurance coverage.

Clinical case managers enrolled in this program learn how to assess, evaluate, and analyze patient care outcomes in the *Clinical Outcomes* course. They also learn about the development, implementation, and evaluation of case management plans/critical pathways. Care mapping as a quality improvement mechanism and evaluating case management plans through variance analysis are also discussed.

Patient Education: Principles and Strategies is another important course that prepares case managers in their role as patient and family educators. Patient teaching across the lifespan; the teaching/learning process; identifying the learner needs, barriers, and readiness for learning; and motivational factors are some of the topics discussed. Case managers also learn how to incorporate patient and family teaching into the case management plan. The effective use of teaching strategies and tools is explored.

In the *Practicum in Clinical Case Management* course, students get the opportunity to apply the theory, knowledge, and skills they learned in class to practice settings. With the help of a clinical case manager as a preceptor, students select a practicum site in which they operationalize their future role in case management into a particular care setting. During this practicum, they practice the clinical case manager role, test their skills and knowledge, and refine them as needed.

This degree program in case management provides case managers with a wide understanding of case management models and systems and prepares them for success in the role of case manager in a variety of settings.

CERTIFICATION IN CASE MANAGEMENT

In addition to case management certificate, noncertificate, and degree programs, national certifications also exist. There are multiple certifications in case management; however, the two major ones are as follows:

1. That sponsored by the CCMC, which has been offered since July 1, 1995. Before then it was sponsored by the Certification of Insurance Rehabilitation Specialists Commission (CIRSC). The certification confers that the holder is a specialized person in the practice of case management (CCMC, 2001). This certification targets all professional providers such as nurses, social workers, physical therapists, and counselors.

2. That offered by the American Nurses Credentialing Center (ANCC), Commission on Certification, since 1996. The American Nurses Association (ANA) initiated a taskforce for the establishment of a credentialing examination that provides certification in nursing case management (NCM). However, this offering is limited only to nurses.

There are tens of thousands of certified case managers today; however, the majority (approximately 35,000) are certified by either the CCMC or the ANCC. The content of the certification examinations correlates with the elements of case management discussed in this book: content, context, processes, aims, outcomes, and role relationships. It is also reflective of the content of the curricula in case management educational programs.

Certifications are offered through national testing. One must obtain a passing score on a case management certification examination to be considered certified and be able to use the designated case management credential; that is, CM if offered by the ANCC, or CCM if offered by the CCMC. A nationally recognized certifying body, such as the ANCC or the CCMC, provides the testing for certification. Currently, certification for case managers is not mandatory as it is for other specialties such as midwifery, nurse anesthetists, and nurse practitioners. However, employers are increasingly requiring a certification in case management as a prerequisite credential for hiring case managers, especially in the managed care, occupational health, and **workers' compensation** areas of case management practice.

Importance of the Case Manager Certification

Certification in case management is important because it affirms that the case manager possesses the knowledge and skills required to render appropriate, quality, and safe case management services to potential clients. Certifications can be used for professional growth and development or as a means for advancing one's career. They are a measure of knowledge, skills, expertise, and competence. In addition, they testify that one has achieved special/advanced competence; that is, expanded knowledge and skill in a particular area of practice, such as healthcare quality, utilization review and management, or managed care. Furthermore, they allow the public to have more trust and faith in case managers and the services they provide. Certifications also make case managers more marketable; provide them with better job opportunities, financial rewards and compensation; and increase their chances of recognition and celebration by their employers. Certified case managers are more likely to get promoted compared with those who are not certified. In addition, certifications in case management assist healthcare organizations in meeting the quality management and improvement standards of accreditation agencies. They also keep case managers current with their knowledge and healthcare trends.

Differentiating Licensure, Certificate, and Certification

It is important to differentiate certification from the terms *licensure* and *certificate*. These terms should not

be used interchangeably because they mean different things. Box 11-2 contains the definitions of these terms. **Licensure** is a restrictive form of regulation. It is also mandatory before pursuing practice, whereas certificate and certification are voluntary. Currently, all case management certifications require a basic professional licensure as a prerequisite to certification. Both certification and licensure are obtained by achieving a passing score on an examination. Licensure recognizes basic performance, knowledge, and skill, whereas certification recognizes exceptional performance and advanced knowledge and skill. Generally, certificates do not require any form of testing and do not reflect one's level of competence but rather attest to one's participation in a particular learning experience.

Choosing a Certification

As more professional organizations provide certification opportunities for case managers, certifications have gained significant meaning and recognition. They may ultimately be used for regulation and accreditation of case management programs; entry into case management practice; validation of knowledge, skills, and competence; and recognition and achievement of excellence. Today there are more than 15 different organizations that provide certification in case management (Table 11-1). These organizations are mostly related to specialties such as rehabilitation and **disability case management,** utilization management, healthcare quality,

TABLE 11-1   Certifications in Case Management

Certification	Organization and Website	Fee*
Certified Case Manager (CCM)	Commission for Case Manager Certification www.ccmcertification.org	$290
Nurse Case Manager (RN, CM)	American Nurses Association www.nursingworld.org	$130-$370 based on membership
Case Manager, Certified (CMC)	American Institute of Outcomes Case Management www.aiocm.com	$200
Case Manager Administrator, Certified (CMAC)	National Association of Healthcare Quality www.cphq-hqcb.org	$300-$350 based on membership
Certified Professional in Healthcare Quality (CPHQ)	The Center for Case Management www.cfcm.com	$300
Continuity of Care Certification, Advanced (A-CCC)	National Board for Certification in Continuity of Care www.nbccc.org	$300
Certified Disability Management Specialist (CDMS)	Certification of Disability Management Specialists Commission www.cdms.org	$290
Certified Rehabilitation Registered Nurse (CRRN)	Rehabilitation Nursing Certification Board www.rehabnurse.org	$195-$285 based on membership
Certified Social Work Case Manager (CSWCM)	National Association of Social Workers www.naswdc.org	$100
Certified Managed Care Nurse (CMCN)	American Board of Managed Care Nursing www.abmcn.org	$225
Certified Occupational Health Nurse/Case Manager (COHN/CM)	American Board for Occupational Health Nurses www.abohn.org	$185
Care Manager Certified (CMC)	National Academy of Certified Care Managers www.naccm.net	$225-$264 based on processing fees
Certified Professional in Utilization Review (CPUR) and Certified Professional in Utilization Management (CPUM)	InterQual www.interqual.com	$235

Modified from a review published by the American Health Consultants: *Hosp Case Manag* 9(suppl 2):1-8, 2001.
*Based on the fees at the time this chapter was written. Fees are subject to change.

case management, nursing, managed care, gerontology, and workers' compensation and occupational health.

The decision as to which case manager certification case managers must pursue can be a confusing and frustrating undertaking. One must make the decision based on one's field of practice or specialty, discipline, and the requirements or criteria of the certifying body. When making the choice, case managers must answer the following questions first:

- Is the certification a prerequisite for my current or potential job?
- What is the benefit of the certification for my career advancement and professional development?
- Is the certification a mandatory expectation for credentialing in my role or for accreditation of the case management department?
- What are the specific standards of care, practice, and performance that govern my practice setting/

environment (e.g., acute care, managed care organization, workers' compensation)?
- What are the eligibility criteria for the different certification examinations? Which one am I able to meet?
- What is the cost of the certification?
- For how long is the certification valid?
- What are the criteria for certification renewal?
- How much information is available from the certifying bodies regarding the examinations?
- Which certification is nationally recognized? (American Health Consultants, 2001)
- Is the certification more general in focus, or is it highly specialized?
- Will there be any financial compensation if I obtain a certification?
- Is the certifying body a for-profit or not-for-profit organization/agency?
- Is the certifying body accredited by the National Commission for Certifying Agencies?

- Is there any published research about the validity and reliability of the certifying examination? How current is such research?
- Do the certifying bodies abide by the codes of ethics?
- Does the certifying body have a clear review and appeal or grievance process? (American Health Consultants, 2000)

Answers to these questions assist case managers in determining which certification is best to pursue. It is important not to make such decision arbitrarily or hastily. A well thought out decision prevents oversight, problems, and unnecessary trouble. It also allows case managers to find the certification that fits their needs, abilities, and aspirations.

THE COMMISSION FOR CASE MANAGER CERTIFICATION

The CCMC (2001) advocates for case management as a specialized area of practice rather than a profession. Case management experts who developed the eligibility criteria for the certification agree that case management services can be provided by a variety of professionals from different health and human services professions (e.g., nursing, social work, physical therapy). As a result, these professionals, when certified as case managers, use the credential "certified case manager" (CCM) in conjunction with their professional licensure (e.g., registered professional nurses use the credentials RN, CCM; certified social workers use the credentials CSW, CCM).

The certification examination of the CCMC is accredited by the National Commission for Certifying Agencies. The examination is offered twice every year, during the months of June and December. The initial certification is valid for 5 years, and renewal of the case manager certification is required every 5 years. It can be achieved through reexamination or demonstration of professional development, which entails participation in approved continuing education programs. In addition, certified case managers applying for certification renewal should also provide evidence that they continue to hold the same license or certification they held at the time of the initial certification (e.g., registered professional nurse, certified social worker, certified physical therapist). More information on the certification is available at http://www.ccmcertification.org.

Eligibility Criteria for the CCMC Case Manager Certification

The CCMC has established two eligibility criteria that have to be met by all applicants at the time applications for the examination are submitted (Case Manager's Tip 11-2). One criterion is licensure/certification, and the other is employment/experience. In addition, all applicants "must

 CASE MANAGER'S TIP 11-2

Eligibility Criteria

All applicants for the Commission for Case Manager Certification examination must meet the following two eligibility criteria:

1. Licensure/certification: completion of a postsecondary program in human and health services
2. Employment/experience in the area of specialty indicated by the license or certificate

be of good moral character, reputation, and fitness for the practice of case management" (CCMC, 2001, p. 3).

The licensure/certification criterion requires the applicant to have completed a minimum education of a postsecondary program in the field of human and health services that promotes the physical, psychosocial, or vocational well-being of the persons being served. For example, registered professional nurses at all levels of education (diploma, bachelor's, master's, or doctorate degrees) are eligible for participation in this certification. The CCMC only honors the educational programs that provide a license/certificate that permits the holder to legally practice without the supervision of another professional (e.g., registered professional nursing programs).

In addition to meeting the licensure/certification criterion, the applicant for the case manager certification examination must provide verification of employment and experience in the area of specialty as indicated on the license or certificate. To be eligible, one must provide evidence of either (1) 12 months of full-time employment under the supervision of a certified case manager, (2) 24 months of full-time case management employment without supervision of a certified case manager, or (3) 12 months of full-time employment as a supervisor of case management services and/or case managers. Applicants should demonstrate that their employment experience entails the components of case management services as defined by the CCMC, which are assessment, planning, implementation, coordination, monitoring, and evaluation.

CCMC Examination Content Topics

The certification examination consists of 300 multiple-choice questions that address six different broad activities related to the job description and roles and responsibilities of case managers and the case management process. These include, as they appear in the CCM Certification Guide (CCMC, 2001): assessment, planning, implementation, coordination, monitoring, and evaluation. The examination also addresses six

CASE MANAGER'S TIP 11-3

Topics to Review for the CCMC's Certification Examination

1. Patient's bill of rights
2. Legal and ethical issues
3. Patient's privacy and confidentiality
4. Continuum of care
5. Clinical information systems and communication of information
6. Public benefit programs
7. Patient assessment and data-gathering procedures
8. Disease processes and treatment modalities
9. Psychosocial assessment of patients and families
10. Assessment of support systems
11. Coping with and adaptation to illness
12. Evaluation of patient responses to treatments and quality of care
13. Advocacy
14. Negotiation of services
15. Managed care
16. Insurance principles, policy coverage, inclusions/exclusions
17. Cost/benefit analysis
18. Cost-containment strategies
19. Precertification for services
20. Healthcare delivery systems
21. Screening and intake of patients for case management services
22. Coordination and facilitation of care activities
23. Patient and family education
24. Discharge/transitional planning and levels of care
25. Case management plans
26. Community resources and services
27. Documentation of case management services
28. Role of the case manager
29. Consultation
30. Legislation and public policy related to case management
31. Liability issues/concerns of case management
32. Outcomes management; variances and variance analysis
33. Utilization review and management
34. Americans with Disabilities Act
35. Durable medical equipment
36. Evaluating the effectiveness of case management services
37. Interpersonal communication and relationships
38. Clinical pharmacology
39. Aspects of acute and chronic illness and disability
40. Job analysis and modification
41. Work adjustment and transitions
42. Life care planning
43. Mental health and psychiatric disability management

---

core components of case management. These are as follows:

1. Processes and relationships
2. Healthcare management
3. Community resources and support
4. Service delivery
5. Psychosocial intervention
6. Rehabilitation case management

These core components must be evident in the applicants' practices, and their focus must entail the continuum of care, address the ongoing needs of the individual patient being served by the case management process, and be applied in multiple settings and environments. Furthermore, these activities must deal with the broad spectrum of the patient's needs and must involve interactions with relevant components of the patient's healthcare team such as the physician, family members, third-party payers, employers, and other providers (CCMC, 2001).

Case Manager's Tip 11-3 presents a suggested list of topics that may aid case managers in their preparation for the CCMC's certification examination.

THE AMERICAN NURSES CREDENTIALING CENTER'S CASE MANAGEMENT CERTIFICATION

The ANCC is the credentialing arm of the ANA. It offers the nursing case management certification through its Commission on Certification. Although the ANA's certification program has been in existence since 1973, the certification in nursing case management is less than a decade old. Unlike the CCMC, but similar to all the other ANCC's certifications, the case management certification is offered only to licensed nursing professionals. When certified as case managers, nurses use the credential "certified case manager" (CM) in conjunction with their professional licensure; that is RN, CM. The goals of the ANCC are to promote and enhance public health by certifying nurses using the ANA's scope and nationally recognized standards of nursing practice. Passing the ANCC's certification in case management affirms that the case manager has demonstrated knowledge, skills, and abilities within a defined area of specialty (ANCC, 1999).

The ANCC Commission on Certification's case management examination is accredited by the National Commission for Certifying Agencies. It is offered twice every year, during the months of June and October. The initial certification is valid for 5 years, and renewal of the case manager certification is required every 5 years and is contingent on maintaining registered nurse (RN) licensure and meeting all recertification requirements. It can be achieved through reexamination or by obtaining the specified number of contact hours of continuing education. Other options for recertification requirements are related to academic credits, publishing in refereed media, or conducting research (ANCC, 1999). More information on the certification is available at http://www.nursingworld.org.

Eligibility Criteria for the ANCC Case Manager Certification

The ANCC has established the nursing case management examination based on core clinical skills and standards of practice that are evident in any of the ANCC certifications or that of the American Association of Critical Care Nursing. Therefore a core nursing specialty certification is one eligibility criterion that is required for taking the case management examination. Candidates must submit proof of a current certification when applying for the examination. However, to help candidates fulfill this eligibility criterion, the ANCC Commission on Certification allows those who do not meet this criterion to complete an additional 50 questions related to the ANA's Standards of Clinical Nursing Practice (ANCC, 1999). There are three additional criteria that must be met by candidates before they are deemed eligible to take the examination. These are as follows:

1. An active RN license in the United States or its territories.
2. A baccalaureate or higher degree in nursing (required to submit proof of degree).
3. Practice within the scope of an RN case manager for a minimum of 2,000 hours within the past 2 years. Those who do not already hold a core nursing specialty certification are required to have practiced as an RN for 4,000 hours, with at least 2,000 of these hours in the capacity of a nurse case manager in the past 2 years (ANCC, 1999).

ANCC Examination Content Topics

Content of the nursing case management certification examination is based on clinical skills and standards of nursing practice. It is provided in two forms: one with the additional core nursing specialty section (i.e., the 50 questions) and one without. Nurse case managers who

elect to take this examination and do not already have a core nursing specialty certification, such as certification in gerontology, oncology, medical-surgical, or critical care nursing, are obligated to take the core specialty section as well. Those who are certified are exempted from this section. Passing the certification is dependent on passing both sections of the examination where applicable: the case management and the core specialty nursing sections. Topics addressed in the examination are based on the views and philosophies of nursing case management as defined by the ANA. Case Manager's Tip 11-4 presents a suggested list of topics that may aid case managers in their preparation for the ANCC's certification examination. These topics focus on the five components of the framework of nursing case management, which are as follows:

1. Assessment
2. Planning
3. Implementation
4. Evaluation
5. Interaction

FORECASTING THE FUTURE OF CASE MANAGEMENT CREDENTIALING

Credentialing of case managers by the organization that employs them is a vision for the future, but not far from being a reality. It can be employed by healthcare organizations as a process for deeming that a professional possesses appropriate credentials to practice in a particular role such as that of case manager. It is very likely that credentialing will become the norm for three reasons: (1), because more professionals become case managers, especially those with advanced degrees and education; (2), healthcare providers and executives are pursuing practitioners with advanced preparation for the role of case manager; (3), accreditation agencies are starting to include credentialing in their accreditation standards and expect providers to have a process for credentialing case managers. Advanced practitioners who assume the case manager's role are licensed professionals and mostly have graduate educational degrees in a particular discipline such as nursing, healthcare management, or social work.

Credentialing is a peer review process one undergoes to provide evidence of continued competence, advanced knowledge and skills, and good standing. It is important for demonstrating that one's certification, license, and practice privileges are current and that one's performance satisfactorily meets the standards of competence. The successful completion of this process results in the endorsement of case managers for continued practice; that is, the authority, responsibility, and accountability to perform certain duties and clinical activities as designated

CASE MANAGER'S TIP 11-4

Topics to Review for the ANCC's Certification Examination

1. **Assessment**
   - Case screening
   - Identification of target population for case management services
   - Validation of clinical and demographic data
   - Assessment tools and risk screens
   - Barriers to availability, accessibility, and affordability of treatment
   - Motivational and adherence issues
   - Review of client history and current condition
   - Health promotion and illness prevention
   - Educational needs and patient/family teaching
   - Evaluation of support and social systems
   - Overutilization and underutilization of resources

2. **Planning**
   - Prioritization of needs
   - Setting outcomes and goals
   - Selecting resources
   - Treatment options
   - Designation of appropriate levels of care
   - Designation of appropriate settings
   - Ascertaining appropriate providers
   - Identification of gaps in care
   - Advocating for client services
   - Negotiating and managing financial aspects of care

3. **Implementation**
   - Communication of progress toward outcomes
   - Coordination of services
   - Referrals to other providers
   - Cost-effective interventions
   - Compliance with regulation, standards, and legislation
   - Utilization of community resources
   - Documentation of the nursing case management process
   - Accountability for implementing the plan of care

4. **Evaluation**
   - Achievement of clinical goals
   - Customer satisfaction
   - Financial analysis and management
   - Data collection, aggregation, and analysis
   - Resource utilization
   - Collaborative practice

5. **Interaction**
   - Advocacy
   - Facilitation of services
   - Liaison and collaboration with other disciplines and providers
   - Coordination of care
   - Brokering of services
   - Negotiation of services
   - Communication
   - Risk management
   - Mentoring

in their job description and scope of practice. The process of credentialing must be planned and operationalized in a systematic way. Credentialing can be implemented as an annual or biannual formal peer review process and may include the examination of the following:

- Professional license
- Certification/recertification status
- Educational background
- Competence
- Knowledge and skill of current practice trends
- Professional conduct
- Demonstrated quality outcomes in performance/practice

Currently, credentialing is not mandatory. It is carried out by individual healthcare organizations voluntarily for ensuring public interest, consumer protection and safety, ethical practice, and professional development. Mandatory credentialing of case managers cannot occur until a nationwide standardization of the case manager's role, scope of practice, and education are established.

Consumers of case management services demand the assurance that case managers are properly licensed, certified, and credentialed. Credentialing through a peer review process helps organizations to meet such consumer demands.

 KEY POINTS

1. Case management programs are of different types. They either are college/university-based, institution-based, or independent agency-based.
2. Case management programs are available as certificate or degree programs.
3. Regardless of their preparation or background in case management, case managers are eligible to sit for the case manager certification examination.
4. Certification in case management is important because it affirms that case managers possess the knowledge, skills, and competence required for rendering case management services to their clients.

5. It is important for case managers to examine all of their certification options before they select a specific certification. Case managers must select the certification that best fits their field of practice.

REFERENCES

American Health Consultants: Tips to help you research credentialing programs, *Case Manag Advisor* 11(11):191-192, 2000.

American Health Consultants: Navigating the maze: how to choose and get the CM credential you need, *Hosp Case Manag* 9(1):1-4, 2001.

American Nurses Credentialing Center: *Modular certification examination catalog,* Washington, DC, 1999, American Nurses Association.

Commission for Case Manager Certification: *CCM certification guide,* Rolling Meadows, Ill, 2001, The Commission.

Falter E, Cesta T, Concert C, et al: Development of a graduate nursing program in case management, *J Care Manag* 5(3):50-78, 1999.

Haw M: State-of-the-art education for case management in long-term care, *J Case Manag* 4(3):85-94, 1995.

Haw M: Case management education in universities: a national survey, *J Care Manag* 2(6):10-23, 1996.

New England Healthcare Assembly: *New England healthcare assembly's case management certificate program,* marketing brochure, Boston, 1996, New England Healthcare Assembly.

Seton Hall University, College of Nursing: *Seton Hall University's nurse case management certificate program,* marketing brochure, South Orange, NJ, 1996, Seton Hall University.

Simmons F: Developing the trauma nurse case manager role, *Dimens Crit Care Nurs* 11(3):164-170, 1992.

Sowell R, Young S: Case management in the nursing curriculum, *Nurs Case Manag* 2(4):173-176, 1997.

Spenceley S: The CNS in multidisciplinary pulmonary rehabilitation: a nursing science perspective, *Clin Nurse Specialist* 9(4):192-198, 1995.

Toran M: Academic case management, *Case Manager* 9(1):43-46, 1998.

Villanova University, College of Nursing Graduate Program: *1996-1997 graduate nursing catalog,* Villanova, Pa, 1996, Villanova University.

Wells N, Erickson S, Spinella J: Role transition: from clinical nurse specialist to clinical nurse specialist/case manager, *J Nurs Adm* 26(11):23-28, 1996.

12

Developing Case Management Plans*

There is no doubt that the current healthcare delivery system is experiencing massive and revolutionary changes. With the increased infiltration of **managed care** and managed competition and the interest of consumers in quality, safe, and cost-effective care, healthcare administrators, nursing executives in particular, are pressured to seek intelligent changes to the way care is delivered. Most healthcare institutions, whether acute, ambulatory, long term, or home care, have undergone some sort of reengineering and redesign. Regardless of the setting, **case management** continues to be the best way to deliver high-quality, efficient, and cost-effective care.

Case management delivery systems have been proven successful in various care settings (Guiliano and Poirier, 1991; Zander, 1991, 1992; Hampton, 1993; Tahan and Cesta, 1995; Cohen and Cesta, 1997). They rely heavily on **case management plans** (CMPs) that delineate the best/ideal practice. In this chapter a 10-step process for developing these plans is discussed. The process provides a template for healthcare professionals who are interested in implementing CMPs and a step-by-step guide to developing them, with practical examples to simplify the process.

Although CMPs are not new to many healthcare organizations across the **continuum of care,** the lack of a deliberate and systematic process to develop these plans holds these organizations back from creating timely and efficient results. This chapter is highly beneficial for healthcare providers, case managers in particular, who are involved in the development of CMPs. They may acquire new knowledge and strategies to simplify the task of developing CMPs, or even choose to implement the proposed process if they currently do not have a formal one in place.

OVERVIEW OF CASE MANAGEMENT PLANS

Similar to case management delivery systems, CMPs became popular because of the economic and political characteristics and pressures of the healthcare environment. Some of the driving forces of CMPs are as follows:

1. Changes in reimbursement methods: **prospective payment system** and case rates
2. The advent of managed care and managed competition
3. Consumerism and industrialization of the healthcare market
4. Standards of regulatory and **accreditation** agencies and their requirements of a quality, collaborative, and seamless approach to care provision
5. Disparity in the use of resources as a result of variations in practice patterns of providers
6. Demand of consumers for quality, safe, and cost-effective care
7. Increase in lawsuits and healthcare **litigation**
8. Increasingly complex and costly innovations in healthcare technology and treatment options

Since their inception, CMPs have been used as tools to define the standards of care and practice and as guides for patient care activities for all members of the healthcare team alike. Whatever they are called, "they define the optimal schedule of key interventions done by the various disciplines [and providers] to achieve desired patient outcomes for a particular diagnosis or procedure" (Dykes, 1998, p. xiii). They are systematically developed as statements, guidelines, and strategies for patient care management. CMPs are important tools developed to assist providers in delineating the desired sequence of

---

*Part of this material first appeared in Tahan HA: A ten-step process to develop case management plans, *Nurs Case Manag* 1(3):112-121, 1996.

interventions and treatments and in making decisions about appropriate and necessary interventions that effectively address particular clinical situations. They usually incorporate the best scientific evidence of effectiveness with expert opinion and recommendations of governmental, professional, or specialty organizations.

CMPs have been in use for over 50 years; however, they have been known as **practice guidelines** (PGs) and were originally developed by physician groups mainly for malpractice and **risk management** purposes. The label *case management plans* has only been popular for the past 2 decades, after the discipline of nursing introduced the use of **clinical pathways** as a strategy to address the nursing shortage of the 1980s. With the demand for quality and safe healthcare services, the Agency for Healthcare Research and Quality (AHRQ), formerly known as the Agency for Health Care Policy and Research (AHCPR), advocated for the development and implementation of PGs as a strategy for **quality improvement** and evidence-based practice. This took place in the late 1980s and is still a major focus for AHRQ today; in fact, the agency has developed and published multiple PGs and has made them available to healthcare organizations free of charge.

This development has encouraged healthcare providers of different disciplines and specialties to implement the AHRQ's guidelines in their practice. However, because of the complexity of the guidelines, it was essential for AHRQ to pursue other strategies for implementation, among which is the development of clinical pathways/CMPs. This resulted in a shift in focus of the nursing clinical pathways to interdisciplinary plans as we know them today. Because of this development, CMPs and PGs should not be used interchangeably as they are not one and the same. There exists some differences between the two and these are presented in Box 12-1.

The format of the CMPs is basically known as a "time-task" matrix that applies either an abbreviated, one-page version or a comprehensive, detailed booklet (Tahan and Cesta, 1995; Cohen and Cesta, 1997). CMPs have been developed based on the Gantt chart process and design. They are available in paper or electronic form. However, their purposes, the way they are used, and the process in which they are developed are approximately the same (Thompson et al, 1991; Ferguson, 1993; Katterhagen and Patton, 1993; Esler et al, 1994; Bozzuto and Farrell, 1995; Hydo, 1995; Ignatavicius, 1995; Ignatavicius and Hausman, 1995; Meister et al, 1995).

CMPs are labeled differently in different institutions. Some are copyrighted, such as CareMaps; some are not, such as **multidisciplinary action plans (MAPs)**.

BOX 12-1 Differences Between CMPs and PGs

1. CMPs focus on quality and efficiency; PGs focus on appropriateness of care.
2. CMPs are multidisciplinary in nature; PGs are medically focused.
3. CMPs are healthcare organization–specific; PGs are national standards.
4. CMPs may be used for documentation; PGs may not and are not written with that purpose in mind.
5. CMPs follow a specific timeline; PGs do not.
6. CMPs are less costly than PGs.
7. CMPs are less complex and time-consuming to develop than PGs.
8. Variance identification and tracking is an integral part of CMPs but not PGs.
9. CMPs apply a "time-task" matrix in format; PGs follow a text or algorithm format.
10. CMPs consider the recommendations of PGs in their development; PGs are developed based on a thorough literature review.
11. CMPs are used by providers, payers, and consumers; PGs are limited to providers.

Examples of CMPs include critical path, anticipated recovery path, clinical pathway, care guide, collaborative plan, coordinated plan, integrated plan of care, or action plan. Throughout this chapter, these plans will be referred to by using the generic term *case management plan*. Case Manager's Tip 12-1 lists the characteristics and benefits of CMPs.

The use of CMPs has created a multitude of advantages. Among the most important are cost-effectiveness and reduction in **lengths of stay,** readmissions to acute care settings, or home care visits; consistency and standardization in care provision; implementation of best practices and evidence-based treatment options; improved quality of care and customer satisfaction; better allocation of resources and coordination of services that result in eliminating redundancy, fragmentation, and duplication of care activities; clearly defined plans of care and delineation of responsibilities; and improved communication systems among the various disciplines and providers (Guiliano and Poirier, 1991; Zander, 1991; Ignatavicius, 1995; Ignatavicius and Hausman, 1995; Tahan and Cesta, 1995; Cohen and Cesta, 1997).

TYPES OF CASE MANAGEMENT PLANS

CMPs link the processes and **outcomes** of care. They are used as structured and formal plans that delineate the delivery and management of patient care services

CASE MANAGER'S TIP 12-1

Characteristics and Benefits of CMPs

1. Each plan addresses a specific diagnosis, medical problem, surgical procedure, or phase in the care needed.
2. The plans represent a timeline of patient care activities based on the clinical service. This could be minutes or hours in the emergency department, days in the acute care setting, weeks in the neonatal intensive care unit, months in long-term facilities, or number of visits in ambulatory or home care settings.
3. The plans include well-defined milestones or trigger points that aid in expediting care and indicate an impending change in care activities (e.g., switching from intravenous to oral antibiotics when temperature is within normal range for 24 hours) or readiness of patients for different care setting (e.g., criteria for transferring a patient from an acute to a subacute or nursing home care setting). The triggers are discipline- or provider-specific.
4. The length of each plan depends on a predetermined length of stay based on the diagnosis/procedure and reimbursement rules, guidelines, and mechanisms.
5. The plans prospectively delineate the necessary interventions in a way that eliminates fragmentation, redundancy/duplication, and use of unnecessary resources.
6. The plans clearly delineate the responsibilities of the various healthcare team members as they relate to each particular department.

7. The plans identify the outcome indicators or quality measures used to evaluate the appropriateness and effectiveness of care.
8. Each plan may include a specific variance tracking section to evaluate any delays in care activities/processes or outcomes.
9. The plans may be used as one strategy for ensuring compliance with the standards of care of regulatory and accreditation agencies.
10. The plans are interdisciplinary in nature—a mechanism that reinforces a seamless approach to the delivery of care and standardizes and ensures consistency in the care provision processes.
11. The plans can be used as an educational tool for housestaff, student nurses or nurses in training, and newly hired employees.
12. The plans help improve performance in the areas of patient and family teaching, coordination of services, collaboration and communication among the healthcare team members, and discharge planning.
13. The plans may also be developed in a "patient version," which can be given to the patient and family at the time of admission into the hospital or community care setting. This helps the patient understand what is projected to take place during the course of treatment.
14. The plans may be used for negotiation of managed care contracts and reimbursement rates as they prospectively define practice and identify the critical steps in the care of patients with a specific diagnosis or procedure.

and outcomes. They also are used to identify best practices, standardize care activities, promote consistency and continuity in practice patterns across providers and levels of care, enhance interdisciplinary collaboration and a seamless approach to patient care delivery, and provide a mechanism for measuring outcomes of care and addressing variances and deviations from the standards. Healthcare organizations have designed and implemented many different types of CMPs (Box 12-2). Some of the plans include more details than others, some are multipurpose, and some may address the responsibilities of multiple disciplines and providers.

Generally, there are three main areas of focus when CMPs are developed and implemented. These are as follows:

1. To standardize old or current practice; that is, to ensure consistency and continuity in care delivery, services, among providers, and across settings. CMPs are developed for this purpose when there are no

other innovations, knowledge, or better ways/ideal practices for the provision of care.

2. To implement evidence-based practice or state-of-the-science care; that is, to change the current methods and strategies of care delivery and management through the use of knowledge gained from outcomes of research and clinical trials. CMPs are developed for this purpose when the latest research outcomes

---

BOX 12-2   Types of Case Management Plans

1. Issue-specific recommendations
2. Algorithms
3. Protocols
4. Preprinted order sets
5. Guidelines
6. Clinical/critical pathways
7. Multidisciplinary action plans

about new treatments and interventions have proven to be more beneficial to patients and cost-effective.

3. To innovate and develop new practices; that is, to implement new strategies, treatments, and interventions where there are no known ideal or evidence-based practices. CMPs are developed for this purpose when experts in an organization are interested in testing different treatment options that are still considered to be controversial or have not been tested before. Such CMPs usually result in identifying ideal and evidence-based practices after the period of experimentation is concluded.

Issue-Specific Recommendations

Issue-specific recommendations are statements of care and decisions and are usually limited to clinical situations in their format and content. They also are clear, concise, and direct to the point. They tend not to address the total aspects of care of a patient with a specific diagnosis but rather an individual aspect or a related process of care, such as prescribing medications for a patient with pneumonia (Box 12-3). In addition, they identify the role of a particular discipline, and in that regard they define the responsibility of a specific care provider to the clinical situation they address. For example, an issue-specific recommendation regarding the discharge of patients who are receiving intravenous (IV) antibiotics while hospitalized and who are known to be IV drug users may indicate that the prescriber of care and treatments (e.g., physician, nurse practitioner) should switch an IV antibiotic to its oral form before these patients' discharge from the hospital. Another

example is the need to measure the temperature of a febrile patient rectally, or to send a blood specimen for microbiology/bacteriology testing when the patient's temperature is greater than or equal to 103.5° F.

Issue-specific recommendations may stand alone as policy statements or be part of the standard of care. Sometimes they are incorporated in the CMPs to enhance quality and safe practice, prevent errors and medical litigation, and promote adherence to the standards of accreditation and regulatory agencies. Issue-specific recommendations are not as popular today; however, healthcare providers used to develop and implement them more often before the advent of other more detailed types of CMPs such as clinical pathways, **algorithms,** and MAPs. Healthcare providers have used them to proactively delineate the responsibilities and practices of the various disciplines involved in patient care and in specific situations.

Algorithms

Algorithms are problem-based procedures of care that are developed by healthcare providers as consensus statements to delineate the process(es) of caring for a patient with a specific medical condition or health problem such as asthma (Figure 12-1). They include a step-by-step guide to the care of patients and usually focus on the clinical decision-making process regarding the patient's assessment and the required diagnostic and therapeutic interventions and treatments. Usually, algorithms are written in an "if ... then" style (Cole and Houston, 1999); however, the use of the "if ... then" may not always be explicit. Sometimes, arrows (indicating direction) and boxes (containing the recommended care options) are used instead of "if ... then," such as in the example presented in Figure 12-1. Regardless of the method used, algorithms apply a stepwise format that is systematic, chronological, and outcomes driven.

Algorithms focus on the logical progression of intervention options that are driven by the patient's response to treatment (Cole and Houston, 1999) and aim at resolving the patient's problem. They are rules-based and leave little room for decision making and judgment because they are prospectively developed as explicit interventions for managing specific conditions. These decisions are specified in the content of the algorithm and follow the style described above. As with CMPs, it is appropriate to deviate from the algorithm; however, the healthcare provider deviating from the plan must have a logical reason for such actions and must document the rationale of the deviation in the patient's medical record. Sometimes documentation flowsheets/tools (Figure 12-2) are developed in conjunction with the algorithms to simplify the process of

---

BOX 12-3 Example of an Issue-Specific Recommendation: Treatment of Community-Acquired Pneumonia

Recommendations for Initial Antibiotics for Patients with Pneumonia

Less severe pneumonia
- Cefuroxime, Ceftazidime, Timentin (one of these drugs) and/or
- Erythromycin

Severe pneumonia
Patients with symptoms/treatment such as respiratory rate >30/min, PaO_2/FIO_2 <250, mechanical ventilation, bilateral or multiple lobes involved, increase in size of >50% in 48 hours, shock, on pressors, oliguria
- Ceftazidime, Imipenem, Ciprofloxacin (one of these drugs) and
- Erythromycin

DR/PA/NP: _____ ALLERGIES: _____ DATE: ____/____/____

INITIAL: OBTAIN:
0-15 mins. Brief history, COR/lung assessment, PF **before** Treatments, Pulse oximetry.

Consider: Oxygen per Nasal Cannula/Face Mask Ensure patient is stable enough to stay in Asthma Treatment Area.

HIGH-RISK PTS FOR RESPIRATORY FAILURE:
History of Intubation. Multiple Hospital Admissions. Psychiatric History, Pregnancy, Respiratory Rate >30, Peak Flow <100, Multiple Diagnoses.

0-20 Minutes:
#1 Treatment: Inhaled Beta Agonist = Albuterol Sulfate Omja; atopm Solution diluted in NS with ≥5L Oxygen via hand-held/FM Nebulizer.

Repeat Heart Rate/Respiratory Rate/Peak Flow/Physical Exam after first treatment and document findings

20-40 Minutes:
#2 Treatment: Albuterol treatment (as above)
Obtain History: Full physical assessment of patient and document on Emergency Department chart (care provider). Obtain temperature.
Repeat Heart Rate/Respiratory Rate/Peak Flow, documentation

GOOD RESPONSE
Peak Flow ≥70% of predicted, respiratory status improved, reduced wheezing, shortness of breath. Patient able to ambulate x 2 around Emergency Department (ED) without respiratory discomfort.

DISCHARGE PATIENT
• Consider brief course of Oral Corticosteroids; Oral Prednisone if Solumedrol given in ED.*
• Triamcinolone (Azmacort) if patient requires ≥2 Albuterol treatments in the ED.

ORGANIZE FOLLOW-UP APPOINTMENT
Provide clinic numbers. Consider Asthma Team Consult for patients needing fast track Asthma Clinic.

POOR RESPONSE
Little change in Peak Flow/Respiratory Rate and respiratory status/quality. Signs and Symptoms persist

MODERATE RESPONSE

Peak Flow <70% predicted, Signs and Symptoms persist (see Nomogram)

If IV access is needed: place Saline Lock; Draw Chemistry and Hematology bloods; hold for PRN use.
Consider: CXR/ABG/labs: CBC/SMA7/Theophylline depending on Signs/Symptoms and patient needs.

GIVE CORTICOSTEROIDS 40 mg PO/IV
(Prednisone PO, Methylprednisolone IV)
*See notation at bottom
40-60 Minutes: Albuterol treatment and repeat Vital Signs/Peak Flow/Physical Exam/Pulse Oximetry

Hour #2
#4 Treatment: Albuterol Treatment and repeat Vital Signs/Peak Flow/Physical Exam
Consider: CXR/ABG/labs: CBC/SMA7/Theophiline

Hour #3:
#5 Treatment: Albuterol Treatment and repeat Vital Signs/Peak Flow/Physical Exam

Hour #4
#6 Treatment: Albuterol Treatment and repeat Vital Signs/Peak Flow/Physical Exam
Evaluate test results/Clinical Outcome/Signs and Symptoms
Disposition: Decision should be made: Discharge vs. Hospitalize

FOR DISCHARGE HOME
CRITERION: Evaluation of patient's response to Asthma Treatment:
Peak Flow ≥70% predicted improved respiratory status, minimal wheezing. Patient able to ambulate around ED x 2 without respiratory discomfort. Improved general assessment.

• **MEDICATIONS: Prescription refills, Metered Dose Inhaler/Spacer with specific instruction and demonstration of use.**
• **Oral Steroids and individualize as per patient needs.**
• **Arrange for a Follow-Up Appointment:** Provide clinic numbers. Consider Asthma Team consult for patients needing fast track Asthma Clinic.

DISPOSITION

FOR HOSPITAL ADMISSION
Follow admission procedure
Initiate Inpatient **Asthma MAP**
Reassess patient in 12 hours to F/U on Steroid effectiveness, then reevaluate for potential discharge.

Until admission, ED orders must be written to continue the following:

1. Albuterol treatments continued 1-2 hours.
2. Continue Steroid treatment 6-8 hours.
3. Repeat Vital Signs/Peak Flow/Physical Exam/Pulse Oximetry as indicated.

*NOTE: Prednisone 5 mg, Triamcinolone 4 mg, Methylprednisolone 4 mg

Figure 12-1 Algorithm for the care of patients with acute asthma exacerbation in the emergency department.

DR/PA: _____   ALLERGIES: _____

RN: _____   DATE: _____ / _____ / _____

••• CARE PROVIDERS MUST INITIAL NAMES IN COLUMN AND SIGN BELOW TO OFFICIATE ORDERS •••

TIME	B.P.	PULSE	R.R.	PEAK EXPIRATORY FLOW	PULSE OX MEASURE-MENT	PULMONARY EXAM	TREATMENT	CARE PROVIDER INITIALS	
								Nurse	Dr/PA
ADM TO ED Time _____							Consider O$_2$: _____		
0-20 MIN. Time _____							#1 *Albuterol Sulfate Inhalation Solution = 2.5 mg diluted to 3 ml in N.S. with > 5LO^2 (i.e., Dosepks.)		
20-40 MIN. Time _____	■				■	T^0 _____ PO/R	#2 *Albuterol Treatment EVALUATE RESPONSE/DISPO STEROID TREATMENT: _____ _____		
40-60 MIN. Time _____							#3 *Albuterol Treatment Consider: labs, CXR, ABG		
HR. #2 Time _____	■						#4 *Albuterol Treatment Consider: labs, CXR, ABG		
HR. #3 Time _____	■						#5 *Albuterol Treatment		
HR. #4 Time _____							#6 *Albuterol Treatment DISPO. DECISION—D/C vs HOSP.		

TIME	ADDITIONAL ORDERS	Nurse	Dr/PA

•• CONT VS AND ASSESSMENTS ON ED. NSNG. FLOW SHEET WITH ADMISSION AND INITIATE ASTHMA MAP ••

VARIANCE/ASSESSMENTS

ASTHMA TEAM CONSULTED:	INITIALS	PRINT NAME	TITLE	SIGNATURE
YES____ NO____ TIME:_____				

Figure 12-2   Documentation tool algorithm for the care of patients with acute asthma exacerbation in the emergency department.

patient care provision and documentation. In this case the algorithm and the documentation tool are implemented as a package; one is not used in the clinical setting without the other.

Protocols

Protocols are similar to algorithms in their systematic and logical progression format. They are usually specific to a patient's problem and mainly used as integral components of clinical trials and research. They also are used as formal guides to delineate all of the steps for the application of a particular procedure or intervention (Cole and Houston, 1999). In addition, protocols provide a standardized approach to meeting desired outcomes of care. An example is an acute coronary syndromes protocol that classifies chest pain and angina into different levels of intensity or seriousness and details the appropriate and necessary treatments/interventions for each level. In this example the protocol guides the healthcare providers in the assessment, diagnosis, and treatment of chest pain.

Preprinted Order Sets

Preprinted order sets are prospectively prepared by one or more disciplines or healthcare providers to delineate a standardized process for the diagnosis and treatment of patients with particular problems. These orders focus mainly on medical/physicians' practice. However, they may also address the responsibilities and expectations of other providers, including nurses and other allied health professionals (e.g., social workers, physical therapists). They are developed based on research outcomes and the latest recommendations of professional societies such as the American Heart Association. The purposes of preprinted order sets are to standardize and expedite care, provide evidence-based care, and prevent variation in the practice patterns of providers. Sometimes preprinted order sets are used alone or in conjunction with CMPs. They are a positive way of increasing physician buy-in to CMPs.

Guidelines

Guidelines are statements of specific recommendations for the care of patients with a particular health problem such as heart failure. They are written in a narrative or outline format to provide guidance for the care and management of patients, especially in the areas of diagnostic and therapeutic tests and procedures. Unlike issue-specific recommendations, they make reference to time and may include specific timeframes for the implementation of designated actions or the achievement of certain outcomes. Guidelines have been used in anesthesia for many decades; however, they only became popular in other specialties and disciplines with the advent of case management and managed care. They are thought to reduce legal risk and are adopted by healthcare organizations and professional societies for that purpose.

Guidelines are systematically developed recommendations for care to assist healthcare providers in making decisions regarding the appropriateness and necessity of care and services. Similar to the other types of CMPs, guidelines provide practitioners with advice that is based on expert opinion, consensus statements, and research outcomes. Moreover, they intend to reduce practice variations and improve patient care outcomes (Figure 12-3). Today guidelines are developed and advocated for either internally in a healthcare organization or nationally by federal agencies such as the AHRQ and professional organizations such as the American Medical Association. They may be broad or specific depending on their source of origin. Those developed or adopted by a healthcare organization tend to be based on the nationally acceptable guidelines and more specific in content and timeframes, taking into consideration the systems and process of care present in the particular organization.

Clinical/Critical Pathways

Clinical/critical pathways are specific guidelines of care developed to delineate the contributions and responsibilities of the various disciplines and specialists for the care of specific patient populations. They are problem-based and discipline-focused in content (Figure 12-4). The clinical/critical pathway format is based on the Gantt chart used by engineers and architects. Karen Zander was the first to use clinical pathways at the New England Medical Center in Boston, Massachusetts, in the mid-1980s. They were called CareMaps then, applied a one-page format, and focused almost exclusively on nursing. They were originally used as a strategy to address the nursing shortage; however, they grew to become of multidisciplinary focus and today are adopted for use by all disciplines and providers.

Similar to the other types of CMPs, clinical/critical pathways are developed based on national standards and research outcomes and are best used for evidence-based practice. However, they differ from the other types of CMPs, except MAPs, in that they include specific timeframes for all of the recommended activities. They also are used as cost-effective tools for the delineation of key and critical resources and activities; to specify the order, timeliness, and progression of these activities; and to provide a mechanism for the evaluation of patient care outcomes and for meeting the desired outcomes.

Clinical Practice Guideline: EMERGENCY DEPARTMENT–BASED MANAGEMENT OF GERIATRIC FALLS ORIGINATING IN THE COMMUNITY

Purpose:	The appropriate management of the elderly (age >70) brought to the Emergency Department as a result of a fall.
Diagnostic Considerations: *This guideline reflects expert opinion nationally and locally regarding the initial management of patients presenting to the ED as a result of a fall. It may not be applicable for all patients.*	• Obtain history of past medical problems (e.g., diabetes, cardiac) and details of events before the fall (e.g., level of consciousness, chest pain, dizziness), including home environment, social support systems, prior falls, substance abuse (alcohol and drugs), and use of assistive devices. • Review all medications—especially psychotropics, benzodiazepines, antihypertensives, and over-the-counter drugs. • Full physical assessment with special attention to: 1. "Mini-mental' cognitive exam 2. Depression scale 3. Functional ability (activities of daily living) 4. Neurological exam (including standing, rising from bed to sitting, turning and walking, and special attention to tremors) 5. Blood pressure and pulse (lying, immediately after standing, and 10 minutes after standing) 6. Cardiac exam with special attention to carotid and abdominal bruits, and murmurs 7. Examination of feet for lesions or deformities, gait 8. Labs: CBC, basic or comprehensive panels, VDRL, B_{12}, urine analysis, pulse oximetry, thyroid functions 9. Radiographic studies: If indicated, x-rays of chest and all areas involved in injury, CT scan to rule out subarachnoid or subdural hemorrhage 10. ECG

ASSESS PATIENT FOR ACTIVITY AND SIGNS AND SYMPTOMS AT TIME OF FALL

ACTIVITY AT TIME OF FALL*	SIGNS AND SYMPTOMS AT TIME OF FALL*
1. *Head extended backwards:* posterior circulation insufficiency 2. *Turning head suddenly:* carotid artery compression 3. *Shaving:* carotid sinus hypersensitivity 4. *Dizziness when standing or with different position:* orthostasis, vertigo 5. *Coughing, urinating, bowel movement:* valsalva-induced syncope 6. *Climbing stairs:* proximal muscle weakness, joint instability, poor footing, poor vision, environmental factors 7. *Slipping when walking:* slippery floors, poor steppage height, poor footwear, poor balance 8. *Was patient using assistive devices at time of fall?* faulty equipment or improper use of device 9. *Transfers bed to chair:* proximal muscle weakness, orthostasis, high/low furniture, improper technique 10. *Toilet/bath:* incontinence, no grab bars, slippery floors, toilet seat too low, micturition/defecation syncope 11. *Eating:* postprandial syncope	1. *Dizziness:* arrhythmia, hypotension, drug reaction, dehydration, middle ear infection, vertigo, seizure, drug and alcohol withdrawal. 2. *Loss of consciousness:* arrhythmia, seizure, aortic valve disease 3. *Chest pain:* arrhythmia, myocardial infarction 4. *Proximal muscle weakness:* hypothyroidism, hypokalemia, immobilization, polymyalgia rheumatica 5. *Confusion:* drug reaction/overdose, depression due to drug and alcohol withdrawal, dementia, hypoxemia, pneumonia, urinary tract infection, sepsis 6. *Impaired hearing:* ear wax, Meniere's disease, acoustic neuroma, hearing aid malfunction 7. *Impaired vision:* glaucoma, cataracts, macular degeneration, incorrect eyeglass prescription 8. *Difficulty walking:* proximal muscle weakness, hypnotic/sedatives, arthritis, parkinsonism, paraplegia, cerebellar dysfunction, improper shoes and assistive devices, dragging clothes, foot problems 9. *Neuro deficits:* transient ischemic attack, cerebrovascular accident, head trauma, seizure 10. *Metabolic disorders:* infection, electrolyte imbalances 11. *Hypotension* 12. *Poor judgment:* dementia, psychiatric disorder

SEE REVERSE SIDE FOR "CLINICAL MANAGEMENT" AND ADDITIONAL REFERENCES

Figure 12-3 Example of guideline, care of patient with a fall (emergency department). (Courtesy St. Vincent's Hospital and Medical Center, New York City, New York.)

IF ETIOLOGY CANNOT BE DETERMINED, FURTHER WORK-UP IS NEEDED			
Emergency Department Management of Suspected Etiology	Metabolic lab work as indicated if positive findings: *Infection (treat/consider) admission electrolyte abnormality/lab work abnormality* • Treat abnormality accordingly • Alter medications • Consider admission	Cardiac Continue cardiac monitoring if positive findings: *Cardiology consult* • Consider admission	Neuro CT/MRI if head injury if positive findings: *Neuro/Neurosurgery consult* • Consider admission

	ACUTE MEDICAL PROBLEM IDENTIFIED	
NO ACUTE MEDICAL PROBLEM IDENTIFIED **(Environmental cause)** • Home evaluation needed • Outpatient follow-up with RN, SW, PT/OT • Referral to case management for home care evaluation	If no admission to the hospital is needed: • Referral to case management for home care evaluation • Home evaluation needed (yes/no) • Outpatient follow-up (RN, SW, PT/OT)	• Admission to the hospital as needed
ALWAYS REMEMBER: • Falls/risk assessment implementation • Cognitive status assessment (Is the patient able to follow the discharge instructions?)	**THINK:** • Symptoms • Prevention • Location • Activity • Time • Trauma	

Figure 12-3, cont'd   Example of guideline, care of patient with a fall (emergency department). (Courtesy St. Vincent's Hospital and Medical Center, New York City, New York.)

Multidisciplinary Action Plans

MAPs (Figure 12-5) are similar to clinical pathways in their purpose, focus, and process of development. However, they are more detailed, several pages in length (sometimes they are developed in a booklet format), allow room for documentation, and have medical orders embedded in them. In addition, they provide evidence of a collaborative and seamless approach to care for accreditation agencies and result in opening the lines of communication among the various providers.

MAPs specify both the actions/interventions necessary for the care of patients and the related and expected outcomes. They detail outcomes in relation to progression toward recovery; that is, the outcomes follow a specific sequence that is temporal and allows practitioners to easily evaluate the patient's condition and progress in relation to recovery or problem resolution and to determine the appropriate next step in care. This is done by prospectively delineating the intermediate outcomes that must be met first so that the care and the patient can progress in the desired direction. The outcomes are presented in the MAPs using specific timeframes similar to those applied for the interventions and treatments. This characteristic, as it pertains to outcomes,

tends to be lacking in clinical/critical pathways. Another differentiating factor between MAPs and clinical pathways is that MAPs may include algorithms and preprinted order sets, whereas pathways usually do not.

PROCESS OF DEVELOPING CASE MANAGEMENT PLANS

CMPs are developed best through an interdisciplinary team that is granted the authority and responsibility by a higher administrative structure, usually a steering committee charged with implementing case management systems, to develop a specific plan for a particular diagnosis or procedure. The interdisciplinary team is given the responsibility of developing the actual content of the plan. The steering committee, however, provides the team with ongoing expert and administrative support throughout the process.

Team members meet numerous times to discuss and develop the CMP. Sometimes they work individually in between meetings. The length of time needed for the development and completion of one CMP usually depends on the complexity of the diagnosis or procedure; the number of physicians and practitioners who will use the plan; the extent of the disagreements

Clinical Pathway: Open Reduction Internal Fixation of Femur

	Admission	Day of Surgery (Hospital Day #1)	Post-Op Day #1 (Hospital Day #2)	Post-Op Day #2 (Hospital Day #3)
Consults	Medicine service as indicated Anesthesia service	Physiatry service Pain management service as per MD	Pain management follow-up	Pain management follow-up
Tests	CBC, UA ECG (if male >40; or female >50 years of age) Chest x-ray (if >60 years of age) Per clinical need or pre-op variance	CBC Post-op x-ray	CBC PT (if on anticoagulants, e.g., coumadin)	CBC PT (if on anticoagulants, e.g., coumadin)
Treatment	Skin assessment Neurovascular check Heel pads	Auto reinfusion per MD Venodynes Knee immobilizer per MD V/S: q4h x 24 hrs Neurovascular check q4h Cryotherapy per MD Intake and Output x 24 hrs Check hemovac drain	Physical therapy Venodynes Knee immobilizer per MD V/S: q4h x 24 hrs Neurovascular check q4h Heplock Check hemovac drain	Physical therapy Venodynes Knee immobilizer V/S: q8h Neurovascular check q4h Discontinue IV/Heplock Remove hemovac drain Dressing change/evaluate by MD
Medication	Pre-op medications Additional medication per MD and patient history	Antibiotics: surgical prophylactics Analgesia: IM or per pain management Anticoagulant per MD	Antibiotics: surgical prophylactics Analgesia: IM or per pain management Anticoagulant per MD	PO analgesics Anticoagulant per MD
Diet	NPO after 12 MN	NPO Clear liquids as tolerated	As tolerated	As tolerated
Activity	Bed rest	Bed rest turn and posture Isometrics 10 x/hr	OOB (check weight-bearing status) Turn and posture in bed Isometrics/active exercises Begin ambulation with walker	Increase ambulation with walker Isometrics/active exercises ORIF safety precautions Transfers to all surfaces
Teaching	Orientation to unit, PT, and rehab	Discuss signs and symptoms of infection Instruct re: dressing change and pain management	Prepare for discharge Arrange for follow-up appointment Provide prescriptions as needed	Reinforce discharge instructions

Figure 12-4   Example of a clinical/critical pathway.

Major Thoracic Surgery
(Thoracotomy, Lobectomy, Wedge Resection)

Clinical Service: Thoracic Surgery	Primary Nurse:

Admitting Diagnosis:

Secondary Diagnosis:

Patient Problem List/Nursing Diagnosis

Addressograph

#1	Knowledge deficit	#4	Potential for wound infection
#3	Alteration in comfort related to pain	#5	
#2	Ineffective breathing pattern related to thoracic surgery	#6	

Allergies   (* = Variance)

ELEMENTS OF CARE	Date: __/__/__ Peri-Op/Day 0	O R	E V E	N G T	Unit:_____ Date: __/__/__ POD #1	N G T	D A Y	E V E	Unit:_____ Date: __/__/__ POD #2	N G T	D A Y	E V E
Assessment/ Monitoring	• Vital signs q4h (Telemetry) • Admission weight • Assess/pre-op site • Complete nursing admission data form • Peri-op nursing assessment and care plan part I, II, III completed • Consent signed **Outcome:** • **Stable cardiac/ pulmonary status**				• Vital signs q1h • See PACU post-op orders • Telemetry • Assess thoractomy wound **Outcome:** • **Bleeding WNL** • **Patient maintains pulmonary/cardiac status, heart rate, MAP-WNL, and ECG**				• Vital signs q4h • Telemetry • I & O q4h • Weight • Assess thoracotomy wound site • Dressing change **Outcome:** • **Chest tube site dry and intact** • **Balanced I & O**			
Lab Tests/ Procedures	• Admission panel • U/A • PTT/INR • CXR ☐ PFTs				• CBC • ABGs • Chem 7 ☐ CPK—MB x 3				• CBC • Electrolytes • ECG • CXR **Outcome:** • **CBC, electrolytes, and coagulation profile WNL/ baseline**			
Treatment	• Betadine shower • Lab work completed in preparation for OR **Outcome:** • **Patient can successfully demonstrate use of incentive spirometer**				• See Critical care sheet flow sheet (PACU) • Evaluation for extubation • Venodyne boots • Pulse oximetry q30 minutes—1 hour • Nasal oxygen PRN **Outcome:** • **Patient extubated** • **Patient transferred to CTICU when pulmonary/cardiac status stable**				• Evaluate removal of tubes: ☐ Chest tube ☐ Foley ☐ Epidural **Outcome:** • **Good bilateral aeration** • **O₂ Sat WNL** • **Chest tube drainage <100 cc/24 hours** • **Chest tube, (-) air leak**			

The CMP was developed as a suggested interdisciplinary plan of care. This is only a guideline, which may be changed and individualized according to patient condition and assessment data. This CMP is not to be used as a substitute or replacement for clinical assessment.

Figure 12-5   Example of a multidisciplinary action plan.   *Continued*

ELEMENTS OF CARE	Date: __/__/__ Peri-Op/Day	D A Y	O R	5 C	Unit:_____ Date: __/__/__ POD #1	N G T	D A Y	E V E	Unit:_____ Date: __/__/__ POD #2	N G T	D A Y	E V E
Medications/ IV	• Peripheral line inserted ☐ Pre-op antibiotics				• See Post-op orders PACU ☐ Pain management protocol ☐ Post-op antibiotics ☐ Begin digitalization protocol				• Provide pain medication as indicated (Epidural PCA) **Outcome:** • **Patient maintained on oral medications** • **All lines discontinued** • **Adequate pain control**			
Nutrition	• NPO after MN				• Diet progression **Outcome:** • **Tolerates diet**				• Progression to clear liquid diet **Outcome:** • **Tolerates clear liquids**			
Activity	• OOB Ad lib				• Turn q2h • ROM q4h • Incentive spirometer q1h				• Dangle with OOB-chair • Assist ADL • Evaluate activity progressive • Evaluate for PT **Outcome:** • **Patient tolerates OOB-chair**			
Consults	• Anesthesia dept. ☐ Pulmonary								Evaluate for referrals: ☐ Home care ☐ PT ☐ SW ☐ Other			
Psychosocial	• Evaluate psychosocial needs of family and patient **Outcome:** • **Patient verbalizes acceptance of need for surgery and is prepared for OR**				• Evaluate psychosocial needs of family and patient **Outcome:** • **Primary nurse meets with family/caregiver and provides support**				• Evaluate psychosocial needs of family and patient			
Patient/ Family Education	• Share and discuss patient/family pathway • Evaluate need for referrals • Check pre-op home services **Outcome:** • **Patient verbalizes understanding of the surgical procedure and expectations**				• Review CMP with patient/family • Answer any questions **Outcome:** • **Family able to verbalize activity progression**				• Coughing/deep breathing exercises (ICS) • ROM/activity progression • Discuss disease process and risk factor modification **Outcome:** • **Patient/family able to verbalize activity progression and instructions**			
Discharge Planning	• Expected 5 days LOS reviewed with patient/ family **Outcome:** • **Patient/family understands pre-op teaching**				• Assess postdischarge needs				**Outcome:** • **Patient clinical status and discharge plan discussed**			
MD Approval Sign:												
Print Name:												
DICT. Code:	Time:				Time:				Time:			
RN Review:	Time:				Time:				Time:			

Figure 12-5, cont'd Example of a multidisciplinary action plan.

Signature	Title/Initials	Signature	Title/Initials
	MD / ____		RT / ____
	RN / ____		CSW / ____
	RN / ____		RD/ ____
	RN / ____		NP/ ____

Addressograph

Signature	Title/Initials	Signature	Title/Initials	Signature	Title/Initials
	RN / ____		PA / ____		___ ___ / ____
	RN / ____		PT / ____		___ ___ / ____
	RN / ____		OTR/ ____		___ ___ / ____
	RN / ____		___ ___ / ___		___ ___ / ____

ELEMENTS OF CARE	Date: __/__/__ POD #3	N G T	D A Y	E V E	Date: __/__/__ POD #4	N G T	D A Y	E V E	Date: __/__/__ POD #5	N G T	D A Y	E V E
Assessment/ Monitoring	• Vital signs q4h (telemetry) • Daily weight • Review CBC, SMA6 Assess thorocotomy wound daily • I & O q4h • Evaluate removal of tubes **Outcome:** • **O₂ SAT WNL** • **No significant bleeding**				• Vital signs q4h (telemetry) • See critical care flow sheet • Assess thorocotomy wound daily **Outcome:** • **O₂ SAT WNL** • **Free of dysrhythmias**				• Discontinued telemetry • DC orders written **Outcome:** • **Thorocotomy Wound site clean and healing** • **Temperature within normal/afebrile**			
Lab Tests/ Procedures	• Assess blood tests needed M-W-F • CXR as needed				• Review lab data for discharge **Outcomes:** • **WBC, WNL** • **CXR sign negative for severe pleural effusion or pneumonia**				• Review labs before 8 AM			
Treatment	• O₂ Therapy PRN • Remove tubes ☐ Chest tube ☐ Foley ☐ Epidural/PCA • 1st dressing change by PA • Incentive spirometer **Outcome:** • **All tubes removed** • **Chest tube drain <100 cc/24 hours** • **Chest tube, (-) air leak**				• Incentive spirometer **Outcome:** • **Patient has no complaints of dyspnea and tolerates room air**				• Incentive spirometer **Outcome:** • **Patient has no complaints of dyspnea and tolerates room air**			

Figure 12-5, cont'd   Example of a multidisciplinary action plan.   *Continued*

among physicians regarding the content of the plan that may arise while attempting to build **consensus;** the number of disciplines involved; the experience of the team members involved in the process; the availability of team members, their commitment, their productivity, and how well they can work together (i.e., group dynamics); and the presence or absence of a support person or an expert in CMP development. One CMP may take as long as 6 to 9 months for completion, particularly if the team is developing a CMP for the first

ELEMENTS OF CARE	Date: __/__/__ POD #3	N G T	D A Y	E V E	Date: __/__/__ POD #4	N G T	D A Y	E V E	Date: __/__/__ POD #5	N G T	D A Y	E V E
Medications/ IV	• Daily assessment of oral medication **Outcome:** • **All lines discontinued** • **Patient controlled on oral medications**				• Evaluate discharge meds • Prescriptions written				• Prescriptions given by 9 AM at the latest			
Nutrition	• Diet progression				• Regular diet				• Regular diet			
Activity	• Ambulate 100 ft bid ADLs minimal assist OOB-chair tid Incentive spirometer q1h				• Stair climbing • Ambulate 200 ft tid • Incentive spirometer q1h • ADLs independent **Outcome:** **ADLs independent**				**Outcome:** • **Patient is able to provide self-care and demonstrates independence with ADLs**			
Consults	• Daily evaluation for referral by care team ☐ Oncology				• Daily evaluation for referral by care team				Fast track referral to home care: Y____ N____			
Psychosocial	**Outcome:** • **Patient asks appropriate questions about discharge activity plan** • **Questions are answered**				• Provide emotional support as needed				**Outcome:** • **Patient/family expressed needs met**			
Patient/ Family Education	• Wound care • Signs and symptoms of infection • Discharge instruction • LOS reinforced • Stress management • Thoracic surgery booklet • Risk factors				• Home exercise program given to patient • Prescriptions explained • Discharge notice given • Home services in place **Outcome:** • **Patient verbalizes and understands discharge meds**				**Outcome:** • **Caregiver/patient repeats/demonstrates instructions and can verbalize knowledge of medication, activity and exercise plan, and signs of wound infection**			
Discharge Planning					• Implement discharge plan • Clothes in room • Arrange for transportation or pick-up				Discharge order written by 8 AM • Leave unit 10 AM • Discharge lounge 10 AM if needed			
MD Approval Sign:												
Print Name:												
DICT. Code:	Time:				Time:				Time:			
RN Review:	Time:				Time:				Time:			

Figure 12-5, cont'd Example of a multidisciplinary action plan.

time, or as little as a few weeks if team members are well experienced in the process and the topic of the plan is less controversial.

Steering Committee

The steering committee is composed of professionals who hold executive-level positions in the organization. The departments represented on the steering committee may include, depending on the sophistication of the healthcare organization, operations, finance/cost accounting, marketing, nursing/patient care services, information systems, medical records, legal and **risk management**, quality improvement and **utilization management**, managed care and case management, data management, research, and other **ancillary services** as deemed necessary. Members of the steering committee may be the high-ranking officers of each of these departments or their designee. It is not always necessary to have a representative from each of these departments. Some institutions may choose not to create a new stand-alone committee for this purpose. Responsibilities of a steering committee, in this case, may be added to a preexisting committee such as a quality council or a length-of-stay or cost-reduction taskforce.

The major role of the steering committee is to put together a strategic plan for the implementation of case management systems. This plan describes the processes of training and educating those involved in the process; selecting and prioritizing the diagnoses and procedures for which CMPs are to be developed; and providing support for the teams charged with developing CMPs. Members of the steering committee provide leadership, support, and direction for the development, implementation, and evaluation of the case management system.

Most institutions have established a standardized process for the development of CMPs. The steering committee is responsible for the development of this process. Having an established formal process is important because it provides the interdisciplinary team with the foundation for successful development and implementation of CMPs, simplifies the work, and lays out the expectations. An ideal process is a simple one that clearly identifies the steps in a systematic way and makes it easier for the team to follow.

This chapter includes an example of such processes (Figure 12-6) for healthcare administrators to adapt to their organizations and adjust as needed. This example follows a 10-step process that differentiates between the work and responsibilities of the steering committee and the interdisciplinary team.

The steering committee is responsible for the first four steps because they require higher administrative authority in decision making. They are related to the logistics of case management systems and plans and are part of the overall case management implementation plan put together by the steering committee and approved by key executive personnel in the institution. The remaining six steps are the responsibility of the interdisciplinary team and address the actual work of the team and the creation of the CMP.

Step 1: Design the Format of the Plan

Deciding on the format is crucial, because the format guides the development of the content of the plan (Case Manager's Tip 12-2). The format should be made easy for all healthcare professionals to follow and use. This step is integral to the establishment of case management systems because it affects clinical practice and other care activities and processes (e.g., documentation, **performance improvement** processes, coding of the medical record, presentation of the standards of care and practice).

The CMP should be designed in such a way that includes the various elements of patient care (Box 12-4) (Ferguson, 1993; Ignatavicius and Hausman, 1995). Some of these elements are related to the medical/surgical care of the patient, whereas others are nursing in nature. In addition, there may be elements related to support or administrative services. Specific sections of the CMP should be allotted to quality indicators, outcome measures of care, **variances** tracking, and data collection. The number of the different care elements for each CMP depends on the diagnosis or surgical procedure addressed. For example, a plan for chest pain evaluation may include a pain management section but not occupational therapy. However, speech pathology and physical and occupational therapy are important when addressing a stroke CMP. A CMP to be used in a subacute care facility designated for ventilator-dependent patients should always include a respiratory care section that stresses the institution's protocol for weaning patients off mechanical ventilation.

The final format of the CMP (see Appendix 12-1 for an example) should be presented to the institutional medical records committee, legal/risk management department, and medical board for review and approval before it is made official. A decision regarding the format should be in place before authorizing any interdisciplinary team to start working on a CMP. The approved format becomes the desired CMP's template that is followed by all interdisciplinary teams to maintain consistency and uniformity of plans. The format also provides the framework based on which the team can construct the content details of the CMP. The steering

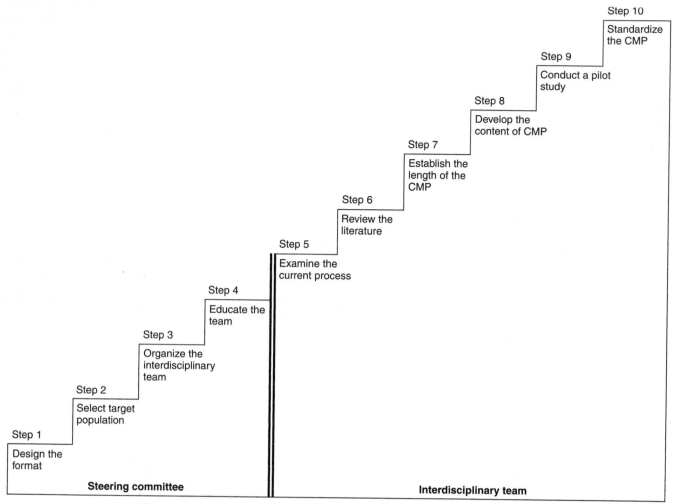

Figure 12-6 The process of developing case management plans (CMPs).

committee then develops guidelines for the use of the template/final format of the CMP. The guidelines explain in detail how the template should be followed or used, the definitions of each of the care elements, and examples of the various patient care activities that could be listed under each care element (Box 12-5). This is important because it maintains continuity and consistency of CMPs across the various interdisciplinary teams. When a team is established, a copy of the template/format and a copy of the guidelines should be presented to and discussed with the team members.

Step 2: Identify/Select Target Population

The mechanism for selecting target populations can be done at any time during the design phase of the CMP format. The steering committee studies the patient populations/groups served by the institution. It then selects the groups that need improvement regarding cost and quality, present a risk for financial loss, or are a potential for revenue.

There are several criteria that must be considered when selecting target populations for which to develop CMPs. These include volume of the patient group, cost of care, complexity of care needed, institutional length of stay compared with other **benchmarks,** variations in practice patterns, the need for multiple services/care settings or providers, feasibility of developing the plan, potential revenue (i.e., control of resources, fragmentation and duplication of care), opportunity for improvement in quality of care and outcomes, reports from payer groups, problem-prone/high-risk diagnoses or procedures, and results of internal and external quality management monitoring (Ignatavicius and Hausman, 1995; Tahan and Cesta, 1995; Cohen and Cesta, 1997).

It is important to evaluate the number of patients seen in a particular **diagnosis-related group (DRG)** when selecting a target population. The decision of which DRG should be targeted is made based on the number of patients seen in a particular DRG during a whole year. The larger the number of patients seen, the better the opportunities for improvement.

CASE MANAGER'S TIP 12-2

Factors That Affect Choosing a Particular CMP Format

1. Whether the CMP will be used for documentation
2. The number of disciplines that need to be represented in the plan
3. Complexity of the diagnosis/procedure
4. The clinical area or service or care setting
5. Whether the plan will replace any existing preprinted physician orders or protocols
6. The appropriate timeline
7. Forms that must be eliminated from the patient's record on implementation of the plan
8. Related risk management and legal issues
9. Whether the plan will be a permanent part of the medical record
10. Existing standards of regulatory and accreditation agencies
11. Plans for automation of the medical record
12. Whether the plan will integrate physician orders and algorithms or guidelines

---

BOX 12-4   Elements of Patient Care as They May Appear on the Plan

1. Assessment of patient monitoring
2. Tests and procedures
3. Care facilitation and coordination, including care milestones
4. Consultations and referrals
5. Medications
6. Intravenous therapy
7. Activity
8. Nutrition
9. Patient/family teaching
10. Treatments: medical, surgical, and nursing interventions
11. Wound care
12. Physical therapy and occupational therapy
13. Pain management
14. Outcome indicators and projected/desired responses to treatments
15. Safety
16. Discharge planning
17. Psychosocial assessment

The established CMP will then be applied to a larger population, which maximizes the benefit.

Because a DRG is too broad and may include several procedures that require different resources, whereas the International Classification of Diseases, Ninth Revision, Clinical Modification **(ICD-9-CM)** is very specific, evaluation and analysis of patient populations should be made at the ICD-9-CM code level. Consider DRG 112 (percutaneous cardiovascular procedures) as an example. It includes several different procedures, with each designated a separate ICD-9-CM code (Table 12-1) (St. Anthony Publishing, 1992). The treatment plans for each of these procedures are different—cardiac catheterization is a diagnostic procedure, whereas angioplasty is a therapeutic procedure, and electrophysiological cardiac stimulation is a diagnostic procedure but very different than catheterization, which makes developing a CMP for DRG 112 more difficult. However, developing a separate CMP for each procedure/ICD-9-CM code is more feasible and desirable. As a result, it is better to consider developing a separate CMP for each ICD-9-CM code than for the DRG.

Another example is DRG 96: bronchitis and asthma, age greater than 17 years with **complications** and **comorbidities** (Table 12-2). There are major differences between treating these two disease entities. It is best to deal with this DRG based on ICD-9-CM codes (St. Anthony Publishing, 1992). Sometimes it is appropriate to combine two or more ICD-9-CM codes in one CMP. For example, combining asthma ICD-9-CM codes 493.20, 493.21, 493.01, and 493.11 in one CMP that delineates the standard of care of adult asthma is relevant because there exist minimal to no variations in the treatment of asthma in the different ICD-9-CM codes. However, combining ICD-9-CM codes 493.20, 493.21 and 491.1, and 491.2 is not appropriate because treating asthma is different than treating bronchitis, and the standard of care for both diagnoses cannot be combined into one standard.

The volume of patients seen in one DRG should not be considered in isolation from other measures, such as cost per case, cost per day, consumption of resources (e.g., the number of x-ray examinations, blood tests, or electrocardiograms in one hospitalization or episode of care), average length of stay, outcomes, and profit and loss ratios. Patient populations that exert financial loss on the institution are considered the best target for CMP development.

Table 12-3 is an example of one administrative report that can be used to identify a target population. Examining the data presented, one can see that DRGs 88 and 127 have longer lengths of stay and at the same time have profit losses. Thus considering the development of CMPs for these two DRGs is worthwhile because the opportunities for improvement and profit are high. To address these two DRGs requires the establishment of two different teams for CMP development because the DRGs are related to two different services—pulmonary and cardiology.

Conversely, DRGs 90 and 143 are not a high priority for CMP development because the length of stay is

BOX 12-5 Guidelines for the Placement of Patient Care Activities in the Case Management Plan

Each patient care activity should be indicated in the appropriate "care element" category. The following is a master list that should be used as a guide by interdisciplinary teams during the process of developing a case management plan.

Assessment and Monitoring

1. Physiological assessment measures (e.g., blood pressure, temperature, pulse[s], respirations, hemodynamic monitoring)
2. System assessment (e.g., cardiac, pulmonary, gastrointestinal)
3. Intake and output
4. Drainage of bodily fluids
5. Weights

Tests and Procedures

1. Laboratory tests (e.g., blood work, urine, sputum, pathology)
2. Unit tests (e.g., glucose fingerstick, guaiac, urine dipstick)
3. Routine diagnostic tests (e.g., electrocardiogram, chest x-ray examination, ultrasound)
4. Diagnostic/therapeutic procedures (e.g., operations, cardiac catheterization, angiogram, angioplasty, gastrostomy tube placement)

Treatments (Preventive and Therapeutic)

1. Dressing change and wound care
2. Intermittent compression device
3. Chest physiotherapy
4. Oxygen therapy and ventilator-related care
5. Central line site care
6. Tracheostomy care

Medications

1. Routine medications necessary for the particular case type (standing, as required [prn], and single dosages; premedication needs when preparing a patient for a particular procedure)

Pain Management

1. Pain management protocol
2. Frequency of evaluating pain status and response to medications
3. Indications/recommendations for nonpharmacologic actions
4. Medications for pain management

Intravenous Therapy

1. Intravenous fluids (e.g., D_5W, D_5NSS)
2. Blood and blood products

Nutrition

1. Type of diet/meal
2. Instructions for diet progression

3. Fluid restrictions
4. Tube and supplemental feedings
5. Parenteral nutrition

Activity

1. Activity limitations/ambulation
2. Safety instructions
3. Physical and occupational therapy
4. Fall risk assessment
5. Skin integrity risk assessment
6. Functional measures

Consults

1. Routine consults (e.g., infectious disease, anesthesiology)
2. Specific consults (e.g., speech pathology for a stroke patient)

Psychosocial Assessment

1. Coping and adjustment to illness and hospitalization
2. Support system
3. Anxiety level

Patient/Family Teaching

1. Assessment for readiness to learn
2. Assessment of limitations/barriers to learning
3. Assessment of learning needs
4. Education plan, including areas of teaching (e.g., medications, disease process, activity/exercise, dietary limitations, specific medical/surgical regimen after discharge)
5. Need for particular equipment (e.g., glucometer for diabetic patients)

Discharge/Transitional Planning

1. Assessment of discharge needs
2. Referrals of high-risk patients to home care, social work, nutrition
3. Completion of any necessary paperwork for nursing home placement
4. Transitioning patients from one level of care to another

Outcome Indicators (Expected Outcomes of Care)

1. Intermediate outcomes
2. Discharge outcomes

Variance Tracking

1. Instructions on the use of variance section of the case management plan
2. Classifications/coding
3. Action plan
4. Date and time

Patient Problems

1. Delineate how patient problems should be stated (i.e., medical/nursing language)
2. Actual and potential problems

TABLE 12-1   Different Procedures in DRG 112

Percutaneous Cardiovascular Procedures	ICD-9-CM Codes
Angioplasty, coronary, PTCA, multiple vessel with or without thrombolytic agent	36.05
Angioplasty, coronary, PTCA, single vessel with thrombolytic agent	36.02
Angioplasty, coronary, PTCA, single vessel without thrombolytic agent	36.01
Catheterization, heart, lesion, or tissue	37.34
Mapping, cardiac	37.27
Removal, obstruction, coronary artery, other specified	36.09
Valvuloplasty, percutaneous	35.96
Simulation, cardiac, electrophysiological	37.26

PTCA, Percutaneous transluminal coronary angioplasty.

TABLE 12-2   Different ICD-9-CM Codes in DRG 96

Bronchitis and Asthma, Age Greater Than 17 with Complications and Comorbidities	ICD-9-CM Codes
Bronchitis, chronic, mucopurulent	491.1
Bronchitis, chronic, obstructive	491.2
Bronchitis, chronic, simple	491.0
Asthma, extrinsic	493.01
Asthma, intrinsic	493.11
Asthma, chronic obstructive, with status asthmaticus	493.21
Asthma, chronic obstructive, without status asthmaticus	493.20

TABLE 12-3   Example of Administrative Report Used to Identify Target Populations

DRG	Description	Total Cases*	Average Length of Stay	Excess Days†	Profit (Loss)‡
88	Chronic obstructive pulmonary disease	150	6	2	($1,145.43)
89	Simple pneumonia and pleurisy, age greater than 17 years with complications and comorbidities	165	7	2	($989.56)
90	Simple pneumonia and pleurisy, and age greater than 17 years without complications and comorbidities	100	3	(1)	$1,120.56
127	Heart failure and shock	200	7	3	($1,895.62)
143	Chest pain	116	3	(1)	$460.75

*Total number of patients seen annually in each DRG.
†Total number of days above or below average length of stay at comparable institutions.
‡Amount per case.
NOTE: The figures in this table are hypothetical and are presented for clarification purposes only.

lower than that in comparable institutions and they are financially profitable. The institution may decide to develop CMPs for these diagnoses based on other factors and improvement efforts, such as quality of care, practice patterns, and allocation and use of resources.

Deciding which CMPs must be developed is not always the decision of the steering committee. Some healthcare organizations leave such decisions open and encourage the various departments and specialties to decide on the topics that are appropriate for them. Other organizations may purposefully leave such decisions to the clinicians and address the development of CMPs as a department-based quality improvement plan. In either case, the steering committee may institute the use of a communication tool/form so that it is kept abreast of the developments in each department (Figure 12-7). The use

of this tool is beneficial to the organization. It helps keep the steering committee informed of the activities and improvements taking place at the department level. It also ensures that the departments are kept focused and on target and that their efforts are not being wasted. Furthermore, it allows the steering committee to evaluate the level of responsibility, accountability, and initiative assumed by the department.

Step 3: Organize an Interdisciplinary Team
Traditionally, members of the interdisciplinary team were selected by the steering committee, and recommendations from department heads were usually considered when organizing the team. Today, however, most healthcare organizations defer this responsibility to the various departments and clinical specialties. In

this case, the departments and the steering committee communicate constantly. The department may also seek the advice of the steering committee when problems arise or challenging decisions need to be made. The selection of members is based on their communication skills and ability to work in a team, their clinical competence and past experiences, and their commitment to their work. Becoming a member of an interdisciplinary team and contributing to the development of processes that improve patient care can be a rewarding experience for staff members.

Based on the type of the CMP to be developed, members from the various disciplines involved in patient care are selected to serve on the team. It is important to include all disciplines so that the completed plan is thorough and well written. Every team should include representatives from various departments or disciplines such as medicine (including house staff), nursing, case management, quality improvement and **utilization management,** social services, home care, and nutrition. Members

from other departments may participate on a consultation basis. These departments may include pharmacy, medical records and coding, finance, patient representative, materials management, laboratory, and radiology. Some departments may be represented as needed based on the diagnosis being worked on. For example, representation from rehabilitation, occupational therapy, and speech pathology is essential for a team working on a stroke CMP, respiratory therapy for asthma, chronic obstructive pulmonary disease, or pneumonia plans.

The interdisciplinary team should be moderate in size (i.e., 6 to 10 members). A larger team reduces its productivity, increases the risk for disagreements, and delays the process. The team is empowered by the steering committee to make independent decisions. The steering committee may designate one of its members to act as a sponsor for the team. The sponsor's role (Case Manager's Tip 12-3) includes coaching the team through the process, removing obstacles and answering unresolved questions, acting as a liaison between the team

---

When a CMP topic is selected, please complete this form and send to the steering committee. This will allow us to maintain a database of CMPs in development and ensure that work does not commence in an area where another CMP is in development or already in existence.

Medical service involved: _____

Suggested case management plan title: _____

Projected volume of cases per year: _____

Rationale for development: (Mark "X" all that apply)

_____ LOS outlier   _____ High variance in practice

_____ Cost outlier   _____ High volume

_____ Quality issues   _____ Legal risk

_____ Research   _____ Clinical trial

Other: _____

Physician Co-Leader: _____

Tel. #/Beeper: _____

Nurse Co-Leader: _____

Tel. #/Beeper: _____

Team Members: (List all involved discipline categories, or names if members already selected)

_____   _____
_____   _____
_____   _____
_____   _____

Figure 12-7   Case management plan, predevelopment communication form.

CASE MANAGER'S TIP 12-3

Roles and Responsibilities of the Team Sponsor
1. Provides the team with administrative support and power
2. Acts as a resource
3. Answers any unanswered questions or, when unable, facilitates obtaining the answer
4. Acts as the team's liaison with the steering committee
5. Ensures that work is on track
6. Helps the team with problem solving
7. Alerts the team to not make decisions regarding issues that are beyond their realm of responsibilities or power
8. Brings feedback about the team to the steering committee

 CASE MANAGER'S TIP 12-4

Roles and Responsibilities of the Team Leader and Team Facilitator
Team leader
1. Chairs the meeting
2. Prepares the agenda
3. Introduces team members and explains the charge and goals of the team
4. Guides team members through the process of developing CMPs
5. Keeps the team focused on its goals
6. Stimulates discussion regarding treatment modalities and patient care activities and seeks different opinions
7. Encourages active participation of members
8. Helps members reach a common understanding and resolutions on disagreements
9. Builds consensus of members regarding ideal/best practice to be included in the CMP
10. Guides members through problem-solving process when necessary
11. Elicits information, ideas, opinions, comments, and recommendations
12. Ensures that every member gets the opportunity to contribute
13. Obtains commitments for actions
14. Follows up on unresolved/unconcluded issues
15. Clarifies and summarizes conclusions and decisions
16. Collaborates with the facilitator of the team
17. Collaborates with the sponsor of the team

Team facilitator
1. Coaches the team leader and the members
2. Serves as a role model
3. Ensures the participation of every member
4. Monitors group processes and relieves tension when it arises
5. Interjects as needed
6. Keeps the team focused
7. Maintains a positive and collegial atmosphere during meetings: openness, acceptance, trust, respect, support, cooperation, collaboration, listening, cohesiveness, and teamwork
8. Makes suggestions to keep the team moving forward
9. Confronts interpersonal or process problems
10. Serves as a liaison with team members between meetings
11. Offers support and training sessions as necessary
12. Clarifies ideas and decisions and makes recommendations during meetings
13. Collaborates with the team leader and the sponsor

and the steering committee, and overseeing the administrative activities that keep the team functioning. In addition, it is important that the steering committee appoint two members of the interdisciplinary team to act as the team leader and the facilitator (Case Manager's Tip 12-4). Most healthcare organizations designate a physician and a nurse to assume these roles. These two members play an important role in keeping the work of the team progressing and ensuring that the goals and objectives of the team are met within the established timeframe. Some institutions may require the team to present its recommended CMP before the steering committee when it is completed and ready for implementation.

Direct care providers should be well represented on the team as team members (Case Manager's Tip 12-5) because they are instrumental in sharing their firsthand experiences with the day-to-day patient care activities. To prevent physicians' resistance to the use of CMPs, it is recommended that they be involved in the process from the beginning and given the leader or co-leader role on the interdisciplinary team (Tahan and Cesta, 1995; Cohen and Cesta, 1997). Past experiences show that physicians who participate on a team act as champions in promoting case management systems and CMPs in their institutions and continue to be the best supporters and sellers.

Step 4: Educate/Train the Team in the Process
Before the team launches the development process for a CMP, members should be trained in the process. Formal training must include topics such as general overview of case management systems and plans; the process of developing CMPs; the responsibilities of the team leader, facilitator, and member; and tools and

CASE MANAGER'S TIP 12-5

Roles and Responsibilities of the Team Member

1. Participates actively in meetings
2. Attends meetings
3. Provides relevant information
4. Collects data
5. Supports the team's charge and goals
6. Cooperates in achieving consensus when needed
7. Completes assignments
8. Maintains a positive and collegial atmosphere during meetings
9. Respects the team's ground rules
10. Represents co-workers
11. Seeks guidance when needed
12. Acts as a recorder
13. Collaborates and cooperates in the team process

strategies for success. Examples of the work of other teams, if they exist, should be shared (Ignatavicius and Hausman, 1995; Tahan and Cesta, 1995; Cohen and Cesta, 1997). It is in this forum that the expectations from the team, the administrative support available to the team, and the role of the sponsor and the steering committee as they relate to the role of the interdisciplinary team should be discussed. The team should be given the opportunity to ask any questions or raise any concerns. It should also be informed of the ongoing support of the steering committee throughout the process. After completing the required training, the team starts its work on the plan.

One may ask who prepares the steering committee regarding case management systems and how members of the steering committee acquire their related knowledge. Most healthcare organizations hire an outside consultant (an expert in case management systems) to help and guide them through the process. The consultant plays an important role in helping the steering committee develop the best case management system for the organization. The consultant also develops an education packet specific to the institution's policies, procedures, and operations to train members of the steering committee and the interdisciplinary teams that will be developing CMPs. Sometimes organizations may prefer to hire a full-time employee (instead of a consultant) who is an expert in the area of case management to assume full responsibility for the program. The employee is usually responsible for coordinating all the activities of the program; educating committee members, interdisciplinary team members, and staff; and acting in place of the consultant.

Developing the Plan's Content
Step 5: Examine the Current Practice

This step represents the start of the work on the actual content of the plan. The team members usually begin with brainstorming regarding the care of a patient. Members are asked to concentrate on the routine rather than the exception (i.e., the normal recovering patient and not exceptions or extraneous situations) because exceptional patients usually represent a small number of cases. During brainstorming, members attempt to list any quality barriers regarding patient care and any experienced delays in the past. Discussing the quality barriers helps members better understand the current situation and identify the improvement efforts the CMP will address.

After brainstorming is exhausted, team members move on to developing a flow diagram for the current process. A flow diagram that highlights the most important steps in the process of caring for a patient is recommended to prevent the team from getting bogged down with the unnecessary details. The flow diagram (see Figure 1-1, p. 13, for an example of a flow diagram) should reflect the projected care of the patient from admission until discharge and in some cases until after discharge or from the beginning to the end of the care episode.

There are several ways to examine current practice patterns. The two most important ones are review of medical records and interviews of care providers. In medical record reviews, members concentrate on the critical elements of care presented in Box 12-4, such as assessment, tests and procedures, treatments, consultation and referrals, care facilitation and coordination, medications, IV therapy, activity level, nutrition, patient and family teaching, wound care, physical and occupational therapy, pain management, **outcome indicators** and projected desired responses to treatment, and **discharge planning.** Data collection regarding the critical elements and the associated timeframes of delivery of patient care activities is essential in the development of CMPs. Mostly, tools to simplify and standardize the process of collecting data are developed by the team members before starting the data collection process.

Particular attention is given to the care activities considered as critical milestones of care or trigger points for a change in the treatment plan. For example, it is important to collect data about when an IV antibiotic is switched to its oral form during the hospitalization of a patient with pneumonia or when an IV corticosteroid is switched to an oral form while caring for a patient with asthma. These milestones are important because they affect the length of stay and are considered outcome measures or **quality indicators.** It is recommended that a thorough chart review be done regarding the most significant care activities that are required for a case type, with particular evaluation of their timeframes for completion. For example, caring for a patient hospitalized for a coronary intervention procedure may require healthcare professionals (physicians, nurses, and others) to ensure the successful completion of several different care activities (Box 12-6) preprocedure, intraprocedure, postprocedure, and at the time of discharge. These activities, as specified in Box 12-4, should be the center of medical record reviews when developing a CMP for coronary interventions.

Practice patterns of individual physicians should be assessed for variables such as length of stay and cost per case (Table 12-4) by examining the effect of starting time of antibiotic therapy on length of stay (Figure 12-8) or by reviewing the use of resources per case (e.g., counting the number of electrocardiograms, x-ray examinations, scans, blood tests). In the example seen in Table 12-4, physician B has the lowest average length of stay and the lowest cost per case. This physician appears to be providing care differently from the others. Medical records for this physician's patients must be reviewed and compared with other physicians' records to identify

TABLE 12-4   Example of Physicians' Practice Patterns for DRG 89: Simple Pneumonia and Pleurisy, Age Greater Than 17 Years with Complications and Comorbidities

Physician	Number of Patients	Average Length of Stay	Cost per Case
A	55	6.5	$9,280.56
B	50	4.5	$6,985.44
C	34	7.0	$9,986.53
D	30	7.0	$9,895.32
E	25	6.9	$9,643.50
F	18	5.8	$7,856.64

NOTE: The above data are presented for clarification purposes only.

differences and determine appropriate practice patterns for the CMP.

Using the example in Figure 12-8, one can see that the earlier the first dose of antibiotic is started in a pneumonia patient, the shorter the average length of stay will be. Based on this conclusion, the interdisciplinary team might recommend that the antibiotic to be used to treat pneumonia should be started as early as the time of admission. This recommendation should be reflected in the timeline of the CMP for pneumonia.

After completing the medical record reviews, team members interview representatives of the healthcare team who provide care for the patient population in question. This includes physicians, house staff, nurses who provide direct patient care, and ancillary and professional staff. Similar to the medical record reviews, the interviews concentrate on the critical elements of care and their attached timeframes.

Other important documents available in the organization are also reviewed by the team and are studied carefully for their relation to and impact on the delivery of care. These may include any data reports on file in the institution (e.g., utilization, financial, **quality assurance** and improvement, and medical record reviews),

---

BOX 12-6   Indicators for Data Collection from Medical Records Review of Patients: Postcoronary Intervention Cases

1. Demographic data: age, sex, risk factors related to coronary artery disease, and insurance coverage (e.g., Medicaid, Medicare)
2. Comorbidities
3. Resource utilization (tests): blood work, chest x-ray examination(s), electrocardiograms, angiograms, and echocardiograms
4. Medications (preprocedure and postprocedure): cardiac medications, anticoagulants
5. Length of stay (preprocedure, postprocedure, and total) and time spent in the cardiac catheterization laboratory (during procedure)
6. Length of stay in the coronary care unit and in the telemetry unit
7. Ionic/nonionic contrast use
8. Sheath: arterial, venous, or both; time spent with sheath in place; timing of sheath removal; use of vascular hemostasis device (e.g., Vasoseal/collagen)
9. Ambulation: length of time on complete bed rest after sheath removal
10. Need for community services after discharge
11. Patient/family teaching regarding disease, procedure, medications, diet, prevention, and exercise
12. Complications: hematoma, pseudoaneurysm, bleeding

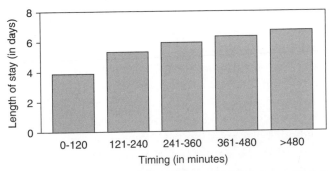

Figure 12-8   Example of physician's practice pattern: timing of first antibiotic dose and length of stay for patients in DRG 89. (NOTE: The data in this figure are presented for clarification purposes only.)

the standards of care and practice, the preprinted physician orders, protocols, and guidelines (Ignatavicius and Hausman, 1995; Tahan and Cesta, 1995; Cohen and Cesta, 1997).

As members of the CMP development team review the practice patterns of providers and a sample of the medical records, they may find that there is no consistency in treatment plans. An important strategy to address such situations is a review and evaluation of related literature (see step 6 below). This helps the team to decide on which plan of care to adopt. However, the literature may not always provide the answer. In this case the team's next strategy is to pursue consensus building on a desirable treatment approach with key and influential providers in the organization to resolve this dilemma. Situations such as this are common, especially in areas in which treatment options are controversial, no research is available to support one type of treatment versus another, or no national standards/recommendations are made by professional and specialty organizations. When the CMP development team encounters such a situation, it must look at it as an opportunity for a change in practice and for innovation; that is, developing new care methods and treatment options. The team must then test the new methods and evaluate their outcomes. If the outcomes achieved are not desirable, the new methods must be altered as indicated and then retested. If found to be favorable, they should be adopted on a larger scale as the normal practice and standard of care. Such a process results in the development of new ideal/best practices in areas that otherwise might be considered controversial.

Step 6: Review the Available Literature

A thorough review and evaluation of the literature is essential because it raises awareness of team members to the latest trends and technology in patient care. The available research should be studied carefully and used to validate the recommendations made in the CMP. This creates an opportunity to provide patient care that is research/evidence-based. Without consideration of the relevant outcomes of research and clinical trials, the CMP developed becomes specific to the healthcare organization and may not reflect the ideal/best practice, or the state-of-the science care (Janken, Grubbs, and Haldeman, 1999). To promote the development of a CMP that is evidence based, research utilization methodologies must be incorporated in the process of developing the content of the plan. This is achieved through a critical review, analysis, and evaluation of the literature. Therefore it is important to merge the processes of CMP development and research utilization. This can be achieved by applying the following steps

(Janken, Grubbs, and Haldeman, 1999):

1. Review the research literature as it pertains to the topic of the CMP or the clinical practice problems.
2. Evaluate and critique the research for its strengths and weaknesses.
3. Evaluate the appropriateness of the research outcomes for application in practice.
4. Apply the outcomes that are considered ready for implementation in practice by incorporating them as an integral part (i.e., care activities and interventions) of the content of the CMP.

Review of the literature should also include an examination of any published related quality improvement efforts, CMPs, and existing standards of care that are developed by professional organizations such as the Joint Commission on Accreditation of Healthcare Organizations (JCAHO), physician groups and societies such as the American Medical Association, nursing organizations such as the American Nurses Association, or governmental agencies such as the AHRQ, formerly known as the AHCPR. Other essential literature to be used in the development of CMPs is the literature on **transitional planning** and managed care guidelines. It is necessary to examine transitional planning to obtain information on the latest regulations about the various care settings across the continuum and their related admission and discharge criteria and associated **reimbursement** methods. The managed care literature relates to the Milliman & Robertson Guidelines (Schibanoff, 1999) and InterQual criteria (InterQual, Inc, 1998). These guidelines play an essential role in ensuring that the CMPs developed adhere to the managed care reimbursement standards by including appropriate interventions and care progression activities and reinforcing the provision of quality care and services.

Step 7: Determine the Length of the Plan

The length of the CMP is based on several factors, including institutional administrative reports regarding the average length of stay and reports of length of stay per physician, the DRG's length of stay for **Medicare** and non-Medicare populations, managed care contracts and their respective organizations, variations in practice patterns as they relate to the length of stay, physician preference, reimbursement reports, benchmarks from other healthcare organizations, and improvement targets (Ferguson, 1993; Esler et al, 1994; Bozzuto and Farrell, 1995; Ignatavicius, 1995; Ignatavicius and Hausman, 1995; Tahan and Cesta, 1995; Cohen and Cesta, 1997). The team should study the length of stay issue very carefully, and it should seek the steering committee's support and guidance as needed. The length of the CMP, as decided by the team, should be within the reimbursable range and lower than the institution's current average length of stay for that particular diagnosis or DRG. Also, it is crucial that improvement targets regarding length of stay, mostly decided by the steering committee, are made known to the interdisciplinary team before launching the development process of the CMP.

Step 8: Write the Content of the Plan

This step involves compiling all of the data collected in the previous steps. Representatives from each department are asked to write a draft of their respective part in the provision of care following the approved format of the plan and based on the results of the data collected from chart reviews, interviews, and review and evaluation of the literature and research outcomes. All drafts are then put together on one form to be discussed and finalized by the team members.

The content of the plan should reflect the state-of-the-science care and the ideal/best practice that were agreed on by the team, in realistic timeframes. For example, expecting to complete an echocardiography by day 2 of the hospitalization of a chest pain patient, knowing that the system requires a turnaround time of 72 hours from ordering to completion, is not realistic. Such an unrealistic expectation will result in delays in care, compared with the plan, every time a patient with chest pain is admitted for treatment. However, the team may make a recommendation to the steering committee that the process for completing an echocardiography in 72 hours be evaluated so that a 2-day turnaround is possible. It then becomes the responsibility of the steering committee to make a final decision regarding the timeframe.

When the team finishes the plan, it should be circulated for review by a group of physicians, nursing leaders, ancillary department heads, and support services involved in the care of the specific patient population. The CMP also must be sent to the pharmacy department to review whether the medications selected are cost-effective and to the coding division of the medical records department for a review of word choices that may enhance coding and improve reimbursement. This review must be done before concluding the content of the plan, and it could be done earlier in the process.

The CMP will then undergo a final review by the team with regard to the recommendations of the reviewers. The final draft of the plan is then presented to the steering committee for approval. The steering committee may suggest the use of an approval form (Figure 12-9). In case such a form is used, the multidisciplinary development team will be required to

---

This form must be completed by the facilitator of the CMP development team. The purpose of this form is to provide the steering committee with a concise record of CMPs. The completion of this form is essential for archival of all plans, a system to expedite updates to the tools on an annual basis, and a checklist to ensure policies and procedures for CMP development have occurred.

Case management plan title: _____

Medical service/department: _____

Date completed: _____

Development group: (Attach list with names and titles or the Predevelopment Communication Form)

Suggested implementation date: _____

	Yes	No
Physician order set attached:	____	____
Patient/family version of the pathway attached:	____	____
Variance indicators outlined on tracking sheet:	____	____
Is this a revision of a current CMP?	____	____
(If yes, attach old CMP)		
Current CMP attached:	____	____

Signature/Date

Reviewed by: _____

Medical/Department Chairman: _____

(approval of clinical content and use in practice)

Director of Nursing: _____

(consistent with clinical standards)

Medical Records Staff: _____

(approved format and abbreviations)

Pharmacy: _____

(review the drugs suggested for accuracy of dosage, if formulary, etc.)

Figure 12-9 Case management plan communication and approval form.

submit the final draft of the CMP attached to the approval form for the steering committee review and approval. The use of this form is important for record keeping with regard to the review and approval process. The team clarifies any questions asked and presents the reasons a particular practice pattern was recommended. Finally, the CMP is put into practice.

Step 9: Conduct a Pilot Study of the Plan

In this step the team implements the use of the CMP. Training and education regarding the CMP for all healthcare providers involved in the particular specialty or diagnosis should be completed before implementation of the plan (Box 12-7). The CMP is then evaluated for quality, feasibility of use, appropriateness of timeline and clinical activities and interventions, length of stay, any delays or variations in care, practice patterns of physicians and other care providers, and compliance. For the CMPs that include state-of-the-science care and are considered research/evidence-based, it is important for the team to evaluate the appropriateness of such content to the patient population addressed in the CMP. Therefore it is necessary for the team to evaluate the patient outcomes achieved by the CMP to ensure that they are consistent with those reported in the original research or clinical trials. If outcomes are found to be consistent, the CMP is then finalized as the standard of care. However, if the outcomes are not similar, the team must reexamine the interventions, evaluate the possible causes, and revise the content accordingly. Such process must continue until the team is pleased with the results.

The CMP is piloted on a group of patients. In addition to evaluating the content of the CMP, it is as important

to survey the providers using the CMP for their perception and satisfaction with its use. Figure 12-10 contains an example of a tool that can be used for this purpose. The results of the pilot are then analyzed and discussed by the interdisciplinary team, and revisions are made accordingly. The plan is then printed in the final version for official use.

Step 10: Standardize/Normalize the Plan

After completing the pilot study of the CMP and making the required changes, the interdisciplinary team meets to develop policies and procedures regarding the use of the plan. It should be made clear to all involved healthcare professionals that the CMP represents the standard of care for that particular population and should be followed when caring for the patient. It should also be made clear that some patients might not fit the CMP and that it is appropriate not to use the CMP in these situations (Case Manager's Tip 12-6). It is common knowledge that CMPs do not apply to every type of patient because they are developed based on the care of the average patient (i.e., for 80% of the population) and not the exceptional cases. The final plan is then added to the master manual of CMPs and circulated in the final format to key people in the institution. The plan can be shared with various healthcare providers in different forums such as grand rounds, newsletters, and administrative and departmental meetings.

Policies and procedures on the use of CMPs, particularly documentation of patient progress and variances, what to do when a patient does not fit the CMP, and why it is important to individualize the CMP, are extremely important and should be in place before implementing the use of CMPs. Such policies and procedures serve as a guide and reference for any healthcare practitioner required to use the CMPs.

PATIENT AND FAMILY CASE MANAGEMENT PLANS

The design and use of CMPs is not limited to those used by providers of care. Patient- and family-focused plans (for use by the lay public) are popular today and are viewed as essential tools for patient/family education about necessary treatments and care expectations. Patient and family CMPs have become an integral component of case management systems. They are developed as an essential progression of provider's CMPs and packaged together as a set of plans that delineate the care of patients for both providers and consumers alike.

Patient and family CMPs (Figure 12-11) are defined as tools for educating the consumers of healthcare. They are patterned after provider's CMPs and include basic information about the plan of care using lay terminology,

---

BOX 12-7 Education and Training of Staff and Providers on the Use of CMPs

The education and training of staff and providers must address the following objectives:
1. Present an overview of CMPs
2. Discuss the purpose and benefits of CMPs
3. Define CMPs
4. Describe the roles and responsibilities of the various professionals and providers affected by the use of CMPs
5. Explain the elements of care, definition of outcomes, variances and their classifications, and the format of the CMP
6. Explain the use of the variance tracking tool
7. Review an example of a CMP using a case study
8. Perform documentation using a CMP
9. Review the standards of care practice and policies and procedures pertaining to CMPs

CMP title: _____

Date: _____

Instructions: Please check Y, N, or No Opinion for each statement.

	Y	N	No Opinion	Comments
1. Format				
a. Is easy to read and follow over time				
b. Is easy to document on				
c. Provides adequate space to write modifications				
2. Documentation				
a. Improved with the use of the CMP				
b. Time has decreased				
c. On the CMP is not redundant with other requirements. If no, comment why				
3. Education				
a. Prepared staff adequately to use the CMP				
b. Clearly defined each discipline's role in the use of the CMP				
4. Variance tracking				
a. Form was easy to use				
b. Codes were adequate for describing variance				
5. Outcomes				
a. Evaluation was easier than with a traditional plan of care				
6. Collaboration				
a. CMP enhanced the interdisciplinary team communication				
7. Facilities				
a. Interaction with patients and families				
b. Timely completion of patient education				

What did you like best about the CMP?
_____

What did you like least?
_____

What would you like to see added to this CMP?
_____

Figure 12-10 Assessment of staff's perception and satisfaction with the CMP.

a language that patients and their families are able to understand easily. Similar to provider's CMPs, they are diagnosis, procedure, or problem specific; apply a timeline that is appropriate to the care setting they are used in; and may follow a "time-task" matrix format. Furthermore they are written in simple language (i.e., fourth to sixth grade reading level), concise, clear, and characterized by the use of graphics and clip art. The graphics are pictures and symbols used to make the plan more valuable, meaningful, attractive, and interesting to read and use for patients. This is especially important because the plans are directed to those without a medical background.

Patient and family CMPs are used to facilitate the following:
1. Educate patients and their families about the normal course of treatment
2. Communicate to patients and their families realistic expectations of the care and their timeline
3. Answer patients' and families' questions
4. Enhance informed decision making
5. Empower patients and enhance their ability to assume more responsibility toward their care
6. Reinforce the role patients and their families play in their care as integral members of the healthcare team (Parker, 1999)

Dear Patient and Family,

During your hospital stay, the healthcare team at the _____ Hospital will be using a *guideline* known as the Asthma Patient/Family Pathway to assist in the evaluation and treatment of your asthma. We have outlined the various steps that will be involved in your care. Specially designed for patients with asthma, this guideline allows you to participate in your recovery and prepares you for going home. However, your treatment may vary somewhat because of your unique needs. In most cases, we will also provide you with continuing assistance and guidance after going home, through a home care program. If you have any questions about this Patient/Family Pathway or your progress, please speak to your doctor or nurse.

WE ARE HERE TO HELP YOU GET BETTER!
WE WANT YOU TO BECOME PART OF THE TEAM—TO KEEP YOU WELL.

CARE PROVIDERS	• A team of doctors, nurses, and respiratory therapists will work together to evaluate and treat your asthma. 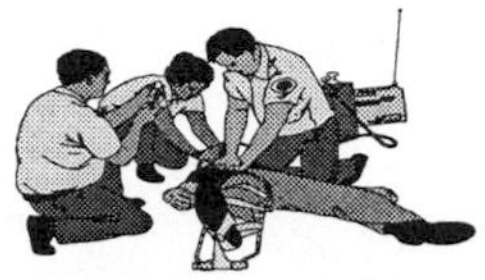
TESTING	• Peak flow: You will have a simple breathing test one or more times daily. • Blood tests and x-rays: These may be needed one or more times during your stay. • Oxygen measurements with a machine that has a probe for your finger may be done.
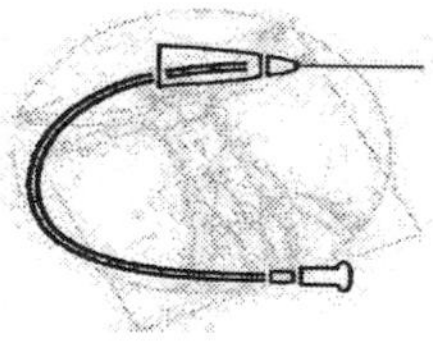 **TREATMENTS**	• Intravenous cortisone is usually given for the first 24 hours, sometimes longer. This will be switched to cortisone (prednisone) by mouth as you improve. • Bronchodilator medicines to open up your airway will be given with the nebulizer, frequently at first. As you improve (usually after 24 hours), the bronchodilator will be switched to a metered-dose inhaler (MDI). • Inhaled cortisone will also be started with the MDI as you improve. • You may require oxygen through nasal prongs or mask until your asthma improves.
NUTRITION	• The nutritionist will advise you concerning your diet. • Taking extra fluids is helpful. 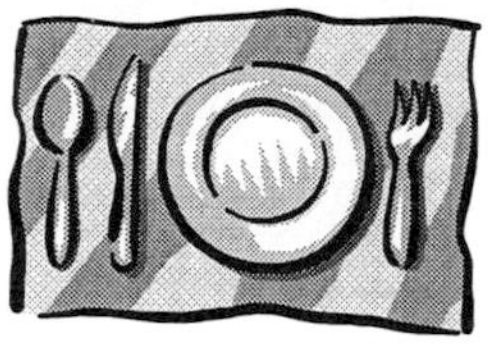
TEACHING	• Learning about asthma is absolutely necessary for you to remain healthy. • Asthma is a preventable and controllable condition. • Your healthcare team will start soon after admission to teach you about avoiding "triggers" for asthma, the correct use of medications, and your MDI. • They will develop a plan of care for you to use at home. • Instructions will be given to you in writing.
GOING HOME	• Most people are ready to go home by the third day. • Your healthcare team will coordinate your plan of care at home. • Many patients will receive several visits at home from specially trained nurses and/or other healthcare providers. • Follow-up visits in your doctor's office will be arranged. 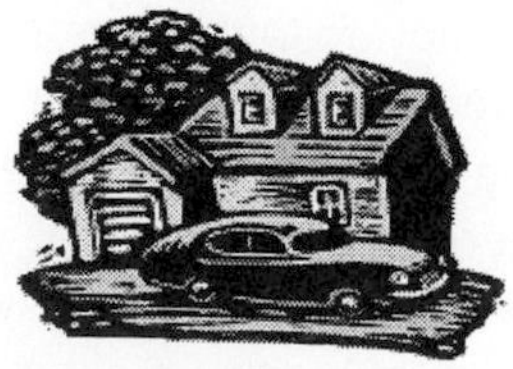

Figure 12-11 Example of patient and family pathway, adult asthma.

CASE MANAGER'S TIP 12-6

Implementing CMPs

It is important for the interdisciplinary team developing the CMP to identify the inclusion/exclusion criteria to guide healthcare providers in the implementation of the CMP. It is also important to identify the conditions under which the CMP may be discontinued. Examples of situations when a CMP may be discontinued are as follows:

1. A change in the primary diagnosis of the patient
2. Significant change/worsening in the patient's condition
3. Failure to meet the expected clinical outcomes within the designated timeframe, which results in a serious delay in progressing the patient as specified in the CMP

Patient care plans can also be used as a tool for contract development between a provider and a patient/family. The expected outcomes of the plan are reviewed with the patient and family and given to them in writing. The patient is then asked to sign the plan, indicating that he or she agrees with it. In this way the contract is developed between patient and provider and the patient becomes an active member of the care team, participating in the development of the goals of care and the expected outcomes and timeframes for achieving the goals.

The plan is reviewed with the patient and family at the appropriate time intervals; that is, at times related to milestones of treatments, as specific outcomes are achieved, or when decisions about treatment options are needed. For example, if the plan consists of daily goals of care, then it should be reviewed with the patient on a daily basis. If the patient achieves a goal sooner than expected, then that achievement should be reviewed and the plan altered accordingly.

Patient and family CMPs are developed by a multidisciplinary team of providers that represent the various specialties and disciplines involved in the care of patients with a particular diagnosis. They are also reviewed and approved by a steering committee similar to the provider-based CMPs. The process of developing patient and family CMPs differs from that of provider's CMPs in that the development team includes a patient advocate or representative whose role is to bring the perspective of patients to the development process. The process is similar to the way patient education materials are developed. In fact, most institutions integrate the patient's CMP development team with the patient and family education committee because of their common aspects and objectives. The skills, knowledge, and expertise of members of the patient/family education committee make it easier for the team to develop patient-focused CMPs. They also enhance writing plans that are personal and conversational in nature. For example, it is common to see patient and family CMPs with phrases such as "you will need to," "you will be asked to," "your physician," or "your nurse." Another characteristic related to style is the use of words that are nonmedical in nature, such as "walk" instead of "ambulate," "going home" instead of "discharge," or "low blood sugar" instead of "hypoglycemia."

The type and number of care elements included in a patient and family CMP varies based on the diagnosis or procedure it addresses. Usually the number is kept to a minimum; that is, limited to those that are essential. The most common elements are tests and procedures, activity and exercise, diet, medications, pain control, teaching and instructions, and preparing to go home. The content included in these elements relates to what is predictable, essential, and standard. "Less is more" is the rule of thumb. It is important to focus on activities the patient is able to handle and control. Refraining from the use of content that patients are unable to comprehend is desirable because it may make them feel frustrated, anxious, or fearful.

STRATEGIES FOR PHYSICIAN PARTICIPATION AND BUY-IN

Physicians play a key role in the success of the interdisciplinary team charged with developing a CMP for a particular diagnosis or procedure. Physician participation in developing the plan is integral to improving consistency (i.e., eliminating variations in physician practice patterns) in the care of patients with similar diagnoses who are cared for by different physicians. Obtaining physician support is a prerequisite to achieving the identified goals of the team. Physician buy-in to the use of CMPs before their development and implementation is a key to compliance in their use afterward. Case Manager's Tip 12-7 lists some strategies that can be employed to obtain physicians' buy-in and increase their participation in the interdisciplinary teams for CMP development.

ORGANIZING THE WORK OF THE INTERDISCIPLINARY TEAM

The steering committee may provide the interdisciplinary team members with policy/guidelines that define what is expected from the team and how the work should progress in each meeting. These guidelines are used to facilitate, simplify, and expedite the process of developing and implementing CMPs (Case Manager's Tip 12-8). The steering committee assigns the team's

CASE MANAGER'S TIP 12-7

Gaining Physicians' Support of CMPs

Strategies and benefits that can be communicated to physicians to gain their buy-in and increase their participation in the interdisciplinary teams to develop CMPs include the following:

1. Involve physicians in the process of developing CMPs from the beginning. Find a champion(s) and capitalize on his or her participation to influence others.
2. Approach influential physicians who are interested in improving the quality of care and reducing the related cost for participation.
3. Demonstrate the benefits of CMPs to physicians' personal practice.
4. Educate physicians about the use of CMPs and share with them related published materials (e.g., evaluative research, description of case management systems, physicians' opinions from other similar institutions). Also share similar information with their office staff.
5. Emphasize that CMPs are recommendations for treatment rather than rigid guidelines or standing orders. Make clear to all physicians that the CMP should be individualized for each patient on initiation and that changes are possible.
6. Delineate how CMPs enhance quality of care:
   a. Clearly and proactively defined care expectations and physicians' preferences
   b. Improved continuity of patient care, especially if a patient requires care across different patient care units within the same institution
   c. Detailed patient/family education requirements
   d. Open communication patterns among various disciplines involved in the care
   e. Care-related variance data tracking; the use of variance data for continuous quality improvement efforts

7. Delineate how CMPs enhance cost of patient care:
   a. Predetermined patient care activities that are sequenced in a timely manner to achieve appropriate length of stay and expected outcomes
   b. Modifications of physicians' practice pattern
   c. Consistency in patient care across physicians
   d. Improvement in patient care as a result of variance tracking
   e. Benefits of the CMP in reducing risk management issues
8. Communicate how CMPs improve compliance with the standards of regulatory and accreditation agencies.
9. Explain how the plan could be used as an education/training tool for residents, house staff, nurses, and students.
10. Emphasize that the plans may be used as marketing tools to attract more participation from managed care organizations.
11. Stress opportunities for research and creativity in patient care delivery.
12. Emphasize that data from tracking variances facilitate changes in hospital systems to eliminate inefficiencies in patient care.
13. Share an individual physician's performance data/practice pattern and how it compares to that of other physicians in the hospital and in comparable institutions.
14. Avoid a punitive approach. Reward those who are willing to participate and address the concerns of those who are hesitant.
15. Use data and not emotions to gain cooperation.
16. Educate physicians about the reimbursement methods, their impact on practice behaviors, and the role CMPs play in managed care contract negotiations.

leader and facilitator before the team's first meeting. These two members are specially trained to assume these roles. Interdisciplinary team members are also trained in the roles they play. Preparing all members of the team, including the facilitator and leader, is important because training improves the team's productivity and increases members' skills in teamwork and CMP development.

Despite the popularity of CMPs, there still exists some confusion about how to maintain a multidisciplinary focus while encouraging all disciplines to use CMPs. Selling the use of CMPs to a diverse and large group of providers is not an easy task. Obtaining buy-in from the

different disciplines requires special tactics and political correctness. Using multidisciplinary teams for the development, implementation, and evaluation of CMPs is a move in the right direction. However, this is not the answer to all concerns. Tahan (1998) described 14 strategies that can be used for enhancing the multidisciplinary nature of CMPs and the participation of the different providers in their development. These strategies are summarized in Box 12-8.

Interdisciplinary teams need an average of six to eight meetings, 1 hour each, to complete a CMP. The following sections outline an example of how the work of the team should be planned.

CASE MANAGER'S TIP 12-8

How to Compile a CMP Policy/Guideline

1. Define a CMP using a template/an example.
2. Use a glossary of terms.
3. Provide direction for content of the CMP using a standard set of patient care elements to be included in the plan. Define each element and include examples.
4. Identify the steps to be followed by the team in the development process of a CMP (i.e., selection of the case type, how to identify opportunities for improvement [e.g., high risk, high volume, cost outlier, length of stay outlier, problem prone, quality issue, physician preference], how to identify the need for data and where to obtain them [internal and external mechanisms], and the process of consensus-building associated with defining the content of the CMP).
5. Define the approval process of the CMP and the role of the steering committee.
6. Define the use of a disclaimer. State an example. Clarify whether a standard statement is to be used on all CMPs. Include the statement in the guidelines and in the CMP template.
7. Define the use of outcomes and their types: intermediate and discharge or process, structure, and patient-related. Include examples of each in the guidelines.
8. Clarify the documentation process associated with the CMP. Review daily the process of the plan during the time it is in use/applied in patient care. State the implications for all providers and disciplines.
9. Explain the use of preprinted physician orders and algorithms.
10. Describe the functions of members of the CMP development team, including the roles and responsibilities of the team leader, facilitator, and member.
11. Explain the process of variance (outcomes) data collection and tracking and the mechanism of reporting and feedback. Define the relationship between variance data and quality improvement initiatives.
12. Identify the implementation process. Pilot the CMP before standardization and wide use.
13. Define the education process: who should teach, who should attend, and how should teaching/training be conducted (e.g., area/discipline-based, centralized).
14. Address the issues of patient and family confidentiality associated with the use of CMPs.
15. Discuss the use of patient and family pathways. Define the reading level to be followed, the format, the use of pictures, their process of implementation, and so on.

From Tahan H: *Nurs Case Manag* 3(1):46-51, 1998.

BOX 12-8 Strategies for Enhancing the Multidisciplinary Nature of CMPs

1. Every discipline is equally important regardless of the degree of its involvement in the delivery of patient care.
2. Membership in CMP development teams should be reflective of the patient population being addressed.
3. Every team member should be empowered as a champion in advocating the use of CMPs in their own discipline/department.
4. Communication to the various clinical, administrative, and support providers/staff members on all levels cannot be overemphasized.
5. Clear, concise, and crucial guidelines for the development, implementation, and evaluation of CMPs are significant factors that must not be ignored.
6. The various sources of data available in the organization are integral for making multidisciplinary decisions and building consensus and must be shared with the team.
7. Documentation in the CMP should not be limited to nursing.
8. Ensuring compliance with standards of regulatory and accreditation agencies, especially a seamless approach to patient care.
9. The role of the ancillary departments (allied health and support services) is an important element of successful CMP development and must not be ignored.
10. Resource allocation and management is every department's benefit.
11. The multidisciplinary nature of CMPs increases the chances of obtaining new managed care contracts and maintaining or enhancing old ones.
12. Multidisciplinary CMPs are documented standards of care and practice for all disciplines and help reduce the risk for legal liability and malpractice litigation for all disciplines.
13. CMPs help establish an interdisciplinary outcomes- and research-based practice environment.
14. CMPs may be used as a strategy to enhance patient and family satisfaction.

Preparation Meeting

The steering committee assigns the team leader and facilitator based on the specific case type/CMP to be developed. A meeting is then held between representative(s) from the steering committee and the leader and facilitator, during which the goals and expectations of the interdisciplinary team are discussed. During this meeting the following issues are finalized:

■ Membership of the team, including physicians
■ Length of stay of the CMP

- Training and education of the team members
- Date, time, and place of the team's first meeting
- Finalizing the agenda of the first meeting
- Notifying team members of their participation on the team
- Establishing a timeline for the team's work and a target date for completion of the CMP
- Sharing of the available data (previous administrative, length of stay, and **utilization review** reports) related to the CMP type

Interdisciplinary Team's First Meeting

During the first meeting, the interdisciplinary team leader discusses the team's goals and expectations and the timeline for completion of the expected work. A list of all team members and their phone numbers is distributed. If the CMP development form is not already completed and submitted to the steering committee, it is finalized during this meeting. This meeting is geared toward educating the team members. The issues discussed include the following:

- The process of developing a CMP
- Goals for improvement
- Specific discussion regarding the responsibilities of each member in the development of the CMP
- The template of the CMP as provided by the steering committee
- The available data related to the particular case type and examples of CMPs from other institutions
- Assignments for the next meeting (plan of care related to each discipline)
- Finalizing the meeting's schedule (date, time, location, and frequency)

Second Meeting

During the second meeting, team members conduct a medical records review and discuss the following:

- The preliminary plan of care prepared by each member of the team as it relates to the discipline he or she represents
- The timeline placement of the recommended interventions
- The assignment for the next meeting (finalize the plan of care of each discipline)

Third and Fourth Meetings

During the third and fourth meetings the team finalizes the recommended plan of care, compares the ideal/best practice with the review of literature available, and makes changes as needed. The team starts to discuss the expected outcomes of care and does the following:

- Finalizes the interventions and the treatment plan

- Starts discussing the **intermediate and discharge outcomes** of care
- Begins looking at the preprinted physician order set
- Ensures that the patient's actual and potential problems are included in the plan

Fifth Meeting

In the fifth meeting members of the interdisciplinary team present the intermediate and discharge outcomes of care related to their portion of the CMP. A discussion takes place on whether these outcomes are feasible within the timeline recommended. If any problems are identified, adjustments are made. The preprinted physician order set and the list of patient's problems are also confirmed. At this point the CMP is near completion. The team starts to discuss variance tracking and what types of data are to be collected.

Sixth Meeting

The sixth meeting is spent finalizing the significant data for variance tracking. The team also prepares the final CMP to be shared with the chief of the department in which the CMP will be implemented. It is important to also obtain the steering committee's feedback on the recommended CMP before it is finalized. In addition, the team starts planning for pilot testing of the CMP.

Seventh Meeting

During the seventh meeting, the interdisciplinary team discusses the recommendations made by the chief of the department and the steering committee. The CMP is revised accordingly. The pilot-testing plan is finalized, and the CMP is confirmed in its final version that is ready for testing.

Eighth Meeting

The last meeting is spent reviewing the pilot data. Data are analyzed, and a decision on whether the CMP is ready for wide implementation is made. Based on the data collected during the pilot period, the CMP is revised and finalized. At this point the CMP is ready to become the standard of practice. It is usually submitted to the steering committee in its final version with recommendations for implementation. The report generated by the interdisciplinary team, which is based on the pilot of the CMP, is also given to the steering committee. In this meeting the work of the interdisciplinary team is completed. The team may also decide on follow-up dates for meetings to evaluate the use of the CMP and the variance data collected to determine if any changes should be made in the CMP.

The interdisciplinary team members work on their assignments in between meetings. The actual meeting

CASE MANAGER'S TIP 12-9

Strategies for Running Effective Meetings

1. Identify the purpose of the meeting.
2. Prepare an agenda before the meeting, distribute it to the members, and allow them to add items/issues to it.
3. Be sure that all agenda items are necessary and appropriate.
4. Allocate in advance the time needed for discussing each agenda item.
5. Start and finish the meeting on time.
6. Stay on schedule during the meeting. Adhere to the allotted time for each item. If discussion is not concluded within the allotted time, follow up on the item in the next meeting.
7. Assign subgroups to work on certain issues in between meetings to maximize the utility of the meeting time. Ask these subgroups to report back with the outcomes/decisions during the next meeting.
8. Allow and encourage participation of all members.
9. Clarify and summarize discussions/decisions before an issue is concluded.
10. Ensure that the environment is conducive to the meeting: room, ventilation, temperature, seating.
11. Keep interruptions to a minimum.
12. Record minutes.
13. Maximize the use of visual aids (e.g., handouts).
14. Prevent disagreements. Use consensus building when issues arise.
15. Generate a sense of team spirit.
16. Ensure normal group dynamics because they are essential to accomplish the purpose.
17. Limit participation in the meeting to the necessary players.
18. Schedule the meeting on a date and at a time when all necessary attendees are available.
19. Be sensitive to organizational politics.
20. Avoid mixing business with pleasure.
21. Keep conversations relevant and discussions balanced.
22. Avoid editorializing.
23. Promote active listening.
24. Recognize individual expertise and talent.
25. Do not dominate the discussion.
26. Avoid value judgment statements.
27. Allow for difference of opinions.
28. Negotiate win-win resolutions.
29. Conclude the meeting with a summary of accomplishments and follow-up work.
30. Express appreciation.

---

time is used for follow-up on work progress and for discussions around identified concerns or issues. Case Manager's Tip 12-9 presents strategies for holding effective meetings. These strategies can be applied by case managers when being involved in running meetings, whether related to developing CMPs or not.

The use of CMPs has become more popular in virtually all patient care settings. The standardization of the process of developing these plans is extremely important. The previous discussion provides healthcare and nursing administrators and case managers with a practical, step-by-step approach to developing CMPs. It can be used as a tool to train members of interdisciplinary teams involved in developing CMPs. The method presented is flexible and can be tailored to any organization or care setting across the continuum. It can be used to develop CMPs for the care of patients in acute, ambulatory, long-term, or home care settings. The process to be followed in these settings is the same, but the content and format of the plans may vary.

The use of CMPs has successfully contained healthcare costs, reduced lengths of stay, improved quality of care, streamlined use of resources, and opened communication lines among the healthcare team members.

Formalizing the process of developing CMPs is the first step toward ensuring that these benefits will be met. The proposed process is beneficial to all healthcare providers in any care setting, particularly case managers, whether they are involved in developing CMPs or are planning to get started. It can be used by interdisciplinary team members as a blueprint to develop CMPs. It serves as a guide or safety mechanism to ensure that all bases are covered during the developmental process and before the plan is concluded.

 KEY POINTS

1. It is necessary for each institution to have a steering committee to oversee the development, implementation, and evaluation of CMPs.
2. It is more effective to have a formal process and structure for developing CMPs.
3. CMPs should be developed based on the literature, particularly research and evidence-based practice, expert opinion, and recommendations of professional organizations and societies.

4. It is important to seek the input of all healthcare providers involved in the care of a particular patient when developing a CMP.

5. The CMP, after it is piloted and approved, should become the institution's standard of care and applied by all practitioners.

6. The interdisciplinary team charged with developing a particular CMP should be given enough guidance by the steering committee and provided with appropriate training and education regarding the process.

7. CMPs should have the Milliman & Robertson Guidelines and InterQual criteria built in to ensure cost-effective and quality outcomes.

REFERENCES

Bozzuto B, Farrell E: A collaborative approach to nursing care of the open heart surgical patient, *Case Manage* 6(3):47-53, 1995.

Cohen EL, Cesta TG: *Case management: from concept to evaluation,* ed 2, St Louis, 1997, Mosby.

Cole L, Houston S: Structured care methodologies: evolution and use in patient care delivery, *Outcomes Manage Nurs Pract* 3(2):53-59, 1999.

Dykes P: *Psychiatric clinical pathways: an interdisciplinary approach,* Gaithersburg, Md, 1998, Aspen.

Esler R, Bentz P, Sorensen M, et al: Patient-centered pneumonia: a case management success story, *Am J Nurs* 94(11):34-38, 1994.

Ferguson LE: Steps to developing a clinical pathway, *Nurs Adm Q* 17(3):58-62, 1993.

Guiliano HH, Poirer CE: Case management: critical pathways to desirable outcomes, *Nurs Manage* 22(3):52-55, 1991.

Hampton DC: Implementing a managed care framework through care maps, *J Nurs Adm* 23(5):21-27, 1993.

Hydo B: Designing an effective clinical pathway for stroke, *Am J Nurs* 95(3):44-50, 1995.

Ignatavicius D: Clinical pathways: the wave of the future, *Healthc Travel* 2(5):23-25, 46-47, 1995.

Ignatavicius DD, Hausman KA: *Clinical pathways for collaborative practice,* Philadelphia, 1995, WB Saunders.

InterQual, Inc: *System administrators guide,* Marlborough, Mass, 1998, InterQual.

Janken J, Grubbs J, Haldeman K: Toward a research-based critical pathway: a case study, *OJKSN* document no. 1C, July 1, 1999 (clinical column). Available online at http://www.stti.iupui.edu/library/ojksn/cc_doc1c.pdf.

Katterhagen JG, Patton M: Critical pathways in oncology: balancing the interests of hospitals and the physician, *J Oncol Manage* 2(4):20-26, 1993.

Meister S, Rodts B, Gothard J, et al: Home Care Steps protocols: home care's answer to changes in reimbursement, *J Nurs Adm* 25(6):33-42, 1995.

Parker C: Patient pathways as a tool for empowering patients, *Nurs Case Manag* 4(2):77-79, 1999.

Schibanoff JM, editor: *Health care management guidelines,* New York, 1999, Milliman & Robertson.

St. Anthony Publishing: *DRG: working guide,* Alexandria, Va, 1992, St. Anthony.

Tahan H: The multidisciplinary mandate of clinical pathways enhancement, *Nurs Case Manag* 3(1):46-52, 1998.

Tahan HA, Cesta TG: Developing case management plans using a quality improvement model, *J Nurs Adm* 24(12):49-58, 1995.

Thompson KS, Caddick K, Mathie J, et al: Building a critical pathway for ventilator dependency, *Am J Nurs* 91(7):28-31, 1991.

Zander K: Care maps: the core of cost and quality care, *New Definition* 6(3):1-3, 1991.

Zander K: Physicians, care maps, and collaboration, *New Definition* 7(1):1-4, 1992.

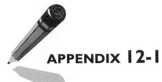

APPENDIX 12-1

CASE MANAGEMENT PLANS

This appendix presents a template for case management plans. Case management plans usually delineate the standards of care; identify patients' actual and potential problems, the goals of treatment, and the necessary patient care activities; and establish the projected outcomes of care.

Things to Remember About Developing Case Management Plans

- Establish an interdisciplinary team.
- Identify team members based on the diagnosis or surgical procedure in question. Members should be chosen based on their clinical experiences, leadership skills, communication skills, tolerance to hard work, and commitment to the institution and the project.
- Identify a team leader and a facilitator.
- Provide the team with administrative and clerical support.
- Establish a project work plan (timeline of activities) before the team's first meeting.
- Train team members in the process of developing CMPs.
- Team members should prepare their work in between meetings. Meetings should be held to review the work and determine the next steps.
- Regardless of the format of the CMP, it should always include the patient care elements as identified by the organization, the patient problems, projected length of stay and outcomes of care, a variance tracking form, and patient care activities and interventions.
- Create a timeline for the CMP as indicated by the care setting. For example, minutes to hours in emergency departments, number of visits in clinics and home care, days in acute care, weeks in areas of longer length of stay such as neonatal intensive care area, and months in nursing homes and group homes. The timeline of CMPs in subacute care and rehabilitation centers can be established based on the length of stay, goals of treatment, and intensity of activities. For the most part, it is daily or weekly.

- Preestablish the expected (acceptable) length of stay.
- Determine the mechanism for tracking variances and define the variance categories to be evaluated.
- Ensure that the CMP is the standard of care applied by all healthcare providers, including physicians.
- Include patient and family teaching and discharge planning activities in all CMPs.
- Determine whether CMPs are a permanent part of the medical record.
- Maximize documentation on the CMP. Require all patient care services to use the CMP for documentation.
- Develop CMPs based on the latest recommendations of research and professional societies.
- Avoid being rigid in recommending treatments. For example, use words like "consider" when including treatments, medications, or interventions that may not be applicable to every patient, completion may not always be possible within the indicated timeframe, or progress may be dependent on the patient's condition.
- Identify the intermediate and discharge outcomes of care in each CMP.
- Delineate the ICD-9-CM code or the DRG number of the CMP on the cover page.
- Include all disciplines involved in the care of patients as indicated by the diagnosis or surgical procedure considered.
- Stress the importance of patient care activities that historically were identified as problem areas or requiring improvement.
- Establish a timeframe for reviewing and revising the CMP.

TEMPLATE OF A CASE MANAGEMENT PLAN

Diagnosis: _____ ICD-9 code: _____ DRG#: _____ Expected LOS: _____

Admit Date: ___/___/___ Discharge Date: ___/___/___ Actual LOS: _____

Attending MD: _____ Primary Nurse: _____

Date: ___/___/___ Day ___ of ___

Care Elements	Respons. Party*	Expected Outcomes	Initials	Comments/Notes
Assessment/ Monitoring				
Lab Work				
Tests/ Procedures				
Treatments				
Medications				
Consults				
Activity				
Nutrition				

Care Elements	Respons. Party*	Expected Outcomes	Initials	Comments/Notes
IV Therapy				
Respiratory Therapy				
Physical Therapy/ Occupational Therapy				
Wound Care				
Pain Management				
Patient/ Family Education				
Psychosocial Assessment				
Discharge Planning				

Initials	Signature	Initials	Signature

*Responsible Party: Registered Nurse (RN), Attending Physician/House Staff (MD), Nurse Practitioner (NP), Social Worker (SW), Home Care Intake Coordinator (HCIC), Physical Therapist (PT), Occupational Therapist (OT), Nutritionist (NUT)

13 Quality Patient Care

Perhaps the most important topic in healthcare today is quality. Although healthcare organizations have always had quality at the top of their priority list, especially when the **prospective payment systems** began, only recently has it been recognized that continuously improving and managing quality can make a difference. The difference can be as vital as survival or providing the healthcare organization with a competitive advantage in the marketplace. Today the healthcare industry recognizes that a focus on quality is the best way to ensure that revenues equal or exceed expenses. This approach is particularly important because it prevents healthcare providers and administrators from paying more attention to cost than quality and allows them to attain an acceptable balance between the two entities. Measuring and evaluating quality of care, therefore, has become more and more imperative in this era of healthcare. In addition, quality patient and organizational **outcomes** have become necessary components of the process of care delivery and management.

IMPORTANCE OF QUALITY

Today's competitive healthcare environment demands constant attention to improvements in quality. Consumers are demanding that they receive full value for their healthcare dollar. The goal of any healthcare provider is to have consumers desire to return if necessary for their healthcare needs. If healthcare organizations fail to strive for quality, they will fall behind in the highly competitive marketplace. Focusing on quality allows healthcare organizations to achieve many benefits, which include the following:

- Efficient use of resources
- Meeting the demands and needs of consumers
- Enhancing patient and family satisfaction

- Provision of compassionate, ethical, and culturally competent care
- Ensuring patient safety through reduced risk for injury and avoidance of medical errors
- Professional and satisfactory performance by providers (Powell and Ignatavicius, 2001)

MEANING OF QUALITY

Probably the most difficult hurdle is to agree on what quality means. What are the properties, characteristics, and attributes of care that lead us to a judgment of good or bad quality? Quality means different things to different people: the providers and consumers of healthcare. Historically, the providers of care have defined quality. However, since the mid-1980s consumers of care have become more and more involved in defining quality and influencing the perception of providers and payers of healthcare. This shift has necessitated that organizations incorporate quality into their strategic plans, mission, and vision.

The Institute of Medicine defined quality as the degree to which healthcare services increase the likelihood that desired outcomes are consistent with professional knowledge available at the time care is provided to individuals and populations (Vladeck and Shalala, 1997). However, customers' definition of quality is dependent on their needs and values. Although these may vary from one customer to another, what is important to customers is feeling welcome and made comfortable by healthcare providers and being understood. In addition, customers appreciate providers with a friendly, compassionate, and supportive attitude and with technical skills and knowledge, and they appreciate cleanliness and comfort in the physical environment of care. Although the customers' and providers'

CASE MANAGER'S TIP 13-1

Perception of Quality

A patient's perception of quality is only as good as the last encounter.

---

definitions of quality are not the same, it is important for providers to define quality and desired outcomes of care based on the needs, values, and interests of customers. This match is important so that the individuals accessing healthcare experience the services provided to them as being of good quality.

Quality of care may include, but is not limited to, available healthcare services, standards of providers, comprehensive assessment and documentation, collaborative and informed relationships with patient and family, minimal injuries or complications for hospitalized patients, evaluation of new technology and resources, and effective management of healthcare resources (McCarthy, 1987). Along with patient satisfaction, the patient's view of what is important in his or her care may be seen as one aspect of quality when defining indicators of quality. The overall quality of healthcare will be judged on the entire package, including health outcomes, accessibility, timeliness and efficiency of services, interdisciplinary communication, and the direct and indirect costs of illness and care (Case Manager's Tip 13-1).

CHARACTERISTICS OF QUALITY

From the customer's point of view, there are three types of quality characteristics: "take it for granted" quality, expected quality, and exciting quality. Take it for granted quality is what a healthcare setting must offer to be acceptable (e.g., staff competency). Expected quality includes those things that are necessary and expected (e.g., food quality). Exciting quality pertains to those items that are nice to have but are not necessary (e.g., environmental features) (Larson and Nelson, 1993). The customers' needs and values as they relate to quality are of the necessary and expected type of quality. Healthcare providers and organizations cannot ignore them, otherwise the customer will view the services provided as being of "bad" quality. Effective case management must work within a framework that demonstrates quality improvements while taking the patient's perceptions, values, and expectations into account.

Characteristics of quality are also available based on the perception of providers. One approach to describing the characteristics of quality includes the following

attributes Donabedian (1980) outlines when assessing for quality:

1. *Effectiveness:* The ability to provide care in the correct manner, given the current and available knowledge, and the ability to attain the greatest improvements in health now achievable by the best care
2. *Efficiency:* The ability to lower the cost of care and resources without diminishing attainable improvements in health
3. *Balance:* The balancing of costs against the effect of care on health so as to attain the most advantageous balance
4. *Acceptability:* Conforming to the wishes, desires, values, beliefs, and expectations of patients and their families in the care decision-making process
5. *Legitimacy:* Conformity to social preferences in care delivery as expressed in ethical principles, values, norms, laws, and regulations
6. *Equity:* Conformity to a principle that determines what is just or fair in the distribution of healthcare, its effect on health, and its benefits among the members of the population

The Joint Commission on Accreditation of Healthcare Organizations (JCAHO) (JCAHO, 2001) defines other attributes of quality, some of which are similar to those of Donabedian. These attributes are as follows:

1. *Efficacy:* The degree to which care has been shown to accomplish the desired outcomes
2. *Availability:* The degree to which appropriate care is made accessible to meet the patient's and family's needs
3. *Optimality:* Ensuring the most advantageous balance between benefits and costs of care delivery and services
4. *Timeliness:* Ensuring that care is provided with no delay and when needed
5. *Continuity:* The degree to which care activities and services are coordinated among providers, settings, and over time
6. *Safety:* The degree to which the risk of an intervention or care environment is reduced for patients and providers
7. *Respect and caring:* Providing care with sensitivity and respect for the patient's values, beliefs, expectations, and cultural differences

Healthcare providers historically have been concerned with the maintenance and improvement of quality of care for hospitalized patients (Dash et al, 1996). Most healthcare organizations have a mission statement that tends to incorporate the institution's emphasis on quality and its culture or values and beliefs. Phrases usually include honesty, commitment to patient/customer satisfaction, and commitment to employee satisfaction in an environment that is conducive to the provision of best care and ensuring the best outcomes. The values are what the organization regards as important. They are the principles that the organization upholds and defends, the fabric that holds the organizational structure together, and the foundation on which it rests.

SETTING THE STANDARDS FOR QUALITY

Everyone is interested in the quality of healthcare, how it is measured, and the results of these measurements. There are many groups that are involved in setting the standards for quality (Box 13-1). Providers, **payers,** and customers of healthcare services, as well as governmental and nongovernmental agencies, are all interested in quality. Each, individually and as a group, influences the national standards against which performance is measured and evaluated. Each of these players is interested in quality for different reasons. For example, providers' interest in quality pertains mainly to being competitive, and marketable; however, payers' interest is in ensuring cost-effectiveness and balancing between cost and quality. On the other hand, customers focus on the delivery of appropriate and safe care, whereas governmental agencies' regard for quality relates to keeping control of healthcare legislation and

promoting what is in the public interest. Moreover, nongovernmental agencies and associations play a role in advocating for patients and lobbying for a change in legislation.

The motivation behind the interest of these groups in healthcare quality can be summarized in two ways. Some have pursued quality-related information to make better and more informed decisions regarding healthcare choices, whereas others have sought out such information for political reasons. Regardless of these interests, the variation in the motivation creates a healthy pursuit of, and competition for, what is best for the customer. To survive in the healthcare market of today, healthcare executives and providers must maintain current knowledge of the interests of these groups, particularly the interests of customers, governmental agencies and politicians, and public advocates and lobbyists. They must also use this knowledge to ensure that their practices and care delivery systems are updated and altered to meet the expectations of these groups. If they fail to do this, they are at risk for causing customer dissatisfaction, decreased quality, increased costs, and unnecessary use of resources.

A HISTORICAL REVIEW OF QUALITY
Quality Assurance

Until the mid-1980s, quality in healthcare was measured by concepts and processes categorized under the rubric of **quality assurance** (QA). This all-encompassing phrase, *quality assurance,* comprised the healthcare industry's breadth and width of understanding as to what quality was about as it related to the management and treatment of individuals receiving healthcare services. The name described the underlying philosophy behind it in that quality assurance programs were designed to assure or maintain a particular predetermined level of expectation, activity, process, or standard of care. QA focused on errors and problems, and most of the time it applied a retrospective process of evaluation. Therefore QA, by definition, was a mechanism for developing predetermined standards of care, implementing strategies for assuring that those standards were met (Coyne and Killien, 1983), and designing an action plan to address staff/provider noncompliance.

Following a QA approach to measuring quality and evaluating compliance, providers applied certain levels of expectation that were also known as *thresholds.* These thresholds identified a minimal level of performance that the organization would expect to accomplish. For example, the threshold for patient falls in the hospital setting might be that less than 3% of all patients would experience a fall while hospitalized. As long as the organization did not exceed that threshold,

---

BOX 13-1 Examples of Groups That Set the Standards for Quality

1. Consumer advocacy groups
   - Coalition of independent groups
   - Public advocates
   - Lobbyists
2. Governmental agencies
   - Health Care Financing Administration/The Centers for Medicare and Medicaid Services
   - State Departments of Health
   - Agency for Healthcare Research and Quality
3. Nongovernmental agencies
   - Joint Commission on Accreditation of Healthcare Organizations
   - Commission for Accreditation of Rehabilitation Facilities
   - National Committee on Quality Assurance
4. Professional associations and organizations
   - Healthcare providers
   - American Nurses Association
   - American Hospital Association
5. Media
   - Journalists
   - Reporters
   - Television news programs

it was satisfied and confident that quality care was being provided.

Unfortunately, QA did not provide an infrastructure for improving performance or exceeding these thresholds. Organizations consistently measured their performance against those thresholds and did not expect to do any better if they were met.

Transforming Healthcare

As the cost of healthcare continued to rise in the 1980s, healthcare organizations began to recognize that they could no longer continue to conduct business as they always had and that they had to begin to search for mechanisms that would not only maintain quality but improve it as well. Healthcare tends to lag behind other industries by 5 to 10 years so that changes in industry will often be indicators of changes that will eventually occur in healthcare (Marszalek-Gaucher and Coffey, 1990). This was no less true for the quality initiatives undertaken by the healthcare industry in the late 1980s and early 1990s. Industry began to focus on total **quality improvement** (QI) in the 1970s, with healthcare following suit about a decade later.

Other changes were also taking place. Society and consumers of healthcare services were becoming more educated and aware of the changes occurring in other industries. They became less tolerant of the inefficiencies they traditionally had experienced from the healthcare industry such as lack of coordination of care, fragmentation and duplication of services, and long waits to see physicians or get results of diagnostic tests. This growing sophistication led to greater expectations on the part of the public, which had to be responded to by the industry.

Healthcare expenditures were becoming a priority in the United States in both the public and private sectors. Diminishing **reimbursement** and the changes in its methods forced care providers to reassess how they were doing business and to begin to look for new ways to become more cost-effective and efficient. As industry had before it, healthcare began to adopt strategies such as **total quality management (TQM)** and **continuous quality improvement (CQI)** as vehicles to help improve quality of care (Box 13-2).

The ability of the healthcare industry to make this shift in focus would be dependent on its ability to redefine itself, particularly in terms of how it measured its own quality. One consistent theme before the 1980s was "more is better." This related to the fact that healthcare organizations were rewarded for being bigger with lots of hospital beds and lots of staff; for providing unlimited services; and for doing more and more tests, treatments, and procedures. But the rewards were

---

> ### BOX 13-2 Definitions of Quality Assurance, Quality Improvement, and Performance Improvement
>
> **Quality Assurance**
> - Designing a product or service and controlling its production so well that quality is inevitable
> - In healthcare, the activities and programs intended to guarantee or ensure quality of patient care (JCAHO, 1994)
>
> **Quality Improvement**
> - Involves improving current processes and is normally accomplished with a series of projects to improve quality (Marszalek-Gaucher and Coffey, 1990)
>
> **Performance Improvement**
> - Ongoing system focused on high-risk, high-volume, and/or high-prone issues that affect patient care quality used to identify and resolve problems (Claflin and Hayden, 1998)

---

changing. Reimbursement structures were changing with fixed price strategies such as the prospective payment system (see Chapter 2). This kind of reimbursement scheme motivated healthcare organizations to manage fixed dollar amounts; therefore the notion of doing more and more with little concern for appropriateness was no longer financially rewarded. The new measure of success became how the organization was able to manage those dwindling returns and still come out even in the end.

Dwindling returns meant that healthcare organizations had to maintain their customer base. Therefore it became increasingly important for them to attract and to retain patients. Patients needed to feel that they were receiving quality, efficient, and effective care of the highest possible level.

Quality Improvement

It became clear that CQI had to replace QA as a process for not only maintaining quality but also continuously improving the level of quality. This is accomplished by continuously learning about the processes and outcomes of care delivery and then using this knowledge to reduce variation and to make these processes less complex. By reducing variation and streamlining the processes of care, the overall level of performance of the organization is improved (Claflin and Hayden, 1998). The organization begins to shift from a focus on individuals to a focus on systems, processes, and outcomes. In fact, outcomes become the drivers of the care delivery processes and systems.

QI adds a number of dimensions to the traditional approaches of QA. It not only identifies levels of quality but also expects the organization to meet and exceed these levels. It focuses on the processes and systems that affect quality rather than on individuals (i.e., staff or providers). It also uses data as an important tool in understanding variations in performance and seeks mechanisms to improve and reduce them. In addition, it avoids being punitive or relating the primary source of errors and variations to staff and their actions. QI, therefore, approaches quality from a much broader perspective than that of QA and, most importantly, its work never ends. The organization does not put a stop to its strive toward continuously exceeding its own level of performance over time.

Performance Improvement

Performance improvement becomes the mechanism or infrastructure for CQI. It follows a logical series of steps in the process of continuous improvement:

1. Identify a system, process, or outcome needing improvement
2. Determine the strategies or elements that need to be implemented to improve the problem identified
3. Implement the improvement strategies
4. Monitor the effects of the improvement strategies over time
5. Change or amend the strategies as needed

Regardless of the specific improvement plan implemented, the ultimate goal is for the organization to never become stagnant but to always be moving forward in its systems, processes, thinking, and philosophy. Another goal is to identify defective areas and opportunities for improvement and to implement an action plan for improvement, applying the CQI methodology.

USING STRUCTURE/PROCESS/ OUTCOMES TO MEASURE QUALITY

One of the biggest obstacles affecting the performance improvement strategies of any healthcare organization is the difficulty in linking structure, process(es), and outcome(s). **Case management** has been defined as a

structure and process model because it links both of these elements to the outcomes of care.

The Structure of Care

The structure of the organization has to do with the characteristics of the systems of the organization and its environment (Box 13-3). The structure is also concerned with the characteristics of the providers of care and the patients themselves. Structure characteristics relate to the setting/level of care, the nature of the care delivery system/model (e.g., interdisciplinary approach), the credentials, competencies, and educational levels of the providers, and the health status and condition of the patients.

The system characteristics of any organization are complex and diverse. Those listed in Box 13-3 are just a small sample of the types, elements, or characteristics that make up the healthcare system. Each of these, either individually or in a group, has an effect on how care delivery is structured and how it ultimately affects patient and organizational outcomes.

The provider characteristics demonstrate the diversity of the care providers in any organization. It is clear from this list that each provider brings unique characteristics (i.e., skills, knowledge, and competencies) to the care delivery model, and based on the differences, each may approach a particular patient or clinical problem in a different way. The provider's years of experience will also affect how the group of providers may address a particular problem or patient situation. The varied experiences of the providers will ultimately impact how the group may problem solve a complex or challenging situation (see Chapter 8 for more on this topic).

Finally, the patients and their families/caregivers bring a unique view of themselves, of the care providers, and of what they may believe is quality care. Their participation in their own care may be dependent on the providers' ability to engage the patients in ways that are relevant to them and that are consistent with their values, beliefs, and needs. Ultimately these characteristics shape the patients' responses to care activities, their participation in the care processes, and finally the outcomes of the care interventions.

BOX 13-3 Elements of the Structure of Care		
System Characteristics	**Provider Characteristics**	**Patient Characteristics**
Organization of services	Age	Socioeconomic status
Financial incentives such as payer mix	Gender	Educational level
The workload	Beliefs/attitudes/prejudices	Age
Specialty mix	Level of experience	Gender
Access and convenience for patients	Job satisfaction	Ethnicity, including health habits and beliefs

BOX 13-4	Elements of the Processes of Care
Technical Style	**Interpersonal Style**
Coordination	Manner and demeanor
Continuity	Communication
Medication administration	Patient participation
Physician ordering systems	Counseling and support
Scheduling	

The Processes of Care

Healthcare is delivered using specific and predetermined processes. These processes are the procedures providers use, the methods they deploy, and the various styles and techniques they may render in the delivery of healthcare services. The processes of care (Box 13-4) are concerned with the functions and responsibilities of the healthcare providers and how they fulfill them. The processes can be divided into two groups, the technical and interpersonal styles employed as healthcare providers care for patients and their families. These, when combined with the structural characteristics described previously, will ultimately affect the organization's ability to assist patients in their transition toward expected outcomes of care.

The processes of care are applied within the structural elements listed in Box 13-3 and discussed previously. The structure can be thought of as the skeleton, and the processes as the muscles. The processes are what get one from point A to point B. They move patients from one destination to the next. To provide quality care, therefore, it is necessary to have both the structure and the processes. The list in Box 13-4 is only a sample of the possible processes in any healthcare organization. Case managers will find themselves interfacing with virtually any and all kinds of processes in the course of their work. The providers' and case managers' technical styles may be affected by the organization they work in and their personal (i.e., structural) characteristics as described previously. Have you ever walked onto a patient care unit and been able to feel something? You may have had an immediate sense that the environment was positive, negative, or apathetic. You may not have

known why you felt that way but there was something present in the environment that gave you that specific impression. What you were sensing was the interpersonal style and dynamics of the setting you were in.

Case Management Links Structure and Process

Case management transcends all of these structural and process variables as it attempts to move patients toward their expected outcomes of care. The **case manager** must consider all of the elements in the structure and in the processes while creating care plans; planning for discharge; and interacting with patients, physicians, and other healthcare providers. Case managers must consider and assess all of the variables to make cogent and appropriate plans of care. Finally, the case managers must, in conjunction with members of the interdisciplinary team, identify expected outcomes that are consistent with the characteristics within the structure of care and compatible with the processes of care.

Outcomes of Care

Outcomes of care can be thought of as the goals or objectives of the care rendered and the services provided. Like structure and process, outcomes too can be categorized and thought of in various subsets or classifications. They are the end results and consequences of care delivery and processes and the effects of the structural variables/characteristics of the healthcare delivery system (Box 13-5).

A quality **case management plan** usually includes the structure and processes, as well as the expected outcomes of care. Each process should include an expected outcome as illustrated in Chapters 9 and 12. Each intervention should also include an expected outcome that is prospectively identified.

Typically, case managers will use the clinical endpoints as indicators for when a patient has completed a particular stage in the care process and can be moved on to the next. The outcomes can be linked to those found in the InterQual criteria (InterQual, Inc, 1998) and Milliman & Robertson Healthcare Management Guidelines (Schibanoff, 1999). For example, a drain might be removed postoperatively after the drainage

BOX 13-5	Categories of Outcomes			
Clinical Endpoints	**Functional Status**	**General Well-Being**	**Satisfaction with Care**
Signs and symptoms	Physical	Health perception	Access
Laboratory values	Mental	Energy/fatigue	Convenience
Deaths	Social	Pain	Financial coverage
Educational	Role	Life satisfaction	Quality
			General

has decreased to a predetermined and acceptable amount/volume per hour.

Outcomes can also be used very effectively when linked with discharge/transitional planning. By moving the patient toward a predetermined set of outcomes, the time for discharge, or transition to the next level of care, is driven by the patient's achievement of those expected outcomes and is not based on arbitrary timeframes. In this way the case manager can defend the time at which a patient should be discharged if the patient, family, and/or physician are resistant. The case manager can also defend the need to extend the hospital stay in the event that a premature discharge is identified based on a review of the patient's progress in achieving the expected outcomes. The case manager can also use the achievement, or lack of achievement, of the expected outcomes for clinical insurance reviews to ensure that reimbursement occurs and, when necessary, that additional hospital days are approved by a **third-party payer.** In these ways outcomes can be a powerful and dynamic tool that provides the case manager with objective indicators for use for a variety of purposes.

The classification of outcomes has shifted over time based on the individuals or groups defining them and also has been influenced by the changing sociopolitical characteristics of the healthcare environment. Traditionally, outcomes have been defined by the providers of healthcare services, particularly physicians. Physicians have always examined outcomes as measures of patient mortality, morbidity, **complications** to treatment, errors, and adverse events or side effects. These types of outcomes were driven by physician practices and reflected the interest of physicians in their own services. Not until the mid-to-late 1980s, but more so during the last decade, did consumers of healthcare become more influential in changing the outlook of outcomes. They were successful in pressuring providers to examine the quality of care using outcome indicators that are consumer-focused rather than provider-focused. This movement resulted in defining a new set of indicators that is considered more contemporary. Examples of these indicators are clinical outcomes such as resolution of disease symptoms; patient's quality of life and well-being; functional ability; satisfaction with care; and financial outcomes such as cost per case/encounter, reimbursement **denials,** and many others. These indicators are most fit today for evaluating the impact of case management models/systems of healthcare.

Using Structure/Process/Outcomes to Measure Quality

Because case management links the three elements of structure, process, and outcome (Case Manager's

 CASE MANAGER'S TIP 13-2

Linking the Structure and Process to Outcomes of Care

Case management has been described as a structure and process model, linking both of these to the outcomes of care.

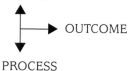

STRUCTURE

OUTCOME

PROCESS

Tip 13-2), case managers can serve an important function in assisting their organizations in the measurement of quality of care. As case managers review the patient's achievement of the expected outcomes of care, they can also review the processes used to achieve those outcomes. The processes, as identified on the diagnosis-specific case management plan, become the standard of care for patients with that diagnosis. The patient's ability to reach the expected outcomes is dependent on the selection of the most appropriate processes for achieving those outcomes. It is also dependent on the organization's processes supporting the care interventions needed. For example, perhaps the case management plan calls for a particular test such as magnetic resonance imaging (MRI) to be done on day 1 of the hospital stay. What are the consequences if day 1 happens to fall on a Sunday when MRIs are not routinely done? The patient's stay will be prolonged, quality care will not be provided as per the case management plan, the patient's satisfaction with care will suffer, and reimbursement may be put at risk. The case manager, by collecting these delays as variances, can provide the organization with meaningful information that may assist in making organizational improvements, which in turn will result in the provision of better quality of care.

Another example is the switch of a patient from an intravenous (IV) antibiotic to its oral form. The case management plan may call for the switch to take place after several prerequisite clinical outcomes have been met. In the case of community-acquired pneumonia, the switch from an IV antibiotic may depend on the patient's achievement of a reduced white blood cell count, a reduction in fever, and the ability to take oral medications. What might happen if the patient achieved these outcomes but the attending physician does not write an order for the switch to take place? This may result in compromising the quality of care, prolonging the hospital length of stay unnecessarily, and increasing the cost of care or sustaining a denial in reimbursement by a commercial insurer.

QUALITY CATEGORIES OF ORGANIZATIONAL VALUES

Commonly, organizational values can be divided into five categories of quality: (1) patient/customer focus, (2) total involvement of taking responsibility for quality, (3) measurement or monitoring of quality, (4) systems support, and (5) CQI (Organizational Dynamics, Inc, 1991). To differentiate the categories, it is necessary to define each more fully and to give examples of a strong versus a weak organizational commitment to quality.

Patient/Customer Focus

The patient/customer focus of quality is related to service, products available, and sharing of information to both internal and external customers of an institution (Case Manager's Tip 13-3). Customer service has become a common buzzword. Determining whether one's external customers received the quality they valued is a powerful tool for an organization to use. In the past, most facilities believed that if they tracked the number of problems or occurrences and they remained within an acceptable level, then the organization was providing quality customer service. More recently, the technique of asking the consumers about their expectations of quality care was found to be much more telling and accurate rather than a hospital making random assumptions as to what the customer needed or considered as quality care. Patient care surveys are now widely used in all types of settings as successful tools for quality care assessment and improvement.

As case management programs become more visible, patient satisfaction surveys may need to be altered so that they capture not only environmental amenities such as food and room comfort but also include the professional care received. Case management should be added to patient care surveys.

It is appropriate to consider an example of an organization's commitment to quality customer service: Patients are called after discharge to hear if their expectations were met. Their suggestions and complaints are

 CASE MANAGER'S TIP 13-3

The Role of Customer Service in Quality
Customer service is what defines quality in today's healthcare market and will more than likely continue to play a major role in a hospital's survival as we become more deeply involved in a managed care environment.

taken seriously, addressed, and responded to. The organization that does not incorporate customer service into its quality program, does not respond to patient complaints, and ignores suggestions made by its customers jeopardizes its reputation, competitiveness, market share, and financial status.

Total Involvement

The total involvement of taking responsibility for quality relates to the fact that management personnel or QA personnel cannot be the sole personnel involved in QA and QI efforts. It is everyone's responsibility to be involved in the achievement, enhancement, and maintenance of quality. Quality is the direct result of positive and desirable employee behavior (Williams, 1994). Positive employee behavior is usually the result of staff job satisfaction. Employees tend to feel ownership of their organization's values when they have been involved in the selection of those values. Productive behavior is evident when an organization's goals are clear and understood by its employees, their role in the organization is defined, and the policies and procedures governing their role are well communicated. For example, the hospital that supports a strong case management team and empowers its members with the permission to solve problems independently and autonomously is an organization with a commitment to quality. The hospital that shows weakness in this area of quality commitment will not address the need for a case management program and will wait for some divine intervention to solve its problems.

Measurement or Monitoring of Quality

Measurement or monitoring of quality must be done to meet the goals. Improvement is impossible without measurement (Organizational Dynamics, Inc, 1991). The case manager's role is to ensure that the patient is moving along in the acute, subacute, or home care level of care in a timely fashion. If any outcomes are not achieved or are delayed, it is the case manager in these settings who is responsible for determining why and for facilitating a corrective action plan. These untoward occurrences are called **variances** (see Chapter 14). By reviewing a patient's progress regularly and anticipating the plan, patient variances will be kept to a minimum and **length of stay** issues will be avoided. Healthcare provider variances are related to omissions or errors made by practitioners. Regulations and policies govern this area. If a healthcare provider omits a medication, this is a variance that could affect the treatment plan and outcomes. Operational variances are those that happen within the healthcare setting. Examples include a patient waiting for a rehabilitation bed, delays in discharge, equipment failures, and scheduling delays. Retrospective analysis and trending of variances result in identification of frequently occurring variances. This analysis will help monitor quality and identify areas for improvement. Outcomes are paramount criteria of good quality either by themselves or as related to costs if efficiency and optimality are to be determined (Donabedian, 1991).

Systems Support

Systems support includes planning, budgeting, scheduling, and performance management needed to support the quality effort. If systems are well coordinated, the time it takes to accomplish the work will be reduced. Everyone should be invested in providing quality work. A team effort should be fostered to accomplish unified goals. A good example of this is a healthcare delivery system called *patient-focused care* that is being adopted in many acute care settings. This system is based on the philosophy that the patient is the center core of focus and that all disciplines involved with the patient must be able to access that patient easily. Patients should not have to seek out the area needed for their treatment; it should come to them. The patient requiring physical therapy should not have to be transported to the physical rehabilitation department; the department's physical therapist should be available in the unit in which the patient resides. This decreases the nonproductive time of transport and can ultimately have the effect of shortening the hospitalization.

Continuous Quality Improvement

Through CQI, organizations foster creativity to do things better tomorrow than they did yesterday. CQI is a way of correcting flaws and making improvements. Well over a decade ago, the industrial leaders of the world realized that to remain competitive and survive in our economy today, CQI techniques were needed. There are three individuals who stand out as pioneers in the development of QI techniques: Philip B. Crosby, W. Edwards Demming, and Joseph M. Juran. Crosby (1979) designed a 14-step approach for his quality improvement process (QIP) (Box 13-6).

Demming's and Juran's work dates back to the 1920s and 1950s, respectively, and was responsible for enormous improvements in Japanese manufacturing. In 1986 Demming's approach to QI came to America. He is best known for involving the employee in the QI effort, applying a never-ending cycle of continuous improvement and eliminating rework and non-value adding processes to reduce cost. This approach involved groups of employees coming together to discuss problem identification and problem solving. When this process is

---

> **BOX 13-6   Quality Improvement Plan: A 14-Step Approach**
>
> 1. Management commitment
> 2. Quality improvement plan
> 3. Measurement
> 4. Cost of quality
> 5. Quality awareness
> 6. Corrective action
> 7. Zero defects planning
> 8. Employee education
> 9. Zero defects
> 10. Goal setting
> 11. Error cause removal
> 12. Recognition
> 13. Quality councils
> 14. Do it all over again

From Crosby PB: *Quality is free: the art of making quality certain,* New York, 1979, McGraw-Hill.

---

applied to healthcare, it involves strategies not only to improve quality but also to reduce costs.

In the United States the concept of quality has matured first from the early quality control or inspection and testing effort to the middle ground of QA, in which selected specialists monitored quality, identified errors or incidents, and kept report cards on each individual blamed for the problem. The QA specialists tend to lack the authority or clout necessary to change the way work is performed. Moreover, QA and its inspection techniques never catch the real issues affecting patient care. The fully mature quality effort is known as *continuous quality improvement* or *total quality management.* The organizations that embrace this concept are those advanced in the ability to empower their employees to be responsible for quality. For the past decade the JCAHO (JCAHO, 1996, 2001) has set forth the charge to integrate QI endeavors that focus on actual performance and outcomes.

The JCAHO has designed the quality cube (Figure 13-1) to depict a model for assessing quality. It illustrates the relationship of performance and important functions to a range of patient populations and services provided. The cube is a tool that stimulates thought related to improvement priorities.

Health professionals have successfully shifted their efforts from QA to QI and most recently advancing to such terms as *continuous quality improvement (CQI), total quality management (TQM),* and JCAHO's latest term: *process improvement (PI).* QA, as stated earlier, tends to focus on reduction of errors, meeting standards set up by regulatory agencies, and measuring defined outcomes. This model functions in response to problems and has a retrospective view of tracking

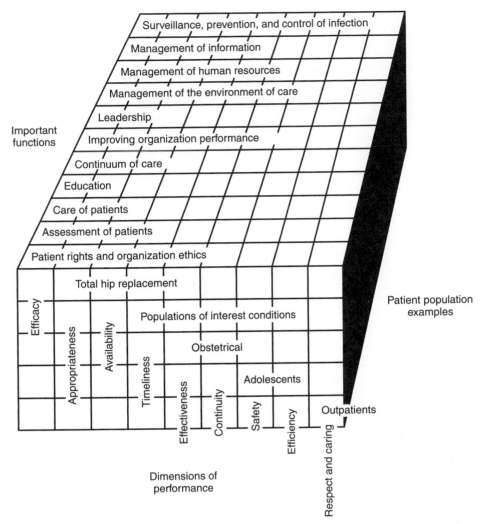

Figure 13-1 The quality cube: a model for assessing the quality of healthcare. (Redrawn from the Joint Commission on Accreditation of Healthcare Organizations: *The 1996 accreditation manual for hospitals,* Oakbrook Terrace, Ill, 1996, JCAHO.)

occurrences after they have happened. QI, on the other hand, focuses on improving a process to effect improvements in the outcomes, meeting customer needs, and measuring customer-identified outcomes. It is a continuous proactive process that avoids focusing on employee and punitive approaches and involves all employees at all levels. The QI approach is one in which the advantage is clear, and it assumes that most people want to do the right thing and do it well. According to the Health Outcomes Institute (1994), quality in healthcare is achieved by "doing the right thing right," where "the right thing" is outcome management and one does it "right" by controlling the process.

We have moved from the paradigm of QA, where provider-defined outcomes (such as morbidity, mortality, and clinical endpoints) rule, to QI, which relies on customer-defined outcomes (such as cost of care, health-related quality, and patient satisfaction). QI focuses on the continued improvement of all processes

rather than just those identified as a problem. This type of approach can improve quality of care of the majority of patients and also decrease statistical outliers. **Outlier thresholds** are set by the Centers for **Medicare** and **Medicaid** Services (CMS), formerly known as the Health Care Financing Administration (HCFA). This is the range of days a patient may stay hospitalized at the maximum reimbursement rate. Outliers are those who exceed the set range of days. In contrast, QA governs itself by the 80/20 rule (or "Pareto Principle"), which states that 80% of costs are generated by 20% of the patients. Therefore those who abide by this principle will only address a small percentage of issues. Table 13-1 provides a snapshot summary of QA versus QI activities.

CASE MANAGEMENT AND CQI

How does the QI approach to healthcare fit in with a case management model? Case managers' skills and role characteristics, as discussed in previous chapters,

TABLE 13-1 Summary of Quality Assurance Versus Quality Improvement

Topic	Quality Assurance	Quality Improvement
Drivers	Licensure satisfaction	Strategic planning
Focus	Errors	Outcomes
Approach	Top-down	Top-down/bottom-up
Process	Retrospective	Proactive
Goals	Reduce errors	Satisfy the customer
Actions	Track outliers	Improve processes and outcomes
Type of change	Incremental	Incremental and continuous
Employees	Not invested	Participation in quality improvement teams

Modified from Newell M: *Using nurse case management to improve health outcomes,* Gaithersburg, Md, 1996, Aspen.

exemplify many of the descriptive elements of QI: problem solving, negotiation, mentoring, quality monitoring, customer relations, and outcome analysis. Usually the first function for a case manager is to select those patients who would benefit from case management. The next function is to facilitate patient treatment goals and discharge plans. In a successful case management program all patients should be monitored for quality, use of resources, and length of stay. Once a patient is identified as one who would benefit from case management, a case management plan of care is designed. The plan is developed to optimize the treatment plan and outcomes, streamline the care to avoid delays or roadblocks, and avoid any compromise in quality. By following these **guidelines,** quality issues are easily tracked. Two tools that are commonly used to track issues of quality are indicator reports and variance reports. Indicator reports are usually geared more to physician practice patterns and untoward occurrences as sequelae to their practice (e.g., an unplanned return to the operating room during the same hospitalization, postoperative complications, or abnormal laboratory results not addressed)—simply put, identifying anything that does not happen when it should. Variance reporting is discussed in much more detail in Chapter 14.

In general, the case manager is the driving force behind the success of quality patient care through case management. The case manager who checks on quality indicators (outcomes) and variances not only identifies problems but also must find remedies for the patient's care to continue to successfully and efficiently move through the hospital system.

A case management program has a major importance to any quality effort. Case managers have the potential to reduce readmissions and the ability to evaluate the possibility of meeting a patient's healthcare needs in an alternative and probably less-costly setting. The case manager must ensure that a patient receives adequate and appropriate care while acute and must provide adequate quality follow-up and postdischarge care. By doing this efficiently case managers reduce premature discharges at healthcare facilities and help to guarantee that patients' discharge plans are adequate, safe, and meet their needs, with the ultimate goal of quality care, patient satisfaction, and avoiding unnecessary readmissions.

You can quickly conclude after reviewing Case Study 13-1 that had all the healthcare disciplines involved in the discharge plan of Mrs. Lopez been consulted, the undesired outcome could have been avoided. By simply reviewing with the home care agency the equipment that the patient was using in the hospital versus the equipment being used at home, the undue anxiety of the patient's family would not have occurred. Had the home health nurse and case manager assessed the ventilator and related supplies that would be used in the home, the patient's well-being could have been maintained by altering the education of the caregivers in the home.

CONSUMER/PATIENT SATISFACTION

An important outcome of any case management program is customer satisfaction. Patient and family satisfaction are essential outcomes to measure; physician, team members, and other involved agencies, as in the previous example, are also important customers. Case managers must work closely with all members of the healthcare team to assess, monitor, and analyze the delivery of care, the case management plan, and the patient/family response to the care to continuously improve the organization's quality of performance (Flarey and Smith-Blanchett, 1996).

A case management plan is designed typically through a multidisciplinary process; when executed correctly, the team's collaboration designs the single best treatment plan for a specific patient type. The plan also provides for a collection and ongoing evaluation of potential quality issues. These issues are usually identified through variances or complications. The entire process enables a focus on quality by continually assessing and identifying opportunities for improvement (Flarey and Smith-Blanchett, 1996).

Case management's efforts for improvement must be accomplished case by case. Case management plays a crucial role in evaluating and monitoring a patient's case management plan and outcomes such as discharge goals. Case managers are the professionals most aware of the patient's functional, physical, and

CASE STUDY 13-1 ■ Example of Unnecessary Readmission to Hospital

Mrs. Lopez is a 68-year-old woman who was admitted with a diagnosis of congestive heart failure. She developed acute respiratory problems and was placed on a ventilator. Her family was very involved in her care and met with the case manager regularly to organize a quality-of-life discharge plan. The case manager worked diligently to provide this patient and her family with all the necessary tools and provisions to meet their needs for going home. The plan was to go home even if Mrs. Lopez remained on the ventilator. A respiratory company was closely involved and worked with the case manager and family to teach the necessary skills to the family and prepare the home for a ventilator. The case manager worked with Mrs. Lopez's daughter to teach her basic respiratory care and Ambu bagging techniques and to improve her confidence when dealing with her mother's ventilator. After many weeks of preparation, the doctor, case manager, patient, family, and respiratory

therapy company all believed they provided a high-quality discharge plan. Within 3 days of discharge Mrs. Lopez was readmitted in respiratory distress. The family was devastated and complained that the visiting nurse from home care was much delayed and did not provide the same information taught to the family in the hospital. The Ambu bag that they were using in the hospital did not work like the one provided at home; the daughter became distraught and called an ambulance. What went wrong with the quality of this care plan? Was this the most effective discharge plan? Did the case manager include all caregivers in this plan, including those involved in follow-up care? If the case manager had included the skilled home care agency in the discharge plan, could this outcome and readmission have been avoided? Were costs, patient satisfaction, and caregiver needs affected by this incomplete plan?

✓ CASE MANAGER'S TIP 13-4

Customer Service Rule of Thumb
A customer service rule of thumb says that a satisfied customer will tell 3 people, but a dissatisfied customer will tell 20.

---

cognitive abilities and know best how these abilities will affect and determine a patient's level of functioning after discharge/transition from an acute care setting or an episode of illness. Offering the best possible discharge/transitional plan is vitally important because of the potential for reducing readmissions and providing alternative care methods for less cost—and thus the ultimate outcome of heightened patient, family, physician, and payer satisfaction.

Being able to exceed customers' expectations for quality service must be the driving force; this central concern is a primary reason a registered nurse or social worker becomes a case manager. Quality service should be a way of life for any case manager on a day-to-day basis, and it is one of the standards necessary today for healthcare to prosper and survive (Case Manager's Tip 13-4).

COST/QUALITY/CASE MANAGEMENT

As healthcare costs increasingly become a public issue and managed care organizations spend more and more time examining documentation of healthcare expenses

and charges, it is more apparent that quality monitoring must also include elements of not only practice patterns and patient satisfaction but also cost-containment strategies.

In healthcare organizations problems that go undetected can have devastating effects that involve wasted time and money. When a problem is not fixed at the time it occurs, it will only become more costly to fix later (Organizational Dynamics, Inc, 1991) (Figure 13-2).

Costs usually involve the necessary expenditures and those that are avoidable. A *necessary cost* is one that is needed to sustain a certain standard. *Avoidable costs* are those that occur whenever things are done wrong or when unnecessary steps are applied in the process. Necessary and avoidable costs can be further defined by prevention, inspection, and failure costs. *Prevention costs* are those intended to ensure that things will not go wrong. *Inspection costs* are the costs of finding an error or variance and fixing it. *Failure costs* are those incurred when outcomes and patient or customer satisfaction are negatively affected. Any institution pays a big price for a marred reputation, rework, waste, legal penalties, extra charges, or loss of business.

Poor quality is very costly. To help reduce the potential costs poor quality incurs, it becomes imperative that case managers facilitate QI by making sure that they get involved and have the confidence and skills required to do their job well. This does not mean that case managers are solely responsible for the cost of quality. They must work in concert with all of the members of the

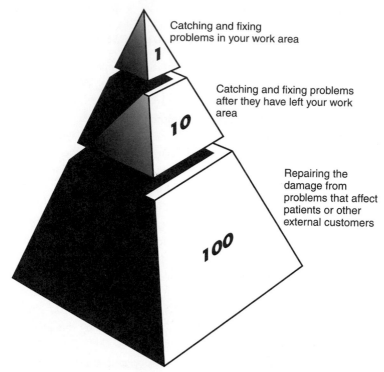

Catching and fixing
problems in your work area

Catching and fixing problems
after they have left your work
area

Repairing the
damage from
problems that affect
patients or other
external customers

Figure 13-2 The 1-10-100 rule. It makes a difference when a problem is fixed. The 1-10-100 rule states that if a problem is not fixed when it occurs, it will only become more costly to fix later in terms of both time and money. (Redrawn from Organizational Dynamics, Inc: *The quality advantage,* Burlington, Mass, 1991, Organizational Dynamics, Inc.)

interdisciplinary team. For example, a physician writes an order for a medication that the patient has an allergy to. If the nurse notices this error as the order is picked up, it would involve a simple solution of ordering another medication that is more appropriate for the patient. However, if the order goes to the pharmacy and the allergy is not noted, the pharmacist fills the order, and the nurse administers the drug; it could end in terrible tragedy. The cost of the incorrect drug is only the tip of the iceberg for this error. The dollars alone cannot fully measure the impact of such an avoidable error on the patient and the hospital. The real cost of this undetected problem shows the heightened damage as illustrated in the 1-10-100 rule. Not only has a medication occurrence added increased cost, but patient satisfaction is at stake as well.

The obvious key to reducing costs and maintaining quality is prevention. The case manager, in the daily review of patient care, works toward preventing errors, delays, problems, and bottlenecks to care. The next best strategy after prevention is early detection and treatment of the problem. Again consider the scenario of the drug error. If the immediate physician order error goes undetected, then the first level of prevention fails unnecessarily. However, if the nurse detects the problem before administration of the drug, then early detection prevents the potential full impact of the error. On

the other hand, if the nurse administers the incorrect drug, then early detection is not employed. To compound this error, perhaps the patient is aware that a mistake has been made, and this is ethically necessary. Now the confidence in the physician and hospital staff has been marred. The case manager is now involved in identifying this quality issue and must now get the physician and perhaps a hospital representative in to speak with the patient and attempt to make amends. It now becomes clearer that the cost of quality in this example could have the worst effect of all no matter how simple the issue may be—a dissatisfied patient who will never return to that healthcare facility.

A second area in which cost and quality intertwine is the cost associated with misuse of personnel or equipment resources. For example, a case manager specializing in cardiac care began to notice a strange occurrence on the unit. Many of the cardiac patients were being monitored simultaneously on both the telemetry units and physician-ordered Holter monitors. The case manager began to ask the obvious question, "Why?" The Holter monitors were an added expense for the hospital not only because the equipment was costly but also because of the misuse of personnel required to read the Holter monitor data and generate and file a report. The same data were available on the telemetry monitors.

The case manager decided to investigate the problem by analyzing the cost of the Holter monitoring. In addition, the case manager met with various physicians and the medical director to troubleshoot the rationale behind ordering the Holter monitoring for telemetry patients. What was discovered by the case manager was that new telemetry technicians had been hired by the hospital and the physicians did not have the confidence that their patients' monitors were being read with the same caliber as they were with the previous telemetry team. The case manager then set out to reassure the physicians of the qualifications, training, and orientation of the new telemetry technicians and personally reviewed a number of cases in which the Holter and telemetry were used, comparing the diagnostics of both to show the physicians that the quality of their patients' care had not been compromised. Because of the perseverance of this case manager, the additional use of Holter monitors with telemetry units was diminished. By analyzing this problem the case manager identified an opportunity for QI through the most cost-effective method available to the patients.

The last area is the cost of delays. There is much at stake when quality is affected by a delayed service. All of the issues mentioned thus far come into play here. The cost associated with delays, the impact on patient satisfaction, and the misappropriation of resources and personnel will significantly affect the cost of outcomes. Delays are very costly to hospitals and can negatively influence how they are judged by managed care companies, other physicians, customers, and patients.

The example of the ventilator-dependent patient is useful here as well. Suppose that the patient appears to have the potential to be weaned from the ventilator. Weaning can be an arduous task, but the ultimate payoff is so exciting and cost-effective that if done successfully it can save the hospital many costly dollars. The challenge of weaning a patient from a ventilator lies with an experienced team who follows the patient very closely. This involves the efforts of case management, as well as social work, dietary, respiratory therapy, speech therapy, the physician, nursing staff, the patient, and the family. The multidisciplinary approach to this complex patient's care management plan is essential to its success.

First the case manager and social worker must work with the family to help them adjust to the idea that weaning their loved one may take some time and may or may not be successful. This alone is difficult and at times frustrating and disappointing for a family. Once the case manager has established that the patient and family are emotionally prepared, the next step is for the other disciplines to educate the family on the care required at home. The timing and availability of the other departments can make or break the length of time it takes to wean a patient. It becomes crucial for the case manager to stay on top of the whole process from start to finish so that everything is in place at the right time. The social worker must work on applications for personal care attendants or any financial arrangements that need to be finalized before discharge. The dietitian must be closely involved with the patient, watching all food intake. The right balance of protein, fat, and carbohydrates must be monitored because weaning cannot take place without the proper caloric intake. A negative nitrogen balance from inappropriate intake can significantly delay the weaning process.

The speech therapist has the vital role of training the patient in different speech and swallowing techniques. If this is attempted with a dedicated positive approach toward the patient's progress, the odds of success are greater. Not all patients are able to meet the criteria for successful speech therapy. It is the case manager who will discuss the potential with the speech therapist and physician to see if the patient is a good candidate. Successful speech and swallow training can make the difference between a patient who will require tube feedings and the patient who can go home on oral food intake. Imagine the delays that can occur in this area alone if no one takes an aggressive risk in attempting to train the patient. Should this area not be explored or attempted with strong expertise, the patient will require tube feedings, which will surely cause a delay because of the added teaching required. The family will need to learn the tube feeding procedures, and the patient will have an additional psychological hurdle to get over.

This is an area in which the case manager can again be involved. A patient-teaching checklist can assist all disciplines in tracking the progress of the family and their ability to learn various tasks such as tube feeding. Without the use of such a tool an additional delay can occur because there will be no record of the progress or lack of progress a family is making in learning the necessary skills required. Another discipline that must coordinate its intervention when weaning a patient is respiratory therapy. The therapists must monitor all of the oxygen saturation data and be willing to try the patient on and off the ventilator for periods, knowing that this is a tedious task that requires patience and perseverance. Any missed opportunities to try the patient off the ventilator could delay the ultimate weaning process and may even cause a failed weaning of the patient. Obviously if the attempts are failed the medical costs of this patient's care increase dramatically.

All interdisciplinary efforts should be to work toward keeping the cost of this patient's care as low as possible. It is very important for the physician to have a trusting

CASE MANAGER'S TIP 13-5

The Importance of Keeping the Physician Informed

An informed physician is better equipped to intervene appropriately and not react to inconclusive data.

 CASE MANAGER'S TIP 13-6

Key Elements to Help Avoid Delays in Patient Care Planning

1. Make sure that family/patient education is begun early.
2. Maintain open physician communication.
3. Include all disciplines on the team.
4. Use case management to guide progress.
5. Use patient teaching tools to assist disciplines in tracking progress.
6. Include outside agencies such as home care or respiratory therapy companies early.
7. To achieve your goals, be persistent, persevere, and have patience.

---

relationship with all of the involved disciplines in the patient's discharge plan. If the physician becomes discouraged with the progress being made, the chances are that he or she will make the decision that the patient is not weanable. The physician must be kept well informed by the nursing staff whenever progress is being made (Case Manager's Tip 13-5).

The case manager again has the important role of assisting the physician in making educated decisions regarding whether the patient is making significant enough progress to be weaned off the ventilator. The case manager must also have the expertise to know when to call the skilled nursing agency to begin the preparations for discharge from the hospital setting. If the timing is off on this phase of the discharge plan, a major delay will be incurred. As in the scenario discussed earlier in this chapter (see Case Study 13-1), if the skilled nursing piece is not included in the discharge plan the risk of an unnecessary readmission is significant. Similarly, if the outpatient home respiratory therapy company is not brought into the loop at the right time, the home may not be properly prepared for a ventilator if this patient cannot be weaned. It behooves the company to check the home electricity for the ability to accommodate the ventilator. Thus if the patient does not come off the ventilator, the potential delay of wiring the home for appropriate electricity can be avoided.

There are other tools that can assist the case manager's efforts toward a successful weaning and cost-effective quality discharge plan. The use of a **clinical pathway** or **multidisciplinary action plan (MAP)** that is specific to weaning a patient off the ventilator will serve as an excellent guideline for all disciplines involved in the case to help track areas of strengths and weaknesses. It will help to standardize the process and yet individualize it to specific patient needs. Patient teaching pathways or patient education tools can help to include the patient and family in the plan. The teaching guidelines can assist as a resource for the patient and family at times when the information being taught becomes overwhelming. Anything that can help to reinforce teaching will ultimately be a benefit to the patient/family and ultimately lead to a timely discharge not hindered or

delayed by lack of understanding on the patient's or family's part (Case Manager's Tip 13-6).

CASE MANAGEMENT AND OUTCOMES MANAGEMENT

Outcomes management is a process that focuses on cost and quality of healthcare. It is defined as a method for the implementation of ideal and desirable patient care services that ultimately enhance patient and organizational outcomes. Case management provides the mechanism by which effective and efficient outcomes are provided, ensured, enhanced, and facilitated. Both outcomes management and case management processes are interested in quality patient care. This makes their marriage desirable and feasible. Almost all of the case management programs today include an outcomes management component whose purpose is to measure the effectiveness of the program. Other benefits of having an outcomes management program are as follows:

- Ability to identify improvement opportunities so that enhancements in patient care delivery and outcomes can be made
- Enhancing practitioner practice patterns and maximizing consistency and standardization
- Collecting pertinent and timely data
- Focusing on strategies that result in reducing complications, morbidity, and mortality
- Optimizing the provision of quality healthcare that meets the interests of consumers, providers, and payers
- Determining what treatments are effective, how much they cost, and whether the results are valued by consumers
- Assisting healthcare organizations in meeting the standards of regulatory and accreditation agencies

BOX 13-7 Outcomes Management Process

1. Review strategic goals
2. Match goals to outcome indicators
3. Design clear, measurable, time-oriented outcome indicators
4. Select appropriate outcomes measurement tools
5. Collect data
6. Analyze data
7. Communicate findings
8. Identify, design, and implement improvements
9. Repeat the process

The case manager plays an important role in monitoring and managing outcomes of care. The outcomes management process consists of a series of steps (Box 13-7) that guide the case manager toward measuring/assessing, monitoring, and managing patient outcomes over time.

Outcomes measurement is conducted by a systematic and quantitative observation and assessment of an outcome at one point in time. It is the measurement of what happens or does not happen after an action or intervention is implemented or not implemented. This is followed by the **outcomes monitoring** process of specific outcomes, during which repeated measures take place over time. This process allows the case manager to identify what characteristics (structure) of the patient care delivery system and processes resulted in the observed outcome; that is, making a causal inference that allows an understanding of what happened and the design of a more effective improvement plan. Finally, the outcomes management process results in optimal outcomes through improved administrative and clinical decision making and service delivery. It takes place as the case manager and other members of the interdisciplinary healthcare team use the information and knowledge they have gained during the assessment and monitoring processes to improve care. **Outcomes indicators** measured can be classified into many categories, such as clinical, functional, and cognitive abilities (of patients); financial; knowledge; quality of life; and satisfaction with care and services (see Chapter 14 for more details).

The case management plan of care is one tool used in this process. The case management plan prospectively determines the interventions and expected outcomes or goals of care. For example, the case management plan may call for an asthma patient to be switched off IV Solu-Medrol/hydrocortisone when the peak flow reading is greater than 250 ml/min. The case manager would measure the point at which this outcome was met in the population of asthma patients and continue to monitor

the achievement of this outcome over a period. The case manager might determine that on evenings and weekends a timely switch off the IV medication did not routinely take place. The interdisciplinary team would then need to identify strategies for improving this process and thereby improving the quality of the care the asthmatic patients were receiving.

By effective outcomes management, the case manager facilitates the achievement of quality patient care. The case manager assists the interdisciplinary team in the development of the plan of care, including the identification of patient outcomes of care for specific case types. The case manager then monitors the achievement of those outcomes over time and works with the interdisciplinary team to improve processes so that the quality of patient care is continuously improving. For these reasons, it is difficult to separate out the functions of case management from those of quality/outcomes management. The two are fundamentally linked and dependent on each other for the provision of quality, safe, and cost-effective patient care.

Case management and CQI are connected very closely in terms of the basic philosophy and process. The asset that case management has is the ability to simultaneously consider quality and cost. The tracking methods used by case management help to measure the cost of good quality versus inferior quality.

The ongoing goal of any formal case management program is to identify the optimal treatment plan and most cost-effective discharge/transitional plan achievable. If such plans are developed, quality is sure to follow. A case manager's quality effort takes place case by case. Case management is an organized approach to improving quality and efficiency in patient care and cost.

In the face of today's perceptions and expectations of healthcare consumers, it is an ongoing challenge for case management to significantly impact quality and cost-effectiveness; the challenge must be accepted if we are to survive this tidal wave that the healthcare industry is experiencing.

KEY POINTS

1. Today's competitive healthcare environment demands constant attention to improvements in quality and performance.
2. There are three types of quality: take it for granted quality, expected quality, and excited quality.
3. Organizational values consist of five categories of quality: patient/customer focus, total involvement for taking responsibility for quality, measuring/monitoring quality, systems support, and CQI.

4. It is everyone's responsibility to be involved in the achievement of quality.
5. Quality assurance focuses on reduction of errors, whereas quality improvement focuses on improving a process of care and its outcomes.
6. The key to reducing costs and maintaining quality is prevention.
7. Case management focuses on integrating the structure, processes, and outcomes of care.

REFERENCES

Claflin N, Hayden CT: *Guide to quality management,* ed 8, Glenview, Ill, 1998, National Association for Healthcare Quality.

Coyne C, Killien M: A system for unit-based monitors of quality of nursing care, *J Nurs Adm* 17(1):26-32, 1983.

Crosby PB: *Quality is free: the art of making quality certain,* New York, 1979, McGraw-Hill.

Dash K et al: *Discharge planning for the elderly,* New York, 1996, Springer.

Donabedian A: *Exploration in quality assessment and monitoring, vol 1: the definition of quality and approaches to its assessment,* Ann Arbor, Mich, 1980, Health Administration Press.

Donabedian A: *The role of outcomes in quality assessment and assurance,* Miami, 1991, excerpts from Annual Conference on Nursing Quality Assurance.

Flarey DL, Smith-Blanchett S: *Handbook of case management,* Gaithersburg, Md, 1996, Aspen.

Health Outcomes Institute: *Introduction to outcomes,* Bloomington, Minn, 1994, The Institute.

InterQual, Inc: *System administrators guide,* Marlborough, Mass, 1998, InterQual.

Joint Commission on Accreditation of Healthcare Organizations: *Lexicon dictionary of health care terms, organizations, and acronyms for the era of reform,* Chicago, 1994, JCAHO.

Joint Commission on Accreditation of Healthcare Organizations: *The 1996 accreditation manual for hospitals,* Oakbrook Terrace, Ill, 1996, JCAHO.

Joint Commission on Accreditation of Healthcare Organizations: *The 2001 accreditation manual for hospitals,* Oakbrook Terrace, Ill, 2001, JCAHO.

Larson-Nelson C: Patients' good and bad surprises: how do they relate to overall patient satisfaction? *QRB* 19(3):89-94, 1993.

Marszalek-Gaucher E, Coffey RJ: *Transforming healthcare organizations,* San Francisco, 1990, Jossey-Bass.

McCarthy C: Quality health care inches closer to precise definition, *Hosp Peer Rev* 12(2):19-20, 1987.

Organizational Dynamics, Inc: Excerpts from conference presentation, Burlington, Mass, 1991, Organizational Dynamics, Inc.

Powell S, Ignatavicius D: *CMSA core curriculum for case management,* Philadelphia, 2001, Lippincott Williams & Wilkins.

Schibanoff JM, editor: *Health care management guidelines,* New York, 1999, Milliman & Robertson.

Vladeck B, Shalala D: Medicare and Medicaid programs: use of the OASIS as part of the conditions of participation for home health agencies, 42 CFR, Part 484, *Federal Register* 62:11035-11064, 1997.

Williams RL: *Essentials of total quality management,* New York, 1994, American Management Associates.

14 Measuring the Effectiveness of Case Management

As a **case manager** or an administrator of a case management program in your organization you may be called on to participate in the evaluation of the **case management** model, its effects on the organization, or its effects on patient **outcomes.** You may have direct responsibility for evaluating the effectiveness of the model, the outcomes of the case management plans in use, the success of the case manager's role, or the case manager's performance. Some of the evaluation criteria to be discussed in this chapter may require an organizational effort in terms of data collection and/or analysis. Some you may be able to facilitate as part of your own daily job activities.

Whenever possible, it is important to have an evaluation process and a plan set up before implementation of the model. This is particularly true for those outcomes that affect the organization. Categories such as **length of stay** (LOS), patient and staff satisfaction, clinical care outcomes, and costs of care should have baseline **benchmarks** against which the hospital can judge success or failure. Additional measurement points will be identified prospectively during the course of the hospital stay or course of treatment or intervention and then at the point of discharge or completion of services, depending on the care setting. Other indices, particularly those related to clinical or patient outcomes, will evolve over time.

OUTCOMES AS INDICES OF QUALITY

Broadly speaking, outcomes can be grouped by those that have an effect on the organization versus those that have an effect on patients. These indicators may be the best measures of quality because they provide an understanding of the functioning of the organization and its effects on the product of services and patient care. Outcomes are the result of actions or processes. In patient care they are defined as the goals of the healthcare process. A good outcome is one that has achieved the desired goal.

Case management, through the use of tools such as **multidisciplinary action plans (MAPs)** and **clinical pathways,** and through case management team conferencing, allows healthcare providers to prospectively identify the expected outcomes or goals of care. There are no organizational or clinical processes or tasks that are carried out that do not have an expected outcome attached to them. Therefore outcomes in their narrowest sense allow us to understand the effects on an individual patient and in their broadest sense provide us with an understanding of the functioning (i.e., efficiency and effectiveness) of an organization or the healthcare system at large. These linkages provide us with an understanding of the structure (the organization), the process (the delivery system), and the expected outcomes (goals of care).

Expected outcomes of care are of different types. Some are related to the organization's performance but are not directly related to the patient's health. Others are related to the patient's health but are not directly related to the organization's performance. Still others are solely related to the clinical processes, meaning they are purely clinical in nature.

OUTCOMES NOT DIRECTLY RELATED TO THE PATIENT'S HEALTH

Not all outcomes are related to the patient's health. Some are related to the organization's performance, such as those presented in Box 14-1.

Patient Satisfaction

Understanding patients' satisfaction with the care and services we provide helps us to improve those services

---

BOX 14-1   Expected Outcomes Not Directly Related to the Patient's Health

1. Increase patient satisfaction
2. Increase staff satisfaction
3. Improve the turnaround time for tests/treatments/procedures
4. Reduce the cost of care
5. Reduce length of stay
6. Improve interdepartmental and interdisciplinary communication

---

over time and to continuously improve patients' level of satisfaction with the care they receive. Patient satisfaction data are either collected toward the end of the hospital stay or soon after discharge. All hospitals and many other healthcare organizations collect and monitor data on patient satisfaction. Unfortunately there may not always be a mechanism for feeding that information back for the improvement of system processes or expected clinical outcomes.

Patient satisfaction data collection instruments must be carefully analyzed to determine whether the instrument is valid and reliable. Some instruments, if not tested and determined to be valid and reliable, can be used only to monitor trends and not for statistical analysis. Some organizations mail questionnaires to patients after discharge. Some administer them just before discharge while the patient is still on the institution's premises. The advantages and disadvantages of both methods are summarized in Table 14-1.

Whether organizations mail their customer satisfaction surveys to patients after discharge or distribute them on-site with discharge papers or through some other means, there exist some pros and cons with either method. Mailing questionnaires means that patients can respond at home, where they may feel safer to share their true feelings. Unfortunately the majority of responses will reflect those patients who had either a very positive or a very negative experience. Those who had a positive experience will want to share. Those who had a negative one will be lodging a complaint. This

skewing of the responses may mean that the sample of people responding does not reflect the experiences of the average patient. To reduce the effect of such bias and concern, some organizations mail the customer satisfaction surveys to a randomized sample of patients.

On-site distribution can be accomplished in various ways. Some organizations include the survey as part of the discharge process. Some may include it on the patient's meal tray sometime before discharge. These methods also have pros and cons. On-site responses may not reflect the patient's candid and true feelings because the patient may fear retribution from the hospital staff if responding negatively. On the positive side, the patient's immediate feelings can be captured and addressed accordingly.

On-site collection is the more labor-intensive process. It requires the distribution and collection of the surveys, whereas the return process is built in when the questionnaires are mailed in. One method of collecting on-site responses that may reduce fear of retribution is to manually distribute the questionnaire to the patient at the bedside 24 to 48 hours before discharge. Along with the questionnaire, provide the patient with a pencil and an envelope. Give the patient a short period to complete the questionnaire and ask him or her to seal it in the envelope when finished. Tell the patient that sealing the envelope ensures there will be no association made between patients and their responses, the sealed envelopes will be retrieved at a later time, and responses will be anonymous. Come back and pick up the envelope later. This technique is effective in getting a more representative sampling of patients, and the responses are then timelier. Unfortunately, it is a labor-intensive process and may require a dedicated employee or volunteer. Not all organizations may have such resources at their disposal. In addition, make an effort to randomize the sample of patients chosen to be included in studying customer satisfaction. Randomization may be applied to both procedures that are followed in the distribution of the questionnaires, on-site and mailed.

Whenever possible, use a questionnaire that is scientifically valid and reliable. One such instrument is the Hinshaw and Atwood Patient Satisfaction Instrument (Hinshaw and Atwood, 1982). *Validity* indicates that the instrument is indeed measuring what it is supposed to be measuring; *reliability* is a measure of the instrument's consistency, meaning that the results are consistent from one data collection time to the next. It is advisable for an organization to select an instrument that is widely used so that benchmark data are available for comparison. An example of such instruments is the Press Ganey Patient Satisfaction Survey that is available

TABLE 14-1   Advantages and Disadvantages of Mailing Versus On-Site Distribution of Questionnaires

Method	Advantages	Disadvantages
Mailing	Greater reflection of patient's true feelings	More satisfied and dissatisfied patients respond
On-site	Timely, "live" responses; face-to-face interactions	Patient may fear retribution; labor intensive

in different versions that are specific to the patient care setting, including ambulatory, acute, and emergency department, or specific to the patient population, such as pediatric and obstetrics. Using the Press Ganey instrument allows an organization to benchmark its results to national and regional databases.

Staff Satisfaction

Measuring and monitoring staff satisfaction carry many of the same issues in interpretation of the data as those presented by the patient satisfaction data. It is difficult to prove a direct correlation between changes in staff satisfaction scores and the use of the case management model. There are so many variables at play in an organization at any one time that only relationships may be concluded from any data. Care must be taken in measuring staff satisfaction by using instruments that are valid and reliable whenever possible. If the results are statistically significant, a stronger and more powerful argument can be made for the correlation between the implementation of the case management model and the changes in staff satisfaction scores.

Staff to be tested should include all those directly affected, such as registered nurses, physicians, social workers, and physical and occupational therapists. Staff should be questioned before implementation of the model and then consistently thereafter in appropriate intervals that reflect change over time. Generally a minimum of every 6 months or once annually is sufficient. Unfortunately, during these longer periods, staff members may leave their position and new staff members may be added. Matching samples over a long period will be difficult to maintain because of staff attrition and turnover.

Turnaround Time for Tests, Treatments, and Procedures

Turnaround time (TAT) can be used as a measure of the organization's process improvement and efficiency after the introduction of case management. Facilitating care and managing the patient through the health-care system should improve the TAT for completion of tests and procedures. The TAT should be measured from the time the physician places the order until the order is completed and results are recorded in the medical record. Acceptable timeframes should be decided in advance. For example, the completion time for computed tomography (CT) scans may be 24 hours from the time the order is written until the results of the CT scan are placed in the medical record.

Monitoring of these periods can be done concurrently or retrospectively through the medical record. Concurrent data collection is always preferred because it is both more accurate and timely. If any problems or delays are identified, they can be addressed immediately. Retrospective data collection, on the other hand, may be more difficult because of lapses in documentation in the patient's medical record or simply the inability to obtain the necessary information. In addition, when problems are finally identified, it is rather late to try to resolve them.

Finally, relationships should be shown between the reduction in TAT and the LOS. As before, it may be difficult to prove sound relationships between LOS reductions and TAT because many other factors may have an effect on the LOS.

Cost of Care

Clinical cost accounting methods are being used more and more as a means of understanding not only hospital charges but also the true costs of care. This information can be used to negotiate realistic and appropriate **managed care** contracts because the hospital understands exactly what costs are associated with the care of a specific population of patients. Cost accounting can also be used as a way of measuring the financial impact of case management on the organization. Although understanding that reduction in LOS of a particular patient population is clearly important, it is also important to determine the amount of resources consumed in the management of that population. Organizations often focus on reducing the LOS but neglect coupling this act with an effort to improve the practice patterns related to tests, procedures, and treatments (pharmaceuticals and others) and eliminating the unnecessary activities. Sometimes they even distribute the same number of tests and procedures across the days left after reducing the LOS. This act keeps the cost of care the same even though the LOS is reduced. Reducing the LOS but consuming the same amount of resources is not as valuable and should be avoided. This will not have the same long-term benefits of shortening the LOS but also reducing the amount of resources used in the care of that case type of patient (Cohen, 1991).

The two main goals of clinical cost accounting are first to identify the organization's standard use of materials for a particular **diagnosis-related group (DRG)** and then to define the standard cost of each clinical service. An understanding of these costs allows the organization to assess its costs relative to the normal **reimbursements,** such as **Medicare, Medicaid,** and other payers. This information also provides a frame of reference or benchmark against which the organization can compare itself with competitors. This can be particularly useful during managed care contract negotiations when the hospital wants to make the most competitive bid possible (Schriefer et al, 1996). Using standardized case management plans allows an organization to calculate the expected cost of care for a particular case type and facilitates the comparison of the actual cost to the expected cost. Such efforts enhance the development of an action plan for improvement.

Internally, clinical cost accounting helps the hospital measure its internal treatment patterns. This information can be linked to the medical staff to determine which physicians are rendering the most cost-effective care. Allowing the physicians to compare their cost per case with the expected cost or that of their colleagues may provide them with information they can use to improve their practice and in the revision of **case management plans** (see Chapter 12).

In the fictitious example in Table 14-2, Physician C has the greatest LOS and the highest cost per case compared with other physicians caring for the same type of patients. This report reflects the intensity of Physician C's use of resources such as medications, antibiotics, radiology, blood products, and other related supplies. This information might be used by Physician C and his colleagues to develop standard **protocols** that address the use of resources and how it can be reduced or controlled.

Clinical cost accounting can be used by physician department heads or chiefs of services as part of staff education programs. The cost information can be used to help them gain a better understanding of the costs of clinical services and their contribution to those costs. Where differing treatment patterns exist, they can review the patient outcomes and relative costs.

On a managerial level, clinical cost accounting can be used as a component of departmental performance reports, providing administrative staff with financial information related to the efficiency of their departments. Medical staff reports such as that shown in Table 14-2 can provide clinically related information to guide physicians in changing their clinical practice patterns and can provide information to the finance department

in terms of the cost versus volume versus profit to the organization.

Length of Stay

LOS is a broad umbrella term that can be interpreted in various ways to indicate the amount of time allotted to the care, treatment, or recuperation of a patient. In the inpatient setting (e.g., acute, subacute, or skilled nursing facilities/nursing homes) it can be measured by the number of bed days or the number of days the patient remains in the hospital. In the home care setting it is calculated by the number of visits to the home and the number of hours or minutes per visit or the total number of hours. In the emergency department the LOS may be measured in hours or parts of an hour (15 minutes). LOS statistics are most commonly used in the hospital setting. They are often used as an indicator of the success of case management in conjunction with or in the absence of a cost accounting system.

To determine success or failure of case management and case management plans and their effect on LOS, hospitals must have a clear understanding of what their LOS goals are and compare those with the current LOS statistics in the organization. Comparisons can be made between the hospital and a variety of benchmarks. The first should be the Medicare and non-Medicare DRG average LOS. Although DRGs are not the primary reimbursement system in every state, they are still used for analytical purposes. It is important to understand the history of the organization so that realistic LOS reduction goals can be set. The hospital should also benchmark against comparable hospitals. These hospitals may or may not be close geographically. National **databases** can be used for this purpose, such as the University Health System Consortium.

Interdepartmental and Interdisciplinary Communication

Measuring changes in communication may be difficult to do. The best way to capture such changes is through anecdotal comments from the team members affected by implementation of the case management model. Try to capture these comments before implementation and then at designated intervals after implementation. It is suggested that this be done in the form of focus groups. Questions asked should focus on the team's ability to communicate in a timely fashion, the level of respect afforded them by other team members, and their sense of team spirit or *esprit de corps*. In addition, patient care–related questions should also be asked, such as staff members' perceptions of the effectiveness of case management and case management plans on patient care delivery and efficiency, cost, quality, and so

TABLE 14-2 Example of Physicians' Cost-per-Case Comparisons for DRG 89: Simple Pneumonia and Pleurisy, Age over 17 Years with Complications and Comorbidities

Physicians	Number of Patients	Average Length of Stay	Cost per Case
A	55	6.5	$9,280.56
B	50	4.5	$6,985.44
C	34	7.0	$9,986.53
D	30	7.0	$9,895.32
E	25	6.9	$9,643.50
F	18	5.8	$7,856.64

on. Ask them to identify any barriers to communication, as well as to give their ideas about how to remove those barriers.

OUTCOMES RELATED TO PATIENT HEALTH

Each time a clinical intervention is applied in healthcare, there is an associated expected outcome (Box 14-2). Case management provides the structure for identifying those outcomes prospectively. Clinical outcomes should be interdisciplinary and come as a result of the collective efforts of the entire clinical team.

Avoid Adverse Effects of Care

The hospital environment can be a dangerous place, and one goal of care is always to get the patient in and out of the hospital without doing any harm. Many of the quality indicators traditionally used in healthcare have focused on errors or problems that are associated with the way care was provided. These have included falls, nosocomial infections, medication errors, returns to the operating room, readmissions, morbidity and mortality reports, and deaths. These indicators are focused on the negative, untoward effects of the care provided to the patient and less on the identification of areas for clinical improvement that appear as patterns or trends. Nevertheless, it is important to continue to track these untoward outcomes after implementation of the case management model or case management plan.

Improve the Patient's Physiological Status

The next set of indicators is concerned with the patient's clinical response to treatment. A goal of care is for the patient to be discharged in a better clinical condition than he or she was in at the time of admission or the episode of care. One measure of this is the patient's physiological status, which refers to the functioning of the various parts of the patient's organs and other body parts. The physiological status can be measured by such things as vital signs, laboratory values, and physical assessment. It is anticipated that these measures improve between the time of admission and the time of discharge.

The patient's physical abilities are assessed through a thorough review of the major body systems. These include the cardiovascular, respiratory, gastrointestinal, genitourinary, neurological, musculoskeletal, and integumentary systems.

Improve Signs and Symptoms

Signs and symptoms are the first stage of illness. In this stage three things generally occur: (1) the physical experience of symptoms such as pain, shortness of breath, or fever; (2) a cognitive awareness of the symptoms and a placing of meaning on them; and (3) emotional response to this awareness in the form of fear or anxiety (Ignatavicius and Bayne, 1991). At this point the person may self-treat or seek a medical opinion. In either case it is anticipated that the signs and symptoms will be reduced or eliminated. If this occurs, the patient returns to the optimal level of wellness.

It is therefore anticipated that after the clinical interventions of the case management team, the patient's signs and symptoms will be improved.

Improve Functional Status and Well-Being

Functional status and well-being address the patient's ability to perform in a variety of areas. These areas include physical health, quality of self-maintenance, quality of role activity, intellectual status, attitude toward the world and sense of well-being related to self, and emotional status. Functional ability refers to the patient's ability to perform activities of daily living (ADLs). ADLs include an assessment of the patient's ability to perform personal care, ability to communicate, and perception of needs (Ignatavicius and Bayne, 1991).

There are a variety of tools to measure functional status. Among these is the commonly used Functional Independence Measure (FIM), developed by Granger and Gresham (1984). The FIM helps to quantify what the patient actually can do, regardless of the clinical diagnosis. Assessment categories include self-care, sphincter control, mobility and locomotion, communication, and social cognition. The FIM helps care providers measure the level of dependence/independence of their patients in an effort to decide what kind of help they may need after discharge to the community.

CLINICAL OUTCOMES

When developing clinical outcomes, the previously discussed categories should all be considered. Some will be more relevant to the clinical picture than others. One approach for monitoring the expected clinical outcomes is through the identification of intermediate and **discharge outcomes.** These should be specific to the

---

BOX 14-2 Expected Outcomes Directly Related to the Patient's Health

1. Avoid adverse effects of care
2. Improve the patient's physiological status
3. Reduce signs and symptoms of illness
4. Improve functional status and well-being

clinical issue at hand. **Intermediate outcomes** are those expected goals that occur during the course of the hospital stay. They also are triggers for change or progression in the treatment process and indicate that the patient is progressing toward meeting the discharge outcomes/criteria. Achievement of the goal or outcome should be based on the patient's expected response to treatment. These expected outcomes can occur at any point in the hospital stay and usually trigger the move to the next phase of treatment.

Discharge outcomes are those expected outcomes that the patient must achieve to be discharged from the hospital. The intermediate and discharge outcomes should be the basis for the case management plans/ tools. The expected outcomes must be identified before the clinical course of events can be determined. Determination of the expected outcomes should be based on an assessment of both the appropriateness of the care (a determination of who should receive what care) and the effectiveness of care (how good the outcomes of the care are). This review of the evidence helps to relate the process of care to the expected outcomes. This review should be based on all the available evidence rather than solely on the **consensus** of the practitioners involved in its development (Crosson, 1995). Physicians, when presented with the factual and scientific evidence behind the case management tool or guideline, are more likely to favor it and use it to guide their practice.

Examples of Outcomes

The following examples (Boxes 14-3, 14-4, and 14-5) of expected outcomes are presented to help understand the differences and the relationships between intermediate and discharge clinical outcomes. Each example does not include an exhaustive list of the outcomes related to the diagnosis or procedure under which they are listed. Members of the interdisciplinary team working on developing the particular case management plan are the ones who decide on the expected clinical outcomes. They are finalized after a thorough discussion of their implications on the care of the patient, LOS, cost, and quality and are always included as an integral part of the case management plan.

BOX 14-3 Inpatient Management of Mastectomy Patients

Intermediate Outcomes
1. Ambulation: ambulate when fully awake
2. Encourage ambulation within 2 hours of surgery
3. Encourage regular diet when patient is able to tolerate solids
4. Change/switch pain medication(s) to oral if pain scores are 5 or less for 24 hours

Discharge Outcomes
Patient may be discharged as soon as the following criteria have been met:
1. Proper functioning of drains
2. Site is free of signs of hemorrhage and infection
3. Pain is controlled with oral analgesics
4. Patient demonstrates ability to care for drains or home care is arranged for follow-up
5. Patient is able to ambulate independently

BOX 14-4 Lower Gastrointestinal Surgery

Intermediate Outcomes
1. *Ambulation:* Patient is out of bed and walking with assistance within 12 hours of surgery.
2. *Gastric decompression:* Nasogastric tubes to be removed 24 to 36 hours postoperatively for drainage under 250 ml or less than 100 ml residual; gastrostomy to be clamped using the same criteria.
3. *Diet:* Begin clear liquids 12 to 24 hours after removal of nasogastric tube or clamping of gastrostomy; advance to full liquid diet the same day; begin with full liquid diet and advance to regular diet on the following day.

BOX 14-5 Uncomplicated Myocardial Infarction

Intermediate Outcomes
1. Intravenous nitroglycerin: Taper/convert to oral or topical beginning on second day
2. Supplemental oxygen: Discontinue once patient is hemodynamically stable (usually begins on day 2)
3. Ambulate on day 2 or when free of chest pain and shortness of breath

Discharge Outcomes
1. Absence of chest pain and signs of ischemia (should occur within 48 hours)
2. Resolution of ischemic ECG changes
3. Cardiac enzymes returning to baseline
4. Medications converted to oral/topical
5. Activity progressed to preadmission level
6. Patient/family verbalizes understanding of the following:
   a. Signs and symptoms of heart attack
   b. Risk factors for heart disease
   c. Medications
   d. Diet restrictions
   e. Cessation of smoking (if indicated)
   f. Activity balanced with rest

ECG, Electrocardiogram.

PATIENT CARE VARIANCES

A **variance** occurs when what is supposed to happen does not take place. It is defined as a deviation from a standard or omission of an activity or a step from a predetermined plan, norm, rate, goal, or threshold (Strassner, 1996). Generally, variances are expectations that are not met. According to *Webster's Third New International Dictionary* (1986, p. 2533), variance is defined as "the fact, quality, or state of being variable or variant ... a difference of what has been expected or predetermined and what actually occurs." In relation to patient care, variances are outcomes or healthcare providers' actions that do not meet the desired expectations. In relation to case management, variances are deviations from the recommended activities in any of the care elements delineated in the case management plan (Ignatavicius and Hausman, 1995; Pearson, Goulart-Fisher, and Lee, 1995; Tahan and Cesta, 1995; Cohen and Cesta, 1997). Variances often result from delays, interruptions, additions, or omissions of patient care activities and processes. They may sometimes be related to expediting patient care (e.g., performing a patient care activity before it is due is considered a variance).

In an era of increased competition in healthcare, case management plans have emerged as the most desirable tools for improving patient care quality through the elimination and/or prevention of variances, reduction in duplication and fragmentation of care elements, and the standardization of patient care activities. When followed appropriately, case management plans result in consistency in the practice patterns of physicians, nurses, and other healthcare professionals and thus reduce variations in patient care. With this comes the significance of patient care variance data collection and analysis, which are integral elements of case management. Variance data collection cannot occur until the expected outcomes of care, as they relate to the case management plan, have been identified. These expected outcomes become the benchmark against which variation in patient care can be determined.

Variance data collection is important because it provides the basis for improvement in patient care activities, processes, outcomes, and quality. The mechanism of variance data collection is usually decided on by the steering committee charged with implementing the case management model and the use of case management plans. Some institutions have delegated this responsibility to a case management department or a **quality improvement** committee/council. Regardless of who is responsible, the process should be made consistent across the various care settings that exist in the same institution.

There is no standardization in the method of classifying variances. Variances are classified into different categories in different institutions. Traditionally the most common broad categories used to classify variances are patient/family (Box 14-6), system (Box 14-7), and practitioner (Box 14-8). Patient/family variances are

---

BOX 14-6   Examples of Patient- and Family-Related Variances

Patient-Related Variances
1. Refuses tests/treatments/procedures
2. Unable to decide on treatment
3. Feels unready for discharge
4. Refuses discharge
5. Noncompliance with medical/surgical regimen, medications, treatments
6. Medical status change/complications
7. Postoperative complications
8. Unable to wean from ventilator
9. Secondary diagnosis with admission (e.g., hospitalized for asthma and diabetes)
10. Language barrier
11. Reaction to medications/allergy
12. Reaction to blood transfusion
13. Poor historian
14. Withholding pertinent information
15. Sign out against medical advice (AMA)
16. Refusing discharge because of religious beliefs, holiday, or inconvenience
17. Noncompliant with diet restrictions
18. Unable to self-administer medication (e.g., insulin)
19. Unable to learn about disease
20. Inability to care for self after discharge
21. No clothes
22. No keys for apartment/left keys at home
23. Lost glasses while in the taxi; cannot see well
24. Lost dentures before admission
25. Lost insurance card
26. Pressure ulcer present on admission

Family-Related Variances
1. Unavailable to pick up patient at time of discharge
2. Unable to provide support for care after discharge
3. Language barrier
4. Late to pick up patient on discharge
5. Inadequate level of knowledge regarding patient care
6. Difficulty with compliance
7. Unable to learn
8. Want another opinion
9. Unable to bring patient's clothes until after business hours
10. Cannot be reached
11. Cannot afford to buy necessary medical equipment or medications

---

BOX 14-7 Examples of System Variances

Hospital/Institution-Related (Internal) Variances

1. Unavailable rehabilitation therapy program on weekends
2. Weekend medical coverage delays requiring changes in treatment (e.g., cannot switch intravenous antibiotic to an oral form)
3. Operating room overbooking
4. Cancellation of operative procedure, test, or treatment
5. Unavailable messenger/transport services
6. Machine breakdown
7. Shortage of supplies
8. Laboratory errors/delays
9. Lost requisitions for tests or procedures or treatments
10. Pending infectious disease approval of medications
11. Nonformulary medications
12. Pending results: radiology, pathology
13. Conflict in scheduling tests, treatments, procedures
14. Not enough personnel to perform tests/procedures
15. Prolonged turnaround time for tests/procedures
16. Prolonged turnaround time for referrals, consults
17. Unavailable beds in the intensive care unit
18. Unavailable beds for emergency admissions
19. Specialty patients diverted to nonspecialty beds
20. Hospital-acquired pressure ulcer
21. Hospital-acquired infection (nosocomial)
22. No pneumatic tube/carrier available

Community-Related (External) Variances

1. No nursing home bed available
2. Transfer to another institution
3. Delayed ambulette transportation
4. No home care available over the weekend
5. Inappropriate transfer from another facility
6. No bed available in a rehabilitation facility
7. Child protective services are late to come
8. Company delivered medical equipment late
9. Managed care organization disapproves home care services
10. Managed care organization did not certify patient's admission to the hospital
11. Managed care organization did not certify an extension in hospitalization (increased days)

BOX 14-8 Examples of Practitioner Variances

1. Delay in communicating the plan of care
2. Miscommunication between interdisciplinary team members
3. Physician not communicating to the patient
4. Physician not communicating to the family
5. Medication error
6. Wrong test, treatment, procedure ordered
7. Incomplete documentation
8. Incomplete admission assessment/history
9. Omission of an order
10. Delayed request for a consultant
11. Delayed response by a consultant
12. No consent obtained for treatment
13. Delay in processing forms
14. Delay in initiating treatment, plan of care
15. Lack of coordination of discharge plan among the interdisciplinary team members
16. Inappropriate use of medical equipment
17. Patient teaching not done/completed
18. Delay in scheduling tests
19. Inappropriate/early discharge
20. Nurse busy with other patients
21. Failure to or delay in obtaining preapproval for treatments/interventions or community services
22. Physician did not prepare/inform patient of discharge
23. Failure to conduct financial screening

---

the result of the patient's behavior or activity or the behavior/activity of a family member (family is used here in its generic sense to denote a patient's spouse, caregiver, significant other, or family member). Variances may be refusal of treatments, or they may occur as a result of changes in the patient's condition or complications of a medical or surgical procedure (e.g., refusal to sign a consent for an operative procedure, infection, fluid and electrolyte imbalance, or family unavailable to accompany the patient home on

discharge). Some institutions separate patient variances from the family-related ones. They may classify changes in the patient's condition as they result from the disease process under a separate category (e.g., physiological). The family-related variances may be classified into a separate category and labeled as *community* variances.

Practitioner variances occur as a result of behaviors of healthcare providers. Examples of practitioner variance are omission of a treatment, test, or procedure; giving the wrong medication; incomplete follow-up and documentation of the patient's response to treatments; or a visiting nurse not showing up for a prescheduled home visit. These variances represent the areas that healthcare providers may have the most control over, and if prevented they can influence positive patient care outcomes, lead to timely discharge, eliminate unnecessary work, and reduce cost.

System variances are those related to the way an institution operates, and they result in delays in patient care processes. They occur because of inefficient operations and systems, and they may be called *operational* variances. Mostly these variances require administrative attention or intervention for resolution. System variances can also be classified as *internal* (i.e., within the walls of the healthcare facility [institution-based]) or *external* (i.e., outside the walls of the healthcare facility [community-based]). Examples of system variances are lost laboratory requisition slips or specimen, failure of an infusion pump, no nursing home bed available, payment denial, or a managed care organization not approving certain patient care services.

Variances are also classified as *positive* or *negative* (Bueno and Hwang, 1993; Hampton, 1993; Ignatavicius and Hausman, 1995; Tahan and Cesta, 1995; Mateo and Newton, 1996). A *positive variance* is defined as a desired outcome that occurs before it is expected (i.e., before the timeframe that is indicated/projected in the case management plan). It is also a justified type of variance. Examples of positive variance are switching a recommended antibiotic to a different one because of a patient's allergy, changing the diet of a cardiac patient who is admitted for the management of heart failure from the salt- and fat-restricted diet recommended in the case management plan to include diabetic restrictions because the patient is also diabetic, and a patient's early discharge because all of the outcomes are met earlier than expected.

A *negative variance* occurs when a patient care activity is delayed and the patient does not meet the expected/desired outcomes (i.e., the recommended patient care activities in the case management plan are not achieved within the specified timeframes). For example, a patient was on anticoagulation therapy and required prothrombin time (PT) testing every 6 hours on the initial day of treatment. He was due for a PT test at 12:00 noon, but the test was not completed until 4:00 PM and the result could not be retrieved from the laboratory information (automated) system until 5:30 PM. The result of the PT test was found to be very high, and the patient required an immediate intervention, putting the anticoagulation therapy on hold temporarily. In this example, a delay in performing the prescheduled PT test was identified as a practitioner variance. This variance resulted in a delay in changing the anticoagulation therapy/plan of care, and the patient was required to stay an extra day in the hospital.

Another variance category is an *add-on variance*. It is defined as an unplanned or extra patient care activity or process. This type of variance occurs as an addition to what is indicated in the case management plan. An example of such variance is added laboratory tests. An add-on patient care activity is considered a variance because it may contribute to an increase in cost or a delay in discharge. Most often this type of variance results in duplication of services or performance of unnecessary patient care activities.

Because there is no standardization in classifying variances, it is difficult to share variances across care settings or institutions for the purpose of **benchmarking.** It is even more difficult to conduct a joint trending analysis of variance data from several healthcare institutions located in a particular community, an analysis that could sometimes be important for improving healthcare in a whole community rather than a particular hospital population. To avoid this, Hoffman (1993) recommends that the standardized critical elements of patient care included in case management plans be used as the classification system for variances (e.g., assessment and monitoring, treatments, medications, patient/family education, **discharge planning**). If this classification system is followed, then data become transferable within and across institutions, which is highly beneficial for improving the quality of patient care.

Variance Data Collection and Analysis

Designing an effective method for documenting, collecting, and analyzing variances remains a great challenge for most healthcare institutions. Whether the process of variance data collection is automated or manual, most institutions have made the case manager the one responsible for collecting variances. Variance data could be collected anytime during the patient's hospitalization. However, the best time is at the time the variance happens or when it is identified. Timely identification and resolution of variances result in the delivery of cost-effective and high-quality care and increase patient/family satisfaction. A variety of sources for variance identification can be used, such as the progress notes of physicians, nurses, and other healthcare professionals; verbal communication with other members of the interdisciplinary care team during a case conference or one-on-one; or communication with other departments.

The extent to which variance data should be collected is extremely difficult to generalize and varies from institution to institution. How to collect data and what is needed should be prospectively determined. Some institutions collect data at random or as they relate to every single patient care activity without considering their impact on the LOS and quality of care. In such situations, data might become overwhelming and unmanageable. Because of the volume, collected data can be difficult to analyze, trend, or use to efficiently generate reports that can be used for quality improvement. It is recommended that the interdisciplinary team developing the case management plan spend some time defining the significant patient care activities that need to be evaluated for variance data collection. A decision as to what should be included should be individualized to the specific diagnosis or procedure of the case management plan. In addition, variance data collection should be limited to data that affect the predetermined outcomes of each case management plan. The steering committee overseeing the process of implementing case management systems and developing case management plans is the best group to guide the interdisciplinary teams in this process. Members of the interdisciplinary team may use a set of questions (Box 14-9) as a guiding tool for better decision making when faced with the dilemma of what variance data should be collected.

Variances must be identified and corrected as soon as possible for better-quality patient care outcomes and prevention of unnecessary delays in the patient's discharge or prolongation in the LOS. Regardless of who is made responsible for variance data collection, there should be the following:

- Concurrent medical record reviews
- Immediate communication of any delays in patient care to the appropriate personnel (e.g., physicians, department chiefs, case managers, nurse managers, interdisciplinary team members)
- Immediate attempts to resolve the situation causing the variance
- Prospective plans for what, how, and when variance data should be collected

If the primary nurses are given the responsibility of collecting patient care variances, then they, rather than the case manager, are responsible for responding to the identified variance. However, the ideal way of correcting variances is for the interdisciplinary team member who has identified the variance to immediately begin to try to correct or resolve it. This approach will then result in the timeliest results and should help to avoid delays in the LOS or deterioration of quality. Members of the interdisciplinary healthcare team should be made aware of their responsibilities toward variance data collection and resolution. Open lines of communication should be established to promote effective and timely communication of variances to the appropriate administrative personnel, particularly when direct care providers such as staff nurses are made responsible for identifying and resolving variances as they occur.

Strategies for Handling Variances

When a patient care variance is identified, certain questions should be answered immediately to resolve the situation and improve outcomes. The answers to these questions will determine the urgency and seriousness of the situation and indicate the corrective action plan. The questions appear in Case Manager's Tip 14-1.

After careful collection of variance data, the data are analyzed. The variance analysis process (Figure 14-1) is a systematic and scientific interpretation through categorization/grouping, trending, and statistical analysis of the data collected. Variance data are usually compiled and analyzed over time to allow for better opportunities for quality and patient care process improvement.

BOX 14-9 Guiding Questions to Better Decision Making Regarding Variance Data Collection

1. What are the most important patient care elements/activities that should be monitored?
2. In what format should variance data be collected?
3. Should both intermediate and discharge outcome indicators be monitored?
4. Should any type of variances be collected or only those that affect the quality of care and length of stay?
5. How easy is it to collect the suggested variance data?
6. How accessible are the desired variance data?
7. Where are the variance data located?
8. How can variance data be identified?
9. Who is responsible for variance data collection? analysis? reporting?
10. How will the data collected be used?
11. How will the data collected be interphased with the existing quality improvement efforts, if any?
12. What is the benefit of the variance data collected in revising the case management plan?

 CASE MANAGER'S TIP 14-1

Questions to Help in Handling Variances and Improving Outcomes
1. What is really happening?
2. Is the situation indicative of a variance?
3. How serious is it?
4. What is causing the variance?
5. What is the effect of the variance on the patient's condition?
6. What is the category of the variance?
7. What action must be taken to correct it?
8. Who should be involved in correcting the variance?
9. How urgently should it be corrected?
10. What should be shared with the patient and the family?
11. When should follow-up take place?
12. What should be documented in the medical record?
13. What should be documented on the variance tracking tool?

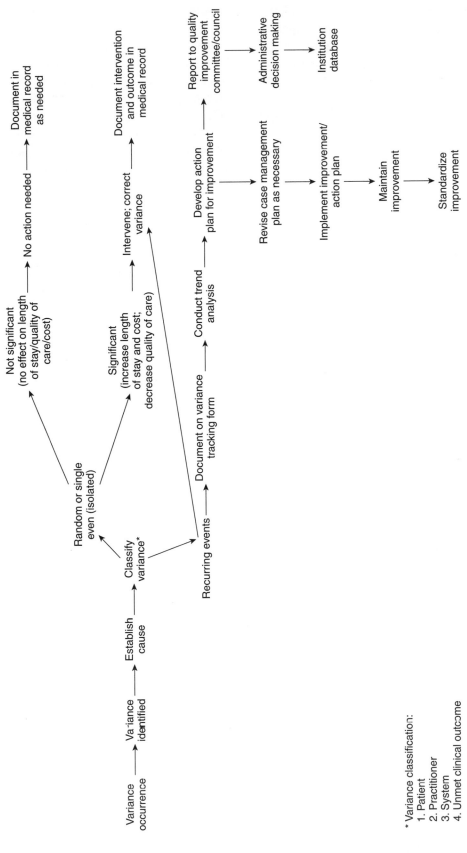

Figure 14-1 The variance analysis process.

* Variance classification:
1. Patient
2. Practitioner
3. System
4. Unmet clinical outcome

The ideal way of dealing with variance data is to link the process to the quality improvement efforts taking place in the institution. Evaluating variances and constructing and implementing an appropriate action plan for improvement ensure better patient care outcomes and prevent the situation from happening again.

Improvement efforts should be spent addressing the recurring variances rather than the isolated, random, or single events because better patient care outcomes are affected by the extent to which the recurring variances are eliminated or prevented. The isolated variances are known to happen as a result of special causes (i.e., not directly related to the systems, operations, or processes an institution has in place). However, recurring variances are the opposite of isolated variances and take place as a result of common causes. These variances require an evaluation and analysis of the systems and processes of patient care the institution follows, as well as the policies and procedures and in some cases the standards of care and practice. It is suggested that efforts to address the isolated variances be decided based on the individual situation, particularly if these

events interfere in the LOS, patient/family satisfaction, and cost and quality of care.

It is not enough to identify and resolve a variance when it occurs. It is equally important to track variances. The purpose of tracking variances is to conduct a trending analysis of each variance category. The results of such analyses are the basis for revising and improving the case management plan, reducing the incidence of variances in the future, and studying the data for necessity of quality improvement efforts, particularly those that are system/operations-related.

Variance data collection and analysis allow healthcare executives to look beyond LOS and cost of care. They are ongoing processes that are helpful in continuously improving the systems of the institution, case management plans, patient care activities, processes and outcomes, and quality of care. It is through this process that standardization of the best/ideal approach to patient care can be achieved and maintained.

Establishing variance data collection tools and formalizing/standardizing the process are integral to the accuracy and reliability of the data collected (Case Manager's

 CASE MANAGER'S TIP 14-2

Strategies for Making Variance Data Reporting Easy

1. If an institution decides to report variance data by source, it is useful to determine these sources (e.g., patient/family, care provider/practitioner, system), standardize them across the various care settings, and include them in the variance tracking tool. It is also helpful to include subcategories for each source. In addition, designating a code for each source and subcategory makes it easier to track, document, collate, analyze, and trend variances.

2. If an institution decides to report variance data by patient care elements applied in the case management plan (e.g., assessment and monitoring, tests and procedures, activity, medications, treatments, nutrition, patient/family teaching), it is important to determine how variances will be tracked and documented in the variance tracking tool. It is not enough to document variances as they relate to patient care elements only. Based on this method, one will only be able to report the frequency (number of occurrences) of variances in each care element. Another clarifying classification should be used in conjunction with this method. One example is the use of positive and negative classification. This way the data could be analyzed in relation to their impact on patient care processes and outcomes.

3. During the process of variance data analysis, some questions may occur that cannot be answered based solely on the data included in the variance tracking tools. In this situation, a review of medical records is suggested. The review should be conducted carefully and in a way that will answer the questions raised.

4. As much as possible, variance tracking tools should include specific places to identify the type (diagnosis, procedure) of the case management plan and the physician in charge of the care of the patient. This information is important for data analysis. It helps in analyzing the data specific to a case management plan and in identifying the physicians with minimal compliance with the plan.

5. Variance data reports should include data on the effectiveness of the case management plans, practice patterns (i.e., how well and how often the case management plan is followed by care providers), and recommendations for improvement opportunities.

6. Making recommendations for improvement opportunities may be made mandatory in each report. Areas to be addressed when recommending improvements may include the processes of care (e.g., improving the promptness of consults, developing patient education materials to be used in patient/family teaching), revisions in the case management plan (e.g., revising a timeframe for an outcome or an intervention, adding a test), and the systems of the institution (e.g., reducing the turnaround time for an echocardiography).

Tip 14-2). Before the initiation of variance data collection, it is imperative to determine what should be measured and how and when assessment and evaluation of care are conducted. It is not uncommon that a variance tracking tool be developed as a part of the case management plan (Figure 14-2). In this case, the tool is made specific and individualized based on the diagnosis or procedure of the case management plan. An institution may elect to use a generic tool (Figure 14-3) that is applicable to any case management plan regardless of the diagnosis or procedure. In both situations, the tool is not made a permanent part of the medical record. It is dealt with as defined in the institutional policy/procedure for variance data collection and analysis.

Providing feedback regarding the effectiveness of case management plans is important. Integral to any strategy for improving patient care is a provision for feedback to the clinicians and administrators who are involved in patient care processes and activities. A formal mechanism for communicating important and appropriate data must be in place in each institution. Reporting variance data should also be done on a regular basis with specific time intervals. Variance data reports should be distributed to members of the interdisciplinary team that was involved in the development of the case management plan and to the related administrators for initiating relevant quality improvement projects.

Patient care monitoring and timely variance identification and resolution are keys to the success of case management plans and are crucial for the delivery of cost-effective and quality care. However, establishing a standardized process for variance data analysis and management remains the best strategy for improving patient care outcomes. In addition, feedback among healthcare administrators and direct care providers is

Long Island College Hospital
Variance Tracking Tool: Adult Inpatient Community-Acquired Pneumonia
Please place a check mark (✓) in the appropriate box

☐ Less severe pneumonia
☐ Severe pneumonia

☐ Initial antibiotic therapy did not meet guideline for severity class

☐ _____
Drug/Dosage

☐ Conversion to oral antibiotic did not occur because of failure to meet:
  ☐ Two consecutive oral temperature readings of <100° F are obtained at least 8 hours apart in the absence of antipyretics
  ☐ Decrease in leukocytosis to <12,000
  ☐ Improved pulmonary signs and symptoms
  ☐ Able to tolerate oral medications
☐ Orders were not written to switch antibiotic
☐ Other:
_____

☐ Oral antibiotic conversion did not meet the guideline selection

☐ _____
Drug/Dosage

☐ Repeat chest x-ray necessary as per guideline
☐ Repeat chest x-ray is <u>NOT</u> necessary as per guideline

☐ Discharge did not occur within 24 hours of conversion to oral antibiotic
☐ Reason documented:
_____

☐ Reason <u>NOT</u> documented

☐ Length of stay
☐ Readmission within 30 days due to failed outpatient management

Figure 14-2 A variance tracking tool specific to a case management plan. (Redrawn from Long Island College Hospital, Long Island, NY.)

MERCY MEDICAL CENTER

Variance Key:
#1—Patient
#2—Process/System
#3—Practitioner
#4—Planning/Discharge

Diagnosis: _____
Date Pathway Initiated: ___/___/___
Date Pathway Completed: ___/___/___
Patient Discharge Date: ___/___/___

Addressograph

Date	Unit	Time	Pathway Day #	Variance Description (See Key)	Action Taken	Signature

MERCY MEDICAL CENTER

A. PATIENT
A1. Patient refusal/noncompliance

A2. Communication barrier
A3. Adverse effects/complications
A4. Comorbidities
A5. Altered mental status
A6. Progression ahead of pathway

B. FAMILY/LIFESTYLE
B1. Noncompliance/unavailability

B2. Environmental barrier
B3. Socioeconomic concerns
B4. Others

C. SYSTEM
C1. Interdisciplinary/transfer issues

C2. Treatment delays
C3. Delayed results reporting
C4. Others

D. CAREGIVER
D1. Physician availability/response time

D2. Physician documentation/orders
D3. Nursing delays
D4. Ancillary delays
D5. Progression ahead of path
D6. Others

House officer: _____   Beeper number: _____   Medical record number: _____

Patient name: _____   Room number: _____

Date of review	Day #	Code	Critical element	Variance explanation	Action if taken

Figure 14-3 Generic variance tracking tools. (Redrawn from Mercy Medical Center, Rockville Center. New York.)

extremely important in refining the use and the effectiveness of case management plans.

OUTCOMES MANAGEMENT AND OUTCOMES CLASSIFICATION

Healthcare providers and administrators are constantly engaged in the evaluation of the outcomes of care and the care delivery system (i.e., the case management model). The interest in outcomes management is integral to case management model evaluation. One must examine both outcomes management and case management to ensure more acceptable care quality and outcomes to the patient and the healthcare organization. Some organizations have made outcomes management as one dimension of the role of the case manager. Other organizations have integrated quality management into the case management department and under the auspices of the administrator/executive responsible for the management of this department. Combining the activities of **outcomes management** and case management results in having the case managers accountable and responsible for outcomes measurement, monitoring, management, analysis, interpretation, and reporting and for **performance improvement.**

Case managers are often found to be collecting data regarding variances (e.g., delays in care), adherence to case management plans, and the outcomes of care activities of both the clinical and administrative processes. This is important for case managers because of their responsibility to "always track outcomes data for the patients in their caseload to determine the effectiveness, efficiency, and efficacy of the case management services provided. It is the ability of ... case managers to use outcomes data intelligently to manage, plan, facilitate, expedite, advocate, coordinate, and evaluate the delivery of patient care that ultimately will result in increasing the degree of success of the case management system" (Flarey, 1998, p. 100).

To facilitate the role of case managers in outcomes management and case management model evaluation, it is important for the healthcare organization to establish an outcomes classification system. Such system must aim at evaluating the case management model and must be standardized across the organization and used by all case managers. It also must identify the outcome indicators to be measured and delineate the process of data collection, aggregation, analysis, interpretation, and reporting. Moreover, such system must adopt the use of predetermined **outcome indicators** reflective of the interest of both the organization/providers of care and the patient population/consumers of care. The classification system must address the standards and requirements of accreditation and regulatory agencies and the expectations of the payers for healthcare, including managed care organizations.

One example of such classification system is shared in Figure 14-4. There is no one best system to be used. However, it is important for an organization to identify the system that works best for its providers and customers. For example, some organizations may consider the patient's functional ability as a separate classification and as independent of the clinical indicators; others may combine the two. The examples presented in Figure 14-4 do not make an exhaustive list of indicators. Others may still be added; however, it is important to define whether the indicator is a patient/family- or healthcare organization–related indicator. The examples shared here are not presented in a measurable format but rather as themes or broad classifications. A healthcare organization to be using this classification system must indicate the outcome indicators in a measurable way, for example cost per case type or an episode of care/illness or managed care reimbursement denial rate. The organization also must delineate the frequency of data collection, the sample, the formulas to be applied in the analysis, and the reporting format. Other ways of classifying outcome indicators are presented in the following sections.

Cost Versus Quality Outcomes

Case managers and case management departments are evaluated in multiple ways. As has been discussed in this chapter, we may choose to look at outcomes in terms of those that directly affect the organization, or we may choose to look at them in terms of those that indirectly affect the organization. Another way to classify outcomes is by those that affect cost versus those that affect quality. We can further break this down to those used to evaluate the case manager versus those that are used to evaluate a department of case management (Case Manager's Tip 14-3).

ORGANIZATION-SPECIFIC OUTCOME MEASURES—EVALUATING THE DEPARTMENT OF CASE MANAGEMENT

When evaluating a department within an organization, certain measures of cost can be selected and used as they relate to the department's goals, mission, and expected outcomes. Examples may include LOS, cost per day/episode of care, cost per case, and cost associated with reimbursement **denials.** As each is selected a frequency for reevaluating each outcome should also be determined. These intervals or frequencies should be appropriate to the selected outcome and should

Classification	Patient/Family-Related Outcomes	Healthcare Organization-Related Outcomes
Clinical	Improved patient care outcomes, such as reduced/controlled pain, morbidity and mortality rates Reduction in signs and symptoms of disease and degree of progression of the disease Prevention of adverse effects of treatments and complications of illness Reduction in practice variation	Standardization of care processes (establishing standards of care/case management plans) Streamlined care processes and delineation of responsibilities Improved turnaround time of tests, treatments, and procedures Increased compliance with standards of regulatory and accreditation agencies
Financial	Optimal and appropriate use of resources and services Provision of care in appropriate setting(s)/level of care Maximal coordination of care among providers Streamlining of diagnostic and therapeutic tests and procedures	Appropriate changes in staff mix/skill mix Reduced cost (e.g., reduction in length of stay, reduction in or elimination of fragmented and duplicate services) Improved reimbursement and revenue Reduction in denials of claims Improved communication among providers and payers (e.g., hospitals and managed care organizations)
Quality of Life	Improved/maximized physical abilities and level of independence Improved psychological, physiological, and social functioning Improved state of well being Improved perception of health status Enhanced self-care abilities/skills Enhanced knowledge of healthcare needs	Prevention of inappropriate hospitalizations Reduction in inappropriate utilization of emergency department services Provision of a safe environment of care Provision of programs that meet patient and family needs Improved accessibility to care/services
Satisfaction	Increased patient/family satisfaction with care Improved continuity of care Improved patient-nurse and family-nurse relationships	Improved staff satisfaction Reduced rates of burnout, turnover, attrition, and absenteeism Enhanced states of communication, collaboration, and teamwork among providers and disciplines (interpersonal, interdisciplinary, and interdepartmental)

Figure 14-4   Classification of outcomes. (From Tahan HA: *Semin Nurse Manag* 6[3]:100-103, 1998.)

 CASE MANAGER'S TIP 14-3

Evaluation Schematic

1. Case manager:
   a. Cost at patient level
   b. Quality at patient level
2. Department:
   a. Cost at organizational level
   b. Quality at organizational level

not be too frequent as to reduce the sensitivity of the data, nor so infrequent as to lose meaning over time.

Cost Measures

Length of Stay

LOS continues to be the most commonly used outcome measure in case management. If your organization or department measures LOS as an outcome indicator then the following factors should be considered:

- By DRG or International Classification of Diseases, Ninth Revision, Clinical Modification (**ICD-9-CM**) code
- By service line
- By physician
- By product line

Cost per Day/Case

Before selecting cost outcomes, consider the following question: Can you access true cost per case using a cost accounting system? If not, other strategies can be used, such as measuring specific resource utilization (e.g., tests, medications, or radiological exams). If you have access to a cost-accounting system then the following are potential measures to be used:

- Cost per physician per day
- Cost per physician per case
- Cost per diagnosis or DRG
- Cost of specific case types by department or specialty
- All of the above

Third-Party Payer Denials

Denial of payment by **third-party payers** is quantifiable and affects the bottom line of the organization; therefore it is commonly used to measure the impact of case management on the organization. The following data elements should be considered when looking at this outcome:

- Reductions in initial denials (whole episode of care or certain hospital days)
- Reductions in final denials (that is after appealing the initial denials)
- Percent of reductions in each of these over time

- Denial reversal rate
- Impact of physician advisor in preventing and/or reversing denials
- Aggregate by physician/payer/department
- As percent of patient days

Quality Measures

Measures of quality are as important as those of cost but may be more difficult to quantify. Measures of quality may include patient and family satisfaction, staff satisfaction, clinical outcomes, and **transitional planning** outcomes. Consider the following examples, knowing that without cost savings attached to them they may carry less weight.

Patient/Family and Staff Satisfaction

- Select a measurement tool
- Select measurement frequency
- For patients—mail-in versus on-site questionnaire
- For staff—which category of staff?
- Which role functions impact satisfaction?

Clinical Quality Outcome Measures

- Achievement of intermediate outcomes—trigger points
- Achievement of discharge outcomes
- Complication rates such as infection rates, returns to the operating room, and so on
- Transitional quality indicators system issues
- Turnaround time for completion of tests/treatments/procedures/consults
- Reporting of test result delays
- Avoidable/preventable mortalities
- Quality improvement initiatives to reduce system delays

Transitional Planning Issues

- Delays in discharge
- Readmits within 24 hours/next day/15 days/ 30 days
- Returns to intensive care units
- Patient complaints regarding discharge planning

ORGANIZATION-SPECIFIC OUTCOME MEASURES—EVALUATING THE CASE MANAGER

In evaluating the case manager, many of the outcome measures are consistent with those selected for measuring the case management department. The only difference is that the data will be aggregated in terms of the case manager; that is, based on the case manager's **caseload** and not the service.

Examples of Cost Measures

- Cost per case
- Length of stay

- Third-party payer denials
- Monitoring of variances
- Variance interventions and analysis
- Transitional planning efficiency and delays

Examples of Quality Measures

- Patient satisfaction scores
- Monitoring of variances
- Variance interventions and analysis
- Transitional planning efficiency and delays
- Performance evaluation
- Competencies
- Clinical outcome measures
- Documentation
- Staff's attendance
- Interdisciplinary relationships
- External professional activities
- Internal professional activities
- Scholarship activities

NATIONAL QUALITY INDICATORS

The focus on quality and outcomes is essential for the survival of healthcare providers, payers, and agencies in today's market. The pressures of consumers of healthcare services have led to a focus on national quality standards through the evaluation and measurement of certain outcome indicators of interest to consumers, payers, and providers. Different national organizations have advocated for national indicators. Although the indicators vary across the organizations, the focus is somewhat similar and to some degree the indicators are the same. The indicators basically focus on access to care and quality and cost of services. It is essential for case managers and administrators of case management programs to be knowledgeable about these national organizations so that they are better able to incorporate their recommended quality indicators in the evaluation process of the case management model.

The indicators of interest to the national organizations are usually related to performance of healthcare providers and agencies. Examples are nosocomial infection rate, fall-related injury rate, cost per episode of care, access to care, consumers' choice of services, patient satisfaction, and qualifications of healthcare providers. The national organizations most interested in quality indicators are the National Committee for Quality Assurance (NCQA); the **Utilization Review Accreditation Commission (URAC);** the Centers for Medicare and Medicaid Services (CMS), formerly known as the Health Care Financing Administration (HCFA); the Joint Commission on Accreditation of Healthcare Organizations (JCAHO); and the American Nurses Association (ANA).

National Committee for Quality Assurance

The NCQA is a national organization comprised of healthcare quality management professionals. Originally established in 1976 to advance the profession of healthcare quality management, today its components include 48 state quality associations; an educational foundation; and an accreditation body for managed care health plans, specifically **health maintenance organizations (HMOs),** and for individual providers in healthcare quality management.

Additionally, NCQA offers a certification to health-care professionals. Individuals certified by NCQA receive certification as a Certified Professional in Healthcare Quality. This certification recognizes professional and academic achievement through participation in this voluntary certification program (Claflin and Hayden, 1998). The national indicators and performance measures identified by NCQA and used in the accreditation standards of managed healthcare plans are known as the Health Plan Employer Data and Information Set (HEDIS). HEDIS focuses on the quality of the systems, processes, care, and services a managed care plan delivers to its clients/**enrollees.** Information collected by NCQA from these health plans is made accessible to both consumers and employers who subscribe to managed care plans. Such information assists the consumer to choose the plan with the best quality performance. Further information about HEDIS is available at http://www.ncqa.org. HEDIS targets the following quality areas:

- Effectiveness of care
- Access and availability to care and services
- Access to preventive services
- Consumer satisfaction
- Health plan stability
- Health plan descriptive information
- Consumer health choice
- Cost of services
- Use of services and **utilization management**
- Credentialing of healthcare providers

Utilization Review Accreditation Commission

The URAC, also known as the American Accreditation HealthCare Commission, was established in 1990 to evaluate the methods of **utilization review** employed by healthcare agencies, particularly the managed healthcare plans because at that time they were widely diverse. As a result of this examination, URAC made health utilization standards available for agencies to use in organizing their utilization review procedures. This acted as a step toward standardization in utilization review practices. In 1994 URAC developed its accreditation program for health plans that were not eligible for accreditation by NCQA, and in 1999 the program was expanded to highly integrated healthcare plans (Kongstvedt, 2001). URAC's accreditation program differs from NCQA's in that it is basically limited to utilization review programs.

URAC's accreditation program is also known today to accredit case management services. More detailed information is available at http://www.urac.org. The quality issues addressed in the accreditation standards of interest to case management are as follows:

- Types of consumers served
- Accessibility to services
- Delivery of case management services
- Provider's qualification and certification
- Case manager's caseload
- Consultation practices with physicians and referrals to other providers
- Quality management program
- Role of support staff
- Privacy and confidentiality practices
- Initiation and termination of services

Outcome-Based Quality Improvement

Outcome-based quality improvement (OBQI) is an approach used by homecare agencies to monitor and continuously improve their quality outcomes. The process relies on clinical, financial, and administrative outcomes data from the Outcome and Assessment Information Set (OASIS) (see Chapter 2 for more information on OASIS) sponsored by the CMS. The goal of OASIS is to improve quality of care delivered to home healthcare patients and to provide data to CMS. Uniform data must be collected on all patients, or on selected patients, in an agency. The data are compared with the same patient outcomes for the previous reporting period and against a reference sample of homecare patients. The data also are risk adjusted to control for any variable that might be affecting them. The outcomes are analyzed to determine whether they are inferior or superior to the previous data collection period. When found to be inferior, the data are then used to spearhead further investigation in the form of a **continuous quality improvement (CQI)** project(s). Further information about OBQI is available at http://www.chspr.org/obqi3.htm. OASIS focuses on the following areas of quality:

- Appropriate patient selection for home care services
- Demographics
- Types of services required
- Follow-up care and/or transfer to inpatient facilities
- Resumption of care
- Disposition status/condition

ORYX—Joint Commission on Accreditation of Healthcare Organizations

The ORYX initiative was implemented by the JCAHO in 1997 as a means to integrate outcomes and other performance measurement data into the JCAHO's accreditation process. The JCAHO's primary mission is to continuously improve the safety and quality of care provided to the public through the provision of healthcare accreditation and related services that support performance improvement in healthcare organizations. Today the ORYX project is known as the *core measures.*

During the initial phase of ORYX, accredited hospitals, long-term care organizations, home care organizations with an average monthly census of 10 or more patients, and behavioral healthcare organizations select two measures from a list of core measures provided by the JCAHO. The measures selected must relate to at least 20% of the patient population. The healthcare organization then collects the data on the selected measures and regularly submits it to the JCAHO. The JCAHO is responsible for analyzing the data and providing performance trends and patterns to the organization in advance of a JCAHO survey. The organization also is responsible for explaining its rationale for selecting the specific performance measures and how the data has been used to improve performance. The JCAHO plans to increase the number of measures and the percentage of patient population gradually each year. Further information about the ORYX project is available at http://www.jcaho.org/perfmeas/nextevol.html.

American Nurses Association

In 1995 the ANA undertook a project (i.e., the nursing **report card** for acute care settings) to explore the nature of the relationships and linkages between nursing care and patient outcomes in acute care settings. This project resulted from the implementation of organizational changes that decreased the numbers of registered professional nurses providing patient care and replaced them with unlicensed personnel. Another factor that led to the demand for such a project was the increasing numbers of reports about incidents of threats to quality and safe patient care delivery. A major purpose of this project was the provision of a framework for educating nurses, consumers, and policymakers about nursing's contribution to inpatient hospital care.

The strategy used to determine the nursing indicators was based on an examination of the nursing scientific literature, consultation with experts and nurse leaders in nursing quality and outcomes research, and conduct of focus groups of nurses from all levels

of practice related to the acute care setting. This project identified three categories of indicators that are still in use today (ANA, 1995). Further information is available at http://www.nursingworld.org. The categories are as follows:

- Patient-focused outcome indicators that include mortality rates, LOS, adverse incidents such as medication errors, complication rates such as pressure ulcers and surgical site infection, patient adherence to discharge plan, and patient/family satisfaction
- Process of care indicators that include nurse satisfaction, documentation of nursing diagnoses and the plan of care, accurate and timely delivery of nursing activities, pain management, skin integrity, patient education, discharge planning, and responsiveness to unplanned patient needs
- Structure of care indicators/nurse staffing patterns that include nurse-to-patient ratio, skill mix, nursing staff qualifications and education, nursing care hours, staff continuity, overtime, use of temporary staff, and staff injury rate (ANA, 1995)

REPORT CARDS

Report cards, also known as *scorecards,* have become a common and popular practice in quality management during the past several years. They are used as a tool for displaying outcomes data in a meaningful, concise, clear, and easy-to-read manner. Report cards can be organized applying the outcomes classification system used by the healthcare organization or the department of case management such as the one discussed earlier in this chapter. They also may include benchmark data and/or targets, which makes the reports more meaningful and valuable (Figure 14-5). An advantage of applying an outcomes classification system to the report card is that it ensures focus on multiple elements of outcomes and not a single parameter such as cost. Adding elements such as consumer satisfaction to LOS and cost outcomes is essential.

Examples of the most common classification categories of outcome indicators are as follows:

- Demographic data and patient descriptors such as age, gender, case mix, insurance, diagnosis, type of surgery, and past medical history
- Clinical outcomes such as use of antibiotics, incision integrity, pain control, and complications
- Financial outcomes/resource utilization such as LOS, intensive care unit LOS, cost per case, and readmission rates
- Functional outcomes/physical ability and mobility such as independence status in ADLs, weight bearing status, ambulation, mental health, and social support system

Outcome Indicators	Benchmark and Target	Actual Outcome
Clinical milestone: Initiation of IV antibiotics therapy	Initiation of antibiotics therapy within 8 hours of arrival	
Clinical milestone: Afebrile × 24 hours WBC decreasing	Switch to PO antibiotic	
Discharge indicators: Afebrile WBC <12,000 Tolerating PO medications	Discharge to home	
Complications: Medical Postoperative	None	
Variance from guideline: System Practitioner Physiological	None	
LOS	4 days	
Cost per case	$6,000.00	
Readmission within 30 days	No readmission	
Third-party payer denials	None	
Reversal of denials	100%	

Figure 14-5 Proposed format for clinical report cards.

■ Satisfaction such as consumer satisfaction, perception of health, and quality of life

Each of these classifications may include several indicators that are measures of the activities, treatments, and outcomes of patient care practices.

Report cards provide healthcare organizations with a mechanism for data collection, aggregation, analysis and trending, benchmarking and comparing, and reporting. Standardizing the way outcomes data are displayed (by applying the above classification, for example) can be advantageous to many audiences, such as healthcare providers, administrators, payers, regulatory and **accreditation** agencies, and consumers. Defining the purpose of the report card and its audience is important because it influences its format, content, and level of sophistication. For example, designing a report card for a case management plan is different from designing a report card for a case management department. The case management plan's report card focuses on the topic of the plan; that is, a homogenous patient population, whereas the case management department is heterogeneous.

Report cards can be generated for a physician or other providers, such as the case manager, or for a disease entity, service or product line, case management plan, or department (i.e., case management department). Regardless of the type of audience the report

card is intended for, Spath (1998) recommends that one first defines the purpose of the report card, delineate the learning opportunity intended by the card, and determine the extent of actions that need to be taken to improve outcomes and performance. It is also important to decide on the frequency of generating the report card and what is expected of those who receive a copy of it. Some organizations distribute the report card on a quarterly basis and as a part of their quarterly **quality assurance**/improvement procedures.

A report card for case management model evaluation or case management plan evaluation is necessary and it is desirable to be made available to key personnel (e.g., senior administrators, physician chairmen/chiefs, case managers, case management plan teams, and finance) in an organization on a quarterly basis. Such a report card may include the elements discussed earlier in the outcomes management and classification and the national quality indicators sections of this chapter. The previous and current improvement activities must also be included as a part of such report. These activities indicate who is responsible for what and indicate the timeframe for completing an improvement activity and its expected outcome. This aspect of the report card ensures the link between the report card and the quality management department or program and communication with the various key players. Report cards that apply this format are looked on favorably by accreditation and regulatory agencies.

KEY POINTS

1. Outcomes can be used as indicators of quality.

2. Outcomes are the goals of healthcare delivery and can be directly or indirectly related to the patient's health.

3. Length of stay is an indicator of the success of a case management model and is often tracked to determine its effectiveness. However, it is not enough to examine it alone; it must be looked at in conjunction with other indicators such as cost of care and those shared in the report card section.

4. Clinical outcome indicators give the case manager a guide for progressing the patient from day to day, episode to episode, or toward discharge.

5. Variance data should be collected using variance tracking tools specific to the institution. Variances should also be classified and coded for ease of tracking. The same classifications should be used across the various care settings.

6. Variance data collection may be made the responsibility of the interdisciplinary team members or the case manager only. Each institution may decide which mechanisms to be followed. Variance data should be tracked, collated, analyzed, and evaluated for improvement opportunities.

7. Results of variance data analysis should be tied into a quality improvement system. Reporting variance data and providing feedback to clinicians and administrators are important and integral to case management systems.

8. Indicators used to evaluate the case management model must be developed based on the recommendations of the national organizations interested in this area such as NCQA, URAC, CMS, ANA, and JCAHO.

REFERENCES

American Nurses Association: *Summary of the Lewin-VHI, Inc., report: nursing report card for acute care settings,* Washington, DC, 1995, The Association.

Bueno MM, Hwang RF: Understanding variances in hospital stay, *Nurs Manage* 24(14):51-57, 1993.

Claflin N, Hayden CT: *Guide to quality management,* ed 8, Glenview, Ill, 1998, National Association of Healthcare Quality.

Cohen EL: Case management: does it pay? *J Nurs Adm* 21(4):20-25, 1991.

Cohen EL, Cesta TG: *Case management: from concept to evaluation,* ed 2, St Louis, 1997, Mosby.

Crosson FJ: Why outcomes measurement must be the basis for the development of clinical guidelines, *Manag Care Q* 3(2):6-14, 1995.

Granger CV, Gresham GE: *Functional assessment in rehabilitation medicine,* Baltimore, 1984, Williams & Wilkins.

Hampton DC: Implementing a managed care framework through care maps, *J Nurs Adm* 23(5):21-27, 1993.

Hinshaw A, Atwood J: A patient satisfaction instrument: precision by replication, *Nurs Res* 31(1):170-175, 1982.

Hoffman PA: Critical path method: an important tool for coordinating clinical care, *Joint Comm J Qual Improve* 19:235-246, 1993.

Ignatavicius DD, Bayne MV: *Medical-surgical nursing: a nursing process approach,* Philadelphia, 1991, WB Saunders.

Ignatavicius DD, Hausman KA: *Clinical pathways for collaborative practice,* Philadelphia, 1995, WB Saunders.

Kongstvedt P: *Essentials of managed health care,* ed 4, Gaithersburg, Md, 2001, Aspen.

Mateo MA, Newton C: Managing variances in case management, *Nurs Case Manag* 1(1):45-51, 1996.

Pearson SD, Goulart-Fisher D, Lee TH: Critical pathways as a strategy for improving care: problems and potential, *Ann Intern Med* 123(12):941-948, 1995.

Schriefer J et al: Linking process improvement, critical paths, and outcomes data to increased profitability, *Surg Serv Manage* 2(6): 46-50, 1996.

Spath P: Nursing performance measures go public, *Outcomes Manage Nurs Pract* 2(3):124-128, 1998.

Strassner LF: The ABCs of case management: a review of the basics, *Nurs Case Manag* 1(1):22-30, 1996.

Tahan HA: Nurse case managers' responsibilities toward patient care outcomes, *Semin Nurse Manag* 6(3):100-103, 1998.

Tahan HA, Cesta TG: Evaluating the effectiveness of case management plans, *J Nurs Adm* 25(9):58-63, 1995.

Webster's third new international dictionary, vol III, Chicago, 1986, Encyclopedia Britannica.

15 Linking JCAHO to Case Management

Marguerite C. Ward, MS, BSN, RN

OVERVIEW OF THE JCAHO STANDARDS

The Joint Commission on Accreditation of Healthcare Organizations (JCAHO) is a private enterprise that sets industry standards for healthcare. These standards are based on current acceptable practices within healthcare with direction toward future industry objectives. The JCAHO is comprehensive in its approach to institutional quality assessment and **performance improvement** and bases its requirements on extensively researched material. It is a voluntary regulatory and accreditation agency in its establishment of standards, but it holds no direct authority over institutions. A JCAHO accreditation of an institution means recognition to reimbursement intermediaries, consumers, and the healthcare industry that acceptable quality standards are maintained and safe, quality patient care is delivered.

The JCAHO conducts nationwide assessments of many types of facilities (e.g., acute care, long-term care, ambulatory care, home care, subacute care, and behavioral healthcare), pointing to a comprehensive approach in evaluating a national standard for review. Each survey incorporates specialty requirements into the overall JCAHO standards to enable the most complete review of a specific healthcare facility.

The JCAHO approaches its review with a focus on **outcomes.** These are measured and evaluated in the following four specific areas:

- Individual: patient/practitioner
- Structure: facility/environment
- Process: delivery of service/systems
- Outcomes: performance assessment and improvement

The intent is to broadly assess the overall institutional performance in meeting quality standards. By weaving its review throughout the many facets of the facility, the JCAHO takes the opportunity to survey if and how well the organization manages itself.

The JCAHO has centered itself around the measurement of quality in an organization. It has defined for healthcare appropriate indications of quality by establishing standards reflective of the best possible practice and providing **guidelines** to indicate the acceptable safety and compliance measures.

The JCAHO standards require a healthcare organization to assess and evaluate its performance on all levels. This begins with the organization's vision, mission, and structure, and it encompasses its actual day-to-day operations and departmental roles. It continues with communication at and between all levels, with careful examination of adequate and planned use of resources and the inspection of the general physical plant facilities.

The JCAHO has organized its standards into two broad categories and a third section dealing with specific healthcare components. There are eleven standards and four structures with functions within these three categories, as outlined in Box 15-1.

Patient-Focused Standards

The JCAHO's patient-focused standards are grouped to reflect the appropriate care and treatment phases for the patient rather than the **caregiver.** The standards cross all departments or divisions, and they are judged to be met when information is obtained and shared by and with other disciplines and appropriate actions are taken based on the data collected.

293

BOX 15-1   JCAHO Standards and Functions

Standards

Patient-focused

1. Patient rights and organization ethics
2. Assessment of patients
3. Care of patients
4. Education
5. Continuum of care

Organization functions

1. Improvement of organization performance
2. Leadership
3. Management of the environment of care
4. Management of human resources
5. Management of information
6. Surveillance, prevention, and control of infection

Structures with Functions

1. Governance
2. Management
3. Medical staff
4. Nursing

From the Joint Commission on Accreditation of Healthcare Organizations: *Comprehensive accreditation manual for hospitals,* Oakbrook Terrace, Ill, 2001, JCAHO.

The JCAHO urges caregivers to reduce the amount of duplication present within the healthcare system. In an effort to promote both efficient use of resources (staff and time) and customer satisfaction, the JCAHO encourages the use of interdisciplinary communication and documentation tools. What is most important is that accurate, validated data be used to plan and evaluate care. Collection and reporting of data may be delegated to the most appropriate caregivers (e.g., case managers) and used by other disciplines once validated (Case Manager's Tip 15-1).

The patient-focused standards guide the patient through an episode of illness back to the most appropriate care setting or level of care. The intent is to

 CASE MANAGER'S TIP 15-1

Promoting Efficient Resource Use and Customer Satisfaction

The JCAHO encourages the use of interdisciplinary communication and documentation tools. What is most important is that accurate, validated data be used to plan and evaluate care. Once data are validated, collection may be delegated to the most appropriate caregivers and used by other disciplines.

efficiently move the patient through the system while meeting the needs of the patient, family, and significant other. Past ideas of only seeing the patient through an episode of illness are gone. The healthcare industry has recognized the need to employ a comprehensive approach to care and treatment. The introduction of cost containment by **reimbursement** parties with payment denials has cautioned the industry to plan appropriately and well but within reason.

Cognizant of these trends, the JCAHO recommends developing an efficient, effective, and safe treatment plan for the patient/family/significant other across the **continuum of care.** Point of entry into the healthcare system, whether hospital, primary care center, or physician's office, is the point of initiation for **discharge planning** and return to the most appropriate care setting. Fundamental in this approach is strong, timely communication of information between and among the various entry points and providers. Meeting the patient-focused JCAHO standards means putting the patient and family/caregiver in the center and allowing the established institutional processes and systems to flow around the patient. The patient should experience hospitalization or an episode of illness in the most seamless way possible. Hospital rules, policies, and procedures should smoothly facilitate this flow. Return to the community care setting should be timely and well planned. Education and medical follow-up care to ensure the patient's ability to manage needed lifestyle adjustments should be outlined and appropriate. Necessary considerations for the cultural diversity of the patient, family, and significant other must be addressed. Each patient must be allowed to participate in planning care and treatments and in addressing specific needs. These include cultural, ethnic, and spiritual considerations.

Organization Functions

The JCAHO patient-focused standards do place the patient, family, and caregiver at the heart of the delivery of services. They clearly delineate the need to adopt a holistic approach in providing care and meeting institutional objectives. In the next group of standards, "organization functions," the JCAHO (2001) establishes requirements to ensure that the facility does the following:

- Designs efficient processes/systems of care delivery
- Examines practice in an organized, planned, ongoing manner
- Identifies opportunities for performance improvements
- Implements cost-effective measures to ensure smooth operations
- Establishes job requirements and measurable criteria for staff performance and competence

■ Maintains a safe, clean, and appropriate environment for all: patient, employee, and visitor

■ Develops effective methods to facilitate the communication of information

■ Proactively examines practice and institutes process changes to reduce medical errors, prevent harm, and promote patient safety

This group of standards focuses on the institution's development of working relationships and systems that allow it to place the patient at the center. The intent in the measurement of these standards is to see strong interdisciplinary teams that are knowledgeable of their individual departmental requirements and those institutional objectives that guide the operations of the facility, always with the patient at the center of the team.

Structures with Functions

The last set of standards governs "structures with functions." These four areas, governance, management, medical staff, and nursing, set the tone for the direction, guidance, and operation of the facility. The JCAHO (2001) requires the organization to clearly define the following:

■ The mission, vision, and ethical code of operations

■ The scope of services provided and the type of populations served

■ The requirements of the practitioners and leaders of the facility, including education, experience, competence, and clinical privileges

■ The involvement of each leader in planning future services of the facility and developing operating budgets

■ The relationship of the governing board in strategic planning, day-to-day operations, and the flow of information within the organization

It is easy to see how the JCAHO has focused and developed its own action plan in guiding organizations toward quality endeavors. It presents the standards manual in order of importance in the same way, as follows:

1. Patient-focused standards
   ↓
2. Organization functions
   ↓
3. Structures with functions

CONTINUOUS SELF-EVALUATION AND IMPROVEMENT

In addition to defining the quality standards, the JCAHO has set an expectation for the organization to continuously evaluate itself and implement measures to improve the delivery of services. A systematic process must be selected by the organization and applied across the board to all areas to ensure a consistent approach. The JCAHO quality assessment and performance improvement methodology is design, measure, assess, improve, and redesign (JCAHO, 2000a). This process is one way to actualize **continuous quality improvement (CQI)** and guide projects/teams through the steps needed to effect sound prioritized change. It asks that each component be examined and defined in relation to the type and amount of services provided, the type of customers served, and the most important components of the services delivered and their associated outcomes. Once the components of service have been outlined, consideration can then be given to assessing and establishing expected performance measures.

Moving through the process, data are collected, aggregated, displayed, and analyzed to determine if performance is satisfactory or needs improvement. If improvement is warranted, a plan is developed, implemented, measured, and evaluated for success. All of this work is then shared within the facility/department to document improvement strides.

The JCAHO further asks the healthcare organization to examine the many facets or dimensions of performance inherent in "doing the right thing" and "doing the right thing well." These include appropriateness, efficacy, timeliness, availability, effectiveness, continuity, safety, efficiency, and respect and caring (JCAHO, 2001).

Finally, the JCAHO asks that the personnel with the most knowledge and those with the ability to implement changes work together in interdisciplinary teams to improve performance and effect better outcomes. Certainly this indicates a most comprehensive approach to reviewing and determining how well an organization meets quality and safety industry standards.

The JCAHO invests resources in developing standards that are future oriented. It strives to incorporate the very best of current practice while anticipating the needs of tomorrow. It is also careful to balance the requirements of the future with the abilities of today. Moreover, it expects to see evidence of current best practice, society guidelines, and recommendations used in consideration of adopting organizational change and setting priorities. This expectation crosses all standards and reinforces the commitment of the JCAHO to the promotion of appropriate, safe, and quality care and outcomes.

The industry's concern with patient safety and medical error reduction has prompted the JCAHO to require healthcare organizations to conduct intense analysis of events (i.e., **root cause analysis** [RCA]) that cause or expose a patient to actual or potential harm. The JCAHO also encourages organizations to proactively examine processes and systems to identify opportunities to reduce risk to patients. Continuous change, evolution of responsibility and accountability, and integration of clinical practice with administrative direction have become the new constants of the JCAHO standards. As standards are adopted and refined, clear emphasis is placed on the relationship, integration, and interdependence of all of the defined JCAHO standards. Selection of care issues (i.e., pain management) and linkage of the issue to all applicable standards define for all members of the healthcare team the quality and optimal outcomes to be achieved when providing care. This concept parallels the intent of practice guidelines and pathways used in **case management** models of patient care delivery.

Examining the requirements to meet standards awakens a realization that systems, processes, manuals, policies, and medical records are not enough to position the organization to achieve the quality outcomes it desires. What is needed is a well-developed cohesive and interactive approach by the organization and its employees to accomplishing its stated goals, objectives, and mission. Adoption of a model and commitment to that model are the first steps in realizing success. Support and encouragement of the model and education regarding the need for change are the next logical steps. Finally, allowing change to occur by empowering those individuals who need to make the change with the ability to do so establishes the model as a working concept. Continually evaluating and improving the model maintains its original intent—to improve care, services, and their related outcomes.

The JCAHO standards direct organizations to consider their primary focus first—the patient, family, and significant other. They proceed with the organizational functions needed to achieve the goal of quality patient care and end with the requirements for knowledgeable, progressive leaders who will demonstrate the ability to encourage and produce change within the organization. However, this is certainly easier to describe than to achieve.

RELATIONSHIP OF CASE MANAGEMENT TO JCAHO STANDARDS

The case management model embodies the same principles as the JCAHO standards. It uses the patient-focused care standards as its base and builds on them with the addition of the organization functions. It is completed by the commitment and acknowledgment of the structures with functions as to its appropriateness, timeliness, effectiveness, efficiency, continuity, efficacy, availability, safety, and attention to respect and caring. The model complements the intent of the JCAHO standards and introduces a practical working approach to ensuring quality in a cost-conscious and safe environment.

Case management reinforces the commitment to doing the right thing and doing the right thing well.

Careful assessment and evaluation of patient needs allow appropriate selection of those patients requiring special attention to move through the healthcare system. Determining complexity of needs allows caregivers to tailor plans of care to meet customer, institutional, and regulatory expectations.

Case management focuses on getting the patient, family, and significant other through the system in the most efficient and safest way possible. An expectation of this is to begin the process upon entry into the system. By beginning with a careful needs assessment on admission, potential patients needing case management and postdischarge services can be identified. Point of entry may be the physician's office, hospitalization, ambulatory care, or **managed care** enrollment. Taking a proactive approach to identifying care and postdischarge needs and to the allocation of appropriate resources allows provisions to be made for a smooth experience through an episode of illness.

By design, case management sets care and outcomes expectations for patient populations with particular diagnoses or procedures for a specific timeframe. It establishes the norm based on industry standards to treat approximately 80% of those patients with the same diagnosis. By defining the norm and establishing sound care paths/clinical **practice guidelines** with delineated outcomes, efficient, safe, and appropriate management of patient care is outlined and can thus be measured. Establishing structure allows providers to maintain control and prepare the patient for the anticipated experience. It makes provisions to begin postdischarge education early during the hospital stay. Allowing for time to evaluate and reinforce critical instructions ensures sound preparation in returning the patient to the appropriate care setting. The intent of case management is to move the patient through the system and necessary **levels of service**/care (acute care, ambulatory care, or home care) with minimal effort, reduced cost, and maximum efficiency and safety. Well-defined outcomes accomplish the following:

■ Provide caregivers an objective determination mark to move the patient to the next level of care

■ Allow objective measures for performance, quality, and variance evaluation

■ Address the overall care needs of the patient while allowing for individualization

The patient remains the focus, the center of case management services. Patient care objectives may include the following:

■ Smooth transition of the patient from one phase of care to the next

■ Providing needed care and treatments in a timely, efficient, and effective manner

- Appropriate resource utilization and management: time, staff, supplies, tests and procedures, costs, and **length of stay**
- Appropriate, timely, and safe discharge/transitional planning and preparation
- Ensuring that patient, family, and significant other have the right tools (equipment, education) to manage lifestyle adjustments while in the community
- Addressing a holistic approach in planning delivery of care by involving the necessary members of the interdisciplinary team

Looking at the JCAHO standards and the case management objectives, it is apparent how well the use of one satisfies the requirements of the other.

The JCAHO has strongly urged healthcare organizations to take a hard look at themselves and to examine both how they provide services and their outcomes. The overall objective is to outline current processes and systems and to assess how well they function. Implicit in the JCAHO intent is to review these functions from the patient's perspective. Organizations are asked to place themselves in the patient's shoes and walk through the process of hospitalization, experiencing it from the consumer's viewpoint. Many hospitals choose to diagram the steps and find that many steps have been added over time to meet departmental needs. Often these additions make the process a little longer and more confusing to the patient. A commitment to improving services and the quality of care delivered leads organizations to ask the following questions:

- Why are things done this way?
- How can the processes of care be streamlined and improve efficiency?
- Which non–value-adding processes can be eliminated, and which ones are necessary to keep?

The basic goal is smooth transition for the patient from one phase of care to the next, each step along the way. Other goals are improved customer satisfaction, a decrease in duplication of services, timely delivery of appropriate and continuum-based services, improved efficiency, reduced cost, a seamless approach to patient care delivery and **transitional planning,** and an improved overall hospital image.

Examining the development of case management, the same principles are seen. A review of current practice outlines the various steps of treatment and care for the patient. Looking at current practice for a diagnosis, outlined by day of stay, allows practitioners to review and decide if services could be scheduled sooner or less frequently. It ensures that practitioners plan needed care efficiently, with attention to cost-effective solutions. It further enables providers to develop standards of practice that address patient care needs and ensure the

delivery of services in a timely manner. This allows each discipline the time to interact with the patient, family, and significant other and to meet specific outcomes.

The flow of hospitalization from one phase/day to the next and from one discipline to the other must be seamless to the patient and family. The JCAHO emphasizes this expectation through its continuum of care/discharge planning accreditation standard (Box 15-2). The continuum of care is defined as an "integrated system of settings, services, healthcare practitioners, and care levels" (JCAHO, 2000, p. 147) along which case managers match patients' needs with appropriate levels and types of care and resources. (See Chapter 6 for more information about the continuum of care and transitional planning.) If the goal of the developed case management model is to place the patient at the center, then the work, care, and treatments must flow around the patient. Use of the case management model to facilitate the process of hospitalization or the management of an episode of care ensures that a plan of care is mapped out and that the care and services are delivered to the patient rather than the patient being delivered to the care and services. The communication and planning processes developed by a healthcare organization are the necessary investments in transitioning from an adopted model to a working plan. This model is a perfect illustration of how to implement the JCAHO standards. The case management model then is an operational approach to meeting the following (JCAHO, 2001):

- Customer expectations by providing a well-planned, seamless approach to care management and across the continuum of care
- Institutional needs by addressing cost-effective solutions to the management of care
- Practitioner needs by allowing timely interventions for the delivery of care within a structured framework
- Regulatory needs by encompassing the principles and standards of the JCAHO in outlining the management of care
- Patient care safety expectations (Box 15-3) by preventing delays in and variances of care delivery processes

The **case manager** is responsible for moving patients with a range of needs through the system and along the continuum of care in a seamless, continuous, and consistent manner. **Case management plans** (see Chapter 12 for more details), proactively developed as baseline tools, facilitate and arrange for an array of care, treatment, and services required in caring for complex patients. The JCAHO suggests the use of clinical practice guidelines for this purpose (Box 15-4). The benefit of the case management model is the provision of an individual practitioner (a case manager) to do this.

BOX 15-2   The Continuum of Care and Case Management

The goal of the continuum of care/discharge planning standard is to maximize the coordination of care activities provided by the various healthcare providers and across the different settings/levels of care. Case managers can enhance meeting this standard by facilitating and ensuring the following activities:

Before admission:
- Assess the patient and family care needs
- Screen the patient and family for the need for postdischarge services and community resources
- Make the information about community resources available and easily accessible to the patients and healthcare team
- Ensure open lines of communication and networks across providers, settings, and facilities

During admission:
- Provide services that are consistent with the healthcare organization's mission and philosophy and that meet the needs of the patient population served
- Provide care and services based on the complexity of the patient's medical and social condition, risk, and staffing levels
- Facilitate the patient's admission and transfer from one level of care to another
- Consult with other providers and facilities for patient transfers or for meeting patient needs

During hospital stay:
- Ensure continuity and consistency in care planning and provision of care

- Facilitate care coordination among all providers and across settings

Before discharge:
- Coordinate postdischarge services based on the patient's assessed needs
- Provide patient and family education in preparation of discharge or transfer to another facility
- Ensure the appropriateness of patients' transfers to other facilities

At discharge:
- Refer patients to other providers and for postdischarge services to ensure that the continuing care needs are met
- Share relevant and necessary information with providers or other facilities to be responsible for the postdischarge care and services

Case managers must coordinate and facilitate patient care throughout all of the phases of care provision; during the patient's entry into the system (e.g., admission to the hospital); and while assessing the patient's needs, diagnosing the problems, planning the treatment and discharge plans, implementing the care, and transferring the patient to other facilities or discharging back into the community.

Discharge planning must focus on the patient's continuing physical, emotional, symptom management (e.g., pain, nausea, shortness of breath, fatigue), housekeeping, transportation, psychosocial, and other needs.

From the Joint Commission on Accreditation of Healthcare Organizations: *Hospital accreditation standards, 2000-2001,* Oakbrook Terrace, Ill, 2000, JCAHO.

The JCAHO does not set different standards for different types of patients. Rather, it outlines high-quality standards for all. The ability to meet the standards for the group of patients with complex needs is challenging. The case management model recognizes this challenge and meets it by placing that complex population in the hands of a dedicated practitioner. The case manager is an additional investment by the organization to meet the increasing demands of today's healthcare population.

Using all of the creativity and know-how necessary to maintain patients "on track" toward discharge, the case manager must plan and intervene as necessary to meet the unique needs of the complex patient. The case management plan/clinical practice guideline provides the necessary vehicle to accomplish this task. Its ability to organize care and treatments, coupled with its outlined progression to outcome achievement, makes it a natural approach for managing care for the patient holistically while meeting regulatory standards. The

ability of case managers to facilitate the process of care for those patients with complex needs is crucial to meeting the needs of the patient, practitioner, institution, and JCAHO standards.

CASE MANAGEMENT AND ROOT CAUSE ANALYSIS

One function of case management models focuses on prevention of untoward events or medical errors and enhancement of patient care safety. This takes place under the umbrella of **quality management** and the delivery of quality patient care services and outcomes. This focus has gained increased attention over the past several years because of the public interest in medical error reduction and the consumer's right for a safe healthcare environment and services. Case managers, by virtue of their role as risk managers, play an essential role in the prevention, investigation, and evaluation of medical errors and **sentinel events.** RCA is the process recommended by the JCAHO for use in the

BOX 15-3   Patient Care Safety and Case Management

The JCAHO introduced a new standard regarding patient care safety and medical/healthcare errors reduction as part of the environment of care and leadership standards. Case managers can facilitate meeting this new requirement because of their role in risk management, variance management, and delays in care activities and error prevention. According to the JCAHO safety standard, the healthcare organization's leadership staff must implement an organization-wide safety program, including activities such as performance improvement, environmental safety, and risk management. The safety program must focus on patients, visitors, and staff. Case managers may facilitate the implementation of the safety program by doing the following:

- Fostering a culture of safety
- Encouraging recognition and awareness of risks and hazards to patient safety
- Acknowledging medical/healthcare errors
- Initiating actions to reduce variances, delays, and risks
- Encouraging voluntary reporting of errors and near misses and promoting a "blame-free" environment of care
- Supporting effective responses to occurrences
- Effecting a proactive approach to errors reduction
- Participating as members of error reduction committees and task forces
- Participating in performance improvement activities that enhance patient safety
- Collecting, tracking, aggregating, and analyzing data on patient safety
- Facilitating communication among members of the interdisciplinary healthcare team to promote a seamless, safe, and effective patient care delivery process

From the Joint Commission on Accreditation of Healthcare Organizations: *Comprehensive accreditation manual for hospitals,* Oakbrook Terrace, Ill, 2001, JCAHO.

BOX 15-4   Clinical Pathways/Practice Guidelines and Case Management

The JCAHO does not mandate but rather recommends the use of clinical practice guidelines for patient care planning and management. It advocates that the guidelines be evidence based, outcome oriented, and interdisciplinary in nature. Case managers can facilitate the development, implementation, and evaluation of these guidelines. To meet the JCAHO accreditation standards, they can ensure that clinical practice guidelines do the following:

- Are developed in an interdisciplinary forum
- Prospectively address the care of patients with particular diagnoses or procedures during hospitalization and across the continuum of care and settings
- Reduce variation in practice by establishing uniform standards
- Anticipate and capture variances and deviation from the plan
- Identify expected outcomes of care and clinical decision points
- Are used for evaluating performance
- Ensure appropriate use and allocation of resources
- Assist clinicians in making decisions on the prevention, diagnosis, treatment, and management of selected medical and surgical conditions
- Are used to identify opportunities for improvement and systems redesign

The JCAHO recommends the use of clinical practice guidelines for designing or improving the processes of patient care delivery. It also encourages healthcare organizations and providers to have in place a standard and formal process for the development, implementation, evaluation, approval, and revision of the guidelines when both clinical and leadership staff are involved and from different departments and disciplines. In addition, JCAHO suggests the use of criteria for the selection and implementation of practice guidelines. Without a doubt, case managers are able to monitor, evaluate, facilitate, and enforce these activities.

From the Joint Commission on Accreditation of Healthcare Organizations: *Hospital accreditation standards, 2000-2001,* Oakbrook Terrace, Ill, 2000, JCAHO.

review and analysis of sentinel events patients may encounter during an episode of care. RCA is a process used by healthcare providers and administrators to identify the basic or causal factors that contribute to variation in performance and outcomes or underlie the occurrence of a sentinel event. A sentinel event is an occurrence that "has resulted in an unanticipated death or major permanent loss of function, not related to the natural course of the patient's illness or underlying condition" (JCAHO, 2000, p. 56). Examples of sentinel events are as follows:

- Suicide of a patient while under the supervision of a healthcare provider (i.e., while in a facility such as a hospital or crisis stabilization center)
- Infant abduction or mix-up
- Administration of wrong blood transfusion (i.e., wrong blood group type)
- Surgery on the wrong patient or body part
- Elopement-related death
- Restraint-related death
- Fall-related death
- Assault/rape while under the supervision of a healthcare provider or while institutionalized

The JCAHO does not require the mandatory reporting of sentinel events; however, the state health departments usually do. Case managers, depending on their organizations and established job descriptions, may be required to facilitate the RCA process, evaluation, and reporting of sentinel events. In such cases, they must be knowledgeable and skilled in this process. They can use the guidelines established by the JCAHO for this purpose.

An RCA is considered acceptable if it does the following:

- Focuses on the system and care processes and not just the provider(s)
- Answers the "why" questions
- Identifies changes that could be implemented to reduce risk and prevent similar incidents in the future
- Is conducted in an interdisciplinary, collaborative manner
- Includes participation by leadership staff, risk management staff, and others as appropriate
- Provides an action plan for implementation, monitoring, and evaluation of the necessary changes, including an identification of the personnel responsible for implementing the changes

DOCUMENTATION STANDARDS

The JCAHO (2001) has challenged healthcare providers to accomplish the following tasks:

- Design and implement efficient patient journeys through the continuum of care
- Decrease duplication through interdisciplinary team work
- Manage information and communication
- Remain cognizant of resource utilization, fiscal responsibilities, and length of stay issues
- Provide quality care based on sound current principles and national standards

Taken at face value, it is easy to see how case management tools fit into the overall scheme of the JCAHO standards. Examining each charge separately reinforces the importance and necessity of carefully developing interdisciplinary plans (also known as **clinical pathways** or *practice guidelines*) to outline specific outcomes to be achieved within specific timeframes (see Box 15-4).

After reviewing the overall intent of the JCAHO standards and seeing the relationship between these standards and case management, it is necessary to look at the documentation tools and their relationship to the standards. This provides further evidence of the efficacy of case management in meeting the JCAHO requirements.

The familiar saying, "If it's not documented, it's not done," holds true when fiscal intermediaries and regulatory agencies review medical records. Any type of

retrospective review that is used to evaluate the quality of care and services provided to patients relies heavily on the evaluation of documentation. Appearances count. Little can be said to give credence to sloppy, illegible, contradictory entries in a patient record. One of the assumptions made when records are not neat, consistent, or complete is that the care rendered is less than adequate, inconsistent, and lacking.

One should always remember that during its survey the JCAHO reviews both concurrent (open) medical records and retrospective (closed) records. Its objective is to see the care and treatment currently rendered and documented and to compare this to past completed documentation (Case Manager's Tip 15-2). Specific diagnoses are chosen for review. The diagnoses chosen usually have high-risk, high-volume, and problem-prone issues or concerns surrounding them and require added interventions—physical, emotional, ethical, psychosocial, or spiritual. This part of the JCAHO survey evaluates the quality of the documentation reflecting the holistic and seamless approach to needed care and treatments for the patient, family, and significant other.

The JCAHO uses a comparison to describe the closed medical record review. It likens the completed record to a book that details a story of patient care. The aim is to see a beginning (assessment and planning for patient care), a middle (interventions, outcomes, and patient responses to the care rendered), and an end (evaluation of services and goals and evidence of a thoughtful and safe discharge plan and preparation). Each phase is necessary in assessing the overall patient outcomes of hospitalization.

The JCAHO has provided structure to assist organizations in resolving issues/concerns related to documentation. It begins by requiring practitioners to base clinical practice on standards of care. These may take many forms, including policy, procedure, and protocol or guideline. The key is that they are based on established and nationally accepted practice. JCAHO requires periodic review and update of care standards to reflect current

 CASE MANAGER'S TIP 15-2

Evaluating the Quality of Documentation: Review of Records

Keep in mind that the JCAHO reviews both concurrent medical and retrospective closed records during its survey. The objective is to compare the care and treatment currently rendered and documented with past completed documentation and to established standards, policies, and procedures.

practice. Changes made must be substantiated with sound reasoning (e.g., regulatory changes, new scientific research outcomes, patient safety, error reduction).

Once standards have been developed and accepted, staff must be educated to expected practice, and the documents must be accessible as reference guides for practitioners. Use of the standard becomes the established norm, and variations in practice must be documented and explained. Once the standard is established and applied in the clinical setting, accountability for individual practice may be enforced with practitioners.

The documentation tools (e.g., case management plans) developed for the case management model are formulated applying the same principles. They serve several purposes (Case Manager's Tip 15-3) and are developed with input from all healthcare providers who will use them. Representation is usually from the various disciplines. They outline current practice for the practitioner based on actual retrospective medical record review and current published evidence-based standards and guidelines. They are designed to facilitate communication by condensing each discipline's plan of care into one document, thereby decreasing duplication and improving timely communication. By outlining care and treatments in an organized manner, an immediate flag is activated when patients deviate from predetermined case management plans. These variations may lead to the following:

- Increased cost
- Prolonged length of stay
- Potential for medical errors or quality issues

 CASE MANAGER'S TIP 15-3

Purposes Served by Documentation Tools

A key point to remember is that the documentation tool (e.g., case management plan) does more than just meet documentation requirements for the JCAHO and other regulatory agencies. It serves several purposes, and it acts as the following:

1. The patient map of care through the system and service delivery
2. The practitioner guide to staying on track when providing necessary care and treatments
3. The communication tool for the multidisciplinary team
4. An evaluation tool for quality management to ascertain variations in practice and project fiscal and quality of care implications
5. A standard of care and practice for regulatory agencies, particularly the JCAHO

- Indication of a need to revise the plan to reflect changes in practice

The basic premise of outlining the pathway and scheduling interventions correlated to length of stay supports the seamless and consistent approach to care. Using the outline, services can be activated for the patient as needed when required. This type of preplanning allows the work to flow around the patient and enhances the patient/family's view of appropriate holistic care. This creates a positive perception of the healthcare team and contributes to improved customer satisfaction.

Another JCAHO contribution toward improving satisfaction with the delivery of care is the charge to decrease paperwork and duplication of data collection. Case management documentation tools support this charge. Objective documentation on the case management plan lets each discipline review what has been done for and accomplished by the patient. Practitioners can then validate required information and patient responses rather than asking redundant questions. Several practitioners all performing the same assessment and data collection suggests to the patient that nobody talks to each other and that each discipline must have to complete its work separate from the rest. Certainly this is neither the intent nor the objective of an interdisciplinary and collaborative team effort. It is, however, a distinct impression imparted to the patient, family, and significant other.

To meet the documentation requirement by the JCAHO of decreasing duplication and fragmentation, documentation tools may be developed for disciplines to build on data collected by the team. Initial assessments may be gathered by one care team member, then reviewed and added to by the next. The purpose is to accomplish the following:

- Reduce duplication, fragmentation, or redundancy
- Organize data logically to support collaboration and access to information for the interdisciplinary team
- Delegate to the appropriate caregiver the appropriate function
- Prepare practitioners for the computerization of clinical data
- Ensure an interdisciplinary approach to care

Building and refining old principles of documentation standards have led healthcare providers to creative solutions for complex issues. Case management is one of those creative solutions. Its ability to meet and support such a wide variety of concerns—fiscal, regulatory, and quality—makes case management a natural selection as a complete model for delivery of care. It blends into the JCAHO philosophy and addresses the requirements of the JCAHO standards. The intrinsic value of case management is its ability to place the patient at the center of the team while supporting collaboration of the interdisciplinary team in meeting stated outcomes. This may be not only one of its most valuable assets but also one of its most challenging to attain.

INTERDISCIPLINARY APPROACH TO PATIENT CARE

Another relationship between case management and the JCAHO to examine is the one involving the interdisciplinary team. How does the organization get individuals and/or departments to move beyond their separate spaces and work together? The answer is to break down the barriers and direct united energies into the delivery of quality patient care. The organization must continuously educate each department (no matter how far removed from the actual delivery of patient care) to the overall hospital mission. This involves commitment and dedication by the leadership team to allow and support necessary collaboration to achieve cohesion among the team.

When the JCAHO revamped and reorganized its approach to the accreditation standards, it collapsed individual departmental requirements into patient-focused and organization functions. The immediate change was felt by all. No longer could nursing or radiology open to a chapter and measure only its individual performance. It was now necessary to work with other disciplines, to know what they did, to determine how and where they overlapped, and to assess the overall organizational performance. The JCAHO pressured hospitals to refocus on their ultimate mission and to seek ways to point each department in the direction of meeting the organizational objectives.

Knowing this to be the sound, correct way for organizations to position themselves, the JCAHO was savvy enough to know that this would require intentional and undivided efforts to achieve desired outcomes. The incentive was the same for each group—to meet the hospital mission. At the center of the hospital mission lie the patient, family, and significant other and the delivery of quality care.

The introduction of quality management and performance improvement concepts enabled organizations to educate staff. These ideas fueled the growth of working teams to assess, evaluate, and improve services, delivery of care, systems, and processes within the organization. What the JCAHO did by revising its quality assessment was to refocus the healthcare organization's way of thinking. It asked healthcare organizations to consider that no matter how well each separate piece of the facility performed, without communication, collaboration, and the ability to work together, inefficiencies

and bottlenecks would occur. The ability to deliver quality services efficiently would be hindered by duplication and miscommunication. What would remain at the center as focus would be the work or the job rather than the patient.

If that approach were moved to the level of the interdisciplinary team, each team member would reiterate the goal of quality patient care, but without the necessary communication and planning to meet patient care needs and with only the immediate needs of the individual disciplines met. This picture is a fragmented approach and does not support a cohesive team image to the patient, family, and significant other.

Case management is a solution to bridging the multidisciplinary team. It provides the walkway or direction the patient needs to take to complete the course through an episode of illness. All team members have the opportunity to identify where and when they need to intervene to accomplish their care goals. Each team member knows who, how, and when to communicate with other team members as progression of the patient along the path takes place. Each member is aware of the involvement of the rest of the team and has access to the specific outcomes and the associated patient responses. The case management model facilitates a holistic approach to patient care. It recognizes the need for the many disciplines to contribute in directing the patient plan of care appropriately and efficiently. It recognizes the need to attend to details, to deal with unexpected issues, and to allow each team member to participate. Case management reinforces the commitment, responsibility, and accountability of the individual disciplines and the interdisciplinary team as a whole to efficient, safe, and timely delivery of care and treatments.

In addition, the case management model assists in educating the interdisciplinary team with regard to necessary concepts and principles for survival in today's healthcare environment. It introduces discussion of the following:

- Cost issues and treatment efficacy
- Appropriate resource utilization and cost containment
- Standards requirements and regulatory needs
- Patient-focused care, reengineering, and redesign
- Care settings and appropriate levels of care
- Interdisciplinary communication and collaboration
- Quality management and performance improvement

The "teams" that previously allowed members to interact independently with the patient, family, and significant other must now interact with each other in helping the patient to journey through the maze of the healthcare system. Based on the developed case management plans, all members contribute their interventions and evaluations, allowing the next phase of care to occur and the work to flow around the patient. This approach is most necessary for providing quality patient care services and keeping all practitioners focused on the seamless transition of the patient through the system.

The case management model provides a strong working model to accomplish many objectives efficiently. It meets patient, practitioner, team, fiscal, and JCAHO needs with its effective and appropriate approach to delivery of quality and safe patient care services. It allows organizations to put action into theory and theory into action.

Implementing a case management model puts a process in place at the level of patient care that parallels the JCAHO standards. It provides a solid infrastructure to move the organization forward in its vision and attainment of delivery of quality services. It recognizes the need to develop patient-centered systems and processes to meet patient needs and institutional objectives. Case management provides the interdisciplinary team with a way to organize standards of care and practice into cost-effective plans that move the patient through the various healthcare settings efficiently. It positions patients and their families at the center, prepares them for discharge appropriately into the community, and helps them to become ready to adopt necessary lifestyle changes and make adjustments. It also positions the healthcare team and organization around patients, supporting them through the episode of illness and assisting them in using documented data regarding practice and outcomes to shape the organization's future.

KEY POINTS

1. Case management models provide a foundation for meeting the requirements of regulatory and accreditation agencies.
2. The use of case management services and plans allows the delivery of efficient, effective, safe, and quality care.
3. The use of both interdisciplinary communication and documentation tools are encouraged by the JCAHO. Case management provides a foundation for both of these.
4. Case management models embody the same principles as those outlined in the JCAHO standards.
5. The interdisciplinary team, such as the case management team, is a focus of the JCAHO standards.
6. Case management ensures that providers do the right things and do them right (i.e., enhance a safe healthcare environment that is free of errors).

REFERENCES

Joint Commission on Accreditation of Healthcare Organizations: *Hospital accreditation standards, 2000-2001,* Oakbrook Terrace, Ill, 2000, JCAHO.
Joint Commission on Accreditation of Healthcare Organizations: *Comprehensive accreditation manual for hospitals,* Oakbrook Terrace, Ill, 2001, JCAHO.

16 Legal Issues in Case Management

Toni Dandry Aiken, RN, BSN, JD
Julie W. Aucoin, DNS, RN,C

Healthcare organizations and providers, in conjunction with the federal government, have been struggling with ways to reduce the cost of healthcare, including costs related to medical **malpractice** insurance and **litigation.** Among the efforts pursued has been the implementation of **case management** systems for patient care delivery and servsices across the healthcare continuum. When fully implemented, these systems rely heavily on the role of **case managers** (discussed in Chapter 4) and the use of **case management plans** (CMPs) (discussed in Chapter 12). This chapter discusses the legal liabilities and malpractice litigation associated with the components of case management systems.

CASE MANAGEMENT SYSTEMS, THE CASE MANAGER, AND THE LEGAL PROCESS

Case management has many wide-reaching effects on patients and their families. Enhanced communication with and education of patients and families allow for a better plan of care and outcomes and more fully informed decisions about the care to be rendered. Because communication is more effective in case management systems, there can be an earlier identification of patients' discharge needs, which may result in the development of improved CMPs to troubleshoot potential problem areas or barriers. Case managers can identify potential problems and barriers within a desired timeframe that can be addressed proactively rather than retroactively. They can prevent overlapping and **overutilization** of many healthcare services through management, coordination, and facilitation of patient care activities, thereby minimizing or eliminating delays in treatments, care, and tests required by patients. Moreover, they can facilitate changes in the provision of care, which may improve cost, timeliness of services, quality, effectiveness, and efficiency of the healthcare system.

Today, case managers are found to assume responsibilities in all care settings (Box 16-1). They are obligated to actively participate in ensuring that patients receive the best healthcare in the most effective and efficient manner. Their autonomy, accountability, and responsibility toward management, planning, delivery, coordination, brokering, facilitation, and evaluation of patient care practices put them at higher risk for malpractice litigation (Nichols, 1996). Because of their position at the hub of the interdisciplinary care team and their role as **gatekeepers** of care, they find themselves increasingly involved in complex situations that require subtle decisions and present higher legal accountability, therefore increasing the chances for malpractice and **liability.**

BOX 16-1 Various Settings Where Case Management Can Be Found

1. Medical and nursing practice (e.g., acute, critical, ambulatory, community, long-term care)
2. Mental health
3. Insurance-based or employee-based programs
4. Independent practice
5. **Workers' compensation**
6. Visiting nurse association and public health practices
7. Social services programs

Several causes of litigation appear repetitively in lawsuits, such as discourteous behavior, communication failures, lack of patient understanding, and lack of information given to the patient and family. For example, patients and/or their families may sue when common complications occur and they claim that they were not informed that such problems could occur.

If the patient is involved in a lawsuit, the case manager may encounter legal terminology that is not commonly used by the layperson. Case managers should become familiar with the legal terminology (e.g., plaintiff, defendant, malpractice suit, standard of care, and **negligence**) that they may come across in the case of a legal claim. The **plaintiff** is the person who brings a claim or lawsuit into court. If the case involves the death of a patient, the plaintiff is the next of kin or the appropriate legal guardian. The defendant in a lawsuit is the person or entity against whom a claim is brought by the plaintiff—in this case, the provider of healthcare services (e.g., the hospital, physician, case manager, registered nurse, social worker, nurse manager).

Most healthcare institutions have provided case managers with the responsibility of managing patient care in collaboration with members of the interdisciplinary healthcare team. Such responsibility increases the risk for malpractice lawsuits against case managers. Malpractice suits are suits filed in court against professional people (e.g., case managers or physicians) who have a level of skill and knowledge that exceed those of a lay or ordinary person. These suits are usually filed against professionals who practice healthcare below the common standards.

STANDARDS OF CARE

In medical malpractice claims, the case manager's care and treatment are judged based on the standards of care applied by other case managers with the same knowledge and experience and who are practicing under similar circumstances in a case management setting. The standard of care is then defined as a scale by which the provider's (i.e., case manager's) conduct is measured to determine if there is negligence or malpractice that has caused damage or injury to the plaintiff and if the provider acted "reasonably" (Nichols, 1996). To avoid malpractice litigation, case managers are advised to practice their duties in a manner consistent with their scope of practice, skills, knowledge, and competence; their job description; and the standards, policies, and procedures defined by their institution.

The sources of standards of care for case managers may include any or all of those issued by professional societies such as the following:

■ National Association of Geriatric Care Managers

■ Case Management Society of America
■ Commission for Case Manager Certification
■ National Institute on Community-Based Long-Term Care
■ National Association of Social Workers
■ American Nurses Association's Steering Committee on the National Case Management Task Force
■ Association of Rehabilitation Nurses
■ American Managed Care and Review Association
■ Agency for Healthcare Research and Quality (formerly the Agency for Health Care Policy and Research)
■ National Institutes of Health
■ The Centers for Medicare and Medicaid Services (formerly the Health Care Financing Administration)

Case managers may also apply the clinical practice guidelines that have been developed by national organizations and associations such as the American Medical Association, American College of Physicians, American College of Cardiology, and American Diabetes Association. If case managers receive certifications, they will be held to the standards of care of the society sponsoring the certification (e.g., the certified case manager [CCM], advance competency continuity of care [ACCC], certified rehabilitation registered nurse [CRRN], certified insurance rehabilitation specialist [CIRS], occupational health nurse [OHN], and certified rehabilitation counselor [CRC]). Other sources of standards include the following:
■ The facility/hospital policies, procedures, and **protocols**
■ Statutes
■ Regulations
■ Regulatory and accreditation agencies
■ Nurse practice act
■ Scope of practice of social workers
■ Equipment manuals
■ Job descriptions
■ Guidelines
■ Authoritative textbooks
■ Expert witnesses

In situations in which the patient is involved in litigation, case managers may be called to testify in court, or the CMP applied for the care of the patient and the medical record may be used to demonstrate the standard of care. Documentation (discussed in Chapter 9) that is thorough, factual, and concrete is essential to aid in the defense of the case manager and to provide a proper "picture" of the care and treatment rendered to the patient.

If there is a claim involving allegations of negligence or breaches of the standard of care, case managers will be held to the standard that was in effect *at the time of the alleged incident*. They will be judged by the "reasonable person's" standard, not the highest standard of care required under the same circumstances.

BOX 16-2   The Four Elements of Negligence

1. A duty (standard of care) is owed to the patient by the practitioner or healthcare organization
2. A breach of duty or a breach of the standard of care by the provider
3. A proximate cause or connection exists between the breach of duty and the patient
4. Damages or injuries incurred by the patient

From Holzer JF: *Qual Rev Bull* 16(2):71-79, 1990; Merz SM: *J Qual Improve* 19(8):306-311, 1993; West JC: *J Health Hosp Law* 27(4):97-103, 1994; Nichols DJ: Legal liabilities in case management. In Flarey DL, Smith-Blancett S: *Handbook of case management,* Gaithersburg, Md, 1996, Aspen.

NEGLIGENCE

If there is an allegation of a breach of a standard based on negligence, then several areas must be evaluated. Negligence is the failure to act as an ordinary, prudent, or "reasonable person" would under similar circumstances. To determine a successful claim against a case manager, four elements of negligence must be evident (Box 16-2).

For example, if a case manager fails to obtain and review pertinent patient records with the managed care organization and as a result the patient is denied the **certification** for surgery or extended hospital stay, causing serious injuries (further unnecessary complications/ deterioration in condition), the case manager and the managed care organization are held liable. The four elements of negligence are evident in this case. The case manager has a duty to obtain and evaluate all medical data so that the patient can receive the appropriate treatment based on needs. By failing to do so, the case manager demonstrated negligence and proximately caused additional injuries to the patient. Breach of the standard of care is also evident. The patient has a valid case.

Damages or injuries can include such things as loss of love and affection; pain and suffering; mental anguish; emotional distress; disfigurement; loss of consortium; past, present, and future medical expenses or lost wages; loss of guidance; loss of nurturance; loss of chance for survival; exacerbation of a preexisting condition; and premature death.

MALPRACTICE

If the case manager is involved in a professional allegation of misconduct or negligent care, then the term *malpractice* is used. Malpractice is defined as professional misconduct; negligent care and treatment; or failure to meet the standard of care, which results in harm to others.

Claims of malpractice or negligence against providers must be brought to the court's attention within a certain period (statute of limitation). The *statute of limitation* is a specific time limit allowed for filing a lawsuit. In personal injury, medical malpractice, and breach of contract claims, state and federal laws vary. Claims should be reviewed to determine the appropriate period within which a claim can be brought against the potential defendant.

INFORMED CONSENT

Case managers are often involved in some way in the process of **informed consent.** Informed consent is consent given for a kind of intervention or service by a patient or the next of kin, legal guardian, or designated person in the **medical durable power of attorney** after the provision of sufficient information by the provider. The elements of disclosure (Box 16-3) are those items that must be discussed with the patient by the healthcare provider performing the treatment, procedure, or surgery.

There are several exceptions to obtaining informed consent and discussing all of the elements of disclosure with the patient. The first exception is if there is an emergency situation and/or a situation in which the client is unconscious or incompetent (e.g., the patient is in a life-threatening situation and there is no time to have a discussion). Second, a therapeutic privilege may be invoked if it is medically contraindicated to disclose the risk and hazards to the patient or if it may result in illness, emotional distress, serious psychological damage, or failure on the part of the patient to receive life-saving treatment. Third, the patient may waive the right to informed consent. Finally, the patient may have had the procedure performed once before and waives the right of informed consent because he or she has already received the information. This information must be documented appropriately in the medical record to protect healthcare providers against malpractice litigation.

LEGAL AND ETHICAL DILEMMAS FOR THE CASE MANAGER

Common legal and ethical issues that are potential areas of exposure and litigation in the area of case

---

BOX 16-3   Elements of Disclosure

1. The type of procedure(s) to be performed (e.g., debridement of knee wound)
2. The material risks and hazards inherent in the procedure (e.g., infection, bleeding)
3. The projected/desired outcome(s) hoped for (e.g., elimination of infected tissue and revitalization of new tissue)
4. Available alternatives, if any (e.g., medication)
5. Consequences of no treatment (e.g., continuation of pain, necrosis, sepsis, or possible amputation)

management may or may not involve case managers directly. Examples of such issues include the following:

■ **Third-party payers** and healthcare facilities can be held legally accountable when inappropriate decisions regarding medical services result from defects in design or implementation of cost-containment mechanisms instituted by the facility or insurance company.

■ Physicians and other providers can be held liable if they comply with the limitations imposed by third-party payers and do not protest when the patient can be harmed by these decisions. Physicians are ultimately responsible.

■ Breach of contract, bad faith, and refusal to provide services and pay **benefits** or **claims** are also issues that may be litigated. A *contract* is an agreement consisting of one or more legally enforceable promises between two or more parties. The elements of a contract are offer, acceptance, consideration, and breach.

■ If there is a breach of implied covenant or good faith and fair dealing, legal actions may be taken.

■ Clients may also allege a failure to exercise due care in the discharge of the contractual duties.

■ A failure to properly investigate an insider's claim is a potential litigation.

■ If standards of medical necessity that are significantly at **variance** with community standards are applied, there may be legal exposure.

■ Failure to properly document care activities and/or **outcomes.**

■ An allegation of good faith violation of duty may be alleged when a subscriber's claim for hospital benefits is denied and the subscriber (an **enrollee** of a managed care organization) is not informed of his or her contractual right to impartial review and arbitration of the disputed claim.

■ Failure to obtain all of the necessary documents/medical records can result in the denial of care needed, which then exerts potential liability.

■ Allegations of negligent referral claims may be filed if there is evidence of failure to properly investigate the qualifications and competencies of the providers and/or facilities to which case managers refer patients for treatment. In addition, if it can be shown that case managers were not reasonable in making a referral to that particular facility or provider, the allegation of negligent referral can be made.

■ Failure of case managers to act as patients' advocates or in the patients' best interest.

■ Failure to apply the "reasonable" standard to the care of patients.

■ Any type of "kickback" or "incentive" program with a provider/payer and the case manager. Such practices are considered illegal (conflict of interest). They also

are unethical behaviors that may result in the patient not receiving the best possible care by the most appropriate provider.

A list of suggestions to help prevent or minimize malpractice litigation appears in Case Manager's Tip 16-1.

Healthcare organizations and case managers should be aware of the reputation and operations of other providers to whom patients are referred for further treatment. Decisions should be made in the best interest of

 CASE MANAGER'S TIP 16-1

Suggestions for Preventing Malpractice Litigation

To prevent malpractice litigation, the healthcare organization and the case manager should do the following:

1. Delineate a referral process for community services and care provision that is in the best interest of the patient and family. The referral process should be accessible in writing to all those involved (i.e., healthcare providers). It should be clear and concise.

2. Ensure that corrective measures are taken and action plans are developed immediately if a healthcare issue arises or if care is questionable. Evaluation and follow-up on such plans should be reflected in the patient's medical record or the hospital's administrative reports as needed.

3. Develop and implement policies and procedures regarding the process of developing CMPs that are easily understood and applied. They should reflect the best interest of the patient and family. In addition, the procedure for documentation of care activities and variance identification and collection should be made easy and explicit.

To minimize malpractice litigation, the case manager should do the following:

4. On admission, and in collaboration with the patient and family and the interdisciplinary team, individualize the CMP to meet the patient's and family's needs.

5. Always consult the treating physician.

6. Review the patient's medical record thoroughly before contacting the representative of managed care organizations.

7. Ensure that **precertifications** for treatments have been obtained in a timely manner.

8. Comply with the law (e.g., patient privacy and confidentiality procedures).

9. Make certain that the patient and family consent to the indicated treatment plan and procedures.

10. Advocate for the patient and family.

patients and their families. Several considerations should be reviewed to determine if the providers to whom patients are referred are appropriate and meet the interests and needs of patients. Examples of these considerations include the following:

- Types of services provided and current practices
- Reports of patient and staff satisfaction scores
- Resource utilization practices
- Practices of quality assurance, assessment, monitoring, and improvement
- Timeliness of delivery of services
- Billing practices (e.g., how they bill, what types of insurance they accept)
- Insurance coverage (i.e., are they properly and adequately insured?)
- Records of any settlements and/or judgments against the facility or healthcare provider (check the courthouse records; do a computer search)
- The allegations of the breaches of the standard of care found in the medical malpractice settlements or judgments (do the allegations pertain to the type of care that would be rendered to the patients to be referred for services?)
- Current **licensure** (check with the state boards)
- Current **accreditation** (check with the appropriate agencies)
- Reports on outcomes of care of patients with similar problems to the ones to be referred

NONCOMPLIANCE/MISMANAGEMENT

If it can be proven that there has been noncompliance with the plan of care (i.e., CMP) agreed on by the family, case manager, and members of the interdisciplinary team, then there may be a claim of mismanagement. It is important for providers, including case managers, to explain to the patient and family that certain complications or undesired outcomes may occur regardless of the efforts made to prevent them. It is also helpful to avoid providing false guarantees regarding outcomes of care, particularly when the situation at hand is considered to be high risk. False guarantees of this kind may be viewed as noncompliance with or mismanagement of the standards of care and practice. When guarantees are provided but not met, and the patient and/or family are able to prove that the guarantees were not met, the situation results in potential breach.

Case managers must practice within the realm of the responsibilities and scope of practice defined by the professional license that they hold and must not infer in any way that they are developing medical treatment plans for their patients. Any evident noncompliance with the regulations governing the practice of nursing

(or the discipline the case manager belongs to such as social work) may present potential problems, which may result in medical malpractice litigation. It may also be a potential problem wherein the case manager is viewed as practicing medicine. This can result in a disciplinary action and an impingement on the license (e.g., revocation, suspension, or probation).

DOCUMENTATION

A case manager must act as the patient's advocate and look out for what is in the patient's best interest. If it is determined that the physician and/or facility that the patient has been referred to is not properly performing or providing the services needed, then action to change the situation must be taken and should be documented so as to protect the provider. Documentation should occur when reviewing and evaluating credentials and performance of practitioners and facilities that patients have been referred to so that the case manager can determine if they are providing the appropriate levels of care needed by patients and families. In addition, follow-up documentation regarding actions taken to correct any identified problems must be evident, along with subsequent documentation of the outcomes of these corrective measures. Moreover, documentation must also include actions the case managers perform in addition to the referrals mentioned previously (e.g., patient/family teaching and counseling) and their related outcomes. Case Manager's Tip 16-2 presents some areas in which accurate and thorough documentation is considered critical in reducing malpractice litigation. Documentation serves multiple purposes, including the following:

- Evidence of the provision of care
- Justification of the need for referrals to specific providers
- Evaluation of the patient's condition in light of treatment
- Evidence that proper investigation of the qualifications, credentials, and competencies of healthcare providers is completed
- Communicating the plan of care of individual patients to the various healthcare team members
- Protection against litigation
- Assistance in determining whether the resources are being used appropriately
- Clarification of continuity of care after the hospital stay
- Summary of nursing and medical history for use in future admissions
- Reporting of data for quality of care review and risk management
- Reporting of data for continuing education and research

CASE MANAGER'S TIP 16-2

Areas in Which Documentation is Critical

1. Plan of care agreed on with patient and family
2. Medical stability of patient within 24 hours of discharge
3. Safety precautions
4. Falls
5. Restraints
6. Third-party (insurance) reimbursement
7. JCAHO accreditation of facility
8. Discharge planning and patient's readiness for discharge
9. Patient/family teaching
10. Informed consent
11. Disclosure of information
12. **Advance directives**
13. **Living wills**
14. Medical durable power of attorney
15. Reportable events (e.g., violent injuries, communicable diseases, abuse)
16. Do not resuscitate orders

- Review of data for billing and reimbursement purposes
- Recording care that forms the basis of evaluation by accreditation and regulatory agencies (e.g., the Joint Commission on Accreditation of Healthcare Organizations [JCAHO], state health departments, National Committee for Quality Assurance [NCQA], **Utilization Review Accreditation Commission [URAC]**)
- Legal evidence for use by the hospital, other healthcare providers, the patient and/or family, and members of the judicial system

CASE MANAGEMENT PLANS

Healthcare providers have raised concerns regarding the admissibility of CMPs as evidence in case of malpractice litigation. It has been noted by lawyers that when CMPs are used for documenting the provision of care (planning, implementing, and evaluating) and are made a permanent part of the patient's medical record, it is most certain that they will be admitted into court as evidence (Nolin and Lang, 1992).

A CMP is an interdisciplinary proactive set of daily prescriptions that has been prepared following a particular timeline to facilitate the care of a specific patient population from preadmission to postdischarge. The CMP identifies patient care activities that are thought to be required for providing care for a specific patient population. These activities are categorized as the assessments, treatments, teaching, **discharge planning,**

diagnostic tests, consultations, and interventions that should be completed for the patient's optimal recovery (see Chapter 12 for a detailed discussion). The CMP holds valuable evidence because it includes information (data and evidence) about the patient's projected and actual course of treatment. It includes the following:

- Patient's actual and potential problems
- Patient's projected and actual outcomes
- Medical interventions
- Nursing and other interventions
- Projected discharge times/target times
- Intermediate and discharge care outcomes

CMPs are usually developed by professional societies, healthcare institutions, insurance companies, or federal agencies. Sometimes they are called *clinical practice guidelines* or *practice parameters*. Professional societies and governmental agencies have developed practice guidelines to counteract or reduce the risk for liability and litigation (Holzer, 1990; Zweig and Witte, 1993). They are developed and used to improve the quality of care and reduce cost through standardizing practice. They are also helpful in reducing the cost of and risk for malpractice litigation through delineating the standard of care (West, 1994).

Once a CMP is admitted into court as evidence, it is thought to be an extremely powerful evidentiary tool used by the jury to determine the sequence of events (treatments and outcomes). If the provider was noted to have been compliant with the projections of the CMP and the documentation justifies the deviation from the CMP's recommendations, then the chances are that the provider's actions will be deemed appropriate and in compliance with the standard of care (Nolin and Lang, 1992). The key in this case is appropriate documentation of variances from the CMP.

The procedure followed in the development of a CMP affects the degree of its consideration by the jury and its reliability in the lawsuit. It is recommended that procedures be developed based on expert opinion, research, and the latest advents of treatment as recommended by professional societies and governmental agencies (Case Manager's Tip 16-3 contains a list of suggestions for CMPs). However, if a CMP is developed poorly and arbitrarily, it will hold no power in court and the standards of care will be judged as inappropriate. As a result the care provider will not be able to defend the case.

PATIENT CONFIDENTIALITY

As is any healthcare provider, case managers are obligated to safeguard the patient's privacy and confidentiality. Unauthorized disclosure of information is considered breach of confidentiality and may result in litigation.

CASE MANAGER'S TIP 16-3

Points to Remember About Case Management Plans

1. Can be presented as evidence if they are made part of the patient's medical record.
2. Improve communication among members of the healthcare team, thus reducing the risk for liability or litigation.
3. Can be determined by the injury as the standards of care.
4. Should allow for deviations. However, documentation in the medical record of variances related to the plan of care, including the medical and nursing plans, is important for reducing liability.
5. Help the jury describe the sequence of events (treatments and outcomes).
6. If developed by one healthcare organization, may be inappropriate for another organization.
7. Will not be admitted as evidence unless proven relevant to the case in question.
8. Should be flexible prescriptions and allow for deviations as long as they are justified.
9. Should be developed following a scientific method.
10. Standardize the care provided by multiple providers.

It is important for case managers to seek the guidance of a legal counsel before disclosing any information. In spite of confidentiality laws, reporting of certain events such as elder or child abuse, contagious disease, death, birth, and animal bites is mandatory and protected by federal laws. Some information requires the patient's permission for release (written and signed release). The release should delineate the name(s) of the party the information is to be released to. Examples of such information include the following:

- Drug or alcohol abuse treatment
- Mental health/psychiatric care
- Sexually transmitted diseases
- HIV or AIDS status
- Abortion
- Specific medical or surgical history

It is important for case managers to remember and respect patients' rights every time they face a legal or ethical dilemma or any challenges related to the provision of care. The patient has several rights that must not be forgotten (Box 16-4).

The case manager can play an important role in advocating on behalf of the patient and family. During such situations, the case manager should always remain aware of the patient's legal rights, as well as issues of confidentiality pertaining to patient care.

BOX 16-4   Patient Rights

1. Right to access to needed health and social services
2. Right to treatment with dignity and respect
3. Right to confidentiality
4. Right to privacy
5. Right to know cost of services
6. Right to self-determination
7. Right to comprehensive and fair assessment
8. Right to notification of discharge, termination, or change of service
9. Right to withdraw from a case management program
10. Right to a grievance procedure
11. Right to choose a particular community services agency or long-term care provider

CMPs can serve an important function in protecting the rights of both the patient and the healthcare provider. Special attention should be paid to the process of their development, their use, and the way documentation is incorporated into them.

 KEY POINTS

1. Case managers can be held liable. They should be aware of the legal process and the legal terminology used.
2. CMPs are admissible in court. They can be reviewed by the jury to determine the standard of care followed at the time care was provided.
3. CMPs should be developed following a scientific and evidence-based process.
4. The use of case management systems in patient care delivery may reduce the cost of malpractice litigation.
5. Thorough documentation in the medical record is extremely important. The patient's medical record and the CMP used can be admissible in court as evidence.
6. Case managers can curtail legal risk by being proactive in their role (e.g., by anticipating and preventing variances or delays in care delivery and outcomes).

REFERENCES

Holzer JF: The advent of clinical standards for professional liability, *Qual Rev Bull* 16(2):71-79, 1990.

Merz SM: Clinical practice guidelines: policy issues and legal implications, *J Qual Improve* 19(8):306-311, 1993.

Nichols DJ: Legal liabilities in case management. In Flarey DL, Smith-Blancett S: *Handbook of case management,* Gaithersburg, Md, 1996, Aspen.

Nolin CE, Lang CG: *An analysis of the use and effect of caremap tools in medical malpractice litigation,* South Natick, Mass, 1992, The Center for Case Management, Inc.

West JC: The legal implications of medical practice guidelines, *J Health Hosp Law* 27(4):97-103, 1994.

Zweig FM, Witte HA: Assisting judges in screening medical practice guidelines for health care litigation, *J Qual Improve* 19(8):342-353, 1993.

17 Application of Legal Concepts to Case Management Practice

Kathleen A. Lambert, BSN, RN, JD

SOURCES OF ANXIETY FOR TODAY'S CASE MANAGERS

Busy case managers can reduce the anxiety associated with the **risk** of legal action by gaining knowledge of the elements of **malpractice** lawsuits, applying the standards of care and **case management** in their practice, being cognizant of the areas that have increasingly been receiving legal attention and scrutiny, and understanding the importance of accurate and timely communication and documentation.

Case managers must "wear many hats" and instantly switch focus in their role as required by the situation at hand. By virtue of the complexity of the role, the **case manager** may end up being everything to everyone: a nurse, social worker, psychologist/counselor, clergyperson, marketing specialist, communicator, translator of medical terminology, navigator of the healthcare system and insurance plans, expert in policies and **coding** practices, accountant, **quality assurance** specialist, lawyer, advocate, mediator, negotiator, educator, and occupational and physical therapist. Because of the diversity of this role and its functions, the case manager must possess creativity, patience, and wisdom. Once all these elements have been artfully combined, the product is then a competent case manager who can be successful in his or her role.

The new paradigm of healthcare management and delivery has grown away from the old paternalistic view of the "doctor knows best," which focused on the treatment of the symptoms, with the goal of achieving a cure. In the old paradigm the patient was dependent, and his or her body, mind, and spirit were viewed as separate entities. The patient chose his or her doctor and hospital, and cost was not a factor in the decision-making process. The new paradigm focuses on the patient as an autonomous human being, with the healthcare professional (e.g., case manager) assuming the role of therapeutic partner and counselor.

Today's emphasis is on promoting healthy lifestyles, with attention paid to patterns, causes, and treatments of illnesses and reduction of their associated risk factors. The body, mind, and spirit are viewed as one integrated entity. Patients are approached for care as total beings rather than the focus being only on the diseased organ. The presence of the case manager in today's healthcare system makes it easier for the patient/family to navigate the systems; survive the challenges; and stay informed of the constantly changing rules, regulations, and demands.

Modern healthcare is a business, and access to care may depend on having health insurance coverage. A patient's choice of physicians or other providers may be limited by coverage restrictions within the patient's plan. Cost-effectiveness is a constant focus of attention for payers and providers alike. A long-term relationship with a particular physician is no longer the norm. Patients cannot be certain that their health plan will continue to include their favorite hospital or physician. Loyalty to healthcare personnel with whom a patient has established a familiar and natural relationship is dwindling, and so is the patient's reluctance to file a lawsuit.

If patients feel that their rights have been violated or that the care they have received is below acceptable standards, they are most likely to sue the healthcare provider or agency (Box 17-1). There exists a mentality in society known today as *lawsuit lottery*—the chance to strike it rich by filing the right lawsuit. Headlines shout

BOX 17-1   The Most Common Reasons for Why People Sue

1. Sense of grief and loss
2. Financial gain
3. Presence of real harm/damage
4. Unanticipated bad results
5. Need to punish the provider or the healthcare facility
6. Suggestions from friends or others who have sued and won

From Blanche NM: *Liability issues for case managers,* Issues and Trends in Nursing Case Management Conference, Princeton, NJ, June, 1998.

about elderly people suing fast food chains for exorbitant amounts of money for hot coffee spilled in their laps (Ruiz, 1995). These types of lawsuits increase the likelihood that patients may sue their provider if they are not satisfied with their care or feel cheated in some way. It is not surprising to learn of patients suing their healthcare provider or organization for astronomical amounts of money for suspicion of harm, even though most of the time these suspicions are unfounded.

Presently, increasing numbers of nurses and case managers are being named in lawsuits. This may be because patients are becoming more knowledgeable about healthcare and therefore their expectations with regard to what type of care they may expect to receive is higher. Healthcare professionals are no longer the sole source of health-related information. It has become common for patients and their family members to show up for their appointments with information they have downloaded from the **Internet** on the signs and symptoms of a specific disease or a variety of treatment modalities that they think might be effective.

Case managers now have greater exposure to potential lawsuits because healthcare systems are increasingly reliant on nurses and other providers, in addition to doctors, to help contain costs and provide responsible care. Furthermore, nurses and social workers are becoming more autonomous in their practice, especially in the area of case management. This autonomy increases the chance that they will be named in a lawsuit.

The nursing shortage is affecting all systems of healthcare delivery. Efforts to contain costs have led many healthcare institutions to downsize while the workloads of those remaining behind have increased, resulting in greater risk for legal action. While the workforce has been downsized, caseloads have increased. Patient caseloads are a primary factor in the quality of case management outcomes. The larger the caseload, the less likely it is for case managers to meet the expectations of delivering high-quality, safe, and efficient healthcare services. Reportedly, the average active monthly case-

load of case managers may range from 16 to 75 cases (Executive Summary Case Management Caseload Data, 2001). This is dependent on the following:
- The organizational vision, mission, and values statements
- The systems and processes of case management
- The goals and the definition of case management services
- The acuity of the client population served
- The experience, knowledge, and training of case managers
- The types of interactions between case managers, providers, and clients
- The resources available to the case manager for handling the daily workload

Many professionals have chosen to leave their practice because of increasing workload, undesirable working conditions and pressures, and high consumer demands. Most often these characteristics of the work environment put the case manager at increased risk for **litigation** and loss of professional license. The laws affecting healthcare are changing, and the threat of lawsuits and disciplinary actions against the professional's license remain a silent threat to those who continue to practice.

Historically the most common causes of legal actions against nurses are patient falls and medication errors. Malpractice payments related to lawsuits brought forth against nurses are relatively rare. According to the National Practitioner Data Bank (NPDB), registered nurses have been responsible for 1.7% of all payments made over the history of the NPDB (U.S. Department of Health and Human Services, 2000). Issues related to undesirable nursing practices in the areas of patient monitoring, treatment, and medication administration are the reasons behind most of the lawsuits and payments. However, these payments do not include the practice of specialized nurses: nurse practitioners, nurse anesthetists, and nurse midwives. No data bank is available yet regarding lawsuits filed directly against case managers because case management is still considered a fairly new area of practice.

According to the American Nurses Association, the average award in a claim against a nurse is $145,000. The highest award has been $5 million against a nurse who gave 10 times the correct dose of lidocaine because she failed to read the label (Catalano et al, 1996). More recently the 2000 Cumulative Data from the NPDB revealed that the median amount awarded in a claim against a nurse was $66,951, and the highest amount was $11 million for an obstetrics case. Other awards were $8 million for improper management of a surgical patient and $6 million for failure to monitor and report on significant changes in a patient's condition (U.S. Department of Health and Human Services, 2000).

Although these types of lawsuits do not relate directly to the practice of case management and the role of the case manager, they have some implications for case managers. As discussed in Chapter 4, one dimension of the role of the case manager is clinical **care management.** This role function focuses on the assessment, coordination, facilitation, monitoring, and evaluation of patient care delivery and outcomes. In this role function, case managers are expected to communicate with the patient and family, physician, and other members of the healthcare team regarding the patient's progress, nuances in medical condition, and responses to treatment. Therefore case managers can be held accountable and responsible for timely communication with the healthcare team. If they fail to do so, they are at risk for litigation, especially if their lack of or delay in communication results in harm to the patient.

The implementation of the case manager's role is thought to reduce the risk for litigation rather than increase it. This is attributed to the fact that the case manager acts as a patient and family advocate, integrator of care and services, and risk manager. Furthermore, the case manager is expected to act proactively to prevent legal risk by exercising his or her established duties as defined in the scope of practice.

BASIS FOR ASSIGNING LIABILITY IN CASE MANAGEMENT

Case managers have duties that derive from the activities in which they are involved and as defined in their job description and scope of practice. Because the law acknowledges that case management is a reasonable activity, case managers can and will be held accountable for their actions in relation to their patients. The law will hold the case manager to the reasonable standard of care for case managers. Case managers must function within the scope of their **licensure,** training, and education, as well as their level of competence. They act as consultants to patients and physicians or other healthcare providers. By virtue of this role, they are able to indirectly reduce litigation risk.

Although they cannot interfere with the doctor-patient relationship, case managers have a fiduciary duty to communicate accurately and in a timely manner to both parties, especially in the situation of changes in the patient's condition that warrant immediate attention and potential change in the treatment plan. If there is contradictory information, the case manager needs to work diligently with the patient and family or **caregiver** and the healthcare team to determine the truth and initiate appropriate action.

 CASE MANAGER'S TIP 17-1

Conflicting Obligations of Case Managers
Liability in the case manager's role arises from the inability to integrate care when conflicting obligations are present. Examples of obligations the case manager has that may be in conflict are as follows:
- Patient advocacy
- Organizational advocacy
- Quality assurance and improvement
- Cost-effectiveness or containment
- Coordination of services
- Brokerage of services
- Contractual obligations to employer
- Contractual obligations to payers
- Laws and regulations

Liability in case management arises from the fact that case managers are integrators of care delivery. As integrators, they are expected to build relationships with the patient, the payer, and the provider (i.e., the physician and/or the healthcare agency). Liability may arise from interrelating these parties (Case Manager's Tip 17-1).

THE DIFFERENCE BETWEEN NEGLIGENCE AND MALPRACTICE

Before reviewing some of the areas of litigation in case management, it is important to differentiate negligence from malpractice (Box 17-2). **Negligence** is an act or conduct that falls below the acceptable standard established by law for the protection of others against unreasonable risk of harm. It is a departure from the conduct expected of a reasonably prudent person under similar circumstances. Claims of negligence can be brought against any member of the case management team. In contrast, malpractice is the failure to render professional services or to exercise that degree of skill and learning commonly applied under all circumstances in the community by the average prudent reputable

---

BOX 17-2   Negligence and Malpractice

Negligence is the failure to act as an ordinary prudent person would act in the given circumstances; applies to the acts of both laymen and professionals.
Malpractice is professional misconduct, improper discharge of duties, or failure to meet the standards of care expected of a reasonably prudent member of the profession in his or her dealings with the patient/family that causes harm to the patient.

member of the profession. However, such an act is considered negligence only if it results in injury, loss, or damage to the recipient of those services or to those entitled to rely on them. Negligence is also defined as any professional misconduct, unreasonable lack of skill or fidelity in professional or fiduciary duties, evil practice, or illegal or immoral conduct.

Only those who are involved in a professional career can have a claim of malpractice brought against them. According to the law, a profession is a vocation or occupation that requires special, usually advanced, education or skill and a confidential relationship with the client. A case manager is considered a professional and is held to professional standards.

The elements of proof are the same for both negligence and malpractice: duty, breach, cause, injury, and damages (refer to Chapter 16 for more details). The difference in proof is in the standard of care. One must establish the "reasonable man standard" first before an action is labeled as negligence. The standard of care for a case manager goes beyond a reasonable man standard and must be established in court so that the jury can determine whether there is liability for the case manager.

ESTABLISHING THE STANDARD OF CARE FOR THE CASE MANAGER

The standard of care measures the competence of the professional. Because a jury is not composed entirely of healthcare professionals, it is necessary to first teach the jury what a case manager does. This is done through a review of certain documents (Box 17-3) that result in establishing or clarifying the standard of care. Once the definition and role of the case manager are established in court, the jury uses this information as a template against which the follow-up information will be compared and contrasted. The jury uses the template to put

---

BOX 17-3 Sources of the Standard of Care Used in a Lawsuit

The standard of care is established by reviewing the following:
- The state nurse practice act or the practice act of other professions if the person involved in the lawsuit is not a nurse (e.g., a social worker)
- The Standards of Practice of Case Management
- Journal articles and books
- Standards from professional organizations
- Certification standards
- Expert witnesses' testimony
- A review of the applicable policies and procedures from the organization for which the case manager works

---

the facts of the case into perspective. This enables the jury to determine if the behavior of the case manager was within or outside the standard of care for case management.

For example, the standard of care requires the case manager to inform the physician of anything significant brought to the case manager's attention by the patient, family, or staff or that the case manager personally observed or assessed. If the case manager fails to meet this expectation, he or she is committing malpractice and can be found guilty of malpractice if a lawsuit is brought forward. To illustrate, the following is an example of what can happen when the patient situation is not fully communicated to the physician. In this Georgia case, the **plaintiff** claimed that the nurse was partially responsible for the baby's resulting lifelong disability because of her failure to fully communicate with the physician. A baby boy who had recently been diagnosed with a respiratory infection spiked a fever of 104° F, became limp, and began panting and moaning. His mother called the after-hours phone number of her managed care plan and spoke to the triage nurse. The nurse advised a cool bath while she contacted the on-call physician. The nurse told the pediatrician that she had ruled out respiratory distress in the baby but neglected to inform the physician of the baby's symptoms of panting and moaning. As a result, the pediatrician did not consider the baby's condition to be critical and directed the nurse to have the mother take her baby to a children's medical center 40 miles from home. The baby had a cardiopulmonary arrest en route to the facility and was diverted to a nearby hospital, where he was revived. However, the color never returned to his extremities. Gangrene developed, and the baby's hands and part of each leg had to be amputated. Meningococcemia was the diagnosis. The baby's family sued the managed care plan, claiming negligence on the part of the nurse and the physician because of the delayed treatment that could have prevented the gangrene. The jury awarded $45 million in this case (Sullivan, 1996).

The nurse has a duty, both to the client and physician, to relay as accurate a description of the patient as possible. If the nurse is in the role of **gatekeeper,** as is the case with many **health maintenance organizations (HMOs),** triage nurses and case managers, clinics, and private practices, the physician must depend solely on the input of the nurse to make his or her own medical judgment (Case Manager's Tip 17-2). This puts the nurse and the case manager in a position of responsibility and accountability not only for their practice but also for the actions taken by other providers based on their actions (Case Manager's Tip 17-3).

CASE MANAGER'S TIP 17-2

Communication Strategies That Reduce Legal Risk

It is the case manager's duty to communicate to the physician any changes in the patient's condition, the plan of care, or the transitional plan. A reasonable and prudent case manager prevents communication breakdown. Examples of strategies case managers can apply to reduce legal risk associated with miscommunication are as follows:

- Convey a message using the exact words used by the patient to describe a situation or symptom(s).
- Share impressions or opinions about the situation.
- Stick to the facts.
- Be clear, accurate, and complete with the message.
- Communicate promptly.
- Communicate anyway, even if unsure.
- Repeat the information if necessary.

The case of *Darling v. Charleston Community Memorial Hospital* (33 Ill 2d 326, 211 N.E. 2d 253, 1965; cert. Denied, 383 U.S. 946, 1966) taught the nursing profession that just reporting observations to the attending physician is not enough. If the treating doctor does not take action in a serious situation, the nurse has the affirmative duty to take that information up the chain of command to get help for the client. What is the chain of command for the case manager? Check your organization for its chain of command. However, normally the chain of command would start with the immediate manager, then the department's supervisor/administrator, and may end with the department's physician advisor, or the chief of medical services for the agency or facility.

CASE MANAGEMENT "HOT SPOTS" THAT HAVE ALREADY RECEIVED LEGAL REVIEW

Case managers are at increasing risk for legal action because of the nature of their role. As the scope of their practice and accountability increases, so does their risk (Case Manager's Tip 17-4). This section reviews some of the areas in case management practice that have been noticed to receive legal attention more than others (Box 17-4). One area that presents increased legal risk is **negligent referral,** which is a **claim** that is usually brought about when there is a large network of providers. Getting the patient into the appropriate case manager's caseload is the best starting point. For example, if a patient is admitted to the hospital and diagnosed with new onset diabetes, the patient may be placed on a diabetes clinical pathway while hospitalized. The inpatient

 CASE MANAGER'S TIP 17-3

Causation

Case managers are rarely involved in actual causation cases. Instead, they are involved in proximate causation that results from dealing inappropriately with many different parties, factors, and/or obligations at the same time, and their acts or behaviors contribute to the harm or damage the patient experiences.

From Blanche NM: *Liability issues for case managers,* Issues and Trends in Nursing Case Management Conference, Princeton, NJ, June, 1998.

 CASE MANAGER'S TIP 17-4

Be Aware of the Law in Your Locality

Healthcare laws and regulations may vary from one state to another. Case managers are advised to remain aware of their state laws and statutes and the latest related changes. Information about the laws and regulations are available and easily accessible on the Internet, on governmental and state-based Websites. Consultation with the risk management and legal departments is recommended if the case manager is unsure about a situation or has any concerns.

BOX 17-4   Areas of Increased Litigation in Case Management

1. Negligent referral
2. Failure to investigate a claim
3. Failure to communicate or document
4. Inadequate or premature patient discharge
5. Fraud and abuse
6. End-of-life decisions and surrogate decision making
7. Denial of services
8. Breach of confidentiality

---

case manager may follow the patient. A referral to the appropriate disease state case manager may then be placed so that he or she can follow the patient after discharge. The patient is also screened for his or her risk level at the **primary care** site to determine the frequency of interactions and follow-up with the disease state case manager. If a patient has a poor **outcome,** all parties involved in the patient's care will come under scrutiny, including perhaps those who made a referral to the contracted provider involved in the claim.

As a patient advocate, the case manager must always act in the best interest of the patient. The case manager must document that a reasonable evaluation was completed to determine the need for a referral, if one is being made. To protect the case manager and the employer from liability related to the provider offering the referred services, the healthcare organization must have a method in place to review the credentials, **certifications,** and documented complaints of all providers used in the referral process. The organization must make sure that the client and family are given several options so that they make the choice that is best for them. An effective strategy is to have a resource manual of providers (e.g., provider panel) available for use by patients and their families or caregivers when a referral is warranted.

Failure to investigate a claim: This usually arises out of contract law. The client has received a **denial** of service and claims that the case manager did not act in good faith when reviewing the medical record. Two cases, *Taylor v. Prudential Insurance Company* and *Aetna Life Insurance Company v. Lovoie*, have been reported (Sturgeon, 1997) in this type of lawsuit. In both cases the jury based its decisions on the case of "incomplete information": sharing of incomplete information with the managed care organization (MCO) and the MCO's failing to examine the claim thoroughly. Both insurers were found liable, and the juries ruled in favor of the clients. To avoid similar lawsuits, an MCO must have a formal process in place for claims review. It also must gather all of the pertinent data before a decision is made (i.e., denial of services) and be able to clearly show the basis of the decision to the client. Applying these strategies diligently assists the case manager and the insurer in the defense against this kind of claim (Powell, 2000).

Failure to communicate and/or document: This is an accusation that should never have to occur. Case managers do so much for their patients and their families, but sometimes they fail to reflect their efforts in the patient's medical record. The medical record must always reflect all of the interventions made on behalf of, or for, the patient. However, case managers must be careful in their documentation and focus only on the facts (Case Manager's Tip 17-5). An easy way to remember what to document is to apply the *ABCs* of documentation: accurate, brief, and complete. This way of documentation includes the following:

■ Identity/role of those involved in the patient's care
■ Consultations and consultants
■ How care decisions are made and incorporated in the plan of care
■ Clarifications about certain conflicting or confusing situations

 CASE MANAGER'S TIP 17-5

Strategies for Better Documentation
■ Document legibly. If the information is in the record but it cannot be deciphered, it is worthless and may even be the source of an error.
■ Record information in the medical record promptly. The lapse of time will increase the margin of error.
■ Make sure that the record reflects the fact that the physician is driving the care and heading up the team.
■ The medical record should reflect every transaction that occurs over the course of case management.
■ Be specific, factual, complete, and accurate.
■ Use descriptive terms for behaviors rather than generalizations.
■ Document the plan of care and the transitional plan, including the postdischarge services arranged for.
■ Document the patient's responses to treatments.
■ Use quotations (exact words used by the patient/ family) when appropriate.
■ Document refusals of treatments and options.
■ Document consents to treatments.
■ Record patient and family education activities.
■ Be clear when recording the goals of treatment and the plan for meeting them.

■ Follow-up on issues, especially those related to changes in the patient's condition
■ Consent to or refusal of treatment

Inadequate or premature discharge: When planning transitional care, make sure that the patient is stable for discharge. The Health Care Financing Administration (HCFA), now known as the Centers for Medicare and Medicaid Services (CMS), detailed six stability markers to note 24 hours before discharge from the hospital. If any of these markers is present at the time of discharge, the discharge is considered inappropriate. These markers are as follows:
1. Parameters for temperature: >101° F orally or 102° F rectally
2. Parameters for pulse: >120 beats/min or <45 beats/ min with or <50 beats/min without beta blockers
3. Parameters for blood pressure: systolic <85 or >180 mm Hg; diastolic <50 or >110 mm Hg
4. Intravenous (IV) fluids and medications after midnight or on the day of discharge
5. Presence of a wound that has bloody or purulent discharge
6. Abnormal test results that have not already been addressed

To prevent the legal risk associated with inappropriate or premature discharge, the case manager must notify the physician in the event that the patient's vital signs fall out of these ranges, test results are abnormal, or there is the presence of discharge from wounds. If the physician still approves of the patient's discharge, documentation of such should be present in the medical record. In this case, the case manager must ensure that plans for follow-up care are arranged for. The case manager must also educate the patient and family about the need for follow-up care and document these interventions and the physician's response in the medical record (Powell, 2000).

In reviewing the transitional care plan, consider whether the plan is appropriate to the patient and that it meets the patient's physical, emotional, social, mental health, and safety needs. Documentation of the discharge plan must include the following:

- Patient/family/caregiver's consent to the plan and communications with patient and family
- Patient responses to interventions
- Contacts with other providers and agencies, as well as names, dates, times, and agreements with them
- Patient limitations and refusals of care
- Any changes in the plan
- Arrangements for the use of **durable medical equipment** (DME) in the home
- Educational needs and instructions provided about medications and other treatments: what to watch for and what symptoms to report immediately to the physician or nurse; also include outcomes such as patient understanding of teaching

A thorough patient assessment at discharge is critical because it prevents a premature discharge from inadvertently occurring. If significant issues or recent changes in the patient's condition were identified, the case manager could then stop the discharge and address them with the physician and the healthcare team.

Close to the claim of premature discharge would be a claim of negligence due to the delay in patient transfer. In the case *Henry v. Felici,* (758 S.W. 2d 836 Texas, 1988) a 3-year-old child died as a result of delay in transfer to another facility for computed tomography (CT) scan and surgery. The court found that the nurses who are given the responsibility to implement a transfer have a duty to see to it that the transfer is made in accordance with the physician's order and as required by the patient's condition. If for any reason beyond the control of the nurses a **complication** or delay in implementing an order is anticipated, the nurses have the clear and unequivocal responsibility to immediately inform the attending physician so that he or she may take whatever action is deemed appropriate under the circumstances. In this case, the nurses failed to inform the physician.

Fraud and abuse: These are claims that can carry severe penalties for the perpetrators. Case managers can prevent fraud and abuse practices by appropriately exercising their responsibility and accountability toward patient care planning, delivery, coordination, and management. Fraud is intentional deception or misrepresentation that could result in some unauthorized benefit. The most common type of fraud arises from a false statement or misrepresentation that is material to entitlement or payment under the **Medicare** program. The violator may be a provider, a supplier of DME, a beneficiary, or some other person or business entity. Fraud in the Medicare program may take the following forms:

- Billing for services or supplies that were not provided
- Altering claim forms to obtain a higher payment amount
- Deliberately applying for duplicate payments
- Soliciting, offering, or receiving a kickback, bribe, or rebate
- Misrepresenting the services rendered
- Misrepresenting the diagnosis of the patient to justify the services or the equipment furnished
- Use of another person's Medicare card in obtaining medical care (HCFA, 1998)

The Healthcare Integrity and Protection Data Bank (HIPDB) is the new data bank created to combat fraud and abuse in health insurance and healthcare delivery. It is a national data collection program for reporting and disclosure of certain final adverse actions taken against healthcare providers, suppliers, and practitioners. The HIPDB is a nationwide flagging system that may serve primarily as an alert to users indicating that a comprehensive review of the provider's, supplier's, or practitioner's past actions may be prudent (Healthcare Integrity and Protection Data Bank, 2001).

The word *abuse* is used to describe incidents or practices of providers that are inconsistent with accepted sound medical, business, or fiscal practices. These practices may directly or indirectly result in unnecessary costs to the services provided, improper payment, or payment for services that fail to meet professionally recognized standards of care or that are medically unnecessary. Examples of abuse include overutilization of medical and healthcare services, unbundled or exploded charges, excessive charges for DME, claims for services not **medically necessary** or not medically necessary to the extent furnished (HCFA, 1998).

A New York judge allowed to proceed a class action suit that claimed that an HMO committed fraud and breach of contract by allowing nonphysicians to make decisions about lengths of hospital stay. Two plaintiffs brought the lawsuit on behalf of themselves and other subscribers to the HMO or its subsidiary. The lead plaintiff alleged that while she was in the hospital being treated for Crohn's disease, her physician recommended that she remain in the hospital for additional tests. However, the HMO denied coverage for the extra hospital stay, and she was discharged. One month later, the plaintiff was hospitalized again for a ruptured intestine. She contended that this condition would not have occurred had she been allowed to remain in the hospital for further tests. The plaintiff claimed that this decision was not made by a physician but by a "concurrent review nurse," or clinical reviewer, based on actuarial guidelines. The plaintiff argued that the HMO's promotional materials had represented that decisions of medical necessity were made by trained physicians *(Batas v. Prudential Insurance Company of America)* (No. 107881/97, NY, Sup. Ct. NY City, May 20). The plaintiff won this lawsuit. In a case such as this the case manager can prevent such legal risk by applying good and responsible **utilization review** and management practices (Case Manager's Tip 17-6).

The National Center on Elder Abuse (Brandl and Raymond, 1997) estimates that nearly 1 million elder Americans were victims of domestic abuse each year over the last decade, and in reported cases of elder abuse, two thirds of the victims were women. Generally, caregiver stress is the root cause of elder abuse, but more recent research has shown that many abusers are not caregivers; instead they are financially or emotionally dependent on their victims. A significant portion of elder abuse is spousal abuse, often occurring for many years. Only one in eight instances of elder abuse and neglect are reported to elder protective services or other authorities (Brandl and Raymond, 1997).

The case manager has an affirmative duty to report known or suspected cases of elder abuse to the local investigating agency. Many times, because of his or her experience in patient assessment and **transitional planning,** the case manager may be able to identify a potentially stressful situation that could lead to abuse and intervene to change the outcome. The agency or facility should have policies and procedures to guide the case manager in reporting and assisting in the investigation of suspected abuse. Protective reporting laws exist to protect the professional against defamation claims when reporting abuse or neglect.

End-of-life decisions and surrogate decision making: These are two topics that have the potential for legal entanglements, especially when the patient's wishes are not followed. The Patient Self-Determination Act of 1991 (Sections 4206 and 4751 of the Omnibus Reconciliation Act of 1990, Public Law 101-508, November 1990) requires that hospitals, nursing homes, HMOs, home healthcare agencies, and other healthcare facilities receiving Medicare and **Medicaid** funds have policies and procedures in place with regard to advance directives. It also requires healthcare providers and agencies to inform their patients of their rights under state law to make decisions concerning treatment or nontreatment. **Advance directives** are legal documents that are drawn up by patients for use in case they become incompetent or incapacitated. The information included in advance directives refers to decisions regarding the execution, withholding, or withdrawing of medical treatment (Perin, 1992).

An advance directive can be a **living will,** a Medical Health Care Power of Attorney, or a document that combines the two. To prevent legal risk, information received from the patient about the existence of the advance directive must be present in the medical record at all times. In addition, all members of the healthcare team must be aware of its presence and act by it as they make decisions regarding the patient's care and treatment options. Healthcare providers, including case managers, are expected to not discriminate against a patient who does or does not have an advance directive (Perin, 1992).

Some states recognize another document known as a Prehospital Advance Directive that directs prehospital caregivers regarding the patient's wishes for resuscitation outside of the acute care setting. In many states,

 CASE MANAGER'S TIP 17-6

Strategies for Better Utilization Review and Management

- Follow the policies and procedures of your organization consistently.
- Apply the criteria of utilization review and transitional planning adequately and in all cases.
- Apply the stipulations of the managed care contract that relate to the case in review.
- Be timely in your review and communications with appropriate parties (e.g., managed care case manager, provider-based case manager, physician, administrators, patient and family).
- Document all transactions.
- When unsure, always ask for clarification or help.
- If you disagree with a denial of service, appeal to review it with the responsible party in a supervisory role.
- Always apply the ethical and legal principles in your practice.

the statutes will identify the persons able to act as surrogate decision-makers in the absence of the written directives and when the patient is incompetent or unable to do so himself or herself. Problems arise when there is disagreement with the patient's directives and the patient is unconscious and failing, when the document cannot be located, or when the surrogate decision-maker is at odds with other family members. Knowing the state law and the institutional policies and procedures about advance directives and surrogate decision making are the case manager's best defenses against these types of legal entanglements. Knowing the client's status regarding resuscitation is another.

In one case, *Allore v. Flower Hospital* (121 Ohio App3d 229, 1997), the client had signed a living will and then went into respiratory distress during the night. The nurse was unaware of the living will and there was no copy on record; therefore the nurse initiated lifesaving measures while trying to reach the patient's doctor. The patient died in the intensive care unit (ICU) later that day, but the patient's estate sued claiming medical malpractice and medical battery arising from wrongful administration of life-prolonging treatment. The court held that the nurse complied with applicable standards of care regarding emergency care in the absence of knowledge of existing directives and that there was no battery because the patient had signed a consent for treatment when he entered the hospital. As a result the estate could not recover any damages. Educating clients on the value of advance directives and making their wishes clear to those involved in their care is an important job of the case manager.

Denial of service: This is never received well by patients. Often the case manager acts as a mediator when dealing with denials of services by an MCO. To mediate successfully and effectively, case managers must be knowledgeable about the denials and appeals processes, patient's bill of rights, and state laws that govern the operations of MCOs. In *Payton v. Aetna U.S. Healthcare,* attorney Robert Payton sought coverage from his Aetna U.S. Healthcare HMO for inpatient rehabilitation for substance abuse in January 1998 while hospitalized for a first-time drug overdose (*Payton v. Aetna U.S. Healthcare,* 100440/99). When the company did not respond, he repeatedly requested coverage and reimbursement, as did his treatment facilities. The requests were denied. In June 1998 he filed a formal complaint with the state attorney general. Within 6 weeks the state attorney general notified Aetna that Payton's individual policy "plainly" covered inpatient substance abuse rehabilitation. Payton also filed a grievance with Aetna. An internal appeals hearing decided that he was entitled to coverage. However, by that time

Payton had been deceased for 8 days after a second drug overdose. Payton's estate sued Aetna, charging that the HMO was responsible for his death as a result of negligently delaying coverage (Riccardi, 2000).

Some of the decisions case managers make may result in professional liability, depending on the outcomes of these decisions and their effect on the patient (Case Manager's Tip 17-7). To avoid legal action related to professional liability similar to the cases discussed, case managers, whether they work for an MCO or a healthcare provider, have an obligation to act as a patient advocate, especially in negotiating decisions regarding services and financial coverage. If a conflict arises, case managers should refer the situation to their superiors so that it can be dealt with appropriately. They may refer the situation to the **risk management** department or the lawyer as a potential litigation situation so that legal risk is avoided or prevented. A proactive approach such as this usually works in favor of both the patient and the healthcare organization.

A judge ordered $120.5 million in the case of *Teresa Goodrich v. Aetna US Healthcare of California* (Robbins, 1999). This is the largest award against a **managed care** company to date. The case dealt with denying payment for treatment that was deemed experimental. No mention or explanation of this term was given in the 20-page handbook that Aetna members were given, even though this was the justification of the denial. *Nelene Fox v. Healthnet* (Thomasma and Marshall, 1997) is another case that involved "experimental procedures" that resulted in an award of $89.3 million to the plaintiff. The final outcome in both cases was the death of the patient. A rule of thumb for preventing such cases of litigation is that case managers must always advocate for their patients. The healthcare community can no longer maximize financial concerns at the expense of patient concerns.

MCOs have a duty to inform patients of their right to appeal insurance denials. Many times it is the case

---

 CASE MANAGER'S TIP 17-7

Case Manager's Professional Obligations and Liability

A case manager is obligated to participate actively in the patient's medical management and care decisions to ensure quality healthcare in the most cost-efficient manner. If the case manager's decisions result in harm to the patient, denial of an essential service (i.e., diagnostic or therapeutic procedure or test), or interference with or corruption of acceptable medical judgment, there may be grounds for professional liability.

manager who informs the patient of the **appeal** and grievance processes. It is not uncommon for a request for service to be denied because of a lack of some important information. Case managers must communicate clearly, thoroughly, and in a timely fashion with regard to the patient's condition and the medical necessity of the service or equipment.

Sometimes a letter from the physician or a conference call with the MCO (e.g., physician-to-physician review) successfully clarifies a point of conflict. In other instances, the sharing of pictures or consumer letters may be needed. Case managers must remember that they cannot resolve every conflict or denial. Sometimes no amount of information is enough to reverse or prevent a denial, and a full appeal process becomes the only option for the patient. In situations where denial of a service is unavoidable and the case manager feels that the patient truly needs the service, the case manager may try to obtain charitable contributions from agencies that provide the needed service. It is advisable that case managers keep information on such resources available for use when needed.

Breach of confidentiality: This is a claim that can sometimes bring severe consequences for the claimant. A former patient of a reputable hospital claims that the medical institution ruined his life by giving information about his psychiatric troubles to a disgruntled former friend without his permission/consent. He is suing the institution for $12 million. The former patient says that the hospital released his medical records to a former friend and business partner who claimed to be him. The former colleague then shared the information about his drug abuse problems with his other friends, family, business associates, and clients (Graham, 2001).

The claim in this case according to the court documents is that the plaintiff has suffered, and continues to suffer, severe injury to his personal and professional reputation and standing in the community, loss of business, physical stress, and mental and emotional anguish and humiliation. This claim is made based on the argument that the plaintiff's suffering is a direct and proximate result of the hospital's unauthorized disclosure of medical records. However, the hospital states that it acted in good faith and that the request for the medical records had all the requisite information. They believe that the signature on the request was a forgery. The trial is currently pending (Graham, 2001). Case managers can safeguard a patient's confidentiality by reinforcing compliance with the law and regulations regarding disclosure of information and the patient's bill of rights (Case Manager's Tips 17-8 and 17-9).

Healthcare is one of the most personal services rendered in our society, yet to deliver this care, scores of

 CASE MANAGER'S TIP 17-8

Confidential Information
Information shared by the patient with the case manager or any other member of the healthcare team is considered confidential and privileged and must not be shared with an unauthorized party without the patient's consent/knowledge. This information is usually shared under circumstances of trust and confidence. Examples of such information are medical history; medications intake; results of the medical/physical examination; information gathered by assessment, observation, and monitoring; and treatments and procedures.

 CASE MANAGER'S TIP 17-9

Safeguarding the Patient's Privacy and Confidentiality
■ Abide by the law at all times.
■ Have the patient/family/caregiver sign a release of information before any information is shared with other parties.
■ Ensure moral and ethical conduct at all times.
■ Exercise the duty to treat patients with decency, respect, and utmost privacy.
Exceptions to the Privacy Rule are as follows:
■ When the patient is a public figure whose actions are considered to be of legitimate interest to the public
■ Duty to communicate communicable diseases, child or elder abuse cases, domestic violence cases, and/or bioterrorism to appropriate law enforcement authorities

From Bernzweig EP: *The nurse's liability for malpractice: a programmed course,* ed 5, St Louis, 1990, Mosby.

personnel must have access to intimate patient information. In return, the healthcare provider must safeguard the patient's confidentiality and right to privacy at all times. In the case of *Hobbs v. Lopez* (645 N.E. 2d 261 OH, 1994), a 21-year-old woman was seen by a physician who diagnosed her pregnancy, discussed options available to her, then sent her home to think over her decision regarding the continuation of the pregnancy. A few days after the visit, the doctor asked the nurse to contact the young woman and find out about her decision. The nurse unwittingly released sensitive information to the young woman's family regarding her pregnancy. She made the parents aware of the girl's consideration of abortion as an option. The young woman later sued based on invasion of privacy, breach of privileged information, and breach of contract.

The Nightingale Pledge states, "... I will do all in my power to maintain and elevate the standard of my profession and will hold in confidence all personal matters committed to my keeping and family affairs coming to my knowledge in the practice of my calling...." The American Nurses Association Code of Ethics for Nurses (American Nurses Association, 1985, p. 3) states that "the nurse safeguards the client's right to privacy by judiciously protecting information of a confidential nature." Maintaining patient confidentiality is not an easy task. Healthcare providers have a strong tradition of safeguarding private health information. However, in today's world the old system of protecting paper records in locked file cabinets no longer applies.

The automation of medical information permits the collection, analysis, storage, and retrieval of vast amounts of medical information that may not only be used but also may be shared with other providers at remote locations. The Health Insurance Portability and Accountability Act of 1996 (HIPAA), came about because of the advent of electronic medical records. The portability aspect of this regulation ensures that individuals moving from one health plan to another will have continuity of coverage and will not be denied coverage under preexisting condition clauses.

The Privacy Rule for the first time creates national standards to protect individuals' medical records and other personal health information. It gives patients more control over their health information and sets boundaries on the use and release of health records. To protect the privacy of health information, the Privacy Rule also establishes appropriate safeguards that healthcare providers and others are required to adhere to. In addition, it holds violators accountable with civil and criminal penalties that can be imposed if they violate the patient's right to privacy.

HIPAA enables patients to find out how their information may be used and what disclosures of their information have been or are to be made. It generally limits the release of information to the minimum reasonably needed for the purpose of the disclosure, and it gives patients the right to examine and obtain a copy of their own health record and to request corrections if they choose to. For the average healthcare provider or health plan, the Privacy Rule requires activities such as the following:

- Providing information to patients about their privacy rights and how their information is used.
- Adopting clear and appropriately communicated privacy procedures in their practice.
- Training employees so that they understand the privacy procedures.

- Designating an individual to be responsible for seeing that the privacy procedures are adopted and maintained at all times.
- Securing patient records containing individually identifiable health information so that they are not readily available to those who do not need them (45 CFR Parts 160 and 164).

Civil penalties for noncompliance with the security standards of HIPAA may range from $100 to $250,000 per person per calendar year. Potential criminal penalties are as follows:

- $50,000 and/or imprisonment for up to 1 year if a person knowingly obtains or discloses individually identifiable health information.
- $100,000 and/or imprisonment for up to 5 years if the perpetrator commits offenses under false pretenses.
- $250,000 and a maximum imprisonment of 10 years when the offender has the intent to sell, transfer, or use individually identifiable health information for commercial advantage, personal gain, or malicious harm (HIPAA, §1177, §1171[b][1], §1171[6], §1177[b][2]).

Implementation of HIPAA is expected by April 2003, and case managers are advised to participate in the implementation process of HIPAA at their facility. There are still changes being made while the administrative simplification mandate of the regulation is being worked out.

ROLE OF THE MEDICAL RECORD REVIEW IN A LAWSUIT

What happens when a patient sees an attorney about a complaint? Usually the medical record is requested for review by the patient and/or his or her legal representative. For "discovery," the attorney or the attorney's appointee will review the record for evidence of negligence, violation of the standard of care, or any other type of violation. *Discovery* is defined as finding legal merit in a case through the collection of evidence and putting the evidence together in the form of elements of the theory that make the case for legal pursuit.

If it is determined that the case has merit and it does go to court, the record is copied and reviewed again right before the court date. The second review of the medical record aims at identifying any additions or changes made to the record that were not there before the action was taken. If there were new entries, this would give the appearance of tampering with the record and would not bode well for the provider or facility named in the lawsuit.

A similar review process takes place by the attorney representing the provider or the facility named in the lawsuit. Case managers may be involved if they had anything to do with the care of the patient suing. If the patient has been discharged and care is no longer being provided, the medical record should be considered closed. Any additional documentation in the record will be considered falsification and will serve against the provider. Case managers can review the medical record for completeness before it is shared with the patient's attorney. However, sometimes they may not have the privilege to conduct a final review because of time constraints and attorney or court pressures.

PROFESSIONAL MISCONDUCT

When a nurse is accused of professional misconduct, the state board of nursing usually investigates the claim by conducting an administrative review. This is a separate appearance from a civil action in court. The state board of nursing can take disciplinary action against a nurse for any violation of the state's nurse practice act. In all states and provinces, the board of nursing has the authority to discipline a nurse if he or she endangers the patient's health, safety, or welfare. Furthermore, the nurse could find herself listed with the NPDB if a violation is confirmed.

The NPDB was created by the Health Care Quality Improvement Act of 1986 and became operational in 1990 (U.S. Department of Health and Human Services, 2000). The NPDB collects information about practitioners who may endanger the public welfare. The data is available to employers in an effort to restrict the ability of incompetent practitioners to move from state to state. Information reported about nurses to the NPDB includes the following:

■ Malpractice payments made by a nurse, including judgments, arbitration decisions, and out-of-court settlements
■ Actions against a nurse's clinical privileges
■ Adverse licensure actions, including revocations, suspensions, reprimands, censure, or probation

A nurse can dispute a report, even if it requires taking his or her claim to the Secretary of Health and Human Services. It is important to note that the NPDB is the repository of information about professionals licensed by states to work in medicine, nursing, pharmacy, physical therapy, occupational therapy, and social work.

PROTECTING THE CASE MANAGER IN THIS LITIGIOUS SOCIETY

Education should be one of the most important values of the professional case manager. Therefore the first piece of advice for case managers to protect themselves from litigation is *Never stop learning!* Other recommendations are as follows:

■ Make it a point to stay abreast of the legislation that impacts healthcare both at the federal and state level.

■ Always review the state professional practice act just to bring to mind what the statutes describe as case management practice.
■ It is not necessary to subscribe to every journal of nursing or other fields, but case managers should review pertinent journal articles that address their clinical area of practice. This can be accomplished relatively painlessly by covering current articles in an executive summary format at department meetings. Several members may review different journals and report to the group.
■ Maintain membership in professional associations. This helps case managers to stay current in their field and gives them a voice in government and in the eye of the public.
■ Network with professional colleagues. This may help the case manager with problem solving and may strengthen the case management profession.
■ Maintain rapport with patients and their families or caregivers. This is one of the simplest and most important things case managers can do to stay out of the courtroom and away from disciplinary action.
■ See and care for the patient as a whole person. The importance of this aspect of care cannot be overstated.
■ Tailor care to meet the specific needs of the individual patient.
■ Follow up on issues with sincere concern—become a touchstone for the patient in a world that has become increasingly impersonal.
■ Establish a connection or a bond with the patient and the family. This will go a long way toward protecting the case manager from litigation.

We do not live in a perfect world, and sometimes, despite everyone's guidance and care, unfortunate things happen to a patient. Reviewing a chart that has carefully and thoroughly documented the case management process will often cause a case to be dismissed during the discovery phase. Remember that the chart is a potential witness in the courtroom—one that the case manager can influence by ensuring that all of the significant information is accurately recorded. The patient's record must reflect communication between the case manager and the following:

■ Patient, family, or caregiver
■ Physician
■ Case management team (i.e., other healthcare providers involved in the patient's care)
■ HMO, health insurance plan, and sources of authorization for care/services

Case management is not a job for the faint of heart. An understanding and appreciation of the legal process, areas of potential liability, and the critical importance of communication support the case manager in giving sound and legitimate care to clients. Those who endure are the crusaders who are leading the nursing, case management, and other professions forward into the challenge of modern healthcare and paving the road for their colleagues with their dedication, creativity, and devotion to the patient.

 KEY POINTS

1. Consumers of healthcare services are most likely to sue providers and/or payers if they feel that their rights have been violated or their care was substandard.
2. Case managers are becoming increasingly exposed to potential lawsuits because of the increased autonomy and independence of their roles.
3. Case management is considered a reasonable activity. It may increase or curtail the likelihood of a lawsuit.
4. Failure to communicate or document an inadequate or premature patient's discharge is more likely today than ever before to result in litigation against case managers.
5. Education, knowledge, skills, and level of competence are the case manager's best defense against legal risk.

REFERENCES

American Health Consultants: *Executive summary case management caseload data survey,* Atlanta, March 2001, AHC.

American Nurses Association: *Code for nurses with interpretive statements,* Kansas City, Mo, 1985, American Nurses Association.

Brandl B, Raymond J: Unrecognized elder abuse, older abused women, *J Case Manage* 6(2):62-68, 1997.

Catalano J, Coltar A, Fiesta A, et al: *Nurse's legal handbook,* Springhouse, Pa, 1996, Springhouse Corporation.

Graham S: Hopkins sued for $12M, hospital released man's medical files, *Baltimore Business J* 19(13):24-30, 2001.

Health Care Financing Administration: *Nationwide Medicare: fraud and abuse,* Baltimore, 1998, HCFA.

National Practitioner Data Bank, Healthcare Integrity and Protection Data Bank: *Fact sheet on the healthcare integrity and protection data bank,* 2001. Available online at http://www.npdb-hipdb.com/pubs/fs/nh017fs.pdf (accessed 12/19/01).

Perin RL: *Arizona statutes affecting nursing practice,* Eau Claire, Wis, 1992, Professional Education Systems.

Powell SK: *Case management: a practical guide to success in managed care,* Philadelphia, 2000, Lippincott Williams & Wilkins.

Riccardi M: Negligence claim against HMO stands, *New York Law J* 223(57):1, 2000.

Robbins DA: Putting care above profit, *Continuing Care* 18(4):18, 1999.

Ruiz P: Crying over spilled coffee: media deform the legal reform debate, *Extra!* 8(3):10-11, 1995.

Sturgeon S: Legal issues in the operation of referral and utilization review systems, *Manag Care Interface* 10(12):66-70, 1997.

Sullivan GH: Legally speaking, when communication breaks down, *RN* 59(4):61-62, 1996.

Thomasma D, Marshall P: *Clinical medical ethics: cases and readings,* Lanham, Md, 1997, University Press of America.

U.S. Department of Health and Human Services, Health Resources and Services Administration, Bureau of Health Professions: National Practitioner Data Bank, 2000, annual report. Available online at http://www.npdb-hipdb.com/pubs/stats/00annrpt.pdf (accessed 12/19/01).

18 Ethical Issues in Case Management

Lynn A. Jansen, PhD, RN

In recent years, Americans have witnessed a well-documented and widely discussed change in their healthcare system. Unlike an earlier era of "unmanaged" health insurance, millions of Americans today are covered by health insurance plans that employ various techniques to curtail rising healthcare costs. These techniques have shifted a considerable amount of decision-making authority from physicians and patients to managed care organizations (MCOs) (Morreim, 1989, 1995; Sulmasy, 1992; Daniels and Sabin, 1997; Hall and Berenson, 1998; Buchanan, 2000; Pearson, 2000). This shift has given rise to skepticism concerning the quality of healthcare patients can expect under **managed care.**

These changes in the American healthcare system also present a number of ethical problems and challenges for healthcare professionals. Professional ethics has to do with standards of "right" and "wrong" conduct as they apply to members of a particular profession. Ethical dilemmas commonly arise when the duty the professional has to act in one way conflicts with a duty the professional has to act in another way. When this happens, the professional must decide which duty takes precedence over the other and on what grounds. **Case managers** sometimes are required to work through these dilemmas alone, without the support or counsel of other members of the organization for which they work. Over time, the stress of making these decisions without organizational support can result in reduced job satisfaction, resentment, or burnout.

This chapter discusses the types of ethical problems that case managers face in their everyday practice. Case managers confront many of the same ethical problems as other healthcare professionals working in provider settings and in MCOs. Nonetheless, these problems are particularly challenging for case managers because nurses and social workers have long defined themselves as patient advocates (Ballew and Mink, 1996; Kushe, 1997; Watt, 1997; Mallik, 1998; Nelson, 1988; Jansen, 2001). By understanding the underlying causes of the ethical problems in some detail, a framework for resolving them can be identified. This framework, known as the *deliberative framework,* is one that case managers are well suited for given their education, training, and experience.

MANAGED CARE AND PATIENT ADVOCACY

Many who have written on ethics in the era of managed care have assumed, either explicitly or implicitly, that the traditional ethics of the profession can and should be simply applied to the new circumstances (Ryden, 1978; Flarey and Blancett, 1996; Donagrandi and Eddy, 2000). It is true that case managers need to be familiar with the code of ethics for their profession. However, it is a mistake to think that the traditional principles of ethics can be easily applied within this context. Although the traditional principles of **justice, autonomy, and beneficence** are important, the meaning of these principles in the context of managed care must be substantially rethought. Moreover, new principles and new ideals need to be articulated and defended for nurses and other professionals who work in this new context.

To understand why this is the case, we need to begin by considering the traditional ideal of the nurse as a patient advocate. This ideal has a strong claim to be the foundation on which traditional nursing ethics rests

(Kushe, 1997; Donagrandi and Eddy, 2000; Jansen, 2001). As this ideal has been commonly understood, the nurse is expected to look out for and promote what is in his or her patient's best medical interests, irrespective of the patient's race, sex, age, or cultural background (Donagrandi and Eddy, 2000).

Relating Patient Advocacy to Beneficence

Patient **advocacy** relates to the ethical principle of beneficence (Case Manager's Tip 18-1). According to this principle, the case manager works with the physician to advance the best interests of their patients. This principle should be distinguished from the virtue of benevolence. The benevolent person is well disposed toward others. He or she cares about their well-being. By contrast, beneficence is an ethical principle that directs the healthcare professional to take action to promote the well-being of his or her patients. The terms *benevolence* and *beneficence* should be distinguished because it is possible for case managers to promote the good of others without being well disposed toward them, and it is possible to be well disposed toward others and yet fail to promote their interests.

The principle of beneficence, at least as it has been understood in medicine, is not general, but specific. It directs the healthcare professional to promote the interests of his or her patients rather than to promote the interests of all patients or of all potential patients (Beauchamp and Childress, 1994). For example, it is sometimes said that a special relationship exists between healthcare professionals and their particular patients and that this relationship grounds the requirement of beneficence (Veatch, 1981; Beauchamp and Childress, 1994).

Finally, the principle of beneficence in medicine has traditionally been understood to be an "interest-maximizing" principle (Veatch, 1981; Morreim, 1989,

 CASE MANAGER'S TIP 18-1

The Case Manager as Patient Advocate

An essential role of the case manager is patient advocate. In this role the case manager may be presented with conflicting choices. Using the principle of beneficence, the case manager should always select the choice that will advance the best interests of the patient. As a patient advocate, the case manager must provide patients and families with the information necessary to help them make better decisions and must support the decisions they make.

1995). This means that it requires healthcare professionals to not just promote their patient's best interests, but rather to do all that can be done to advance these interests.

Accordingly, the traditional ethical ideal of the case manager as a patient advocate is an ideal that directs the case manager to act in ways that will maximize the best interests of his or her own patients. There is little doubt that this ideal is inspiring. It has given, and continues to give, content to the idea that nursing, social work, **case management,** and other healthcare-related professions are moral professions. Yet, notwithstanding its strong appeal, in recent years many have begun to challenge the principle of beneficence that forms this ideal. They have argued that this principle is actually socially irresponsible and that it has contributed to the accelerating costs of healthcare (Veatch, 1981; Pellegrino and Thomasma, 1988; Morreim, 1989, 1995). These doubts have become all the more pronounced as we have moved into a managed care environment.

Given its importance, let us look at this criticism in a little more detail. According to the critics, the traditional principle of beneficence, which forms the traditional ideal of the nurse as a patient advocate, rests on an outdated model of the clinician/patient relationship. This model inaccurately characterizes the clinician/patient relationship if applied in a managed care context. This is true for a number of reasons, among which are the following:

1. The principle of beneficence assumes and takes as its paradigm an overly individualistic relationship between provider and patient (Daniels and Sabin, 1997; Buchanan, 2000).
2. The principle of beneficence assumes that the provider is unconstrained by his or her role in an organization or by organizational policies (Daniels and Sabin, 1997; Buchanan, 2000).
3. The principle of beneficence characterizes the provider's obligation to his or her patient in interest-maximizing terms, which is socially irresponsible given the scarcity of healthcare resources and the need to contain healthcare costs (Veatch, 1981; Morreim, 1989, 1995; Daniels and Sabin, 1997).

These criticisms are compelling. Whatever one thinks of managed care, it is clear that it has transformed the clinician/patient relationship. Through their decisions regarding insurance coverage, MCOs have assumed the authority to decide effectively when and how to limit access to a range of medically beneficial services. These coverage decisions are crucial to the cost-containment techniques characteristic of managed care.

This transfer of decision-making authority has in turn transformed the relationship between healthcare professionals and their patients. Physicians are no longer in

CASE MANAGER'S TIP 18-2

Rethinking Clinical Care Decisions

In the past, clinical decisions were made between the patient and the physician. Managed care has introduced a third party in the clinical decision making process: the insurer. Case managers should always assist patients and families with disputing any decisions made that seem unethical, unfair, or dangerous to the well-being of the patient.

a position to provide their patients with all of the care that might reasonably be expected to benefit them. Before managed care, healthcare professionals could act as if their patients were the only patients there were and they could proceed, at least in many cases, with no concern for costs (Veatch, 1981; Buchanan, 2000). In so doing, it was commonly thought, they discharged their duty of beneficence. But with the emergence of managed care—with its strong emphasis on cost containment—this approach is no longer a viable option (Morreim, 1989, 1995; Buchanan, 2000).

For the same reasons, the traditional ideal of the case manager as a patient advocate is not a viable option in the managed care context. It is an ideal that has a place when the clinician/patient relationship is conceived in individualistic terms and when the need to contain healthcare costs is not pressing. Still, it would be a mistake to conclude from this that case managers working in managed care environments should cease to think of themselves as patient advocates (Case Manager's Tip 18-2). If nursing and social work are to remain as moral professions, then case managers should not abandon the ideal of patient advocacy when they case manage patients in managed care environments. Instead, they must rethink the content of this ideal for these new circumstances.

Rethinking Ethics

Case managers must adjust their ethical self-understanding to fit the managed care environment in which they practice. Like the traditional physician/patient relationship, the traditional nurse/patient and social worker/patient relationship is transformed once cost containment becomes a pressing issue. Under managed care, nurses—and case managers in particular—have conflicting loyalties. They have obligations both to their patients and to the organization for which they work. Balancing these obligations in an ethically appropriate way requires that they cease thinking in terms of maximizing the interests of their patients. Recognition of this

important point is the first step in reformulating the traditional ideal of the case manager as patient advocate.

CASE MANAGEMENT AND NEW ETHICAL CHALLENGES

The emergence of managed care has brought with it an increased need for case management. **Health maintenance organizations (HMOs)** and **preferred provider organizations (PPOs)** have found it necessary to enlist the services of case managers in their efforts to contain costs and maintain quality. According to the American Nurses Association, "the goals of case management are the provision of quality healthcare...enhancement of the client's quality of life, efficient utilization of patient care resources, and cost containment" (Cesta, Tahan, and Fink, 1998, p. 3). These are all important goals under managed care. Done well, case management can reduce the tension between providing quality healthcare and containing healthcare costs. However, it would be a mistake to think that this tension can ever be fully overcome. Accordingly, the ethical challenges confronting case managers who work in managed care settings center on how to manage this tension and what to do when the tension becomes too great.

Balancing Cost and Quality

To understand the nature of this tension, we must clarify the competing goals that can come into conflict. The goal of providing quality healthcare must not be identified with the interest-maximizing principle of beneficence discussed previously. Given the scarcity of healthcare resources, case managers should not view themselves as under an obligation to provide maximal care to their patients. Instead, the goal of providing quality healthcare must be understood to refer to a "reasonable" level of care.

The second goal is cost containment. Managing care with limited resources requires case managers to oversee their patients' journey through the healthcare system with an eye toward eliminating inefficiency and unnecessary expense, especially that which results from duplication and fragmentation of services. Moreover, in organizations with a capitated payment system, case managers must balance the needs and interests of different patients to stay within a fixed budget.

The goal of providing quality healthcare grounds obligations to specific patients. The goal of containing costs grounds obligations to **third-party payers,** provider systems, and society at large (Case Manager's Tip 18-3). This last point is important. Cost containment is often disparaged as a financial rather than a medical goal. This is only partly true because cost-containment techniques are essential to provide members of society—all

CASE MANAGER'S TIP 18-3

Balancing Cost and Quality

When balancing issues of cost versus quality, case managers should always err on the side of quality and/or the best interest of the patient. Reimbursement should always be a secondary consideration.

---

of whom are either patients or potential patients—with affordable healthcare. When case managers function within a legitimate managed care environment to limit costs, they are not merely serving the interests of insurance companies but are serving the interests of society as well.

But what is a legitimate MCO? And when are decisions to limit care "reasonable"? These questions must be squarely confronted if we are to understand the ethical challenges facing case managers under managed care. Unfortunately, these questions are not easily answered. Not only are there no socially accepted standards of reasonable medical care, but also experts disagree among themselves as to what should count as a just healthcare entitlement (Daniels and Sabin, 1997; Buchanan, 2000). In the face of this uncertainty and disagreement, any decision to limit healthcare to contain costs is in danger of appearing ad hoc and arbitrary. A number of writers have proposed procedural standards that must be satisfied if cost-cutting decisions are to be legitimate (Daniels and Sabin, 1997; Buchanan, 2000). These procedural standards can be grouped under the following three principles:

1. The principle of impartiality
2. The principle of publicity
3. The principle of contestability

Case managers need to understand these principles because compliance with them is crucial to responding ethically to the tension between providing quality healthcare and containing costs.

The Principle of Impartiality

The principle of impartiality requires that similar cases be treated alike. At the minimum, this means that case managers should not make cost-cutting decisions that discriminate against groups on the basis of irrelevant differences such as ethnicity, race, age, or gender. The principle also demands that healthcare workers not provide differential treatment to friends, family members, or those who they deem to be socially or professionally more important. When consistently adhered to, the principle of impartiality mitigates the worry that cost-cutting decisions made by case managers will be

arbitrary (Friedman and Savage, 1998; Donagrandi and Eddy, 2000).

The Principle of Publicity

As important as the principle of impartiality is, it is not sufficient for legitimate healthcare decision making. Decisions to limit healthcare must not only be fair, they must also be viewed as fair. This brings us to the principle of publicity (Veatch, 1981; Friedman and Savage, 1998; Buchanan, 2000). Cost-cutting decisions, whether made by case managers or others who work with HMOs and PPOs to contain costs, must be made on the basis of standards and rules that are both publicly known and publicly justified (Buchanan, 2000). This means that these rules and standards must be accessible to healthcare workers and their patients alike. Without this kind of openness, it will be difficult to quell the suspicion that coverage decisions are being made on an arbitrary basis.

In addition to being public, these rules and decisions also should be publicly justified. This means two things. First, it means that the reasons or considerations that justify the rules and standards are themselves made public. Second, it means that these reasons and considerations must be based, as far as it is possible to do so, on needs and values that are widely shared. Norman Daniels and James Sabin have expressed the importance of this last point well. They state the following:

> If the organization shows through the pattern of reasoning (the "case law") reflected in its public reason-giving that its decisions rest on the kinds of reasons all can consider relevant to deciding how to meet varied patient needs under reasonable resource constraints, then even those who disagree with the specific decisions made should acknowledge they are reasonable decisions that are arguably aimed at producing fair outcomes (Daniels and Sabin, 1997, p. 339).

In other words, although compliance with the principle of publicity cannot eliminate disagreement, it may be able to ensure that those who "lose out" in a decision at least will be to able view the decision as one made on grounds that they can recognize to be appropriate.

The Principle of Contestability

The principle of contestability supplements the other two principles. Decisions made by case managers, as well as others in managed care environments, should be contestable. Physicians and other healthcare providers should be encouraging their patients and their families to participate in the decision-making process and to offer constructive public criticism. One way in which this can be accomplished is for decision-making bodies within MCOs and PPOs to establish formal dispute resolution procedures. These would allow those who believed that they had been treated unfairly or improperly to make an appeal for redress without resorting to legal action. Case managers can assist widely in facilitating such processes by teaching and guiding patients and their families as to how to go about filing such appeals.

This is important for at least two reasons. First, in the dispute resolution process, new information or new considerations might come to light. This in turn could result in the formulation of better standards for making coverage decisions in the future. Second, by encouraging criticism of their decisions, case managers and others who must make coverage decisions would ensure that they remain accountable to those who are affected by their decisions. This accountability, and the public recognition of it, is crucial to the legitimacy of the decision-making process (Daniels and Sabin, 1997; Buchanan, 2000).

Legitimate decisions by MCOs must, accordingly, be impartial, publicly justifiable, and contestable. This is particularly true for decisions to limit care on the basis of cost. Earlier in this chapter it was discussed that the traditional understanding of medical beneficence as a duty to maximize the best interests of one's patient—and the ideal of patient advocacy premised on this understanding—must be rethought in the context of managed care. It was stated that medical beneficence and patient advocacy should be understood in terms of providing one's patient with a reasonable, not a maximal, level of care. This suggestion can now be made more concrete. A reasonable level of care can now be understood to be a level of care that is determined by an MCO that makes legitimate coverage decisions, where legitimacy is understood in terms of the principles of impartiality, publicity, and contestability.

Accordingly, when case managers act as patient advocates in the context of managed care, they must attempt to provide their patients with the best possible care that is consistent with legitimate cost-cutting and coverage decisions. By doing so, they will be able to balance their obligation to promote the interests of their patients with their financial and societal obligation to contain healthcare costs and maintain or improve quality.

MAINTAINING ETHICAL INTEGRITY

The three principles discussed in the previous section ameliorate the tension between providing quality healthcare and containing healthcare costs. However, it is doubtful that the tension can ever be completely overcome. This means that even when MCOs make legitimate decisions, healthcare workers may sometimes find themselves in situations in which they cannot support these decisions in good conscience.

When this occurs, how they ought to respond is an important ethical question. For example, consider the following case:

The Problem

A 54-year-old male patient, Mr. X, was being treated with beta-blockers for hypertension. He went to his primary care physician complaining of a dry cough. Mr. X was diagnosed with nasal polyps, and the cough was attributed to postnasal drip. Both Mr. X's physician and the case manager responsible for his care believed that he ought to undergo a total systems review. However, limits set by the insurer precluded this. As a result, Mr. X's symptoms were addressed from a cost-only approach, and a specialist denied him care (Donagrandi and Eddy, 2000).

Ethical Decision-Making Process to Resolve This Problem

In this case, both Mr. X's physician and his case manager confronted a conflict between their obligation to promote his best interests and their obligation to work within the cost-containment guidelines established by the managed care insurer. To determine how they should have responded to this conflict, we first need to distinguish between two scenarios. In the first scenario, the managed care insurer does not make legitimate coverage decisions. In other words, it fails to comply with the principles of impartiality, publicity, and contestability. By contrast, in the second scenario the MCO does make legitimate coverage decisions.

What should Mr. X's physician and his case manager do in the first scenario? One option is for them to adopt the role of the "saboteur," to use a phrase coined by Allen Buchanan (Freeman et al, 1999; Buchanan, 2000). Saboteurs seek to circumvent the coverage limits imposed by managed care. They do this by falsifying diagnoses to get the insurer to cover the services for their patient that they think he or she needs or deserves. In general, this type of response is ethically unacceptable. It requires healthcare workers to engage in deception, and it does nothing to improve the decision-making processes of the MCO.

A better response in this scenario is for Mr. X's physician and his case manager to press for changes in the way in which their MCO makes coverage decisions. For example, they may advise Mr. X to take legal action against the insurer as a way of putting external pressure on the insurer to make changes. They also may consider lobbying the insurer to establish public appeals procedures that would allow patients like Mr. X the opportunity to challenge the coverage decisions that affect him. Finally, if the insurer is sufficiently unresponsive to making changes that would make it legitimate, they should consider limiting their involvement with the insurer as much as possible.

Most insurers are not as illegitimate as the one envisioned in this first scenario of the case under discussion. Let us turn then to the second scenario of the case. Here the insurer makes impartial and publicly justifiable coverage decisions. When it limits coverage, it does so for reasons that all can accept as valid. Moreover, it permits and even encourages physicians and case managers to contest its decisions in public appeals procedures.

Still, even legitimate insurers can make coverage decisions that strike healthcare workers as misguided. In the case we are considering, Mr. X's physician and his case manager may still believe that the coverage decision made by the insurer was incorrect. How then should they respond? Clearly, in this scenario they should be not engaged in sabotage. The role of the saboteur is ethically questionable even when the coverage decisions are illegitimate, and when these decisions are legitimate, it is plainly an ethical mistake to falsify diagnoses. Doing so is deceptive, and it frustrates the legitimate financial and societal goal of containing healthcare costs.

Mr. X's physician and his case manager believed that a total systems review was necessary in his case. After this was denied, they should not attempt to circumvent the legitimate decision-making procedures of the MCO. Instead, they should serve as Mr. X's advocate in the appeals process. Here they should not argue that Mr. X has a claim to all possible medical care that might reasonably be expected to benefit him. They should rather argue either that the cost-containing policies that affect him ought to be revised or that an exception should be made to these policies in Mr. X's case. If they are unsuccessful, then they should explain to Mr. X that they have done all they could do, given the policies of the organization in which they function. They should also explain to him that although they disagree with the decision of the organization, they recognize that the organization has a legitimate interest in containing healthcare costs. Finally, if they are aware that a total systems review for Mr. X would have been provided by an alternative insurer, then they should inform him of this fact.

Acting Responsibly

As this case illustrates, the ethics of managed care involves in large measure an ability to function responsibly in an organizational setting. This requires a shift in perspective from that of an "individualist" who strives to do all he or she can do for his or her patients to that of a "cooperator" who strives to perform his or her role

well within a larger organization (Buchanan, 2000). In turn, this shift in perspective suggests that many ethical problems that arise under managed care cannot be resolved by individualistic or "monological" reasoning (Habermas, 1990). Rather they are problems of "organizational ethics," which require case managers to engage in shared decision making, not just between the physician and patient, but also between patient care representatives, discharge planners, social workers, other providers, and hospital administrators. This highlights an important ethical role for the case manager under managed care. As the person responsible for coordinating the delivery of care to patients, case managers must also assume responsibility for initiating shared decision making to resolve ethical problems that may arise.

THE DELIBERATIVE FRAMEWORK

It was suggested previously that the traditional ideal of the case manager as a patient advocate must be seriously rethought in the context of managed care. We now have seen why this is true. The maximizing ethic of beneficence that supported this traditional ideal has no place in managed care, and the individualistic character of the ideal does not sit well with the need for organizational decision making within managed care. The procedural principles of legitimate decision making that we have discussed, as well as the illustrative case of Mr. X, suggest that we need to develop a new framework for understanding the ethical responsibilities of case management professionals, including nurses, who work under managed care.

The framework used to address these types of dilemmas, known as the *deliberative framework,* consists of two main components:

1. A commitment to shared decision making
2. An account of the nature and purpose of deliberation

Shared Decision Making

Shared decision making has become an important ideal in medicine (Emanuel and Emanuel, 1992; Brock, 1993; Kuczewiski, 1996; Gutmann and Thompson, 1997; Jansen, 2000, 2001). However, for the most part it has been proposed as an ideal for specific types of interactions. For example, shared decision making has been proposed as a model for the physician/patient relationship (Brock, 1993), or for the relationship between genetic counselors and their clients (Jansen, 2001). It has much less often been proposed as a model for healthcare decision making in general (Cape, 1986). With the advent of managed care, this needs to change. Physicians and nurses must work with case managers to come up with comprehensive guidelines for providing care. These **guidelines** should be the product of joint decision making in which physicians, nurses, insurance representatives, and administrators in managed care all are encouraged to participate actively.

This type of shared decision making is not only necessary to arrive at better guidelines and healthcare decisions, but also it is crucial to the legitimacy of MCOs. As has already been pointed out, legitimate cost-limiting decisions must comply with the principles of impartiality, publicity, and contestability. Shared decision making, in which all affected parties are given the opportunity to participate, will make it much more likely that these principles will be satisfied. This is particularly true of the principle of contestability, which requires that patients and their physicians have public opportunities to challenge the decisions made under managed care.

The Nature and Purpose of Deliberation

The second component of the deliberative framework concerns the nature and purpose of the deliberation that should take place among those engaged in shared decision making. The purpose of this deliberation is to arrive at decisions that are both legitimate and seen to be legitimate. For this to be possible, all participants must be open to rational discussion. At the very least this means that participants must consider it a genuine possibility that they will learn something from the deliberative discussion and that they might change their mind about the issues before them.

In addition, participants in the discussion must view one another as equal deliberative partners. This does not mean that they cannot bring their particular expertise, whether it be medical or administrative, to bear on the discussion. However, it does mean that they must not think in hierarchical terms. For example, administrators should not think that physicians must always defer to them and physicians must not think that nurses must always defer to them. In genuinely deliberative discussion, hierarchical relations and attitudes have no place. They obstruct, rather than facilitate, the process of rational discussion.

These conditions for deliberative discussion are fairly demanding. In practice, most of the time they will not be fully realized. However, they can serve as an ideal toward which healthcare workers under managed care should strive. The deliberative framework, then, is an ideal to be approximated; however, it is the main argument of this chapter that this ideal must be realized to a substantial extent if healthcare workers, and in particular case managers, are to make ethically responsible decisions given the new restrictions imposed by managed care.

Clinical Ethics Consults

To illustrate this last point, consider the role and function of the ethics consult. Before managed care, an ethics consult would be necessary only when some relatively well-defined ethical problem presented itself. Most of the time physicians and nurses could proceed as patient advocates, providing all of the care to their patients that could reasonably be expected to benefit them. However, if it is true that the traditional understanding of the ideal of patient advocate must be given up under managed care, then physicians and case managers will often confront a whole new range of difficult ethical questions about what level of care their patients are legitimately entitled to receive. These are not questions they will be able to answer on their own. They will need to consult others about what the managed care cost containment guidelines require and permit and when exceptions can legitimately be made to these guidelines. Often these questions will not have determinate answers until after deliberative discussion has resolved them. Accordingly, under managed care there is an increased need for ethics consults, and these consults, at least when they function well, are instances of deliberative shared decision making.

ORGANIZATIONAL ETHICS

The type of ethics consult that a case manager is likely to call will differ in significant respects from the traditional "clinical ethics consult." In large measure the clinical ethics consult centers on how individual practitioners can best resolve ethical conflicts that arise when they are treating their patients. However, the conflicts that arise in the context of case management and managed care are more *organizational* in nature (Case Manager's Tips 18-4 and 18-5). In some respects these conflicts can better be grouped under a category of "Organizational Ethics" rather than the traditional category of "Clinical Ethics."

Organizational ethics deals with an organization's behaviors as they relate to the individuals represented by that organization (including patients, providers, and other employees), the community served by that

 CASE MANAGER'S TIP 18-4

Organizational Ethics

As a case manager, if your organization does not have an organizational ethics committee, you should advocate for the development of one to assist you in solving ethical dilemmas that you may come across, such as those related to **utilization management,** resource utilization, and **discharge planning.**

CASE MANAGER'S TIP 18-5

Reporting Structure of Organizational Ethics

Organizational ethics committees should be subcommittees of the ethics committee and should report their issues and decisions back to the ethics committee on a regular basis.

> ### BOX 18-1 Examples of the Categories of Organizational Ethics
>
> **Healthcare Business**
> - Cost shifting
> - Billing practices
> - Financial incentives
> - Resource allocation
> - Conflicts of interest
>
> **Societal and Public Health Considerations**
> - Serving the medically underserved
> - Antidumping issues (Emergency Medical Treatment and Active Labor Act [EMTALA])
> - Discrimination against patients
> - Public disclosure of clinical errors
>
> **Healthcare Advertising**
> - Making unrealistic promises
> - Endorsing specific medical products
> - Marketing of healthcare institutions
>
> **Scientific and Educational Issues**
> - Education of future healthcare providers
> - Performing research and clinical trials
>
> **General Business Practices such as Relationships with:**
> - Employees
> - Vendors
> - Payers
> - Outside agencies
> - The public at large

organization, and other organizations with whom that organization may interact. There are a number of different categories of organizational ethics (Box 18-1). However, the types of organizational ethics conflicts that case managers must address will be limited to the unique roles that they play inside the healthcare organization. For example, the roles that case managers play in the following commonly give rise to the types of conflicts for which an ethics consultation would be appropriate:

1. Resolving care-related conflicts
2. Preventing delays in treatments
3. Increasing and facilitating access to care
4. Brokering services within and outside the healthcare organization
5. Obtaining authorizations for treatments from MCOs
6. Advocating for patients while working with MCOs

To illustrate, consider the following case.

Organizational Ethics Consult Case Study

Mr. G was found unconscious. He was admitted out of network to the intensive care unit (ICU) at a nearby inner city hospital. He remained in the hospital for 6 months before being discharged to his home in another state. Two weeks after his discharge, Mr. G experienced another syncopal episode. His wife requested that the ambulance bring him back to the original hospital where he had spent the past 6 months. Because he had full understanding of the patient's condition, had treated him in the past and had developed a professional rapport with him, the physician from the city hospital agreed that this would best serve the patient's medical interests. However, because the patient was "out of network," the case manager was called on to make a decision as to whether the admission was appropriate.

Cases such as this are becoming more common in the era of managed care. In this type of case, case managers best discharge their ethical responsibilities by deliberating with others to determine what response is appropriate. However, the types of people whom the case manager would most likely need to consult will differ from those whom a physician or nurse would consult in a dilemma of clinical ethics. In addition to the patient's family and physician and a trained ethicist, the case manager will also want to deliberate with a member of the managed care department, legal department, patient relations, and social work.

Given their training and institutional role in today's healthcare system, case managers must develop skills for collaborating with physicians, nurses, social workers, patients, and family members of patients on developing comprehensive and integrated healthcare delivery plans for their patients (Jansen, 2001). These collaborative skills are the types of skills that are needed to engage effectively in deliberative decision making to resolve problems of organizational ethics likely to arise under managed care.

With these points in mind, we can finally return to the traditional ideal of the case manager as patient advocate. This ideal can now be understood not to be an individualistic ideal (Case Manager's Tip 18-6) in which the case manager acts to maximize the interests of the patient but rather a collaborative ideal in which the case manager deliberates with others to determine the appropriate type and level of care for the patient.

CASE MANAGER'S TIP 18-6

Ethics Consults

Case managers can function as patient advocates in the following two ways:

1. They can ensure that ethics consults are called when they need to be called.
2. They can ensure that their patients' interests are fully represented and protected in these consults.

Like other healthcare workers, case managers need to adjust to the changing circumstances brought on by managed care. This will require them to rethink some of the traditional ethical ideals that have formed the profession. In particular, an ethic appropriate to managed care must be one that is responsive to the legitimate societal need to contain healthcare spending.

Rather than providing guidance as to how to resolve specific ethical problems, this chapter provides the case manager with strategies that can be used when he or she is presented with any ethical dilemma. These strategies focus on a certain type of process for resolving ethical problems that are likely to arise in the context of managed care (Case Manager's Tip 18-7). The process is deliberative and involves shared decision making between a wide range of professionals. However, to facilitate this process, case managers should also have knowledge of the specific code of ethics for their profession, as well as with the mission, vision, and value statements of the organization in which they work. Boxes 18-2 through 18-6 include a number of professional codes of ethics specific to the field of case management.

 CASE MANAGER'S TIP 18-7

Strategies for Approaching an Ethical Dilemma

- Enforce and promote mutual trust among all parties involved.
- Maintain the patient's confidentiality and privacy.
- Affirm the dignity and worth of each party.
- Project commitment to truthfulness.
- Respect diversity of values and difference of opinion.
- Ensure congruence between verbal and nonverbal messages.
- Avoid task orientation—be person oriented instead.
- Allow sufficient time for each ethical issue.
- Spend enough time with the patient, family, and other healthcare providers, as indicated, for each dilemma faced.
- Interview/meet with patients and families in private rooms and comfortable settings.
- Believe that good communication results in good and desirable outcomes.
- Assume and project a sense of responsibility and accountability for own actions.
- Always involve others in shared decision making regarding the issue at hand.
- Deliberate in accord with a relatively consistent set of values and goals.
- Distinguish ethical problems from other general patient care management issues.
- Seek the assistance of others when unable to address the issue independently.
- Be thorough in gathering information.
- Always apply the institutional policies and procedures; they are intended to support and guide practice.
- Document pertinent information in the patient's medical record.

BOX 18-2   American Nurses Association's Code of Ethics

1. The nurse, in all professional relationships, practices with compassion and respect for the inherent dignity, worth, and uniqueness of every individual, unrestricted by considerations of social or economic status, personal attributes, or the nature of health problems.
2. The nurse's primary commitment is to the patient, whether an individual, family, group, or community.
3. The nurse promotes, advocates for, and strives to protect the health, safety, and rights of the patient.
4. The nurse is responsible and accountable for individual nursing practice and determines the appropriate

delegation of tasks consistent with the nurse's obligation to provide optimum patient care.

5. The nurse owes the same duties to self as to others, including the responsibility to preserve integrity and safety, to maintain competence, and to continue personal and professional growth.
6. The nurse participates in establishing, maintaining, and improving healthcare environments and conditions of employment conducive to the provision of quality healthcare and consistent with the values of the profession through individual and collective action.

BOX 18-2   American Nurses Association's Code of Ethics—cont'd

7. The nurse participates in the advancement of the profession through contributions to practice, education, administration, and knowledge development.
8. The nurse collaborates with other health professionals and the public in promoting community, national, and international efforts to meet health needs.

9. The profession of nursing, as represented by associations and their members, is responsible for articulating nursing values, for maintaining the integrity of the profession and its practice, and for shaping social policy.

From the American Nurses Association: *Code of ethics: the center of ethics and human rights,* Washington, DC, 2001, The Association.

BOX 18-3   National Association of Social Workers Code of Ethics

The following broad principles are based on social work's core values of service, social justice, dignity and worth of the person, importance of human relationships, integrity, and competence. These principles set forth ideals to which all social workers should aspire.

1. *Value:* Service
   Ethical principle: Social workers' primary goal is to help people in need and to address social problems.
2. *Value:* Social justice
   Ethical principle: Social workers challenge social injustice.
3. *Value:* Dignity and worth of the person

Ethical principle: Social workers respect the inherent dignity and worth of the person.

4. *Value:* Importance of human relationships
   Ethical principle: Social workers recognize the central importance of human relationships.
5. *Value:* Integrity
   Ethical principle: Social workers behave in a trustworthy manner.
6. *Value:* Competence
   Ethical principle: Social workers practice within their areas of competence and develop and enhance their professional expertise.

From the National Association of Social Workers: *NASW code of ethics,* Washington, DC, 2001, The Association.

BOX 18-4   Code of Professional Conduct for Case Managers, Adopted by the Commission for Case Manager Certification

The Commission for Case Manager Certification identifies several values of case management practice and rules of conduct expected from certified case managers.

Underlying values are as follows:

1. Belief that case management is a means for achieving client wellness and autonomy through advocacy, communication, education, identification of service resources, and service facilitation.
2. Recognition of the dignity, worth, and rights of all people.
3. Understanding and commitment to quality outcomes for clients, appropriate use of resources, and the empowerment of clients in a manner that is supportive and objective.
4. Belief in the underlying premise that when the individual reaches the optimal level of wellness and functional capability, everyone benefits: the individual being served, their support systems, the healthcare delivery systems, and the various reimbursement systems.
5. Recognition that case management is guided by the principles of autonomy, beneficence, nonmaleficence, justice, **veracity,** and **distributive justice.**

Rules of conduct are as follows:

(These are listed in terms of unethical practices and as violation statements that may result in denial or sanctions on the part of the Commission up to and including revocation of the individual's certification. Those certified through the Commission are expected to always abide by these rules.)

Rule 1: Intentionally falsifying an application or other documents

Rule 2: Conviction of a felony that involves moral turpitude

Rule 3: Violation of the code of ethics governing the profession on which the individual's eligibility for certification as a case manager is based

Rule 4: Loss of the primary professional credential on which eligibility for the case manager certification (CCM) designation is based

Rule 5: Violation or breach of the guidelines for professional conduct (i.e., professional misconduct)

Rule 6: Failure to maintain eligibility requirements once certified

Rule 7: Failure to pay required fees for the Commission for Case Manager Certification (CCMC)

Rule 8: Violation of the rules and regulations governing the taking of the certification examination

From the Commission for Case Manager Certification: *Code of professional conduct for case managers with disciplinary rules, procedures, and penalties,* Rolling Meadows, Ill, 1999, The Commission.

BOX 18-5   Statement of Ethical Case Management Practice from the Case Management Society of America

The following ethical principles are summarized based on the Case Management Society of America's (CMSA) Statement on Ethical Case Management Practice:

1. Case managers must adhere to the code of ethics of their profession of origin (i.e., nursing, social work).
2. Morality and support for right (good) decisions and actions must prevail in the environment of case management practice.
3. Case management practice is guided by the principles of autonomy, beneficence, nonmaleficence, justice, and veracity.
4. The case manager collaborates with the autonomous client with the goal of fostering and encouraging the client's independence and self-determination.
5. The case manager educates and empowers the client/family to promote growth and development of the individual and family so that self-advocacy and self-direction of care are achieved. This means informing and supporting the client in the client's options and decisions related to his or her healthcare.
6. The practice of case management is concerned with preservation of the dignity of the client and family.

7. The case manager is knowledgeable about and respects the rights of the individual and family that arise from human dignity and worth, including consent and privacy.
8. The case manager does not discriminate based on social or economic status, personal attributes, or the nature of the health problem.
9. In case management practice the application of beneficence is balanced with the interests of autonomy in order to prevent paternalism and promote self-determination.
10. The case manager refrains from doing harm to others and emphasizes quality outcomes.
11. The case manager applies the concepts of fairness so as to maximize the individual's ability to carry out reasonable life plans.
12. The case manager advocates for the client to receive needed care and promotes access to service, especially when they are rare or resources are limited.
13. The case manager applies the concept of veracity to case management practice in order to develop a trusting relationship with the client and family and between case managers, healthcare providers, and payers.

From the Case Management Society of America: *CMSA statement regarding ethical case management practice,* Little Rock, Ark, 1996, The Society.

BOX 18-6   Ethical Principles Most Commonly Applied in Case Management Practice

- *Autonomy:* A form of personal liberty of action in which the patient holds the right and freedom to select and initiate his or her own treatment and course of action and to take control of his or her health (i.e., fostering the patient's independence and self-determination).
- *Beneficence:* The obligation and duty to promote good, to further and support a patient's legitimate interests and decisions, and to actively prevent or remove harm (i.e., to share with the patient the risks associated with a particular treatment option).
- *Nonmaleficence:* Refraining from doing harm to others (i.e., emphasizing quality care outcomes).
- *Justice:* Maintaining what is right and fair and making decisions that are good for the patient.
- *Distributive justice:* Deals with the moral basis for dissemination of goods and evils, burdens and benefits, especially when making decisions regarding the allocation of healthcare resources.
- *Veracity:* The act of telling the truth.

 KEY POINTS

1. The traditional ethical principles of justice, autonomy, and beneficence must be rethought in the context of case management and managed care; in most cases, new principles need to be articulated.
2. When case managers function within a legitimate managed care environment to limit costs, they are not only serving the interests of payers of healthcare services but the interests of consumers as well.
3. Applying the ethical principles of impartiality, publicity, and contestability is crucial to responding ethically to the tension of maintaining a balance between access, cost, and quality of healthcare.
4. The case manager as a consumer advocate applies a collaborative idea (collaborates with consumers, providers, and payers) to determine the appropriate type, quantity, level, cost, and quality of care/services for the patient.
5. Those who assume the role of case manager must be familiar with the code of ethics of their professional discipline and those of case management practice. They also must apply the code(s) in their daily function.

REFERENCES

Ballew JR, Mink G: *Case management in social work,* Springfield, Ill, 1996, Charles C Thomas.

Beauchamp TL, Childress JF: *Principles of biomedical ethics,* ed 4, New York, 1994, Oxford University Press.

Brock DW: *Life and death: philosophical essays in biomedical ethics,* Cambridge, UK, 1993, Cambridge University Press.

Buchanan A: Trust in managed care organizations, *Kennedy Institute Ethics J* 10(3):189-212, 2000.

Cape LS: Collaborative practice models and structures. In England DA, editor: *Collaboration in nursing,* Gaithersburg, Md, 1986, Aspen.

Cesta TG, Tahan HA, Fink LF: *The case manager's survival guide,* St Louis, 1998, Mosby.

Daniels N, Sabin J: Limits to healthcare: fair procedures, democratic deliberation, and the legitimacy problem for insurers, *Philos Public Aff* 26(4):303-350, 1997.

Donagrandi MA, Eddy M: Ethics of case management: implications for advanced practice nursing, *Clin Nurs Spec* 14(5):241-249, 2000.

Emanuel L, Emanuel E: Four models of the doctor-patient relationship, *JAMA* 267(16):2221-2226, 1992.

Flarey DL, Blancett SS: *Handbook of nursing case management: health care delivery in a world of managed care,* Gaithersburg, Md, 1996, Aspen.

Freeman VG, Rathore SS, Weinfurt KP, et al: Lying for patients: physician deception of third-party payers, *Arch Intern Med* 159:2263-2270, 1999.

Friedman LH, Savage GT: Can ethical management and case management co-exist? *Health Care Manage Rev* 23(2):56-62, 1998.

Gutmann A, Thompson D: Deliberating about bioethics, *Hastings Center Report* 27(3):38-42, 1997.

Habermas J: *Moral consciousness and communicative action,* Cambridge, Mass, 1990, MIT Press.

Hall MA, Berenson RA: Ethical practice in managed care: a dose of realism, *Ann Intern Med* 128(5):395-402, 1998.

Jansen LA: Deliberative decision making and the treatment of pain, *J Palliat Med* 4(1):23-30, 2000.

Jansen LA: The role of the nurse in clinical genetics. In Mahowald M, McKusick V, Scheurle A, et al, editors: *Genetics in the clinic: clinical, ethical, and social implications for primary care,* St Louis, 2001, Mosby.

Kuczewiski MG: Reconceiving the family: the process of consent in medical decision-making, *Hastings Center Report* 26:30-37, 1996.

Kushe H: *Caring: nurses, women, and ethics,* Oxford, UK, 1997, Blackwell.

Mallik M: Advocacy in nursing: perceptions and attitudes of nursing elite in the United Kingdom, *J Adv Nurs* 28(5):1001-1011, 1998.

Morreim EH: Fiscal scarcity and the inevitability of bedside budget balancing, *Arch Intern Med* 149:1012-1015, 1989.

Morreim EH: Moral justice and legal justice in managed care: the ascent of contributive justice, *J Law Med Ethics* 23:247-265, 1995.

Nelson ML: Advocacy in nursing: how has it evolved and what are its implications for practice? *Nurs Outlook* 36(3):136-141, 1988.

Pearson SD: Caring and cost: the challenge for physician advocacy, *Ann Intern Med* 133(2):148-153, 2000.

Pellegrino ED, Thomasma DC: *For the patient's good: the restoration of beneficence in healthcare,* New York, 1988, Oxford University Press.

Ryden MB: An approach to ethical decision making, *Nurs Outlook* 26:705-706, 1978.

Sulmasy DP: Physicians, cost control, and ethics, *Ann Intern Med* 116:920-926, 1992.

Veatch RM: *A theory of medical ethics,* New York, 1981, Basic Books.

Watt E: An exploration of the way in which the concept of patient-advocacy is perceived by registered nurses working in an acute care hospital, *Int J Nurs Pract* 3:119-127, 1997.

19 Using the Internet for Case Management

The public wants access to healthcare-related knowledge on the **Internet** and at their fingertips. Healthcare providers and other agencies, including those that provide **case management** services, have responded with enthusiasm and have made information available in abundance. In addition, for the past decade the Internet has been increasingly used as an attractive and desirable communication tool and invaluable resource for both healthcare consumers and providers alike. It functions as an easy medium for locating, accessing, exchanging, sharing, and disseminating information. However, posting health-related information on the Internet is not limited to healthcare providers and experts; anyone can post information regardless of one's qualifications. This can make the quality, clarity, credibility, currency, and accuracy of the information questionable.

It is not a simple task for healthcare consumers to evaluate Internet-based information and resources and to make a decision whether to use them. Therefore it behooves healthcare providers to guide consumers in selecting appropriate and reliable information and to educate them about the harms of misinformation. Because of their role in care coordination and management, **case managers** are best positioned to assume the role of guiding consumers in this area. This chapter presents the case manager with a "tool kit" for effective use of the Internet as a medium for locating health-related information for, and communicating with, their patients, families, and other providers and agencies.

Searching for healthcare-related information on the Internet and the World Wide Web (WWW) is essential for case managers' success in the information management and communication dimension of their role. The use of the Internet assists case managers in locating people; telephone numbers; addresses (both regular and electronic mailing addresses); patient and family education materials; and other information about community, governmental, and nongovernmental agencies and resources. This information is most helpful in care coordination, **transitional planning,** resource utilization, and care and **outcomes management.** Ultimately, the Internet serves as an information tool that is essential for both the provider and the consumer of healthcare services. However, because of the virtually limitless amount of information available on the WWW, it presents a great challenge, particularly for the consumer. No wonder patients and their families often express their frustration about the difficulty of accessing information online.

THE INTERNET

The Internet is a public, cooperative creation that operates using national and international telecommunication technologies and networks, including high-speed data lines, telephone lines, satellite communications, and radio networks. The history of the Internet is available on the Website of the Internet Society, which can be accessed at http://www.isoc.org/internet-history/. Most individuals and healthcare organizations and providers connect to the Internet through a local area network (LAN) using a computer. Each computer has a unique Internet protocol (IP) address and connects to the Internet via a local server or host. The local server often connects to a larger server called a *wide area network (WAN).* This can result in connecting many computers and many local and wide area networks into larger networks that ultimately form the Internet and the WWW.

The WWW allows Internet users access to a wealth of information, materials, and documents. The amount of

Internet-based information is growing by leaps and bounds every day. This information is available in many different forms, such as text, pictures, graphics, films, videos, and audio recordings. Compared with film and video, text is the easiest to download and requires the least sophisticated type of technology. Although the Internet has many advantages, it is not free of certain challenges (Box 19-1). Case managers and other healthcare providers must be aware of these and act accordingly to ensure appropriate and safe use of this technology both by providers and consumers alike. It also is important for case managers to have some knowledge of Internet technology and computers so that they can advise consumers of healthcare on patient and family education materials and resources that are easily accessible and do not require extensive Internet and computer knowledge and skills.

Use of the Internet by Case Managers

Case managers can use the Internet (Case Manager's Tip 19-1) in many ways that benefit the provision of patient care and its related **outcomes** (Johnson and Tahan, 2003). These include searching for and downloading information, communicating via individual and group electronic mail (e-mail), and engaging in online chat and support group discussions. Before discussing these benefits, it is important to explain the different types of IPs, also called *Transmission Control Protocols (TCPs),* and how Web pages are named and organized.

Internet Protocols

An IP/TCP is a communication language used by Web clients and servers to communicate with one another. It assembles files, documents, films, and messages into smaller packets for transmission over the network/Internet. Moreover, it allows the distribution of information over the Internet. The IP/TCP ensures that packets reach their intended destination. There are five types of protocols used to access resources on the Internet (Hancock, 1996). These are as follows:

1. The *hypertext transfer protocol,* known as HTTP, provides access to the Internet by defining hypertext links to information on the WWW.
2. The *file transfer protocol,* known as FTP, provides for the transfer or downloading of documents, programs, and files from or to a file transfer server. It is also the method of sending files to and receiving files from remote computers on the Internet.
3. The *Telnet,* known as TELNET, allows one to log on to remote computers.
4. The *simple mail transfer protocol,* known as SMTP, enables the sending and receiving of electronic messages.

BOX 19-1   Advantages and Disadvantages of the Internet

Some of the advantages of the Internet are as follows:
1. It provides almost instantaneous access to information compared with traditional print media.
2. The barriers of time and distance when attempting to access, gather, or disseminate information are resolved by using the Internet.
3. Conducting timely literature or computer searches related to a particular topic. Ease of access to lay information on a variety of healthcare-related topics.
4. The turnaround time for making information (e.g., texts, videos, films) available on the Internet surpasses that required by traditional publication media.
5. Messages can be sent almost immediately by one Internet user to another or to a group of users, regardless of geographical location, distance, or time.
6. It provides the ability to e-mail documents easily and efficiently.
7. Communicating to a large number of people at the same time and using the same message is helpful and desirable.
8. It provides the ability to navigate Web pages that address similar and related topics using hyperlinks.
9. It provides the ability to use the Internet at one's own convenience.

Some of the disadvantages of the Internet are as follows:
1. Accessing the information available on the Internet relies on the availability of the server and the speed and type of the modem.
2. The benefits of face-to-face and personal contact are absent.
3. Not all documents posted on the Internet are refereed/peer reviewed, which threatens their quality and credibility.
4. Information available on the Internet is not thorough and does not replace traditional media and publications.
5. The ease and immediacy of e-mail communication can become a source of trouble and annoyance.
6. The Internet is not guaranteed as a safe medium. Sometimes computer viruses are transmitted intentionally or unintentionally, and hackers may be able to alter the information on some Websites despite password protection activities.
7. Downloading documents from the Internet may present some problems depending on the type of Internet-based services and availability of specific software or technologies.
8. The use of e-mail as a method for distributing "junk" mail may be viewed as a nuisance.
9. Maintaining privacy and confidentiality of information presents a great challenge.

CASE MANAGER'S TIP 19-1

Guide to Using the Internet

There are many Websites that include tips, tools, and other Web-searching resources. Examples are as follows:

1. Finding Information on the Internet
   http://www.lib.berkeley.edu/TeachingLib/Guides/Internet/FindInfo.html
2. Learn the Net: Knowledge When You Need It
   http://www.learnthenet.com/english/index.html (also available in French, German, Spanish, and Italian)
3. Search Engine Watch
   http://www.searchenginewatch.com

---

5. The *hypertext markup language,* known as HTML, produces a hypertext document for display by a WWW browser and uses a standardized set of tags that tells the browser how to display the text and how to specify the hypertext links (Hancock, 1996).

Knowledge of these protocols is not a prerequisite for accessing Internet-based resources; however, it enhances case managers' Internet navigation skills and makes them better able to educate their patients about how to access information via the Internet. If patients present their case manager with certain questions, the case manager can be prepared and ready to answer or he or she can obtain the answers to these questions.

Web Pages

Web pages are named and organized in a specific way to help Internet users to easily locate information on the WWW. The address of a file, Web page, document, or resource available on the Internet and accessed by Web clients is called the *uniform resource locator (URL).* URLs are unique in nature and mutually exclusive. Most Web pages are composed applying HTML. An example of a Web page is http://www.mendedhearts.org/frame-aboutus.htm. This is the address of the home page of The Mended Hearts, Inc., which focuses on healthcare consumers and is designed to offer help, support, and encouragement to heart disease patients and their families. Let us review the specific components of this URL as follows:

1. *http://* is the prefix used to access the file; that is, the hypertext transfer protocol.
2. *www.mendedhearts.org* is the domain name of the server on which the file is located, in this case The Mended Hearts, Inc., main Web server.

3. *www* is the portion of the domain name that specifies the server. In this case, it is the Web server.
4. *mendedhearts* is the subdomain of The Mended Hearts, Inc.
5. *.org* is a suffix that identifies an organization.
6. *frame-aboutus* is the directory in which the file resides.

Suffixes in a URL may include the following types:

1. *.edu* indicates a U.S. educational institution Internet site. An example is http://www.columbia.edu, the Website for Columbia University, New York.
2. *.com* indicates a commercial Internet site. An example is http://www.LWW.com, the home page of the Lippincott Williams & Wilkins publishing company.
3. *.gov* indicates a governmental Internet site. An example is http://www.ahrq.gov, the home page of the Agency for Healthcare Research and Quality.
4. *.org* indicates an organization Internet site. An example is http://www.ncsbn.org, the Website of The National Council of State Boards of Nursing.
5. *.net* indicates a network-related Internet site. An example is http://www.matisse.net, a Website that shares information pulled together from other sites.
6. *.mil* indicates a military Website. An example is http://www.army.mil, the U.S. Army Website.

Understanding the use of different suffixes allows case managers to locate information on the WWW more expeditiously. For example, case managers must know that to locate Websites of governmental agencies, they must use the suffix *.gov* after the acronym of the agency they are interested in locating.

Navigating to Knowledge

The greatest advantage of the Internet is availability and ease of access to information. Case managers and others can use the Internet to obtain any type of information, including professional and scientific literature, research outcomes, latest technologies and therapies, nonprofessional literature, patient and family education materials, health products information, addresses and contact information of medical and consumer agencies, and commercial reports and information. So, how can one search for such information?

To locate information on the Internet, case managers can use search engines. Search engines employ specialized software to query the Internet. The software allows the search engine to constantly acquire new information, documents, files, and other resources and to update the **database** that makes up the search engine. When a person queries a topic, the search engine checks for matches in the database based on the key words used to search the topic. Before you search a topic, it is important to decide whether you need broad,

CASE MANAGER'S TIP 19-2

Differentiating Between Directories and Indexes

Directories, also called *subject catalogs,* are lists of Web-sites that have been filtered by an editor or reviewer or compiled by a person. They are limited to a fraction of the documents available on the WWW. This is because documents are added to the directory only after notification of the document author or the Website owner. Examples of directories are Yahoo, Excite, and Medsite Navigator.

Indexes are large databases of Websites. The entries of an index are usually gathered automatically by search engines des   igned to scan the WWW for any new doc-uments and Websites on a regular basis, usually weekly or monthly, and the resulting new information is then automatically added to the database. Examples of indexes are AltaVista, Infoseek, and the Internet Sleuth.

---

3. Directories are hierarchically organized databases and are best for locating a large amount of information on a topic. Popular Web directories include the following:

Yahoo	http://www.yahoo.com
Galaxy	http://www.galaxy.com
LookSmart	http://www.looksmart.com
OpenDirectoryProject	http://www.dmoz.com
W3 Virtual Library	http://www.virtuallibrary.com

A rule of thumb for the case manager attempting to locate information on the Internet is to use major and meta search engines because the outcomes of such searches will most likely be the information most appropriate and relevant to the keyword used in the search. For example, attempting to search for "case management" using the search engine Metafind will most possibly yield a list of references limited to the topic "case management" and not health management or disease management. Other tips on searching for information are discussed in the following section.

Tips on Searching for Information

Using the Internet to search a particular topic can lead to hundreds or even thousands of Web pages and docu-ments. For example, a recent search of the topic **"managed care"** yielded 378 Websites using the Yahoo directory; 1,979,640 sites using WebCrawler; and 20 sites using the MetaCrawler search engine. However, if you use quotation marks you can narrow down your search and make it more specific. When quotation marks were used for searching the same topic "managed care" applying the same search engines, it yielded 297 sites in Yahoo, 31,810 sites in WebCrawler, and 20 sites in MetaCrawler. Other strategies that can be used to narrow down the search results are as follows:

1. Use AND, OR, NEAR, and NOT between the key-words in the topic.
2. Use a plus (+) sign in front of any word that you want included in the results.
3. Use a minus (–) sign in front of any word you want excluded.
4. Use an asterisk (*) to search for variations on a word.

An additional way to search a topic is by navigating the Web using the hyperlinks included in the results of an initial search. Most of the time Websites related to the topic being searched include hyperlinks to other similar or related Web pages. It is not necessary to review all of the sites displayed in the results of a search. It is common that the first 20 sites displayed are the ones found to be the most useful and most relevant to the topic searched.

Searching the Internet is not limited to locating documents and healthcare information. It can also be used to find newsgroup postings and people. Finding

---

general information or narrow, specific information because this dictates the type of search engine to be applied. Search engines are of three types: major and meta search engines (both also known as *indexes*) and directories (Case Manager's Tip 19-2).

1. Major search engines are comprehensive search tools that are fairly current and used for broad and general topics. The following are some popular major search engines:

AltaVista	http://www.altavista.com
Excite	http://www.excite.com
HotBot	http://www.hotbot.com
Infoseek	http://www.infoseek.com
Lycos	http://www.lycos.com
WebCrawler	http://www.webcrawler.com
Direct Hit	http://www.directhit.com
FastSearch	http://ussc.alltheweb.com
Go	http://www.go.com
Google	http://www.google.com
GoTo	http://www.goto.com
Northern Light	http://www.northernlight.com
Snap	http://www.snap.com

2. Meta search engines are multiengine search sites and are used to search for specific and narrow topics. The following are some popular meta search engines:

DogPile	http://www.dogpile.com
InferenceFind	http://www.wisdomdog.com
MetaCrawler	http://www.metacrawler.com
MetaFind	http://www.metafind.com
All4One	http://www.all4one.com
ProFusion	http://www.profusion.com
SavvySearch	http://www.savvysearch.com
Highway61	http://www.highway61.com
Cyber411	http://www.cyber411.com

newsgroups, or digital discussions and bulletin boards, can be done using search engines that are dedicated to seeking and archiving messages from these forums. Search engines such as AltaVista, InfoSeek, and Excite allow Internet users to locate newsgroups as well; however, there are other sites, such as the following, that are available specifically for the purpose of locating newsgroups:

Google Groups	http://www.groups.google.com
InReference, Inc.	http://www.inreference.com

In addition to locating newsgroups, there are special search engines available for finding people on the Internet. These engines operate through databases that gather people's electronic mailing addresses obtained from the commercial Internet access providers or through tracking the addresses of people who post messages online. If a person has an electronic mailing address but does not use it, it is unlikely for it to appear in the search or for other people to learn of its presence. Examples of these search engines are as follows:

BigYellow	http://www.bigyellow.com
World Wide Yellow Pages	http://www.yellow.com
Yahoo People Search	http://www.people.yahoo.com

Electronic Communication

Electronic communication is the act of transmitting information from one person to another or to a group of people using the Internet and the WWW media/network and technology. This form of electronic communication is completed on demand. However, as with other forms of electronic communication on the Internet, information is posted by individuals or agencies at their convenience and regardless of the specific needs of or requests by others (i.e., Internet users). Examples of electronic communication are e-mail, newsgroups, bulletin boards, and listservs.

The use of e-mail is so widespread and popular today that almost everyone relies on it to conduct regular business functions. E-mail is the most common use of the Internet. It is the act of sending messages from one person to another using electronic media and telecommunication technologies. The transmission of such messages takes place via the Internet or a network. E-mail is also used as a method of communication between one individual and a group of people simultaneously; in this case it is called a *listserv, bulletin board,* or *newsgroup* (Case Manager's Tip 19-3) (Johnson and Tahan, 2003).

Listservs (also called *mailing lists*), bulletin boards, and newsgroups provide a forum for group discussion. These methods of communication consist of a group of people with similar interests (e.g., nursing informatics, case management) or professions (e.g., case manager,

 CASE MANAGER'S TIP 19-3

Using Electronic Communication Tools with Caution

Electronic communication tools such as newsgroups, listservs, chat rooms, mailing lists, and bulletin boards are a rich source of information; however, case managers must caution patients and their families about their reliability. Patients must be advised not to blindly apply the recommendations made by participants of these forums without validating the information first by case managers or other healthcare providers. Case managers must also teach their patients how to differentiate between those that are moderated by a healthcare professional and those that are "free for all."

social worker) who get together to share information through an e-mail–based discussion group. They are asynchronous (i.e., do not need the online presence of people engaged in the discussion at the same time) in nature and allow participants/subscribers to respond to posted messages at their own convenience. Members of these communication forums can be from around the globe; however, they use the same language in their exchange of information.

Another type of mailing list is synchronous discussion groups, or chat rooms, which provide an opportunity for real-time/concurrent conversations and discussions. Each chat room focuses on a specific topic or an area of interest. Not all chat rooms are facilitated by a moderator. Moderators function as a facilitator of the discussion and oversee the content and flow of information. They also possess the authority to disqualify subscribers who are disruptive or use obscene language from participating in a chat room discussion. Some chat rooms are oriented toward professionals such as nurses, physicians, or other healthcare providers; some others are for consumers of healthcare (patients and their families). Provider-based chat rooms focus on the discussion of topics that relate to the delivery of healthcare or the various health professions. Consumer-based chat rooms focus on topics related to health promotion, disease prevention, self-help, emotional support, and sharing of personal experiences. Case managers should be knowledgeable about the advantages and disadvantages of these methods of electronic communication (Box 19-2) so that they become better able to assist healthcare consumers in selecting the most beneficial forums for communication in relation to accessing healthcare services and resources.

BOX 19-2 Advantages and Disadvantages of Electronic Communication

Some of the advantages of electronic communication are as follows:

1. The speed of transfer of information (i.e., communication).
2. The ability to communicate the same message to a group of people at the same time.
3. Being on mailing lists can put information and resources at providers' (e.g., case managers) fingertips.
4. Easy and universal access to patients and healthcare professionals.
5. The ability to transmit files electronically as e-mail attachments.
6. The ability to communicate with healthcare professionals at the patients' convenience and without having to be personally present.
7. Providing patients with easy access to schedule follow-up appointments or request information or advice regarding healthcare issues or treatments.
8. Dissemination of health promotion and prevention information such as newsletters and patient and family education materials.
9. The tendency toward being informal in nature.
10. Participation in moderated discussions with book authors, experts, and authority figures in nursing and patient care.

Some of the disadvantages of electronic communication are as follows:

1. Concern regarding the security and confidentiality of e-mail messages.
2. Dependence on availability of a mail program and an Internet server.
3. The challenge to maintain compliance with the HIPAA standards.
4. The presence of e-mail and Internet hackers.
5. The susceptibility of communicated information to abuse or mishandling.
6. Downloading attachments and files is dependent on comparable/compatible software applications.
7. Similar to regular mail, some e-mail messages are considered "junk" mail.
8. The access of advertising agencies and market researchers to e-mail account subscribers.
9. Misspelling an e-mail address results in returned mail or delivery to the wrong person.
10. Some subscribers of mailing lists/listservs find it easy to respond to posted messages in a flaming or obscene way because there is no face-to-face contact.

From Johnson T, Tahan H: *Improving performance of clinical operations.* In Montgomery K, Fitzpatrick J, editors: *Essentials of Internet use in nursing,* New York, 2003, Springer.

In response to the concerns the public has expressed regarding electronic/online communication and consul-tation, Medem, a national medical society sponsored by more than 50 healthcare organizations, associations, and societies, developed a set of guidelines for "online communication." These guidelines were developed in November 2001 to help healthcare providers enhance the safety and reduce the risk of electronic communication. It is appropriate and important for case managers, especially those who use electronic communication as a case management strategy with their patients, to adopt Medem's recommendations to the best of their ability. These recommendations act as legal, ethical, and professional guidelines that govern communications between the healthcare provider and patients. They may also be applied to e-mail, Websites, listservs, and other methods of electronic communication (eRisk Working Group for Healthcare, 2001). The recommendations are as follows:

1. *Security:* Communicate over a secure network, with provisions for authentication and encryption in accordance with the Health Insurance Portability and Accountability Act (HIPAA) and other appropriate guidelines. Healthcare providers need to be aware of potential security risks, including unauthorized physical access and security of computer hardware, and guard against them with technologies such as automatic logout and password protection.
2. *Authentication:* Take reasonable steps to authenticate the identity of correspondent(s) in an electronic communication and to ensure that recipients of information are authorized to receive it.
3. *Confidentiality:* Take reasonable steps to protect patient privacy and to guard against unauthorized use of patient information.
4. *Unauthorized access:* Establish and follow procedures that help to mitigate this risk. The use of online communication may increase the risk of unauthorized distribution of patient information.
5. *Informed consent:* Obtain informed consent from the patient regarding the appropriate use and limitations of the methods of electronic communication.
6. *Provider-patient relationship:* Do not limit yourself to an online provider-patient relationship. Initiating a provider-patient relationship solely through online interaction can increase the healthcare provider's **liability** exposure.
7. *Medical records:* Maintain a record of the online communications pertinent to the ongoing medical care of the patient and integrate it into the patient's medical record, whether that record is paper or electronic.
8. *Licensing jurisdiction:* Be aware of the state requirements of online communication and licensure. Communicating with patients outside the state the provider is licensed in may subject the provider to increased risk.

9. *Authoritative information:* Make sure that the information you provide or make available via online communication, such as a Website, comes either directly from you as the provider or from a recognized and credible source.

10. *Commercial information:* Avoid Website-based or online communication of advertising, promotional, or marketing products because they may subject providers to increased liability, including implicit guarantees or implied warranty.

PATIENT AND FAMILY EDUCATION RESOURCES

Patient and family education resources are available on the Internet in abundance. Case managers are advised to employ the information searching tips presented in the previous section to locate and access these resources and to educate their patients on how to obtain healthcare-related materials online. Patients and families who are taught how to access Internet resources may feel empowered because of the knowledge they gain in the process. They may also feel a greater sense of control, gain more self-care skills, and assume the responsibility for their own care. Knowing that they are not alone and that other people with similar conditions are accessible via the Internet and online support discussion groups enhances their self-confidence and encourages them to adhere to their medical regimen. Case managers and healthcare consumers may access patient and family education resources through the following:

1. Professional societies such as the American Heart Association (http://www.americanheart.org) and the Oncology Nursing Society (http://www.ons.org)

2. Governmental agencies such as the Centers for Medicare and Medicaid Services (CMS), formerly known as the Health Care Financing Administration (HCFA) (http://www.hcfa.gov) and the National Institutes of Health (http://www.nih.gov)

3. Healthcare organizations such as the Mayo Clinic (http://www.mayoclinic.org) and the Cleveland Clinic (http://www.clevelandclinic.org)

4. Commercial organizations such as WebMD (http://www.webmd.org) or Johnson and Johnson, Inc. (http://www.johnsonandjohnson.com)

5. Consumer-sponsored organizations such as The Mended Hearts, Inc. (http://www.mendedhearts.org) and Health Cite, Inc. (http://www.healthcite.com)

One must be able to differentiate between resources that are developed by healthcare providers and those developed by lay people. Those sponsored by healthcare providers and agencies tend to be more reliable, current, and void of any misinformation. Case managers can assume a significant role in educating their patients in this area and in assisting them to locate the best materials possible. Case managers can be an invaluable resource for streamlining and simplifying available resources for patients and their families in an effort to enhance their adherence to the medical regimen, build their self-care skills, and reduce their anxiety toward their health condition and necessary lifestyle changes. Ultimately, this role enhances the achievement of desirable outcomes.

OTHER USES OF THE INTERNET BY CASE MANAGERS

Case managers may rely on the Internet for the delivery, management, and evaluation of healthcare services. They can also use the Internet to access resources such as directories of healthcare providers of particular managed care companies, information about healthcare **benefits,** governmental program information and guidelines, directories of community resources and healthcare services/agencies, and charitable organizations. These resources are essential for better case management services and outcomes. Case managers may use the Internet in many ways, with the ultimate goal of enhancing the practice of case management. Some of the uses of the Internet for case managers are as follows:

1. Find the latest research outcomes to implement evidence-based practice.

2. Access recommendations of professional organizations and societies.

3. Obtain national standards and guidelines from clearinghouses to use for improving patient care delivery and outcomes.

4. Remain abreast of the latest changes in the standards of governmental and **accreditation** agencies.

5. Share expert knowledge in specific practice areas.

6. Access national benchmark **databases.**

7. Communicate across the globe in a timely fashion.

8. Receive/send announcements and newsletters electronically.

9. Direct questions to authors, researchers, and experts and obtain answers expeditiously.

10. Communicate among settings, levels of care, and different providers. Discuss care issues, make decisions regarding changes in the plan of care, and resolve problems in a timely fashion.

11. Transmit required information (e.g., ORYX data to the Joint Commission on Accreditation of Healthcare Organizations [JCAHO], utilization reviews to managed care organizations, and significant events data to the state health departments) electronically to other public and private agencies and organizations.

12. Participate in continuing educational sessions online.
13. Conduct research and collect data online.

ASSESSING THE QUALITY OF HEALTH INFORMATION ON THE INTERNET

The Internet is a medium of free expression. Some information is accurate, reliable, and credible; some is not and is considered harmful. Maintaining the quality of the information available on the WWW presents a great challenge considering that this medium is volatile and difficult to trace. The reason for this challenge is the fact that the provision of healthcare information on the Internet and the WWW is not regulated. Therefore it is necessary to educate patients and their families about how to examine the quality of the information posted on the Internet to prevent the application of misinformation. Case managers are best positioned to assume the educator role. To be effective they must be familiar with the process of assessing information available on the WWW and must apply specific criteria for this purpose.

As the Internet has become an essential tool for the provision of healthcare services, it is important that healthcare providers, including case managers, play a **gatekeeper** role in ensuring that consumers use only information that is considered of exceptional quality. To avoid any flaws in the process of evaluating the quality of health information available on the Internet, several authors and societies developed and recommended the use of certain necessary criteria for such evaluation. To prevent confusion about which set of criteria is more credible and best to apply, Romano, Hinegardner, and Phyillaier (2000) compared several sets and identified five common and simple-to-use criteria. Case managers may elect to use these criteria as their standard for evaluating the quality of Internet-based healthcare information. The criteria are as follows:

1. *Authority/source:* If it is an author, the Website must include the author's credentials and expertise. If it is an organization, one must question its reputation. The site must also include contact information.
2. *Purpose/objectivity:* The site must clearly state its purpose, its sponsor, and the intended audience.
3. *Content:* The site must disseminate accurate, useful, and relevant information to the need of the users. It must also include relevant and authoritative links to other sites.
4. *Currency:* The site must include the date of posted information and of any updates.
5. *Design:* The site must be well organized, easy to navigate, stable, and free of any clutter.

There are other sets of criteria recommended by other agencies such as the criteria set advocated for by The Health Information Technology Institute of Mitretek Systems (Box 19-3). The Institute developed its criteria by convening a Health Summit Working Group in 1996. It held another Summit in 1998 that resulted in revising the original criteria (Ambre et al, 1999). The set of criteria developed by this Summit is considered credible, is widely used, and is available all over the world. It also has been translated into several languages. The users of these criteria would include policy makers, healthcare information/content developers, providers, consumers, and payers.

Another method for ensuring the credibility and reliability of health information on the Internet is adherence to the "Health on the Net (HON) Code of Conduct." Users of the Internet are able to identify if a site complies with the HON Code of Conduct if the site indicates as such on its home page. This is communicated by including the HON logo/seal on the main page of the Website. The HON Code of Conduct is a self-regulatory solution and voluntary **certification** system applied to address the lack of confidence and problem of distrust in the information available on the WWW. It is the Internet's first and most widely spread ethical standard. It has been available since 1996 in more than a dozen languages, including English (Health on the Net Foundation, 2002). The HON Code of Conduct addresses one of the Internet's main healthcare information-related issues: the reliability and credibility of information made available electronically.

Applying the HON Code of Conduct means quality; that is, the Website follows good standards in the presentation of healthcare information, resources, and advice and strictly abides by the code's principles (Case Manager's Tip 19-4). The code consists of eight principles (Box 19-4): authority, complementarity, confidentiality, attribution, justifiability, transparency of authorship, transparency of sponsorship, and honesty in advertising and editorial policy.

CASE MANAGEMENT-RELATED WEBSITES

The following is a list of Websites that are related to case management practice. This list is by no means exhaustive. Case managers are advised to surf the Internet and the WWW for other sites that may be more relevant to their area of practice. To do this more effectively, they are encouraged to use the tools and tips presented in this chapter. Please note, however, that the URL addresses in this chapter are based on the information available at the time. Websites are constantly being changed by their owners or Webmasters;

BOX 19-3 Criteria for Assessing the Quality of Health Information on the Internet

Credibility

Source

Does the site display the name and logo of the institute responsible for the information and the name and title of the author?

Does the site present the credentials and qualifications of the authors and organizations?

Does the site include any information about the sponsors or other affiliations?

Currency

Does the site display the original document posting date?

Does the site include the date(s) of revisions?

Relevance

Does the content of the documents relate to the information they purport to offer?

Site Evaluation

Does the site apply a peer review process before posting a document?

Does the site share a description of its peer review process?

Content

Accuracy

Does the site identify the data that underlie the conclusions presented?

Does the site include the clinical and/or scientific evidence that supports the position taken?

Disclaimer

Does the site display a disclaimer that describes the purpose, scope, authority, and currency of information provided?

Does the site disclose the sources of information?

Does the site share information in the context of general health information and not medical advice?

Completeness

Does the site present discussions that are comprehensive and balanced?

Does the site include pertinent facts, negative results, and a statement of any information not known about the subject addressed?

Disclosure

Purpose

Does the site display its mission or purpose clearly?

Does the information provided relate to the mission or purpose?

Profiling

Does the site make the user aware of the purpose of the information presented?

Does the site share with the user the process for collecting information and its use?

Does the site present a process for dissemination of information?

Links

Selection

Does the site include any links to other sites?

Does the site employ qualified staff for selecting appropriate and related links?

Does the site include links that are relevant to its mission and purpose?

Architecture

Does the site make it easy for the user to find his or her way backward or forward?

Does the site apply an apparent and logical structure?

Does the site use any meaningful and consistent image-based icons or textual identifiers?

Content

Does the site include links with accurate, current, credible, and relevant information?

Does the site provide information about the linked source before the user clicks to the site?

Back Linkages (Linkages From One Site to Another)

Does the site avoid any bias in the use of back linkages?

Does the site allow for back linkages?

Design

Access

Does the site include graphics and text in its layout?

Does the site allow accessibility using the lowest level available browser technology?

Does the site alert the user to the need for special technology (e.g., real player, multimedia) for access to certain information?

Navigability

Does the site focus on its purpose and target audience?

Does the site allow for simple and easy navigation?

Does the site balance between the use of graphics, text, color, and sound?

Internal Search Capability

Does the site allow for internal search capability?

BOX 19-3 Criteria for Assessing the Quality of Health Information on the Internet—cont'd

Does the site provide search capability by keywords? Retrieve relevant information only?

Does the site's internal search capability apply an easy process?

Interactivity

Does the site provide the users with a feedback mechanism to communicate their comments, criticism, and corrections?

Does the site offer the users access to chat rooms or discussion groups?

Does the site employ a qualified moderator to facilitate the discussion groups?

Caveats

Does the site market products?

Does the site advertise or sell products or services?

 CASE MANAGER'S TIP 19-4

Exercising Caution When Surfing the Internet

Unfortunately, the use of the Health on the Net Code of Conduct does not eliminate incompetence, fraud, or communication of dishonest healthcare information. On the other hand, if a Website is found not to bear the code/seal, it does not mean that it is of poor quality. Users must exercise caution when applying the information available on the Internet and judge for themselves. When in doubt, they must consult with a healthcare provider such as a case manager.

---

therefore some URL addresses may no longer be correct if the Website was altered in some way.

Accreditation Agencies

Joint Commission on Accreditation of Healthcare Organizations	http://www.jcaho.org
National Committee for Quality Assurance	http://www.ncqa.org
Commission for Accreditation of Rehabilitation Facilities	http://www.carf.org
Utilization Review Accreditation Commission	http://www.urac.org

Case Management Organizations

Case Management Society of America	http://www.cmsa.org
The Center for Case Management	http://www.cfcm.com

Case Management Software

HealthShare Technologies	http://www.healthshare.com
Landacorp	http://www.landacorp.com
McKesson HBOC/InterQual Products Group	http://www.interqual.com
Per-Se Technologies	http://www.per-se.com
Threshold Data Technologies	http://www.thresholddata.com
Milliman & Robertson Care Guidelines	http://www.mnr.com/guidelines/index.html
HCIA	http://www.hcia.com
Case Management Resource Guide	http://www.cmrg.com
Advocate 2002 (legal)	http://www.advocate2002.com/advocate/advocate_welcome.htm
Case Tracker	http://www.casetrakker.com

BOX 19-4 Health on the Net Code of Conduct

The Health on the Net Code of Conduct consists of the following eight principles:

1. *Authority:* Medical information is provided only by medically trained and qualified professionals unless a clear statement is made that a piece of information is from a nonmedical person.

2. *Complementarity:* Information provided is designed to support, not replace, the relationship between a patient/user and his or her physician/healthcare provider.

3. *Confidentiality:* Includes users'/visitors' identities. The owners of the site honor the legal requirements of medical/health information privacy that apply in the country/location where the Website is located.

4. *Attribution:* Information included on the site is supported, when appropriate, by clear references and data sources, and dates of the last modifications are clearly stated.

5. *Justifiability:* Balances claims relating to the benefits/performance of a specific treatment, commercial product, or service with appropriate evidence in the manner stated in principle 4.

6. *Transparency of authorship:* Designers of the site provide information in the clearest possible manner and provide contact addresses for visitors who seek further information. The site includes the Webmaster's e-mail address.

7. *Transparency of sponsorship:* Includes the identities of the sponsors of the site and the names of the commercial and noncommercial organizations that have contributed funding to the site.

8. *Honesty in advertising and editorial policy:* Clearly states whether advertising is a source of funding to the site. If that is the case, presents a brief description of the advertising policy adopted by the site. Advertisements are presented in a manner that is easy to differentiate from original materials created by the operators of the site.

Certification in Case Management

Commission for Case Manager Certification	http://www.ccmcertification.org
American Nurses Association	http://www.nursingworld.org
American Institute of Outcomes Case Management	http://www.aiocm.com
National Association of Healthcare Quality	http://www.cphq-hqcb.org
The Center for Case Management	http://www.cfcm.com
National Board for Certification in Continuity of Care	http://www.nbccc.org
Certification of Disability Management Specialists Commission	http://www.cdms.org
Rehabilitation Nursing Certification Board	http://www.rehabnurse.org
National Association of Social Workers	http://www.nasw.org
American Board of Managed Care Nursing	http://www.abmcn.org
American Board for Occupational Health Nurses	http://www.abohn.org
American Academy of Case Management	http://www.aihcp.org/cs%7Emgmnt.htm
InterQual	http://www.interqual.com

Disease Management

Disease Management Forum	http://www.sapien.net/dm/

Ethics

Health on the Net Code of Conduct	http://www.hon.ch/HONcode/

Governmental Agencies

Agency for Healthcare Research and Quality	http://www.ahrq.gov
National Institutes of Health	http://www.nih.gov
Healthy People 2010	http://web.health.gov/healthypeople
National Health Information Center	http://www.nhic.org or http://www.health.gov/nhic/
Centers for Disease Control and Prevention	http://www.cdc.gov
National Institute of Safety and Health	http://www.cdc.gov/niosh/
Occupational Safety and Health Administration	http://www.osha.gov
The Department of Health and Human Services	http://www.dhhs.gov
U.S. Government Statistics	http://www.fedstats.gov
Federal Register	http://www.access.gpo.gov/
Food and Drug Administration	http://www.fda.gov/

Managed Care

Managed Care Information Center	http://www.themcic.com
Health Scope	http://www.healthscope.org
The HMO Page	http://www.hmopage.org
Managed Care Magazine	http://www.managedcaremag.com
American Association of Managed Care Nurses	http://www.aamcn.org
National Association of Managed Care Physicians	http://www.namcp.com
Integrated Healthcare Association	http://www.iha.org
ANA Nursing Quality Report Card	http://www.nursingworld.org
Managed Care Online	http://www.mcol.com

Managed Care—cont'd

National Managed Health Care Congress	http://www.nmhcc.org
American College of Managed Care Medicine	http://www.acmcm.org

Occupational Health

Occupational Safety and Health Administration	http://www.osha.gov

Organizations (Related)

Kaiser Permanente	http://www.kaiserpermanente.org
The Center for Case Management	http://www.cfcm.com
Case Management Society of America	http://www.cmsa.org
Health on the Net Foundation	http://www.hon.ch/
World Health Organization	http://www.who.ch
The Healthcare Advisory Board	http://www.advisoryboardcompany.com
American Association of Managed Care Nurses	http://www.aamcn.org

Patient and Family Education Materials

New York Online Access to Health	http://www.noah.cuny.edu/
HealthFinder	http://www.healthfinder.gov
MedWeb Consumer Health	http://www.gen.emory.edu/MEDWEB/keyword/consumer_health.html
National Health Information Resources	http://www.nhic.org

Patient Rights and Safety

National Coalition of Patient Rights	http://www/tiac.net/
President's Advisory Commission on Consumer Protection	http://www.hcqualitycommission.gov
National Patient Safety Foundation	http://www.npsf.org
Institute for Safe Medication Practices	http://www.ismp.org
VHA National Center for Patient Safety	http://www.patientsafetycenter.com

Quality

National Committee for Quality Assurance	http://www.ncqa.org
MediQual Systems, Inc.	http://www.mediqual.com
The Quality Compass	http://www.ncqa.org/Info/QualityCompass/Index.htm
The Institute for Outcomes Research	http://www.admin@isiscor.com
Medical Outcomes Trust	http://www.outcomes-trust.org
Combined Health Information Database	http://www.chid.nih.gov
Evidence-Based Medicine Tool Kit	http://www.med.ualberta.ca/ebm/
The Center for Case Management Accountability	http://www.cmsa.org/ccma/ccma-main.html
American Institute of Outcomes Case Management	http://www.aiocm.com
InterQual	http://www.interqual.com
National Quality Forum	http://www.qualityforum.org

Workers' Compensation

U.S. Department of Labor, Office of Workers' Compensation Program	http://www.dol.gov/dol/esa/ public/aboutesa/owcpabot.htm
Workers' Compensation Services, Inc.	http://www.workcompaudit.com
U.S. Department of Labor	http://www.dol.gov
U.S. Department of Justice, Americans With Disabilities Act	http://www.usdoj.gov/crt/ada
U.S. Department of Labor, Employment Standards Administration	http://www.dol.gov/esa/
Occupational Safety and Health Administration	http://www.osha.gov

There is no limit to the amount of healthcare resources available on the WWW and the Internet. These resources are constantly changing. Information is updated daily, and in some respects, by the moment. Case managers are encouraged not to fear using the Internet as a resource. If they choose to work with their patients and families, they must do so patiently, starting with the level of knowledge and skill they are at in using the Internet or other electronic communication methods. For some healthcare consumers the Internet may work well, especially for consumers who are enrolled in **disease management** programs or other forms of case management services and programs.

 KEY POINTS

1. The Internet and the WWW allow case managers immediate access to an invaluable amount of health-related information and resources that may facilitate better patient care services and outcomes.

2. Case managers must advise their patients and families not to apply any recommendations of treatments obtained from Internet resources without first consulting their primary healthcare provider or case manager.

3. Applying the tools and tips presented in this chapter on how to surf the Web maximizes search results and increases the chances for obtaining information that is accurate and relevant to the topic of interest.

4. It is important for case managers to apply the criteria of evaluating the quality of healthcare resources available on the Internet.

5. When they are involved in developing resources and information for use via the Internet and the WWW, such as online patient and family education materials, case managers must abide by the Health on the Net (HON) Code of Conduct and Medem's guidelines.

REFERENCES

Ambre J, Guard R, Perveiler F, et al: *Criteria for assessing the quality of health information on the Internet,* Falls Church, Va, 1999, Health Summit Working Group, Mitretek Systems, (policy paper). Available online at http://www.mitretek.org/Home.nsf/Main/Publications (accessed 3/26/02).

e-Risk Working Group for Healthcare: *Guidelines for online communications and consultations,* 2001, Medem. Available online at http://www.medem.com/corporate/corporate_erisk_guidelines.cfm (accessed 3/30/02).

Hancock L: *Physician's guide to the Internet,* Philadelphia, 1996, Lippincott-Raven.

Health on the Net Foundation: *Health on the net code of conduct,* 2002. Available online at http://www.hon.ch/HONcode/Conduct.html (accessed 3/28/02).

Johnson T, Tahan H: *Improving performance of clinical operations.* In Montgomery K, Fitzpatrick J, editors: *Essentials of Internet use in nursing,* New York, 2003, Springer.

Romano C, Hinegardner P, Phyillaier C: Some guidelines for browsing the Internet. In Fitzpatrick J, Montgomery K, editors: *Internet resources for nurses,* New York, 2000, Springer.

APPENDIXES

APPENDIXES A THROUGH F
Case Management Plans

Appendixes A through F present some examples of case management plans (CMPs) that pertain to different care settings or levels of care. The significance of these plans is that they represent an interdisciplinary approach to the plan of care of patients with particular diagnoses,

surgical procedures, or other problems. CMPs delineate the standards of care; identify patients' actual and potential problems, the goals of treatment, and the necessary patient care activities; and establish the projected outcomes of care.

The following examples of CMPs are included here:

NOTE: For an acute care CMP, refer to Chapter 12, p. 217.

Things to Remember When Developing Case Management Plans

Keep the following guidelines in mind when developing a CMP:

- Establish an interdisciplinary team.
- Identify team members based on the diagnosis or surgical procedure in question. Members should be chosen based on their clinical experiences, leadership skills, communication skills, tolerance for hard work, and commitment to the institution and the project.

- Identify a team leader and a facilitator.
- Provide the team with administrative and clerical support.
- Establish a project work plan (timeline of activities) before the team's first meeting.
- Train team members in the process of developing CMPs.
- Team members should prepare their work between meetings. Meetings should be held to review the work and determine the next steps.
- Regardless of the format of the CMP, it should always include the patient care elements as identified by the organization, the patient problems, projected length of stay and outcomes of care, a variance tracking form, and patient care activities and interventions.
- Timeline the CMP as indicated by the care setting. For example, minutes to hours in emergency departments, number of visits in clinics and home care, days in acute care, weeks in areas of longer length of stay such as the neonatal intensive care area, and months in nursing homes and group homes. The timeline of CMPs in subacute care and rehabilitation centers can be established based on the length of stay, goals of treatment, and intensity of activities. For the most part, it is daily or weekly.
- Preestablish the expected (acceptable) length of stay/number of visits.
- Determine the mechanism for tracking variances and define the variance categories to be evaluated.
- Ensure that the CMP is the standard of care applied by all healthcare providers, including physicians.
- Include patient and family teaching and discharge planning activities in all CMPs.
- Determine whether CMPs are a permanent part of the medical record.
- Maximize documentation on the CMP. Require all patient care services to use the CMP for documentation.
- Develop CMPs based on the latest recommendations of research and professional societies.
- Avoid being rigid in recommending treatments. For example, use words such as "consider" when including treatments, medications, or interventions that may not be applicable to every patient, completion may not always be possible within the indicated timeframe, or progress may be dependent on the patient's condition.
- Identify the intermediate and discharge outcomes of care in each CMP.
- Delineate the International Classification of Diseases, Ninth Revision (ICD-9) code or the diagnosis-related group (DRG) number of the CMP on the cover page if appropriate.

- Include all disciplines involved in the care of patients as indicated by the diagnosis or surgical procedure considered.
- Stress the importance of patient care activities that historically were identified as problem areas or requiring improvement.
- Establish a timeframe for reviewing and revising the CMP.
- Make an effort to collaborate with healthcare providers from the different settings/levels of care across the continuum.

APPENDIX G
Preprinted Order Sets

Preprinted physician orders are often developed to accompany CMPs. An example of a physician order set for congestive heart failure can be found in Appendix G (p. 390).

Things to Remember When Developing and Using Preprinted Order Sets

- The order set should match the clinical content outlined in the CMP.
- Have members of the CMP team develop the order set at the same time they are working on the CMP.
- Avoid duplication.
- Obtain approval of the order set from the designated approval body in your organization before using the order set.
- Whenever the CMP is reviewed/updated, the order set must be reviewed/updated at the same time.
- A reference to the order set should be made on the CMP to remind the physician and other staff/care providers to use the order set.

APPENDIX H
Documentation Guides for Physicians

Another useful tool is a preprinted set of documentation clues for physicians to include when documenting in the medical record. The guides are used as tools for informing physicians of the more precise language and the range of options in medical terminology that is required to more accurately code the medical record. Accurate coding depends on the quality and completeness of the physician's documentation. By identifying the specific documentation needed to support a particular case type, the physician can include the necessary verbiage to support the coding of the chart into the DRG that best matches the patient's plan of care and treatments. In this way the organization can have greater assurance that they will receive the most appropriate reimbursement for the patient's care during that episode of illness. Examples can be found beginning on p. 391.

Things to Remember When Writing Documentation Guides

- Be sure to review the coding requirements for that case type with the medical record coding staff.
- Solicit input from physician leaders in a particular clinical area to obtain buy-in and to solicit physician champions.
- Provide periodic updates at various medical staff meetings and in newsletters.
- Use information as appropriate for the care setting/level of care (i.e., from the DRGs, CPTs).

APPENDIXES I THROUGH O
The Manager's Job Description and Performance Appraisal

Appendixes I through O present job descriptions and performance appraisals for various hospital and community case management positions. The case manager's job description should delineate the power and the level of independence granted in the role. It provides a clear description of the role, functions, and responsibilities of case managers. The performance appraisal should always be criteria based. Evaluating performance is important for determining the effectiveness of the case manager in the role. Institutions are advised to incorporate reviewing the job description and the process of evaluating performance in the training and education of case managers when they assume the new role. Goals and objectives of the role and the institution can also be shared.

The following examples of job descriptions and performance appraisals are included here:

- Appendix I: Case Manager—Inpatient (p. 396)
- Appendix J: Case Manager—Admitting Office (p. 398)
- Appendix K: Case Manager—Emergency Department (p. 399)
- Appendix L: Case Manager—Community (p. 400)
- Appendix M: Physician Advisor (p. 402)
- Appendix N: Guide for a Case Manager's Competency-Based Performance Appraisal (p. 403)
- Appendix O: Performance Management Form—Case Coordinator (p. 404)

Things to Remember About the Case Manager Job Description

- Define the scope of practice and describe the role, functions, and responsibilities of the nurse case manager.
- Delineate the role and responsibilities of the case manager and how they relate to other staff and to the various care settings across the continuum.
- Differentiate the case manager job description from that for other staff.

- Delineate the power provided in the role. Define the reporting relationship and indicate to whom the nurse case manager is accountable.
- Define the minimum educational background and experience required for the role.
- Specify the licensure or certification requirements.
- Identify the skills required for the role.
- Establish a job description that fits the institution's operations, systems, and standards of care and practice.
- Establish a job description that reflects the mission, values, beliefs, and philosophy of the institution.
- Specify if it is necessary to belong to specialty professional organizations/associations/societies (e.g., American Nurses Association, Case Management Society of America, National Association of Social Workers).

Things to Remember About the Utilization Review Officer Job Description

- Define the scope of practice and the role functions and responsibilities of the physician advisor.
- Identify the previous experience and skills required for the role.
- Develop a job description that interfaces the physician advisor's role with the case manager's role and the role of other physicians and staff in other departments, such as social work and quality management.
- Define the interface of the physician advisor with managed care organizations, managed care department, board of trustees, and finance.

Things to Remember About Performance Appraisals

- Develop a performance appraisal that is competency-based and reflective of the job description and the case manager's role dimensions.
- Define the rating system used in the performance appraisal.
- Specify the minimum acceptable rating (performance) or the performance threshold.
- Make expectations known.
- Include the skills, knowledge, and abilities required for the job in the performance appraisal.
- Delineate the frequency of evaluating performance.
- Identify the competencies related to the role.
- State the competencies in a measurable and practical way.
- Determine the criteria for merit increases.
- Communicate the percentage of time the case manager is expected to spend in each of the role dimensions. Remember that the percentage for each dimension may vary according to the practice area or specialty (e.g., acute inpatient care setting versus emergency department).

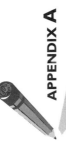

APPENDIX A

COMMUNITY NURSE CASE MANAGEMENT PROBLEM LIST AND PLAN OF CARE

Valley Health System
Community Nurse Case Management
Problem List and Plan of Care

CNCM Name: _____

Client Name: _____

Date	Problem Name	Initial Admit Rating			Goals (Long Term) (See Intervention Flow Sheet for Interventions specific to each client visit)	Problem Resolved, D/C Date or N/A
		K	B	S		

Valley Health System
Community Nurse Case Management
Problem List and Plan of Care

Client Name: _____

CNCM Name _____
(Line through text = NOT APPLICABLE)

Date	Problem Name	Initial Admit Rating K	B	S	Goals and Planned Interventions *(See Intervention Flow Sheet for Interventions specific to each client visit)*	Problem Resolved, D/C Date or N/A
	Medication Management (Potential for alteration in medication compliance)				Goal: Client will take medications as prescribed by primary care provider (PCP).	
					1. RN will obtain PCP orders for medications.	
					2. RN will update medication list as appropriate, including Rx, OTC, and herbal.	
					3. Client will verbalize understanding of medication regimen.	
					4. Client will be able to verbalize possible side effects of medications.	
					5. RN will assist client with obtaining medications, as appropriate.	
					6. Client will utilize medication/pill box appropriately.	
					7. RN will fill medication/pill box with medications as prescribed by PCP.	

Valley Health System
Community Nurse Case Management
Problem List and Plan of Care

Client Name: _____

CNCM Name _____
(Line through text = NOT APPLICABLE)

Date	Problem Name	Initial Admit Rating K B S	Goals and Planned Interventions *(See Intervention Flow Sheet for Interventions specific to each client visit)*	Problem Resolved, D/C Date or N/A
	Respiratory Status (Potential for or alteration in gas exchange r/t inadequate airway clearance)		Goal: Client will exhibit symptoms of optimal gas exchange.	
			1. RN will instruct client in the following: • S/Sx of respiratory infection • Effective coughing and deep breathing • S/Sx of hypoxemia • Energy conservation	
			2. RN will instruct client when to call MD or 911.	
			3. RN will assess lung/respiratory status using stethoscope and pulse oximetry, as appropriate.	
			4. RN will obtain PCP order for pulse oximetry use, as appropriate.	
			5. RN will instruct patient in use of inhalers and/or nebulizer, as appropriate.	
			6. Client will verbalize understanding of S/Sx of respiratory infection.	
			7. Client will demonstrate effective body positioning for maximum airway availability.	
			8. Client will follow prescribed respiratory regimens of care, including medications.	
			9. Client will use O$_2$ as ordered by PCP.	

Valley Health System
Community Nurse Case Management
Problem List and Plan of Care

Client Name: _____

CNCM Name _____ *NOT APPLICABLE*
(Line through text = NOT APPLICABLE)

Date	Problem Name	Initial Admit Rating			Goals and Planned Interventions *(See Intervention Flow Sheet for Interventions specific to each client visit)*	Problem Resolved, D/C Date or N/A
		K	B	S		
	Integumentary (Potential for or alteration in skin integrity)				Goal: Client will have intact skin surface (or absence of S/Sx of infection from skin breakdown).	
					1. Client will verbalize understanding of self-care management of skin.	
					2. RN will provide education on the following: • Proper handwashing • S/Sx of wound/skin infection • Diet and hydration • Activity and/or any limitations	
					3. Client will list at least 3 S/Sx of infection and appropriate PCP notification.	
					4. Client will verbalize importance of adequate nutrition/hydration for maintenance of skin integrity and/or wound healing.	
					5. RN will assess for pain.	

Valley Health System
Community Nurse Case Management
Problem List and Plan of Care

Client Name: _____

CNCM Name _____
(Line through text = NOT APPLICABLE)

Date	Problem Name	Initial Admit Rating K B S	Goals and Planned Interventions *(See Intervention Flow Sheet for Interventions specific to each client visit)*	Problem Resolved, D/C Date or N/A
	Mental Status (Potential for anxiety, depression, or ineffective coping)		Goal: Client will exhibit reduction in S/Sx of anxiety/depression/impaired thought processes with more effective coping abilities to optimize functional abilities in a safe environment. *(Circle those that apply)*	
			1. RN will instruct client on the following: • Disease process, if applicable • Medication compliance • Safety in the home	
			2. RN will give positive feedback to client and reinforce compliance with prescribed regimens of care.	
			3. RN will encourage client to seek appropriate support systems.	
			4. RN will encourage client to verbalize feelings, concerns, thoughts.	
			5. Client will develop a therapeutic relationship with RN.	
			6. Client will identify S/Sx of anxiety/depression/impaired thought processes.	
			7. Client will demonstrate compliance with medications as prescribed by PCP.	

Valley Health System
Community Nurse Case Management
Problem List and Plan of Care

Client Name: _____

CNCM Name
(Line through text = NOT APPLICABLE)

Date	Problem Name	Initial Admit Rating			Goals and Planned Interventions *(See Intervention Flow Sheet for Interventions specific to each client visit)*	Problem Resolved, D/C Date or N/A
		K	B	S		
	Medical Cardiac (Potential for or alteration in cardiac output and/or alteration in fluid volume r/t CHF)				Goal: Client will demonstrate understanding of disease process and self-care management.	
					1. RN will instruct client on the following: • Definition/causes of CHF • S/Sx of exacerbation of CHF • Treatment measure of CHF • Complications of CHF • S/Sx of electrolyte imbalance • Energy conservation • Skin care and assessment of peripheral edema • Prescribed regimens of care, including medications, weight, pulse	
					2. RN will instruct client when to call MD or 911.	
					3. RN will assess cardiac and respiratory status using stethoscope and pulse oximetry, as appropriate.	
					4. RN will obtain PCP order for pulse oximetry use, as appropriate.	
					5. Client will verbalize understanding of CHF.	
					6. Client will follow prescribed regimens of care, including medications, elevation of extremities.	
					7. Client will record daily weights.	
					8. Client will use O_2 as ordered by PCP.	

Valley Health System
Community Nurse Case Management
Problem List and Plan of Care

Client Name: _____

CNCM Name _____
(Line through text = NOT APPLICABLE)

Date	Problem Name	Initial Admit Rating K	B	S	Goals and Planned Interventions *(See Intervention Flow Sheet for Interventions specific to each client visit)*	Problem Resolved, D/C Date or N/A
	Hypertension (Potential for or alteration in blood pressure)				Goal: Client will demonstrate understanding of disease process and self-care management.	
					1. RN will instruct client on the following: • Definition/causes of hypertension • S/Sx of hypertension • Treatment of hypertension • Complications of hypertension • Risk behaviors to alter (e.g., smoking, activity level, diet) • Orthostatic hypotension • Stress reduction • Prescribed regimens of care including diet, medications	
					2. RN will instruct client when to call MD or 911.	
					3. RN will assess blood pressure.	
					4. Client will verbalize understanding of hypertension.	
					5. Client will follow prescribed regimens of care, including medications.	

Valley Health System
Community Nurse Case Management
Problem List and Plan of Care

Client Name: _____

CNCM Name _____
(Line through text = NOT APPLICABLE)

Date	Problem Name	Initial Admit Rating K B S	Goals and Planned Interventions *(See Intervention Flow Sheet for Interventions specific to each client visit)*	Problem Resolved, D/C Date or N/A
	Pain Management (Potential for or alteration in comfort level)		Goal: Client will demonstrate effective level of pain control.	
			1. RN will instruct client on the following: • Use of pain scale and desired level of pain control • Nonmedication methods of pain/symptom control • Activity progression plan • Ways to maintain GI function • S/Sx of constipation and ways to relieve	
			2. RN will assess/reassess client level of pain.	
			3. Client will verbalize intensity of pain on pain scale, frequency, and duration.	
			4. Client will verbalize understanding of nonmedication methods of pain control (e.g., imagery, relaxation techniques, biofeedback).	
			5. Client will alert RN to possible constipation or concerns with GI function (e.g., nausea, vomiting, heartburn).	
			6. Client will follow prescribed regimens of care, including medications.	

Valley Health System
Community Nurse Case Management
Problem List and Plan of Care

Client Name: _____

CNCM Name _____
(Line through text = NOT APPLICABLE)

Date	Problem Name	Initial Admit Rating			Goals and Planned Interventions *(See Intervention Flow Sheet for Interventions specific to each client visit)*	Problem Resolved, D/C Date or N/A
		K	B	S		
	Nutrition (Potential for or alteration in nutritional status)				Goal: Client will follow diet prescribed by PCP.	
					1. RN will instruct client on the following: • Proper diet; • Adequate hydration and/or fluid restriction • Effects of activity/exercise	
					2. RN will assess client compliance with diet.	
					3. Client will verbalize understanding and compliance with diet.	
					4. Client will monitor weight.	
					5. RN will consult/refer to dietician as appropriate.	

Valley Health System
Community Nurse Case Management
Problem List and Plan of Care

CNCM Name _____
(Line through text = NOT APPLICABLE)

Client Name: _____

Date	Problem Name	Initial Admit Rating			Goals and Planned Interventions *(See Intervention Flow Sheet for Interventions specific to each client visit)*	Problem Resolved, D/C Date or N/A
		K	B	S		
	Diabetes (Alteration in metabolism of glucose and production of insulin)				Goal: Client will verbalize/demonstrate understanding of diabetes disease process and self-care management. OR Blood sugars will be within normal limits for patient. *(Circle one.)*	
					1. RN will instruct client on the following: • S/Sx of hypoglycemia and corrective actions to take • S/Sx of hyperglycemia and corrective actions to take • Appropriate diet • Medications that alter blood glucose • Effect of activity/exercise on blood sugar/insulin • Glucose monitoring, including handwashing before fingerstick	
					2. Client will follow prescribed regimens of care, including medications and fingersticks.	
					3. Client will verbalize S/Sx of hypoglycemia and hyperglycemia and actions to take.	
					4. Client will verbalize understanding and compliance with diabetic diet and importance of regularly scheduled meals and snacks.	
					5. RN will assess/review blood sugar fingerstick log.	

Valley Health System
Community Nurse Case Management
Problem List and Plan of Care

Client Name: _____

CNCM Name _____
(Line through text = NOT APPLICABLE)

Date	Problem Name	Initial Admit Rating			Goals and Planned Interventions *(See Intervention Flow Sheet for Interventions specific to each client visit)*	Problem Resolved, D/C Date or N/A
		K	B	S		
	Coronary Artery Disease (Potential for inadequate tissue perfusion r/t decreased circulation)				Goal: Client will demonstrate understanding of disease process and self-care management.	
					1. RN will instruct client on the following: • Definition/causes of CAD • S/Sx of exacerbation of CAD • Treatment measures of CAD • Complications of CAD • Skin care and assessment of peripheral edema • Prescribed regimens of care, including medications	
					2. RN will instruct client when to call MD or 911.	
					3. RN will assess cardiac and respiratory status using stethoscope and pulse oximetry, as appropriate.	
					4. RN will obtain PCP order for pulse oximetry use, as appropriate.	
					5. Client will verbalize understanding of CAD.	
					6. Client will follow prescribed regimens of care, including medications, elevation of extremities.	
					7. Client will use O_2 as ordered by PCP.	

Valley Health System
Community Nurse Case Management
Problem List and Plan of Care

Client Name: _____

CNCM Name _____
(Line through text = NOT APPLICABLE)

Date	Problem Name	Initial Admit Rating			Goals and Planned Interventions *(See Intervention Flow Sheet for Interventions specific to each client visit)*	Problem Resolved, D/C Date or N/A
		K	B	S		
	Safety (Potential for harm, injury, or risk r/t environment)				Goal: Client will maintain safe environment.	
					1. RN will identify safety hazards in the environment (e.g., objects, situations, people).	
					2. RN will remove hazards from the environment and/or modify the environment to minimize hazards (when possible) and with client permission.	
					3. RN will instruct client on the following: • Safe environment • Minimizing safety hazards and risk • Use of protective devices (e.g., side rails, locked doors, repaired fences or gates)	
					4. RN will monitor the client and the environment for changes in safety status.	

Valley Health System
Community Nurse Case Management
Problem List and Plan of Care

Client Name: _____

CNCM Name _____
(Line through text = NOT APPLICABLE)

Date	Problem Name	Initial Admit Rating			Goals and Planned Interventions *(See Intervention Flow Sheet for Interventions specific to each client visit)*	Problem Resolved, D/C Date or N/A
		K	B	S		
	Financial (Actual or potential for financial concerns r/t limited resources)				Goal: Client will have access to appropriate resources.	
					1. RN will identify client resource needs (e.g., medical, financial aid, environmental, access).	
					2. RN will provide information on possible resources to client.	
					3. Client will access appropriate resources. *(List all applicable resources.)*	
					4. RN will make referrals for client, as applicable.	

Valley Health System
Community Nurse Case Management
Problem List and Plan of Care

Client Name: _____

CNCM Name _____
(Line through text = NOT APPLICABLE)

Date	Problem Name	Initial Admit Rating			Goals and Planned Interventions *(See Intervention Flow Sheet for Interventions specific to each client visit)*	Problem Resolved, D/C Date or N/A
		K	B	S		
	Visual Deficit (Potential for or actual vision deficit r/t disease process and/or previous injury)				Goal: Client will accept and learn alternate methods for living with diminished vision.	
					1. RN will assess client's reaction to diminished vision (e.g., denial, depression, withdrawal).	
					2. RN will not move items in client environment without first informing client.	
					3. RN will refer client to appropriate resources (e.g., agency, healthcare provider).	
					4. RN will fill medication box, if applicable.	
					5. RN will instruct patient in maintaining a safe environment.	

Valley Health System
Community Nurse Case Management
Problem List and Plan of Care

Client Name: _____

CNCM Name _____
(Line through text = NOT APPLICABLE)

Date	Problem Name	Initial Admit Rating			Goals and Planned Interventions *(See Intervention Flow Sheet for Interventions specific to each client visit)*	Problem Resolved, D/C Date or N/A
		K	B	S		
	Bowel Management (Potential for or alteration in bowel elimination)				Goal: Client will establish and maintain a regular pattern of bowel elimination.	
					1. RN will monitor client for S/Sx of diarrhea, constipation, and/or impaction.	
					2. RN will instruct client on good nutrition and hydration, as well as specific foods that are assistive in promoting bowel regularity.	
					3. Client will monitor and report changes in patterns of bowel elimination.	
					4. Client will take medications as prescribed.	

Valley Health System
Community Nurse Case Management
Problem List and Plan of Care

Client Name: _____

CNCM Name _____
(Line through text = NOT APPLICABLE)

Date	Problem Name	Initial Admit Rating			Goals and Planned Interventions *(See Intervention Flow Sheet for Interventions specific to each client visit)*	Problem Resolved, D/C Date or N/A
		K	B	S		
	Renal (Potential for or actual renal insufficiency r/t disease process)				Goal: Client will follow prescribed regimens of care to maximize renal sufficiency.	
					1. RN will instruct client on the following: • Definition/causes of renal insufficiency • S/Sx of fluid and electrolyte imbalances • Treatment measures (e.g., dialysis) • Appropriate diet/nutrition (as directed) • Complications of renal insufficiency • Energy conservation • Skin care and assessment of peripheral edema • Prescribed regimens of care, including medications, weight, pulse	
					2. RN will instruct client when to call MD or 911.	
					3. RN will refer client to physician when S/Sx of fluid and/or electrolyte imbalance persist or worsen.	
					4. Client will monitor the following, as appropriate: • Weight • Fluid intake • Peripheral edema • Skin color, turgor • Changes in sensorium/alertness	
					5. Client will verbalize understanding of renal insufficiency.	
					6. Client will follow prescribed regimens of care, including medications, elevation of extremities.	

Valley Health System
Community Nurse Case Management
Problem List and Plan of Care

Client Name: _____

CNCM Name
(Line through text = NOT APPLICABLE)

Date	Problem Name	Initial Admit Rating K	B	S	Goals and Planned Interventions *(See Intervention Flow Sheet for Interventions specific to each client visit)*	Problem Resolved, D/C Date or N/A
	Hepatic (Potential for or actual alteration in liver function 2° to disease process)				Goal: Client will follow prescribed regimens of care to maximize hepatic function.	
					1. RN will instruct client on the following: • Definition/causes of liver disease • S/Sx of fluid and electrolyte imbalances and ascites • Treatment measures (e.g., dialysis) • Appropriate diet/nutrition (as directed) • Complications of liver insufficiency • Energy conservation • Pain management (as applicable) • Skin care and assessment of peripheral edema • Prescribed regimens of care, including medications, weight, pulse	
					2. RN will instruct client when to call MD or 911.	
					3. RN will refer client to physician when S/Sx of fluid and/or electrolyte imbalance persist or worsen.	
					4. Client will monitor the following, as appropriate: • Weight • Fluid intake • Peripheral edema • Ascites and/or girth measurement • Skin color and turgor • Fatigue • Pain management • Changes in sensorium/alertness	
					5. Client will verbalize understanding of liver insufficiency.	
					6. Client will follow prescribed regimens of care, including medications, elevation of extremities.	

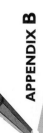

APPENDIX B

COMMUNITY NURSE CASE MANAGEMENT INTERVENTION FLOW SHEET AND PROBLEM RATING SCALE FOR OUTCOMES

Valley Health System
CLIENT NAME _____ MR# _____

INTERVENTION FLOW SHEET
Community Nurse Case Management

Date	Time	V = Visit P = Phone — Dir.	Indir.	Number of Minutes	Problem Name or Number	Inter-vention Number	Rating (K, B, S)	Vital Signs	Pain (if appropriate)	Acuity	Homebound (Y or N)	Next Scheduled MD Visit	Visit Access (Y or N)	Access Code	Initials
							K B S								
							K B S								
							K B S								
							K B S								
							K B S								
							K B S								
							K B S								
							K B S								
							K B S								
							K B S								
							K B S								
							K B S								
							K B S								
							K B S								
							K B S								

INTERVENTION 1 = Assessment 2 = Medication Management 3 = Education 4 = Coordination 5 = Referral 6 = Surveillance
VISIT LOCATION S = Scheduled MD visit U = Unscheduled MD visit E = Emergency room H = Hospital UC = Urgent care F = Free clinic O = Other
ACUITY 6 = ≥1X/week 5 = qo wk 4 = q 3-4 wk 3 = q2 mo 2 = q 3 mo (quarterly) 1 = Phone calls

Problem Rating Scale for Outcomes

Concept	1	2	3	4	5
KNOWLEDGE The ability of the client to remember and interpret information	No knowledge	Minimal knowledge	Basic knowledge	Adequate knowledge	Superior knowledge
BEHAVIOR The observable responses, actions, or activities of the client fitting the occasion or purpose	Never appropriate	Rarely appropriate	Inconsistently appropriate	Usually appropriate	Consistently appropriate
STATUS The condition of the client in relation to objective and subjective defining characteristics	Extreme signs/ symptoms	Severe signs/ symptoms	Moderate signs/ symptoms	Minimal signs/ symptoms	No signs/ symptoms

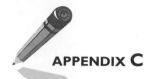

APPENDIX C

COMMUNITY-BASED WOUND CARE PATHWAY AND FLOW SHEET

Winchester Medical Center
WOUND CARE CENTER

WOUND CARE PATHWAY*
(Interdisciplinary—reassess every 30 days)

Patient Name: _____

F = First visit/team evaluation   **S** = No show   **C** = Cancelled   **M** = MD visit   **R** = RN visit   **P** = PT visit

Month/Yr	1	2	3	4	5	6	7	8	9	10	11	12	13	14	15	16	17	18	19	20	21	22	23	24	25	26	27	28	29	30	31

		Visit # _____ Date _____
Elements of Care	**Nursing Diagnosis/ Problems**	1. Alteration in skin integrity 2. 3.
	Expected Patient Outcomes	1. Wound will decrease in size by ____% in ____week(s) **or** 2. Erythema and/or induration will decrease by ____% in _____week(s) 3. Necrotic tissue will decrease by ____% in ____week(s) **or** 4. Wound healed in ____ week(s)
	Assessment	[ ] Improved [ ] Worse [ ] Same [ ] N/A
Plan of Treatment	**Treatment**	[ ] See most current wound care orders
	Patient/Family Participation	
	Activity/Safety	Activity as ordered
	Consults	
	Factors Limiting Progress	
	PLAN	

RN or PT Signature_____ **Date**_____ **Time**_____

Treatment Certification: I certify that I have reviewed the above plan, that the Wound Care Center visits are necessary, that services will be furnished while the patient is under my care, and that the plan will be reviewed every 30 days or more frequently based on the patient's needs.

MD Signature_____ **Date**_____ **Time**_____

This clinical path is a guideline for the patient's care and does not represent a standard of medical care.

Winchester Medical Center
WOUND CARE CENTER

Patient Name: _____

Location: _____

WOUND CARE FLOW SHEET

TYPE OF WOUND: Neuropathic   Arterial   Venous
(Circle appropriate)   Arterial   Surgical   Necrotic
                         Pressure: *Stage II, III, IV*

	Visit # _____ DATE/TIME _____ Wound #_____	Visit # _____ DATE/TIME _____ Wound #_____	Visit # _____ DATE/TIME _____ Wound #_____
Vital Signs (P, R, BP)	P____ R____ BP_____	P____ R____ BP_____	P____ R____ BP_____
PERIPHERAL EDEMA 0 None 3+ 5-10 mm 1+ 2 mm indent 4+ >10 mm 2+ 2-5 mm 5+ tightness (unable to pit)			
DRESSING STATUS 1. Intact 2. Loose 4. Dry 3. Wet 5. Other (specify)			
EXUDATE **A. Amount** 1. None 3. Moderate 2. Minimal 4. Copious			
B. Color 1. Serous 5. Green 2. Sang. 6. Purulent 3. Serous/Sang. 7. Bloody 4. Tan/Brown 8. Other (specify)			
C. Odor 1. Not present 2. Present (specify)			
WOUND BASE 1. Pink 6. Moist 2. Red 7. Epithelialization 3. Yellow 8. Dry 4. Black 9. Tunneling 5. Granulating 10. Other (describe)			
WOUND EDGES 1. Pink 2. Red 4. Undermining 3. Calloused 5. Other (specify)			
SURROUNDING SKIN 1. Intact 2. Macerated 4. Rash 3. Erythematous 5. Other (specify)			
MEASUREMENT (__cm) *Measure each visit* Length (L) Width (W) Depth (D) Tunneling (T) Undermining (U) Surface area = L × W × D Picture taken this visit?	_____ L _____ W _____ D _____ T _____ U _____ Surface area ☐ Picture taken	_____ L _____ W _____ D _____ T _____ U _____ Surface area ☐ Picture taken	_____ L _____ W _____ D _____ T _____ U _____ Surface area ☐ Picture taken
WOUND CARE/TREATMENT	☐ Per wound care orders	☐ Per wound care orders	☐ Per wound care orders
PATIENT REACTION 1. Tolerated well 3. Other (specify) 2. Painful (Use pain scale 0-10)			
PATIENT/FAMILY EDUCATION			
Time spent with patient *(for tracking and billing)*			
RN/PT initials:			

(Use back of page for Narrative Notes.)

Narrative Notes   **WOUND CARE FLOW SHEET**

Date/Time	

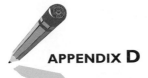

APPENDIX D

HOME CARE PLAN FOR CONGESTIVE HEART FAILURE AND HYPERTENSION

Description of the Pathways

Outcome-driven critical pathways are the key to success for efficient and effective case management. Case managers who use critical pathways or standards of practice and care that are integrated into documentation tools are better able to concurrently define the effectiveness (or ineffectiveness) of care. The pathways improve consistency in care between patients with similar conditions and between different clinicians and agencies. This consistency has led to an increase in episodic resource control with fewer outliers, which is especially important under payment structures such as the CMS prospective payment system (PPS). This standard system increases the predictability of care needs. The format or methodology of the pathway system is the key to achieving these outcomes.

A pathway that offers visit-specific interventions and patient outcomes (that are also used as the documentation tools) results in efficient care, improved continuity of care, patient involvement in care, and improved patient satisfaction. For an example of an outcome-driven pathway, see the congestive heart failure (CHF) *Home Care Steps* protocol sample documents. Some of the components of this pathway system in this sampling include a CHF pathway overview, CHF visit 2, and an HTN CoStep. The Pathway Overview identifies special needs of the patient, normal parameters, and episode-based goals. The visit note provides interventions and outcomes specific to a visit 2 in an episode. These interventions and outcomes are documented as "done or met" or "not done or not met—with the use of a variance code." Variance codes describe the patient reasons why planned interventions and outcomes are not completed or not met. This system also provides an outcome and variance tracking tool that allows for efficient concurrent case management. This tool provides for an at-a-glance view of the home care episode, outcomes that are met, outcomes that are still unmet and the reason why or variance code, and the number of visits completed so far compared with the number of visits planned for the episode. These pathways may be adapted for use in any outpatient setting (i.e., physician office visits or outpatient clinics). The pathways may also be used by insurance case managers for internal use as education tools or as standards of care.

From VNA FIRST Home Care Steps Protocols. For more information about these pathways available for purchase or for educational services, contact VNA FIRST at 1-800-491-9050 or 1-708-579-2292, 47 S. Sixth Ave., Suite 120, LaGrange, Illinois 60525.

CONGESTIVE HEART FAILURE *HOME CARE STEPS* PATHWAY OVERVIEW

Patient Name:_____

Primary Dx _____   ID#:_____
Secondary Dx _____
Date *Home Care Steps* protocols Opened: _____ Closed:_____ Start of Care:_____

PLANNED SPECIAL ASSESSMENTS (Problems/Needs) and TREATMENTS

(Select ✓ items that are currently or recently a problem that are expected
to be outside normal range)
Fill in normal parameters (or where pt *should* be), when known, if applicable:

	OTHER CoSteps or Flowsheets

___ Vital signs _____
___ Blood pressure _____
___ Cardiovascular/angina _____
___ Circulatory _____
___ Respiratory _____
___ Neurological _____
___ Nutrition/Hydration (prescribed diet) _____
___ Weight _____
___ Elimination, Bowel _____
___ Elimination, Bladder _____
___ Edema _____
___ Mobility/exercise/tolerance _____
___ Dyspnea/Fatigue _____

___ ADL _____
___ IADL _____
___ Skin color/integrity/incision _____
___ Vision _____
___ Pain _____
Pain scale ❏ 1-10 ❏ Faces ❏ Other:_____
___ Safety _____
___ Mental health/cognitive _____
___ Labs _____
___ Equipment _____
___ Other _____

NURSING DIAGNOSES: (Choose appropriate diagnoses)

___ 1. Knowledge deficit related to disease process and home care management.
___ 2. Knowledge deficit related to medication use/compliance (# of Medications _____).
___ 3. Pain related to _____.
___ 4. Knowledge deficit related to dietary restrictions.
___ 5. Self-care deficit, bathing/hygiene.
___ 6. Self-care deficit, grooming/dressing.
___ 7. Alteration in activity tolerance.
___ 8. Alteration in lifestyle secondary to disease.
___ 9. Ineffective coping related to diagnosis and prognosis.
___ 10. Potential alteration in skin integrity related to edema.
___ Other: _____

GOALS: (Check appropriate goals)

___ 1. Patient will demonstrate maintenance of stable physiological status, and S/S of improved cardiac output, within normal limits for patient.
___ 2. Patient will demonstrate maintenance of intact skin in edematous areas.
___ 3. Patient will demonstrate ability to maintain medical condition in home without hospitalization, ER visit, or unplanned physician visit.
___ 4. Patient/CG will demonstrate knowledge of disease process, treatment goals, and self-care management.
___ 5. Patient/CG will demonstrate incorporation of treatment principles into lifestyle.
___ 6. Patient/CG will demonstrate compliance with medication schedule.
___ 7. Patient will demonstrate adequate symptom (pain) control through use of medications or other therapies/treatments.
___ 8. Patient/CG will demonstrate compliance with prescribed diet/fluid requirements.
___ 9. Patient will demonstrate optimal level of ADLs/IADLs.
___ 10. Patient will demonstrate progression within planned activity schedule that enables _____.
___ 11. Patient/CG will verbalize S/S to report to RN or physician.
___ 12. Patient will demonstrate ability to maintain safety in home environment without injury/falls.
___ 13. Patient/CG will demonstrate positive health behaviors.
___ 14. Patient/CG will verbalize coping strategies to deal with lifestyle change requirements.
___ 15. Patient/CG will verbalize community resources available and how to contact them.
___ 16. Patient/CG will verbalize plan for follow-up visits with physician or other services.
___ Other: _____

TEACHING TOOLS:

_____
_____
_____

Care Plan Focus
Safety: Visits 1 - 3 (when outcomes are met on these visit protocols)
Disease Control: Visits 4 - 7 (when outcomes are met on these visit protocols)
Health Promotion: Visits 8 - 10 (when outcomes are met on these visit protocols)

LEARNING ASSESSMENT:

Who will be taught ❏ Pt ❏ CG _____ ❏ Understands spoken/written English
❏ Able to absorb/retain info ❏ Willing to learn ❏ Need Interpreter
❏ No available caregiver

SN VISIT FREQUENCY:
Recommended: 3 wk x 1, 2 wk x 3, 1 wk x 1
                    (10 visits total)

ORDERED VISIT FREQUENCY: _____
Planned # Visits: _____

Other Disciplines: _____   _____Signature and Title

Home Care Steps protocols are guidelines designed to address the patient's acute episode of illness. Because each patient presents unique circumstances that must be assessed and evaluated during the provision of home care services, visit intensity and frequency may also be influenced by such factors that include but are not limited to the home environment, resources, the presence of life-supporting therapies, and the presence of chronic illnesses or limiting handicaps.

CHF *Home Care Steps*
Visit 2

Patient Name:_____　ID#:_____

Date: _____

Type of Contact: ❑ Home Visit　❑ Telephone Visit　❑ Other _____

❑ See CoStep: _____　❑ See Flowsheets/Other Forms: _____

Homebound status: ❑ Ambulation　❑ Endurance　❑ Vision　❑ Infection　❑ Respiratory　❑ Mental　❑ Other

Care Elements	Interventions: Use "✓" for complete; variance code for not done.	Comments
DISEASE PROCESS	Perform physical assessment. ___ Assess weight (on patient's own scale if available).___ Evaluate knowledge of disease process. ___ Instruct on definition, ___ S/S of exacerbation of disease process, ___ actions to take, ___ and basic treatment goals.___ Assess for shortness of breath.___ Assess edema.___ Instruct on pacemaker function and care, if applicable.___	T _____ AP _____ RP _____ R _____ Wt:_____ BP R/L Sit _____, Stand _____, Lying _____ Heart: _____ Circulation/edema: _____ Lungs: _____ ❑ Dyspnea ❑ cough ❑ tracheal secretions ❑ cyanosis ❑ hemoptysis ❑ chest pain: _____ Oxygen at _____ liters/min continuous/prn via ❑ nasal cannula ❑ venti-mask at ___ % Skin turgor: _____ Skin color/integrity ❑ Intact ❑ New wound
MEDICATION	Instruct on medication schedule. ___ Evaluate effectiveness of medications/symptom control.___ Instruct on purpose, action, side effects, and interactions of following medication(s):_____ Instruct on medication changes. ___ Demonstrate use of medi-planner and set up if necessary. ___	Pain: ❑ See Pain CoStep ❑ Patient denies pain Location/freq/duration: ❑ Patient rates pain as (___start of visit; ___end of visit) Pain level acceptable to patient ❑ Yes ❑ No, action: ❑ New medications:
NUTRITION/ HYDRATION/ ELIMINATION	Assess fluid and dietary intake. ___ Evaluate knowledge of diet restrictions/fluid requirements. ___ Instruct on diet/fluid requirements as appropriate.___ Provide assistance with meal planning until next scheduled visit.___ Assess bowel and urinary function. ___ Instruct to avoid straining with bowel movements.___	Appetite: good _____ fair _____ poor _____ Diet Intake: _____ Fluid Intake: _____ Abdomen: _____ Bowel: _____ Bladder: _____ ❑ on med for UTI
ACTIVITY	Assess current activity and tolerance levels.___ Instruct to avoid overexertion.___ Instruct on importance of frequent rest periods and pacing activities.___ Assess functional status and ability to perform ADLs/IADLs.___ Evaluate need for assistive devices.___	ADLs: _____ IADLs: _____ Ambulation/Transfers: ❑ Independent ❑ Assist of #___ Endurance:
SAFETY	Evaluate knowledge of how and when to call for help.___ Provide emergency numbers.___ Instruct on basic home safety precautions.___ Assess environment for risk factors.___ Instruct on modification as appropriate.___ Instruct on safe use of oxygen (if appropriate).___	Environment: ❑ safe 　　　　　❑ unsafe/inadequate due to: ❑ Standard Precautions maintained
TREATMENTS	Administer as ordered._____	
TESTS	Perform as ordered._____	
PSYCHO/ SOCIAL	Assess family/social support systems.___ Evaluate caregiver functioning/coping status.___ Evaluate knowledge of Rights and Responsibilities.___	Level of Consciousness/Orientation: _____ Emotional: Sleep pattern: ❑ Cultural impact on care:

_____
Signature and Title

CHF *Home Care Steps*
Visit 2 (continued)

Patient Name:_____ ID#:_____

Date: _____

INTERTEAM SERVICES/ COMMUNITY REFERRALS	Assess ability to purchase necessary supplies, food, etc., for treatment.___ Initiate referrals for agency/community services as needed.___ Evaluate knowledge of plan,___ and barriers of care to home care services.___ Initiate case conference: ___SN, ___MSS, ___PT, ___OT, ___ SLP,___HCA, ___Physician, Other.___ Assess for next physician appointment (Date)._____	Reason for communication/conference: Outcome of communication/conference:

Home Care Aide Supervisory Note: HCA Present? ❑ Yes ❑ No   Following plan of care? ❑ Yes ❑ No
Care Plan Adequate? ❑ Yes ❑ No   Need for continued service? ❑ Yes ❑ No ❑ Pt. Unable ❑ Family Unable
Assessment of Patient/Family relationship with HCA: _____

_____

Changes in plan/goal/update: _____
❑ To HCA Supervisor   Date _____ Initials _____
❑ If Applicable, HCA Name _____ HCA Signature _____ Date _____

Patient/Caregiver Outcomes	Met	Not Met	If necessary, explain Variance Code/Comments.
1. Demonstrates no new, worsening, continued S/S outside normal range.			Condition ❑ improved ❑ unchanged ❑ worsening (see above)
2. Demonstrates ability to maintain medical condition in home without hospitalization, ER visit, or unplanned physician visit since last RN visit.			❑ Hospital, # Days in hospital _____ ❑ ER ❑ Unplanned physician office visit _____
3. Verbalizes purpose, action, and side effects of each medication instructed (as listed above).			
4. Verbalizes general dietary restrictions.			
5. Verbalizes fluid restrictions if ordered.			
6. Demonstrates optimal GI function, i.e., no S/S of N/V, diarrhea, or constipation.			
7. Verbalizes plan to meet basic ADL/IADL needs.			
8. Verbalizes importance of frequent rest periods and pacing activities.			
9. Verbalizes how and when to call for help.			Date of injury/fall:
10. Verbalizes members of support system.			
11. Verbalizes knowledge of plan/barriers to care.			
12. Verbalizes three (3) safety issues regarding use of oxygen.			
13. Other: ❑ Outcomes from previous visit continue to be unmet. Indicate Visit #(s) and Outcome #(s)_____			

❑ If unmet outcomes from previous visits have now been met, write visit and outcome numbers:_____

PLAN (Include next *Home Care Step* Visit # to be completed): ❑ Next Visit Protocol # ___ ❑ Repeat Visit Protocol
Current SN Visit Frequency: _____ ❑ D/C current pathway, initiate _____
❑ Pt/CG involved in POC changes if applicable   ❑ Change primary dx to _____
Supplies/Other to bring for Next Visit: _____

Other Comments/Plans: _____

_____

_____   _____   _____
Signature and Title   Time In   Time Out

HYPERTENSION *CoStep*

This diagnosis is: _____ new

_____ exacerbation

_____ chronic condition

Patient Name:_____

ID#:_____

Start of Care:_____

GOALS					
Patient will achieve adequate symptom control through use of medications or other therapies/treatments.					
Patient will demonstrate compliance with treatment plan (diet, meds, exercise, other).					
PATIENT/CAREGIVER OUTCOMES **Dates:**					
1. Verbalizes importance of slow positions changes.					
2. Verbalizes importance of monitoring daily weight.					
3. Demonstrates correct procedure for taking blood pressure (if ordered).					
4. Verbalizes three (3) risk factors for HTN and how to reduce risk.					
5. Verbalizes sources of hidden sodium in commercial foods.					
6. Verbalizes three (3) foods high in potassium (if applicable).					
7. Verbalizes approved salt substitutes.					
8. Verbalizes bowel program and importance of preventing constipation (if appropriate).					
9. Demonstrates progression within planned activity schedule.					
10. Demonstrates compliance with pacing activities and taking frequent rest periods.					
11. Other:					
Initials:					

Explain each Variance Code when necessary (include date): _____

_____

_____

_____

Outcome Codes

Met = ✓

Not Met = Variance Code

Not Addressed = Blank

V1—Patient too sick

V2—Comorbid Interference

V3—Patient's Cognitive status

V4—Caregiver Difficulties

V5—Lack of Equipment

RN Signatures:

_____

_____

_____

V6—Patient Decision

V7—Other

V8—Not Applicable

V9—Psychological/Emotional Status

V10—Environmental/Community

VNA FIRST *Home Care Steps* Protocols

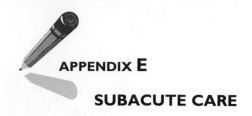

APPENDIX E

SUBACUTE CARE

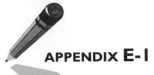

APPENDIX E-I

CLINICAL GUIDELINE FOR SHORT-TERM SUBACUTE ADMISSIONS

NAME:	DOB:
MC:	MA:
OTHER INSURANCE:	
PHYSICIAN:	
DATE OF ADMISSION:	

HEBREW HOSPITAL HOME, INC.
801 Co-op City Blvd, Bronx, New York 10475

CLINICAL GUIDELINES FOR SHORT-TERM SUBACUTE ADMISSIONS

Orthopedics: Joint replacement: specify _____ Fracture: specify
Location/type _____
Neurological: CVA   TIA   Other: _____
Vascular: Amputation   S/P vascular surgery: specify: _____
Wound management: specify: _____
IV antibiotics: specify source of infection: _____

Preadmission data required for the following:
- PRI
- Preadmission assessment form
- Preadmission addendum (for Medicare patients only)
- Hospital data: ECG, laboratory, CXR
- Discharge summary
- Rehabilitation summary
- Rx for treatment
- Financial clearance: Medicare, Medicaid, or managed care authorization

CHECKLIST FOR INITIAL ASSESSMENT OF SUBACUTE PATIENTS
The initial assessment for each subacute patient should include each of the following items:

Present functional capacity
Preexisting functional level
Allergies
Decision-making capacity
Personal or behavioral profile before admission
Use or abuse of drugs or alcohol
Personal preferences related to food, clothing schedules, bathing, and sleeping
Education, occupation, and habits
Strong likes and dislikes
Cultural influences and language
Names of significant others
Educational needs, including those of the family
Motivation for treatment and recovery
Past activities that may be useful to continue in the facility
Types and uses of assistive devices
Equipment needs

Days 1 and 2

Orientation to short-term unit

Introduction to interdisciplinary team

Initial assessment, development, and implementation of treatment plan by physician

Initial assessment and development of plan of care by team members

- RN
- Rehabilitation department: PT/OT/ST
- Nutrition
- Recreation therapy
- Medical social work

Initiation of Minimum Data Set (MDS) for Medicare patients only

Within 5 Days

Clinical care plan meeting with patient, significant other, and team members

Initiation of rehabilitation program

Educational needs identified

If patient is managed care, complete and submit 72-hour report of all clinical evaluations, goals, and treatment plans

Meet with case manager for overview and discussion of goals of care and discharge options

Identification of any potential impediments to the implementation of the care plan

Weeks 1 and 2

Patient receiving services as per treatment plan

Initiation of diagnosis-specific teaching plans

- Specific instruction in use of assistive devices and DME
- Specific medication and dietary instruction
- Specific instruction for home safety

For managed care patients, submission of the weekly progress reports to MCO

For Medicare patients, lock-in of MDS

Initiation of discharge planning process

Weeks 2 through 4

For managed care patients, submission of reports and coordination of services with managed care case manager

Continuation of teaching and treatment plan

- Specific instruction in use of assistive devices and DME
- Specific medication and dietary instruction
- Specific instruction for home safety

Clarification of discharge plan

Identification of any needed home services (i.e., skilled nursing or therapy)

Identification of needed DME and supplies

Discharge Indications:

Patient meets the following criteria:

- Verbalizes understanding of physical limitations imposed by illness
- Independent in ambulation and transfers with or without assistive device
- Able to verbalize appropriate medical follow-up postdischarge
- Independent in self-care management
- Understands options for home care
- Written discharge instructions to be provided

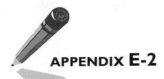

APPENDIX E-2

REFERRAL ASSESSMENT FORM

Hebrew Hospital Home, Inc.
801 Co-op City Blvd., Bronx, New York 10475

REFERRAL ASSESSMENT FORM

Date of assessment: _____

| PRI Classification: _____ |
| RUGs Category: _____ |
| Managed Care Skill Level: _____ |

Hospital: _____ Floor/unit: _____

Date of admission: _____

Name: _____ Insurance: ____ MC ____ MA ____ Other: _____

Age: ____ Sex: ____ Male ____ Female ____   Height: _____ Weight: _____

DIAGNOSIS: _____

____ Cardiac rehabilitation ____ Postsurgery (wound care) ____ Pulmonary ____ Renal ____ TBI

____ Orthopedic rehabilitation ____ Complex medical ____ Neurological ____ IV antibiotics ____ Other: _____

Mental Status: _____ Psyche Hx: _____

CLINICAL COURSE: _____
_____
_____
_____
_____
_____
_____

SPECIAL MEDS/TX (include anticoagulants, antibiotics, and inhalants): _____
_____

Special needs: ____ Private room ____ Contact isolation ____ Oxygen ____ Special DME/supplies (list): _____

Does the patient have a rehabilitation diagnosis: ____ Yes ____ No

Receiving rehabilitation: ____ Yes ____ No   Motivated: ____ Yes ____ No   Needs encouragement: ____ Yes ____ No

Endurance: ____ Good ____ Fair ____ Poor   Weight-bearing status: _____ Assistive device: _____

ADLs (PRI score): Feeding ____ Transfers ____ Ambulation ____ Toileting ____ Foley ____ Colostomy ____

Current rehabilitation program (please check): PT ____ No. of sessions/day ____ No. of days/week ____

OT ____ No. of sessions/day ____ No. of days/week ____ ST ____ No. of sessions/day ____ No. of days/week ____

SUBACUTE rehabilitation goals: No. of sessions/day ____ Treatment plan: _____
_____

DISCHARGE PLAN

Short term/subacute: ____ Long term/custodial: ____

Family contact/significant other: _____ Telephone: _____

Hospital social worker/discharge planner: _____ Telephone/pager: _____

HOSPITAL DATA NEEDED: ____ ECG ____ CXR ____ CBC/ PT/ SMAC ____ Consults ____ PT/OT/ST Notes ____

Culture reports ____ DNR ____ Advance directives ____ Other: _____

Copy of hospital face sheet attached: ____ Yes ____ No

____ ACCEPTED ____ NOT ACCEPTED ____ PENDING (reason): _____

Nurse Case Manager _____ Date _____

HEBREW HOSPITAL HOME, INC.
PATIENT ASSESSMENT ADDENDUM

PATIENT NAME: _____

HOSPITAL LOCATION: _____ **LOS:** _____

NAME OF CONTACT (if applicable): _____

Does the patient have (please check):

❑ Stage 3 or 4 decubiti or multiple-staged decubiti?

❑ Surgical wounds or open lesions?

❑ Foot lesions or infections?

❑ Feeding tube?

❑ Fever with dehydration, pneumonia, or vomiting?

❑ Coma?

❑ Hemiplegia?

❑ Dehydration?

❑ Pneumonia?

❑ Internal bleeding?

❑ Sepsis?

❑ Terminal illness?

SPECIAL TREATMENTS AND PROCEDURES:

A. SPECIAL CARE: Check treatments or programs received during the last 14 days.

Treatments:

1. Chemotherapy	_____
2. Dialysis	_____
3. Intravenous medication	_____
4. Intake/output	_____
5. Monitoring acute medical condition	_____
6. Ostomy care	_____
7. Oxygen therapy	_____
8. Radiation	_____
9. Suctioning	_____
10. Tracheostomy	_____
11. Transfusions	_____
12. Ventilator or respirator	_____

B. THERAPIES:

	Day/min per session
1. Speech: language pathology and audiology service	____ /____
2. Occupational therapy	____ /____
3. Physical therapy	____ /____
4. Respiratory therapy	____ /____

C. PHYSICIAN VISITS:

In the last 14 days, how many times has the physician examined the resident? _____

D. PHYSICIAN ORDERS:

In the last 14 days, how many days has the physician changed the orders (excluding renewals)? _____

RN signature _____ **Date** _____

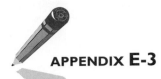

APPENDIX E-3

SUBACUTE DATA COLLECTION TOOL

HEBREW HOSPITAL HOME, INC.
801 Co-op City Blvd., Bronx, NY 10475

SUBACUTE DATA COLLECTION TOOL

Demographic Information
Name _____ Age _____ Unit _____
Date of admission _____ Date of discharge _____
Insurance: _____Medicare _____Medicaid _____Managed care: _____
RUG category _____ PRI classification _____ Managed care skill level: _____
No. of days covered_____ No. of days denied _____ Appeal filed: ____ Yes ____ No
Appeal outcome: ❑ Pending ❑ Overturned ❑ Upheld

Baseline Data
Diagnosis: _____
❑ Cardiac rehab ❑ Postsurgery ❑ Pulmonary ❑ Renal
❑ TBI ❑ Ortho rehab ❑ Complex medical ❑ Neurological
❑ IV antibiotics ❑ Diabetes mellitus ❑ Other: _____
Admission ADLs (PRI score): _____ Feeding _____Transfers _____ Mobility _____Toileting

Services Provided
❑ Skilled nursing ❑ Physical therapy ❑ Occupational therapy
❑ Speech/language pathology ❑ Audiology ❑ Respiratory therapy
❑ Other: specify (i.e., special DME): _____

Summary of Care

(Include specific input from disciplines, weight-bearing status [if applicable], and progress or lack of progress in reaching rehabilitation goals, wound size, labs, and any other pertinent information.)

Was the clinical course interrupted by an unexpected hospitalization? _____Yes _____ No (If yes, please describe):

Did the patient return to the facility? _____Yes _____ No (If no, what was the final disposition?) _____
_____
_____

Patient Education

Were knowledge deficits identified? _____Yes _____ No
Was an individualized teaching plan implemented? _____Yes _____ No
Were expected outcomes identified and documented? _____ Yes _____ No
Were teaching goals met at the time of discharge? _____ Yes _____ No

Discharge Plan

❑ Return to the community without services ❑ Return to the community with services
(describe): _____

❑ Remain in the SNF as a custodial resident

Actual length of subacute stay: _____
Discharge ADLs (PRI score): _____ Feeding _____ Transfers _____ Mobility _____ Toileting

Completed by: _____ **Date** _____

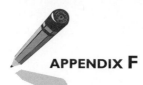

APPENDIX F

LONG-TERM CARE RESIDENT ASSESSMENT INSTRUMENT CASE STUDY AND CARE PLANS

Resident Assessment Instrument Case Study

A. Identification and Background Information

Mrs. M is a 90-year-old Caucasian widowed female (birth date 1-1-12; social security number 100-10-1000) who is being admitted to the nursing home January 12, 2002. She has lived with her oldest daughter for the past 3 years. Recently Mrs. M has been having increased frequency of incontinent episodes. Her daughter can no longer work outside the home and meet Mrs. M's needs. Mrs. M has four children, 10 grandchildren, and has been widowed for 10 years. Her only child living in Missouri is the daughter with whom she has been living. Mrs. M is of German origin and immigrated to the United States when she was 16 years of age. She remains closely tied to the Lutheran church in the community. She was a homemaker and graduated from high school. Mrs. M can still speak German, and when she is upset or becoming ill, she will revert to that language. She usually goes to bed around 9:00 PM and is up at 5:00 AM. She denies sleeping during the day, but her daughter states that she "catnaps." Mrs. M is responsible for her own affairs. She has private funds that she will be using to pay for her nursing home stay. Her medical insurance is Medicare Part A and B. Her daughter is named as Durable Power of Attorney for Health Care and is also named Power of Attorney for Financial Affairs. Mrs. M has made her wishes known: in the event that she should die, she is not to be resuscitated. Her physician supports her position and has written a do not resuscitate (DNR) order and has written a progress note to document her conversation.

B. Cognitive Patterns

Mrs. M is alert and oriented. She was confused at night on one occasion since admission. She became restless and believed her deceased husband was present in the room. Once in the last 7 days she became highly agitated, and the staff sat her up in a chair using a lap buddy to keep her from getting up unassisted. Her daughter reports that this is new behavior and she had not been confused at home before admission. Both long- and short-term memory remain intact. She has not had problems with confusion during the day. She is able to find her own room. She recognizes staff voices but does not always recall names. She can respond appropriately to staff requests. She is currently able to identify the season.

C. Communication/Hearing Pattern

Mrs. M is deaf in her right ear, and hearing aids are not useful. She can hear with difficulty if speech is directed toward her left ear. She is able to make her needs known by speaking. Her speech is clear. There is no speech deficit related to a previous stroke.

D. Vision Patterns

Mrs. M has macular degeneration and is now considered legally blind. She can differentiate between light and dark and can identify objects by shape. She wears glasses to maximize her remaining vision.

E. Mood and Behavior Patterns

Mrs. M has been occasionally tearful since admission. Her daughter states that she was not tearful at home. When asked what is wrong, she states that she misses her daughter and grandchildren. She is very concerned that she will not be able to go to her daughter's house anymore because she is having difficulty making it to the bathroom (BR). These moods are of short duration, and she can be redirected to another activity. She has been taking Prozac since 1997, when she was diagnosed with depression post–cerebrovascular accident (CVA).

F. Psychosocial Well-Being

Mrs. M enjoys activities and attending church services. She has expressed interest in leaving the facility for weekly trips to the mall or an outside activity. She does express concern about having incontinent episodes while on an outing. She enjoys books on tape and occasionally playing bingo with other residents. She has expressed interest in helping with the garden.

G. Physical Functioning and Structural Problems

Mrs. M has residual left-sided weakness. Her left arm is weaker than her right, but she is able to use the left arm to help support ambulation with a walker. Her left leg is also weaker than her right but is only problematic when she is tired or ill. She is able to balance herself using a walker. She became unsteady during the standing portion of the test for balance, but she was able to rebalance herself. Because of her congestive heart failure (CHF), she can only ambulate 20 to 30 feet before becoming fatigued and unsteady. She has limitation in range of motion (ROM). She is not able to use her left arm to touch the back of her head. She is only able to raise her lower left extremities to 70% of normal. She is able to get out of bed and ambulate to the BR unassisted on most days. Limited staff assist (defined as non–weight bearing) of one person is required an average of 3 times per week for transfers and assist to the BR. Limited assist is also required for transfers on and off the toilet 3 times per week. She ambulates with staff to all activities and meals for 20 to 30 feet, then staff will transport her in a wheelchair the remaining distance. She will self-propel in a wheelchair short distances in her room and in the hall on days when she is too fatigued to ambulate. She is able to turn herself in bed at night. She requires limited assistance of one person with dressing daily. She is unable to button her clothing. Occupational therapy (OT) has recommended the use of a large-handled buttonhook. She requires limited assist of one person with transfers in and out of the bathtub. She has fallen four times in the past 6 months. The last fall was 10 days ago and occurred when she was attempting to go to the BR during the night.

Mrs. M is able to perform self-care activities and tasks of daily living. She is very slow but desires to do as much for herself as possible. Her daughter states that her mother was independent at home; however, her slowness in getting around was a problem, especially with incontinence. She will require assistance on outings. (See also physical therapy note.)

H. Continence

Mrs. M is continent of bowel. She easily becomes constipated, leading to fecal impaction, and has had megacolon in the past. Her bowel pattern is daily in the morning with recurrent constipation 3 times a week (constipation diagnosed by presence of fecal smearing, gas, and abdominal pain). She has occasional urinary incontinence (four times in the last 7 days) when she could not get to the BR on time (urgency). A urinalysis was done, showing greater than 30 (white blood cells) WBCs. Because of symptoms of urinary tract infection (UTI) and elevated WBCs, a culture and sensitivity (C&S) was ordered.

I. Disease Diagnoses

Mrs. M has the following diagnoses: CVA in 1997 requiring extensive rehabilitation; anterior wall myocardial infarction (MI) in 1988; CHF related to damage from her MI; arteriosclerotic heart disease (ASHD); osteoarthritis and rheumatoid arthritis (RA); gastrointestinal (GI) bleed and ulcer related to steroid and nonsteroidal anti-inflammatory drug (NSAID) use; hypothyroidism for 10 years; pneumonia twice in the past 6 months; depression diagnosed post-CVA 1997.

J. Health Conditions

Mrs. M has difficulty with joint pain and stiffness in the early AM that resolves after her daily dose of Relafen and movement. She has difficulty moving her fingers in the AM. Her grip is weakened; therefore she uses a large-handled knife and buttonhook. She describes this pain as a 6 on a scale of 1 to 10. She had two episodes of pneumonia this past winter, which has concerned her daughter. Lung sounds on admission were diminished but clear. She sleeps at a 45-degree angle because of orthopnea. Mrs. M is afebrile. Her vital signs on admission were oral temperature 97.6°; apical pulse 68 and irregular; respiratory rate (RR) 18 even and unlabored at rest; and blood pressure (BP) 138/78. She has a grade III systolic murmur, no jugular venous distention, and 2+ pitting edema. She wears bilateral lower extremity Jobst stockings for edema. Her abdomen is soft with active bowel sounds in all four quadrants. She has no complaints of nausea or recent episodes of vomiting, and she has no history of drinking alcohol or smoking cigarettes.

K. Oral/Nutrition Status

The staff noted that Mrs. M was choking on fluids when drinking at meals. A speech therapy consult was ordered to rule out aspiration problems. A bedside swallow examination was performed and showed aspiration with thin liquids only. Speech therapy recommended that she drink only when sitting at 90 degrees with chin tucked and no straws. Her weight is 145 pounds, and she is 70 inches tall. In the past year she has lost 85 pounds. Her daughter reports that, although the weight loss has slowed, Mrs. M has had a 15-pound weight loss in the past 2 months. She is on a 2 g Na therapeutic diet. She does not always eat well, leaving 25% of the food in two out of three meals. She enjoys snacks throughout the day. At home, her daughter supplemented her diet with Carnation Instant Breakfast, increased protein intake to help with her skin, and increased fruit for fiber, and she gave her six small meals daily. Mrs. M feeds herself independently using large-handled utensils but requires staff assist at meals to cut meat and to orient for food location. OT has recommended a Dycem plate and rocker knife to use with meals (see also dietitian note).

L. Oral/Dental Status

Mrs. M has her own teeth and denies oral pain or discomfort. She last saw her dentist 6 months ago.

M. Skin Condition

Mrs. M's skin is intact. She has thin skin that tears easily related to steroid use and has healed skin tears. She has healing bruises associated with past falls. Her Braden scale indicates that she has no impairment with sensory perception; she is able to respond appropriately and can voice discomfort. She does have slight impaired sensory impairment resulting from CVA (score 3). She occasionally has incontinence (score 3). She is able to ambulate independently with her walker for short distances and does so frequently throughout the day (score 3). She is able to move in bed independently (score 3). Her nutritional intake is adequate, although she does have a history of significant weight loss (score 3). She occasionally slides down in her chair or does not completely raise herself up to move. This causes some skin shear (score 2). Mrs. M's total Braden score is 17 out of 23 total points possible. A score of 18 or less in people over 75 years of age indicates that the resident is at risk for skin breakdown.

N. Activity Pursuit Patterns

Mrs. M prefers to be awakened an hour before breakfast (0500) so that she can brush her teeth, comb her hair, and get dressed. She has difficulty moving in the morning because of arthritis; therefore she would prefer to bathe in the evening. A whirlpool bath is used. She has a very firm dislike of showers. Showering "messes up her hair."

O. Medications

Lanoxin 0.25 mg daily, Prilosec 20 mg daily, Relafen 1000 mg daily, Calan 80 mg tid, Prednisone 5 mg daily, Synthroid 0.1 mg daily, Bumex 1 mg daily, Prozac 20 mg daily, Nitroglycerin (NTG) 0.4 mg sublingual (SL) as needed for chest pain (she has difficulty with hypotension after NTG (last used 6/12/01), Peri Colace 100 mg bid, and Metamucil 1 tbsp every AM before breakfast. All medications except NTG are oral (PO).

P. Special Treatments and Procedures

Restorative aide for therapeutic exercise plan 5 times per week.

Q. Discharge Potential and Overall Status

At this time it is not anticipated that Mrs. M will be discharged to return home with her daughter. Her overall status has deteriorated in the last 90 days. A new onset of incontinence and falls has been the most significant change.

NOTE: There are separate physician's orders for laboratory, DNR, speech therapy evaluation, physical therapy evaluation, and therapeutic exercise program.

Care Plans

Problem #1: Acute Confusion

- Hallucinations at night ×1
- Attempt to get out of bed at night unassisted when confused
- Poor vision and hearing contributes to delirium
- Possible acute illness
  - Change in breath sounds, increased edema
  - Abnormal urinalysis (UA)

Goal

1. Will show improvement in delirium symptoms indicated by no confusion at night during next 7 days.

Interventions	Discipline
1. Follow up with physician regarding potential factors causing delirium a. R/O pneumonia, exacerbation of CHF b. UTI	N (nurse)
2. Check hourly between 9 PM and 5 AM; if restlessness noted, check the following and follow up appropriately: a. Vital signs and O$_2$ saturation; if abnormal, notify the physician b. Need to toilet c. Need to eat or drink d. Pain	N, certified nursing assistant (CNA)
3. Offer reassurance if scared or lonely	All
4. Assist up in chair and position at nurse's station	N, CNA
5. Elevate head of bed (HOB) to 45 degrees	CNA

Problem #2: Impaired Mobility/Activities of Daily Living (ADLs)

- Left-sided weakness secondary to CVA that increases with fatigue secondary to CHF (ambulation <20 to 30 feet)
- Pain and stiffness in joints, specifically in AM, secondary to arthritis
- Able to perform self-care but is slow
- Overall poor endurance secondary to CHF
- Desire to do things for herself

Goals

1. Improved ambulation—increase distance to total of 40 feet with walker and stand-by assist (SBA) to minimum assist of 1 by 3/1/02.
2. Maintain ability to dress self with minimal assist to setup during next 90 days.

Interventions	Discipline
1. Therapeutic exercise plan 5×weekly a. Ambulate to dining room (DR)×3 per day with walker and SBA to minimum assist b. If resident becomes tired, wheelchair (w/c) transport remaining distance to DR c. Alternating leg lifts, 5 repetitions each leg: 3 sets daily (see RA manual)	RA, CNA

d. Passive and active ROM to
   left upper extremity (LUE)
   and left lower extremity (LLE)
   q day
2. Promote use of adaptive ADLs   RA, CNA
   equipment
   a. Large-handled buttonhook
      for upper extremity (UE)
      dressing
   b. Dycem for plate stabilization
   c. Large-handled rocker knife for
      cutting
   d. Adaptive foam handles for
      utensils
   e. Keep adaptive equipment in
      tote bag at bedside
3. Assess q AM and prn for arthritis   N
   pain
   a. Offer prn medication in addition
      to routine medication
   b. Offer pain medication before AM
      care and exercises
   c. Provide extra assistance prn
      related to pain and stiffness
4. Promote independence   RA, N, CNA
   a. Provide encouragement and
      reassurance during ambulation
      and ADLs
   b. Allow time as needed to
      complete self-care
   c. Break tasks into shorter
      segments to conserve
      strength

Problem #3: Potential for Injury
- Recent history of falls (four falls in last 6 months; last
  fall within 30 days)
- Poor vision and hearing
- Unsteady gait
- Easily fatigued
- Confusion at night × 1

Goals
1. Fall risk will be minimized as evidenced by no fall with
   injury—immediately with continuous monitoring.
2. Will ambulate with walker safely and independently
   in room by 3/1/02.

Interventions	Discipline
1. Monitor gait, balance and	All
fatigue with ADLs	
a. Encourage resident to	
call for assist when unsure	
of strength/balance	

b. Provide SBA to minimum
   assist prn for ambulation
   and ADLs
c. Consider nonskid socks
   on feet at night
2. Keep light on in room when   All
   awake, night light on at night
3. Keep light on in BR   All
4. Answer call light immediately   All
   because of urge incontinence
   and sensory loss
5. Encourage use of well-fitting,   All
   nonskid shoes
6. Keep bed in low position with   All
   side rails down at all times
7. Use bed alarm, chair alarm   N, CNA
   with periods of confusion
8. Encourage to wear glasses   All
   when awake
   a. Be sure glasses are clean
      at all times
   b. Approach with caution and
      identify self—do not startle
   c. Use wide gestures with
      directions to compensate for
      loss of central vision
9. Speak directly into left ear   All
10. Collaborate with pharmacist/   N
    physician re any medications
    that may contribute to
    falls—review current medications
    and any new medications
11. Monitor and record orthostatic   CNA
    BP on 1/14/02, 1/15/02, and
    1/16/02
    a. Report to physician if >20-point   N
       drop in SBP, >10-point drop
       In DBP
    b. Report to physician if resident   N
       complains of dizziness/
       lightheadedness with position
       change
12. Evaluate all falls per facility   N
    policy; communicate as
    appropriate to physician
    and family

**Problem #4: Alteration in Mood, Risk for Social
Isolation**
- Decreased hearing and vision
- Pain from arthritis, cardiac conditions
- Fatigue from CHF

- Incontinence causing concern about participating in group activities or activities outside the building
- Tearfulness (sad that she may not be able to visit family outside the facility because of incontinence)
- History of depression, post-CVA since 1997

Goals

1. Feelings of loneliness for family will resolve by 3/1/02 as evidenced by the following:
   a. No further episodes of tearfulness
   b. Statements of satisfaction with placement
2. Will demonstrate active participation in facility life ongoing as evidenced by the following:
   a. Socialization with others
   b. Activity attendance of choice, both in and out of facility
   c. Weekly outings out of facility

Interventions	Discipline
1. Meet with resident 2×per week to enhance adjustment and coping skills	Social Service
a. Develop trusting relationship with resident and family	
b. Discuss perceived loss of relationship with family	
c. Allow expression of feelings/concerns	
d. Assist resident to identify choices	
e. Communicate to team members ways to enhance adjustment	
2. Encourage involvement in activities. Resident preferences include the following:	ACT
a. Church activities	
b. Books on tape	
c. Bingo	
d. Gardening	
e. Outings out of facility (check with nursing re toileting)	
• To shopping mall monthly—facilitated by nursing home transportation	
• To own church weekly—facilitated by daughter	
• As requested and facilitated by family/nursing home staff	
3. Encourage family involvement in facility activities	All

	Discipline
4. Monitor for change in mood status	All
a. Tearfulness, statements of sadness	
b. Withdrawal from activities	
c. Change in appetite, sleep pattern	
5. Administer antidepressant medication per medication administration record (MAR)	N
6. See incontinence care plan	All
7. See Potential for Injury care plan for vision and hearing needs	All

Problem #5: Urinary Incontinence

- Inability to reach the BR on time, possibly resulting from UTI
- Use of AM diuretic
- Strengths include the following:
  • Desire to toilet in BR
  • Ability to use call light for assistance

Goals

1. Will achieve urinary continence through routine toileting with staff assist—immediately.
2. Will toilet independently by 3/1/02.

Interventions	Discipline
Offer assistance/cue to BR use as follows:	N, RA, CNA
a. Within 30 minutes of receiving AM diuretic	
b. Immediately after breakfast for bowel movement (BM)	
c. Per facility routine (before and after meals, and at bedtime)	
d. Before activities and outings	
2. Keep call light within reach when in room; leave on bed when resident is out of room	All
3. Answer call light immediately	All
4. If incontinence continues once UTI resolved, follow up for additional causes	N

Problem #6: Altered Nutritional Status and Risk for Dehydration

- Weight loss of 85 lbs in 1 year, 15 lbs in 2 months
- Moderate protein depletion (Albumin of 3.0)
- Requires assist in DR because of vision loss, arthritis—needs help with cutting meat and opening cartons
- Dislikes 2 g Na diet
- Diuretic for CHF

■ Swallowing difficulty, with thin liquids, history of pneumonia

Goals

1. Maintain current body weight of 145 to 160 lbs.
2. Maintain adequate hydration without compromising cardiac stability (CHF) ongoing.
3. Improve albumin level to 3.5 g/dl next 90 days.

Interventions	Discipline
1. Collaborate with physician regarding dietary recommendations	D
a. Change 2 g Na to 4 g Na diet	
b. 5 small meals daily	
c. Carnation Instant Breakfast at 2 PM and bedtime	
d. Albumin level checks monthly ×2 months	
2. Include food preferences of fresh fruit: seedless grapes, oranges, peaches	D
3. Encourage high fiber foods to prevent constipation	D
4. May substitute cold cereal at night	D, CNA
5. Encourage 100% meal consumption	CNA
6. Set up food on plate and orient to clock face	CNA
7. Use adaptive equipment (see ADLs care plan)	CNA
8. Weigh weekly: Tuesdays in the AM before breakfast	CNA
a. If weight is up ≥3 lbs in 1 week, assess for signs/symptoms (s/s) of CHF exacerbation (shortness of breath, rales/crackles, increased fatigue, edema)	N
b. If weight is down ≥3 lbs, assess for dehydration (change in level of consciousness [LOC]; drop in BP, orthostasis, drop in urine output)	
9. Encourage 1500 to 2000 ml of decaffeinated fluids daily	D, N, CNA
10. Follow safety precautions for swallowing	CNA
a. Maintain upright position with chin tuck for fluid intake	
b. Do NOT use straws	
11. Obtain chemistry profile per physician order	N, MD
a. Review values and report abnormal results to physician	
12. Auscultate lung sounds daily and prn if choking noted with liquids	N

Problem #7: Risk for Skin Breakdown; Risk for Skin Tears

■ New onset of incontinence
■ Long-term steroid use causing fragile skin
■ Slides down in wheelchair and does not lift self for repositioning

Goals

1. Will maintain skin integrity ongoing as indicated by the following:
   a. No pressure ulcer development
   b. No skin tears
2. Will have Braden score of 20 by 3/1/02

Interventions	Discipline
1. Complete Braden scale weekly on Wednesday until score reaches 20, then complete quarterly	N
2. Report any changes in skin integrity or signs of breakdown to nurse	All
3. Inspect bed and wheelchair daily for areas that could cause skin tears	CNA
4. Encourage to wear long sleeves	CNA
5. Maintain proper positioning in wheelchair to prevent sliding down (skin shear)	CNA

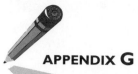

APPENDIX G

PREPRINTED ORDER SETS

 Saint Vincent's Manhattan
153 WEST 11TH ST., NEW YORK, NY 10011

CHF
DOCTOR'S ORDER FORM

DRUG ALLERGIES: ❏ None   ❏ Yes, to _____

PATIENT WEIGHT: _____ KG _____ LB

ADDRESSOGRAPH

ALL ORDERS MUST BE SIGNED AND STAMPED

MEDICATION/IV ORDERS ONLY	NOTED BY		OTHER ORDERS HERE	NOTED BY	
DATE: / / TIME: AM/PM	ED	INPT	**DAY OF ADMISSION**	ED	INPT
			1. Admit to _____		
Lasix ❏ _____ mg IV qd			2. Diagnosis _____		
❏ _____ mg IV bid			3. Condition _____		
			4. Vital signs q4h		
Digoxin ❏ 0.125 mg po qd			5. Diet 2 Gram Na+ _____		
❏ 0.250 mg po qd			6. Allergies _____		
			7. Heparin lock		
❏ Captopril _____ mg po q8h			8. Activity _____		
❏ Aldactone _____ mg po qd (if Cr <1.8)			9. Pulse oximetry q shift		
❏ Enteric coated ASA _____ mg qd			10. O_2 via _____ @ _____		
			11. Strict intake and output—measure and record q. shift		
INFUSION THERAPY FOR CCU PATIENTS ONLY			12. Daily weight before breakfast (same scale please)		
			NOTE: 13-15 to be done only if NOT available from the Emergency Department		
❏ Dobutamine _____			13. ❏ CXR		
❏ Dopamine _____			14. ❏ ECG		
❏ IV NTG (>40 mcg in CCU) _____			15. ❏ CBC, UA, comprehensive panel, PT/PTT/INR (if indicated)		
❏ Enalapril _____			16. ❏ Cardiac enzymes		
❏ Milrinone _____			17. Daily metabolic panel while pt receiving IV Lasix		
			18. ❏ Additional labs _____		
ICCU			19. ❏ ECHO (ext. 8342)		
❏ Dobutamine _____			20. ❏ Heart failure consult ext—CHF1 (2431)		
❏ Dopamine _____			21. ❏ Venous compression device while in bed		
			22. ❏ Telemetry		
			Please have patient's old medical records sent to the floor.		
(PRINT) (SIGN)			BEEPER #		

USE BALL POINT PEN ONLY
PHARMACY IS AUTHORIZED TO DISPENSE GENERIC EQUIVALENT WHEN PROPRIETARY NAMES ARE USED

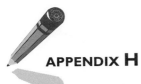

APPENDIX H

DOCUMENTATION GUIDES FOR PHYSICIANS

A Physician Newsletter from the Resource Management Improvement Team

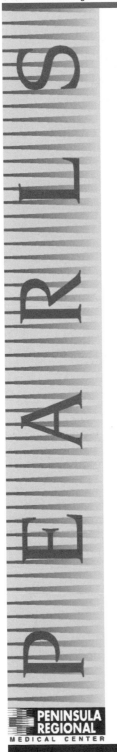

PEARLS PROGRAM

Decrease Denied Days
Through Improved Physician Documentation

PEARLS is a physician newsletter published monthly with a focus on top denial-generating DRGs. Each month's one-page publication eatures a different DRG and includes the following information:

• Summary of hospital's current performance related to number of denied cases and days; our LOS compared to the state's, and the "goal" LOS per payer guidelines

• "Points to Remember"—based on good physician documentation that justifies patients' LOS (based on actual chart reviews)

• List of commonly missed comorbidities

• Payer guidelines

These newsletters are presented by our PEARLS physician team member to the various medical staff department meetings monthly. They are also available in notebooks throughout the hospital and are sent to their office practices for use in their office.

PENINSULA REGIONAL
MEDICAL CENTER

A Physician Newsletter from the Resource Management Improvement Team
©1998 Peninsula Regional Medical Center

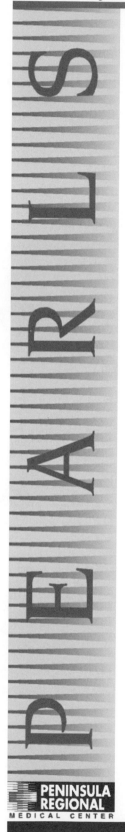

In addition, PEARLS "remeasures" are published monthly. These graphs of improvement demonstrate the decreased denial days over a year period. Along with the graphs, we add reminder pointers and any new payer guidelines that are appropriate for that DRG. Doctors love to see the improvement. Physicians have found the PEARLS newsletters and notebooks to be so helpful that they are requesting that they be available online for quick reference. In addition, members of our medical staff are suggesting other ideas for publication, as well as certain DRGs they would like to have highlighted to improve clinical performance.

The PEARLS Notebook contains an implementation plan and a series of physician newsletters covering the following DRGs:

- 14—CVA
- 358, 359—Uterine Adnexal Procedures
- 79, 89—Pneumonia
- 127—Heart Failure
- 174—GI Bleed
- 143—Chest Pain
- 88—COPD

PENINSULA REGIONAL
MEDICAL CENTER

A Physician Newsletter from the Resource Management Improvement Team
©1998 Peninsula Regional Medical Center

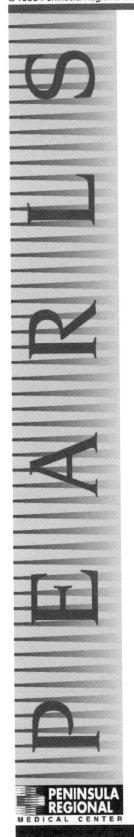

- 182, 183, 184, 296, 297, 298—Dehydration and Gastroenteritis
- 148, 149—Bowel Surgery
- 416—Septicemia
- 124, 125—Unstable Angina
- 107—CABG with Cath
- 430—Psychoses
- 20—Nervous System Infection (Bacterial Meningitis; Guillain-Barré Syndrome)
- 128, 130, 131—DVT
- 141—Syncope

Non-DRG PEARLS:
- Compliance
- Blood Loss Anemia
- Breast Cancer Screening and Diagnosis

As a result of our PEARLS program, in combination with our Patient Care Management Department, we have realized a decrease of denied dollars from $1,609,300 (1998) to $537,250 (through March 2000).

PENINSULA REGIONAL
MEDICAL CENTER

A Physician Newsletter from the Resource Management Improvement Team
© 1998 Peninsula Regional Medical Center

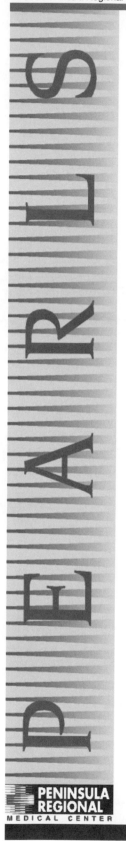

Representatives from the PEARLS team are available for site visits if you are interested. (See price list included.) During our visit, we can provide you with strategies for operationalizing the program at your institution. We look forward to meeting with you.

PRICE LISTING

CD-ROM	$1500
CD-ROM with
PowerPoint presentation	$2500
Site visit:
includes CD-ROM and 3-hour presentation ...	$5000 + our expenses

Dr. Chris Snyder
Dr. Tom Lawrence
Donna Thompson

For more information or to purchase the PEARLS program, contact Donna Thompson, RN, Director of Clinical Quality Improvement, at

Phone: 410-543-7740
Fax: 410-543-7010
E-mail: donna.thompson@peninsula.org

Peninsula Regional Medical Center
100 East Carroll Street
Salisbury, MD 21801

A Physician Newsletter from the Resource Management Improvement Team
© 1998 Peninsula Regional Medical Center

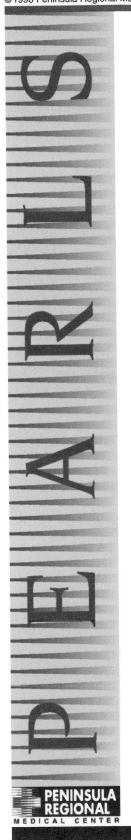

CHEST PAIN

UNSPECIFIED, NONCARDIAC DIAGNOSIS
DRG 143

Denials for FY 97/98: 30 days (15 due to nonacute level of care—15 due to administrative)
PRMC Length of Stay: 1.84   State: 1.50
Per M & R Guidelines: Ambulatory

DOCUMENTATION TO USE

- Document the suspected etiology of chest pain **within** the daily progress notes
- Document your plan every day in your progress notes
- Document daily disposition
- Remember, on the inpatient side, suspected or R/O conditions qualify and may increase LOS
- Signs and symptoms: type and duration of chest pain; constant or intermittent; location, radiation of pain
- Arrhythmias and ECG findings
- History of prior chest pain, MI, angina, or CABG
- Comorbidities
- Patient's functional status
- "Chest pain 2 to esophagitis"
- "Chest pain consistent with unstable angina"
- "Chest pain due to GERD"
- "Chest pain possible GI"
- "Chest pain noncardiac"

Will only optimize your acuity; it will not ↑ your LOS.

WHY IS IT IMPORTANT TO CLARIFY DOCUMENTATION?

- It will ↑ the severity of illness and improve Case Mix Index.
- It will ↑ patient satisfaction by ↓ denial letters that patients receive.
- It reduces physician's day-to-day interaction with payers.

Most common reason for DRG optimization is due to GI etiology.
Document discharge diagnosis in progress notes.
PTCA w/wo stent is an ambulatory procedure per **M & R** and **Payers Guidelines**.

M & R GUIDELINE EXPECTATIONS FOR DOCUMENTATION

Documented Reasons for Admission:
- Pain at rest
- Nocturnal pain
- Prolonged pain
- High risk status
- Inability R/O myocardial ischemia

Inadequate Reasons for Admission—Outpatient Care, Office, Observation Unit, Urgent Care:
- Noncardiac chest pain
- Pneumonia
- Pleurisy
- Esophagitis
- Reflux

PENINSULA REGIONAL MEDICAL CENTER

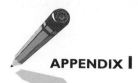

APPENDIX I

CASE MANAGER—INPATIENT

Job Description
JOB TITLE: Case Manager (Inpatient)
DEPARTMENT: Case Management

JOB SUMMARY: The case manager is responsible for facilitating the patient's hospitalization from preadmission through discharge. The case manager coordinates with physicians, nurses, social workers, and other health team members to expedite medically appropriate, cost-effective care. The case manager applies clinical expertise and medical appropriateness criteria to resource utilization and discharge planning. Will advise the healthcare team and provide leadership as needed.

REPORTS TO: Director of Case Management
SUPERVISES: Case Management Support Staff

RESPONSIBILITIES:

1. Within 24 hours of admission, initiates discharge planning by assessing the patient's needs and documenting the assessment on the interdisciplinary plan of care.
2. Within 24 hours of admission, identifies patients and families who have complex psychosocial, financial, and legal discharge planning needs and refers those patients to social work.
3. Ensures that the interdisciplinary care plan and the discharge plan are consistent with the patient's clinical course, continuing care needs, and covered services.
4. Using established criteria, reviews the following:
   a. Appropriateness of patient's admission
   b. Need for continued stay
   c. Information needed for discharge
5. Obtains the following from third-party payer:
   a. Certification due to patient status change
   b. Information needed for discharge
6. Discusses with attending physicians and/or physician advisors the appropriateness of resource utilization, consultations, and treatment plan.
7. Collects data on variances from quality screening criteria approved by the quality assurance committee. Forwards this data to the quality management department for continued support of the clinical departments.
8. Communicates to risk management all incidents that are potentially compensable events.

9. Responds to third-party payer requests for concurrent clinical information.
10. Issues letters of denial and reinstatement within regulatory timeframe.
11. Coordinates activities to ensure patient's appeal right under the discharge appeals program.
12. Ensures that chart documentation supports the need for continued stay.
13. Completes the Patient Review Instrument (PRI) in a timely manner.
14. Conducts daily multidisciplinary rounds (e.g., nursing, house staff, social work) on the assigned units, reviews the patient's plan of care, and focuses on the need for continued hospitalization. Coordinates and leads staff as indicated to ensure the following:
    a. Completion and reporting of diagnostic testing
    b. Completion of treatment appropriate for the acute episode of illness
    c. Modification of the plan to meet the continuing care needs of the patient
    d. Communication of relevant issues and third-party payer information to the team
    e. Assignment of appropriate level of care
15. Discusses estimated length of stay, treatment, and discharge plan with the attending physician, as indicated.
16. Ensures that all critical elements of the plan of care are communicated to the patient and family and are documented on the interdisciplinary plan of care.
17. Coordinates discharge teaching. Ensures that teaching is completed by members of the interdisciplinary team.
18. Consults with physician advisors, nursing staff, and staff in ancillary departments and coordinates the elimination of barriers to efficient delivery of care in the appropriate setting.
19. Resolves and eliminates conflicts in the patient treatment plan.
20. Ensures timely completion of all discharge, transfer, and referral forms.
21. Ensures that discharge prescriptions and discharge orders are written before patient's departure.
22. Ensures that patient follow-up appointments are made before patient's departure.
23. Employs a high degree of skill in all oral and written communications and personal interactions.

24. Uses appropriate resources and methods to resolve conflicts with others.
25. Maintains a calm, rational, professional demeanor when dealing with others, even in situations involving conflict or crisis.
26. Demonstrates active collaboration with other members of the health team to achieve the Case Management programmatic goals.
27. Maintains absolute adherence to hospital and departmental polices and practices regarding confidentiality and patient's rights.

28. Demonstrates knowledge and support of the hospital's mission and values.
29. Maintains clinical competency and current knowledge of regulatory and payer requirements to perform job responsibilities.

SKILLS/QUALIFICATIONS: Licensed as a registered nurse. Baccalaureate degree preferred. At least 5 years of clinical experience as a registered nurse. Supervisory skills required. Utilization review or discharge planning experience preferred.

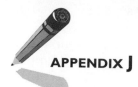

APPENDIX J

CASE MANAGER—ADMITTING OFFICE

Job Description
JOB TITLE: Case Manager (Admitting Office)
DEPARTMENT: Case Management

JOB SUMMARY: The case manager screens all patients referred to the admitting office to determine, through the use of clinical indicators, the patient's severity of illness and the intensity of services required and compares these to the services being requested. The case manager contacts the physician requesting the service to discuss care alternatives when requested services do not meet the clinical indicator requirements.

REPORTS TO: Director of Case Management
SUPERVISES: Clerical Support Staff

RESPONSIBILITIES:
1. Utilizes established criteria for potential admissions to determine the following:
   a. Appropriateness of admission
   b. Appropriateness of setting
   c. Patient placement type (i.e., observation status, outpatient)
   d. Discharge planning needs
   e. Care facilitation need
2. Initiates discussions with attending physician for patients who do not meet appropriateness criteria and for whom alternative care arrangements can be made.
3. Will refer the patient to admitting personnel once appropriateness of setting and care requirements are met to obtain preauthorization/precertification.
4. Intervenes with the payer when needed to assist admitting personnel in obtaining authorization.
5. Initiates discussions with the attending physician if there are anticipated discharge needs apparent at the time of preadmission assessment.
6. Reviews all same-day admissions before the scheduled day of surgery to ensure that authorization has been appropriately obtained and to determine the need for appropriateness of setting or any discharge planning needs.
7. Reviews all requests for transfers from other facilities to ensure that the patient's condition necessitates the transfer and provides feedback to the sending facilities regarding determination.
8. Utilizes an intake assessment form to evaluate patients and families in collaboration with the physician and/or office staff in presurgical testing unit.
9. Documents clinical information necessary to obtain approval from the payer as indicated in the patient medical record and maintains record until patient arrives at the hospital.
10. Notifies the inpatient case manager on issues related to the following:
    a. Coverage limitations
    b. Special patient/family circumstances
    c. Potentially avoidable days (i.e., presurgery, preprocedure days)
    d. Other issues, as appropriate
11. Contacts the patient/family to explore anticipatory discharge planning options, as appropriate, and collaborates with social work as needed.
12. Documents a case manager "preadmit note" in patient record, including discharge planning discussions held.
13. Consults with nursing staff and staff in ancillary departments to eliminate barriers to efficient delivery of care.
14. Refers all potential hospital liabilities/incidents to risk management.
15. Employs a high degree of skill in all oral and written communications and personal interactions and demonstrates collaborative working relationships.
16. Uses appropriate resources and methods to resolve conflicts with others.
17. Meets assigned deadlines and quality standards without reminder from supervisor or others.
18. Maintains a calm, rational, professional demeanor when dealing with others, even in situations involving conflict or crisis.
19. Maintains absolute adherence to hospital and departmental policies and practices regarding confidentiality and patients' rights.
20. Demonstrates knowledge and support of the hospital's missions and values.
21. Maintains clinical competency and current knowledge of regulatory and payer requirements to perform job responsibilities.

SKILLS/QUALIFICATIONS: Licensed as a registered nurse. Baccalaureate degree preferred. At least 5 years of clinical experience as a registered nurse. Leadership experience preferred. Utilization review or discharge planning experienced preferred.

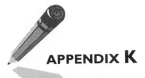

APPENDIX K

CASE MANAGER—EMERGENCY DEPARTMENT

Job Description

JOB TITLE: Case Manager (Emergency Department)
DEPARTMENT: Case Management

JOB SUMMARY: The case manager is responsible for facilitating the patient's hospitalization from preadmission through discharge. The case manager interfaces with physicians, nurses, social workers, and other healthcare team members to expedite medically appropriate cost-effective care. The case manager applies clinical expertise and medical appropriateness criteria to resource utilization and discharge planning.

REPORTS TO: Director of Case Management
SUPERVISES: Case Management Support Staff

RESPONSIBILITIES:

1. Facilitates and expedites the discharge of patients from the emergency department to alternate care settings using established criteria.
2. Facilitates the initiation of diagnostic services, treatment planning, and therapeutic treatment while patient is present in the emergency department of admitted patients.
3. Collaborates with social worker on referrals to alternate levels of care.
4. Collaborates with emergency department physician advisor when unable to resolve issues with the attending physician.
5. Collaborates in the development of clinical practice guidelines and critical pathways for designated targeted diagnosis to ensure staff buy-in.
6. Consults with physician advisor(s), emergency department nursing staff, and staff in the ancillary departments to eliminate barriers to efficient delivery of care.
7. Initiates a mechanism to facilitate communication with other case managers on admitted and observation patients.
8. Identifies issues of clinical resource utilization and/or delays in service/care (based on service standards) with the emergency department staff and refers these issues to the appropriate department head/vice president for resolution.
9. Serves as the first-line clinical responder to payer's clinical questions as required for payer approval for admission/observation.
10. Reports to the emergency department chairman all potential compensable events that need to be reported to risk management.
11. Employs a high degree of skill in all oral and written communications and personal interactions and demonstrates collaborative working relationships.
12. Uses appropriate resources and methods to resolve conflict with others.
13. Meets assigned deadlines and quality standards without reminder from supervisor or others.
14. Maintains a calm, rational, professional demeanor when dealing with others, even in situations involving conflict or crisis.
15. Maintains absolute adherence to hospital and departmental policies and practices regarding confidentiality and patient's rights.
16. Demonstrates knowledge and support of the hospital's mission and values.
17. Maintains clinical competency and current knowledge of regulatory and payer requirements to perform job responsibilities.

SKILLS/QUALIFICATIONS: Licensed as a registered nurse. Baccalaureate degree preferred. At least 5 years of clinical experience as a registered nurse. Leadership experience preferred. Utilization review of discharge planning experience preferred.

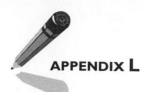

APPENDIX L

CASE MANAGER—COMMUNITY

Job Description

TITLE: Case Manager (Community)
DEPARTMENT: Case Management

JOB SUMMARY: The case manager is responsible for facilitating the patient's care process in the outpatient setting. The case manager coordinates with physicians, nurses, social workers, and other health team members to expedite medically appropriate cost-effective care. The case manager applies clinical expertise and medical appropriateness criteria to resource utilization, referrals to outside agencies, and use of services across the continuum. Will advise the healthcare team and provide leadership as needed.

REPORTS TO: Director of Case Management
SUPERVISES: Case Management Support Staff

RESPONSIBILITIES:

1. Uses high-risk screening criteria to assess patients' level of care needs. Completes this on admission to the outpatient setting and every 6 months, or as needed.
2. Completes a comprehensive physical, social, and financial assessment of the patient/family to determine priorities in developing a plan of care.
3. Coordinates the plan of care with all members of the interdisciplinary team.
4. Identifies patients and families who have complex psychosocial, financial, and/or legal needs and refers those patients to social work.
5. Interacts with patients and families on an as-needed basis to modify and update the plan of care based on the assessment.
6. Obtains from third-party payer certification for use of service across the continuum (i.e., home care).
7. Updates and modifies the interdisciplinary plan of care as needed based on an assessment of the patient's achievement of expected outcomes of care.
8. Collaborates with patients/families to coordinate community services and appropriate resources that meet the patient's/family's needs and goals.
9. Discusses with attending physicians and/or physician advisors the appropriateness of resource utilization, consultations, and treatment plan.
10. Collects data on variances identified in the outpatient setting.

11. Communicates to risk management all incidents that are potentially compensable events.
12. Responds to third-party payer requests for concurrent clinical information.
13. Ensures that chart documentation supports the level of care provided.
14. Conducts multidisciplinary case conferences (e.g., nursing, house staff, social work) as needed to ensure the following:
    a. Completion and reporting of diagnostic testing
    b. Completion of treatment appropriate to the episode of illness
    c. Modification of the plan to meet the continuing needs of the patient
    d. Communication of relevant issues and third-party payer information to the team
15. Discusses estimated length of treatment, frequency of outpatient visits, or other care modalities with the attending physician, as indicated.
16. Ensures that all critical elements of the plan of care are communicated to the patient and family and are documented on the interdisciplinary plan of care.
17. Collaborates in developing, implementing, and evaluating teaching/learning strategies for patient/family in the community.
18. Consults with physician advisors, nursing staff, and staff in ancillary departments and coordinates the elimination of barriers to efficient delivery of care in the appropriate setting.
19. Identifies, resolves, and eliminates conflicts in the patient treatment plan.
20. Performs ongoing evaluation of the plan of care to ensure that current and potential complications are identified and to evaluate the effectiveness of interventions.
21. Ensures that patient appointments are made for follow-up visits.
22. Communicates with other case managers along the continuum, including acute care, home care, managed care, and long-term care.
23. Employs a high degree of skill in all oral and written communications and personal interactions.
24. Uses appropriate resources and methods to resolve conflict with others.

25. Maintains a calm, rational, professional demeanor when dealing with others, even in situations involving conflict or crisis.
26. Demonstrates active collaboration with other members of the health team to achieve the case management programmatic goals.
27. Maintains absolute adherence to hospital and departmental policies and practices regarding confidentially and patients' rights.
28. Demonstrates knowledge and support of the hospital's mission and values.

29. Maintains clinical competency and current knowledge of regulatory and payer requirements to perform job responsibilities.

SKILLS/QUALIFICATIONS: Licensed as a registered nurse. Baccalaureate degree preferred. At least 5 years of clinical experience as a registered nurse. Supervisory skills required. Utilization review and leadership experience preferred.

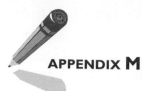

APPENDIX M

PHYSICIAN ADVISOR

Job Description
JOB TITLE: Physician Advisor
DEPARTMENT: Case Management

JOB SUMMARY: The physician advisor is responsible for reviewing all concurrent and retrospective denials brought to his attention by the case management staff. The physician advisor will review the case for medical necessity against established criteria and make a determination as to whether the case is appealable. If the case is appealable, the physician advisor will pursue the case by utilizing the concurrent appeal process or the retrospective appeal process as appropriate.

REPORTS TO: Director of Case Management
SUPERVISES: No one

RESPONSIBILITIES:
1. All potential or actual denials (whether concurrent or retrospective) are referred by the case managers except for the following:
   a. Cases denied because of lack of precertification
   b. Cases denied that are paid based on diagnostic-related groups (DRGs)
   c. Cases that are "technical" denials
   d. Potential denials
2. All concurrent denials are attended to immediately upon, or as soon as possible after, referral.
3. All retrospective denials are prioritized for completion based on the date by which the appeal must be submitted to the payer.
4. A data worksheet is completed for every case reviewed. The worksheet includes patient demographic information and pertinent clinical information. Standardized clinical criteria (e.g., InterQual or Milliman & Robertson) are applied to refute the payer denial.
5. All cases meeting standardized clinical criteria are appealed.
6. Those concurrent cases felt to be medically justified, despite lacking adherence to standardized criteria, will be pursued using the concurrent appeal process.
7. Those retrospective cases felt to be medically justified, despite lacking adherence to standardized

criteria, will be pursued by preparing a clinical justification appeal letter to be included in the appeal packet sent to the payer.
8. For concurrent cases not fitting into one of these criteria, the case is pursued with the attending physician of record to:
   a. Obtain clinical information about the patient that may not be apparent from a review of the medical record but that may be sufficient to justify an acute care stay
   b. Educate the physician on the criteria used to determine the necessity of an acute care stay
   c. Ensure that the patient is in the most appropriate setting or the level of care needed
9. For retrospective cases not fitting into one of these criteria, the case is appealed without a clinical justification appeal letter from the physician advisor.
10. Will prepare a monthly activity report of appealed cases and the outcomes of those appeals. The format and content of the report will be determined by the director of case management.
11. Will participate in physician education programs regarding reimbursement, clinical criteria, and documentation as needed.
12. Will serve as a liaison between the physician staff and the case management staff.
13. Will maintain positive working relationships with the medical directors of the third parties.

EXPERIENCE: Previous utilization management experience preferred. A working knowledge of InterQual and Milliman & Robertson criteria essential.

EDUCATION:
1. Licensed medical doctor
2. Utilization certification preferred

SKILLS: Excellent clinical and administrative skills and judgment. Strong interpersonal and communication skills. Ability to effectively work with other disciplines and departments and outside agencies.

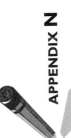

APPENDIX N

GUIDE FOR A CASE MANAGER'S COMPETENCY-BASED PERFORMANCE APPRAISAL

Role Dimension	Relative Weight*	Key Performance Area†	Performance Expectations‡	Performance Level Achieved§	Comments
Clinical/Patient Care	40% 0.4	1. Appraise the need for the case management services through gathering and evaluation of relevant data. 2. 3. 4.	• Assesses patient's condition to identify suitability for case management. • Evaluates the patient based on the selection criteria for case management. • Seeks patient's consent for the services; discusses the goals.	Level: 3 Subscore: ____ $3 \times 0.4 = 1.2$	
Managerial/ Leadership	25% 0.25	1. Advocates for clients through effective partnership with patients, their families, payers, and healthcare team members. 2. 3.	• Establishes an effective relationship with patient, family, and healthcare team. • Communicates with providers and payers in a timely fashion; obtains authorizations. • Facilitates and maintains patients' independence in decision making.	Level: 2 Subscore: ____ $2 \times 0.25 = 0.5$	
Business/ Financial	15% 0.15	1. Integrates factors related to quality, safety, efficiency, and cost-effectiveness in managing patient care. 2. 3. 4.	• Prevents duplication, fragmentation, or the use of unnecessary resources. • Seeks authorization from managed care companies for specific services. • Procures, coordinates, and facilitates healthcare services.	Level: 2 Subscore: ____ $2 \times 0.15 = 0.3$	
Information Management/ Communication	15% 0.15	1. Integrates the quality, safety, efficiency, and cost-effectiveness principles in outcomes management. 2. 3. 4.	• Establishes measurable clinical, financial, and quality-of-care goals/outcomes. • Identifies and manages variances of care. • Maintains open communication with the interdisciplinary team regarding outcomes. • Prepares and disseminates related reports.	Level: 3 Subscore: ____ $3 \times 0.15 = 0.45$	
Professional Development/ Advancement	5% 0.05	1. Maintains a competitive professional status and involves self in professional activities. 2. 3. 4.	• Maintains membership in professional organizations. • Advocates for patients in policy making. • Applies appropriate research findings to the development of policies, procedures, and guidelines for cost-effective/high-quality practice.	Level: 2 Subscore: ____ $2 \times 0.05 = 0.1$	

Total = 100%

Total score = 2.55 (255)
Maximum score = 3 (300)

*The total relative weight per dimension and must be distributed among the key performance areas appropriate to each dimension. These are only examples. Other more detailed expectations must be developed depending on the job description and the practice setting.
†These are only examples. Additional areas may be added depending on the job description. For example, if there are 4 performance areas in the clinical
‡These are only examples. Others may be added depending on the job description. For example, if there are 4 performance areas in the clinical dimension, the total relative weight for the 4 areas must be equal to 0.4.
§Performance level achieved: 1 = does not meet expectations; 2 = meets expectations; 3 = exceeds expectations.
Copyright Hussein Tahan, 2001.

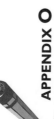

APPENDIX O

PERFORMANCE MANAGEMENT FORM—CASE COORDINATOR

ENGLEWOOD HOSPITAL AND MEDICAL CENTER

SUPERVISORY AND MANAGERIAL PERFORMANCE MANAGEMENT PROGRAM FORM

NAME:

DEPARTMENT: Care Coordination

APPRAISAL PERIOD:

REVIEWER'S NAME:

JOB TITLE: Case Coordinator

APPRAISAL DATE:

JOB TITLE: Director of Care Coordination

PERFORMANCE LEVELS:

5 = Far exceeds expectations—Performance consistently and significantly exceeds job requirements.

4 = Exceeds expectations—Performance frequently surpasses job requirements.

3 = Meets expectations—Performance meets all job requirements.

2 = Meets most expectations—Performance does not fully meet all job requirements.

1 = Does not meet expectations—Performance is below minimum job requirements.

Preparing your performance plan:

• Complete your plan and review with your Vice-President by March 30, 2001.

• Obtain Vice-President's signature in Section Two

• Completed and signed copies to be forwarded to the Organizational Development Department.

*Note: Certain individuals may not have any control over budgeted dollars or directly supervise staff. In those instances, your performance plan will not include the sections of Budget, Turnover/Retention, and Performance Appraisals. However, you should include additional goals as they relate to your management responsibilities in the organization.

SECTION ONE: PERFORMANCE PLAN

SECTION THREE: PERFORMANCE APPRAISAL RESULTS

Job Duty/Responsibility Area and Performance Criteria	Weight (W)	Performance Level Achieved (PLA)	Performance Score (W × PLA)	Comments
Organizational Objectives	%			
• **Service Excellence/Patient Satisfaction** • Achieve overall rating of 81.0 • **Budget** • Surplus as defined by Board • **JCAHO** • No Type 1's				
Departmental Objectives	%			

A. Specific Department Goals
1. Service Excellence
  • Consistently exhibit Service Excellence standards
  • Participate in Service Excellence Performance Improvement initiatives
  • Act as a role model for staff and peers in customer service leadership
  • Support and reinforce those behaviors that are embodied in our Mission and Vision statements
  • Participate in the annual development of overall Service Excellence goals and objectives for the Care Coordination Department
  • Ensure patient's rights to confidentiality, dignity, respect, and involvement in decision making through team rounds
  • Participate in annual Department Open House
2. Monitor Medicare/Medicaid length of stay and identify ways to reduce length of stay through Case Management and identification of safe alternatives to inpatient stay				

3. Implement InterQual and/or Milliman & Robertson Clinical Decision-Making Program on all patients

4. Implement ongoing Care Coordination plan; reevaluate as needed as follows:
   - Assign target length of stay
   - Establish methods to review cases for discharge issues, continued stay needs
   - Develop unit-based mechanisms in conjunction with nurse manager and care managers to communicate anticipated discharge dates and involve care managers in identifying patients who are off guideline or have additional needs

5. Participate in conferences, workshops, and other professional development activities to maintain licensure and/or remain professionally current with advances in field of expertise

6. Ensure ongoing departmental compliance with JCAHO

7. Psychiatric
   - Collaborate and case conference with the multidisciplinary team to provide a complete healthcare delivery system
   - Coordinate on discharge the medical and mental health needs of the patient

8. MSICU
   - Participate in multidisciplinary conferencing to ensure provision of a complete healthcare delivery system for the critically ill patient
   - Facilitate the smooth transition from MSICU to the medical-surgical unit
   - Case conference with the specific unit case coordinator on transfer
   - Assess need for long-term placement for ventilator patients and initiate discharge planning on a timely basis
   - Provide resources to family members
   - Provide emotional support to families of critically ill patients

9. Maternal/Child Health
   - Collaborate daily with the multidisciplinary team to provide a complete healthcare delivery system encompassing the cultural, ethnic, and religious diversity of the clients
   - Maintain open communication with the physician, client, and insurance company to validate length of stay for the high-risk antepartum/postpartum/pediatric client
   - Provide maternal/child community resources for clients on discharge
   - Provide resources for the multiparity client
   - Manage maternity clients lacking prenatal care by providing home care/community follow-up
   - Manage maternity client leaving less than 48 hours after delivery with home care referral
   - Manage teen and single parent
   - Collect data and monitor variances to achieve positive patient outcomes

10. Neonatal Intensive Care Unit

- Collaborate daily with the multidisciplinary team to provide a complete health-care system and smooth transition from hospital to home for the neonate
- Incorporate the plan of care with the insurance company and parent participation
- Provide parents with available community resources and early intervention programs
- Serve as a resource person in providing essential equipment, on discharge, for the high-risk neonate
- Inform parents of outlying costs
- Determine the financial ability of the parents to pay for the necessary equipment
- Know of appropriate transitional care/rehabilitation program for the child with special needs
- Collect data
- Monitor variances to achieve positive patient outcomes

B. Budget

- Maintain an active role in establishing concurrent intervention to facilitate appropriate reimbursement
- Provide ongoing education to physicians regarding the importance of their participation in concurrent stage 1 appeals; facilitate MD to MD communication as required
- Facilitate appropriate and timely utilization of resources
- Ensure that patients are receiving appropriate level of care on a timely basis by tracking system variances
- Ensure cost containment but quality of service in arranging pneumograms

Management				%
A. Turnover				
• To improve turnover and retain staff				
• Use an interdisciplinary team approach				
• Participate in orientation of new staff				
• Participate in interviewing prospective candidates				
B. Communications				
• Maintain regular communication with the multidisciplinary staff to identify patient goals and to facilitate the patient's progression through the continuum of care and needs for safe discharge planning				
• Ensure that care coordination staff are well informed of medical center and department priorities				
C. Participation in medical center committees/events				
Totals:				

SECTION TWO: PERFORMANCE PLAN APPROVAL (SIGNATURES)

APPRAISEE:	DATE:
REVIEWER:	DATE:
SECOND-LEVEL REVIEWER:	DATE:

SECTION THREE: ADHERENCE TO HOSPITAL/DEPARTMENT POLICIES AND REGULATIONS

	MEETS EXPECTATIONS	NEEDS IMPROVEMENT
1. **Attendance/punctuality**		
2. **Dressing/grooming:** Adhere to dress code policy by always exhibiting professionalism in my attire.		
3. **Safety/environmental health**		
4. **Corporate compliance:** Attend annual inservice, sign compliance agreement. Ensure that staff members meet corporate compliance regulations (e.g., attend inservices).		
5.		

COMMENTS:

SECTION FOUR: KNOWLEDGE, SKILLS, AND ABILITIES

Consider the extent to which the employee's demonstrated knowledge, skills, and abilities appear to exceed, meet, or fall short of job expectations.

	EXCEEDS EXPECTATIONS	MEETS EXPECTATIONS	NEEDS IMPROVEMENT
Job knowledge/skills: The understanding of the principles, techniques, skills, practices, and procedures required by the job. The ability to use the materials and equipment required by the job.			
Planning and organizing: The ability to logically and effectively structure tasks, plan the work, establish priorities, and accomplish work activities.			
Communications: The ability to organize and present information clearly and concisely. The ability to keep supervisor, peers, and outsiders (if appropriate) informed about progress, problems, and developments.			
Teamwork: The ability to work effectively with supervisors and co-workers and to appropriately respond to requests for assistance as a productive team member.			
Initiative: The ability to act independently and offer suggestions and new ideas for improving performance and operations.			
Problem solving: The ability to analyze situations, identify problems, identify and evaluate alternative actions, and take appropriate actions.			
Guest relations: The demonstration of a courteous and helpful manner during interactions with others, such as patients, families, visitors, and other employees.			

COMMENTS:

SECTION FIVE: SUMMARY OF OVERALL PERFORMANCE

Total (from **Section Three**): _____

COMMENTS:

SECTION SIX: APPRAISEE DEVELOPMENT

Identify areas for development and specific actions to be taken during the next appraisal period. These may include on-the-job training, special developmental assignments, and off-site training.

COMMENTS:

SECTION SEVEN: COMMENTS AND SIGNATURES

APPRAISEE COMMENTS AND SIGNATURE (The appraisee's signature [optional] indicates only that the appraisal has been discussed with the appraisee and does not indicate agreement with the appraisal.)

COMMENTS:

Signature: Date:

REVIEWER COMMENTS (OPTIONAL) AND SIGNATURE

COMMENTS:

Signature: Date:

SECOND LEVEL REVIEWER COMMENTS (OPTIONAL) AND SIGNATURE

COMMENTS:

Signature: Date:

Glossary

Access to care   The ability and ease of patients to obtain healthcare when they need it.

Accreditation   A standardized program for evaluating healthcare organizations to ensure a specified level of quality, as defined by a set of national industry standards. Organizations that meet accreditation criteria receive an official authorization of approval of their services.

Actuarial study   Statistical analysis of a population based on the utilization and demographic trends of the population. Results used to estimate healthcare plan premiums or costs.

Acuity   Complexity and severity of the patient's health/medical condition.

Admission certification   A form of utilization review in which an assessment is made of the medical necessity of a patient's admission to a hospital or other inpatient facility. Admission certification ensures that patients requiring a hospital-based level of care and length of stay appropriate for the admission diagnosis are usually assigned and certified and payment for the services are approved.

Advance directives   Legally executed document that explains the patient's healthcare-related wishes and decisions. It is drawn up while the patient is still competent and is used if the patient becomes incapacitated or incompetent.

Adverse events   Any untoward occurrences, which under most conditions are not natural consequences of the patient's disease process or treatment outcomes.

Advocacy   Acting on behalf of those who are not able to speak for or represent themselves. It is also defending others and acting in their best interest.

Algorithm   The chronological delineation of the steps in, or activities of, patient care to be applied in the care of patients as they relate to specific conditions/situations.

Alternate level of care   A level of care that can safely be used in place of the current level and determined based on the acuity and complexity of the patient's condition and the type of needed resources.

Ambulatory payment classification (APC) system   An encounter-based classification system for outpatient reimbursement, including hospital-based clinics, emergency departments, observation, and ambulatory surgery. Payment rates are based on categories of services that are similar in cost and resource utilization.

Ancillary services   Other diagnostic and therapeutic hospital services that may be involved in the care of patients other than nursing or medicine. Includes respiratory, laboratory, radiology, nutrition, physical and occupational therapy, and pastoral services.

Appeal   The formal process or request to reconsider a decision made not to approve an admission or healthcare services, reimbursement for services rendered, or a patient's request for postponing the discharge date and extending the length of stay.

Appropriateness of setting   Used to determine if the care needed is being delivered in the most appropriate and cost-effective setting possible.

Approved charge   The amount Medicare pays a physician based on the Medicare fee schedule. Physicians may bill the beneficiaries for an additional amount, subject to the limiting charge allowed.

Authorization   See **certification**.

Autonomy   A form of personal liberty of action in which the patient holds the right and freedom to select and initiate his or her own treatment and course of action, and taking control for his or her health; that is, fostering the patient's independence and self-determination.

Benchmark   See **benchmarking**.

Benchmarking   An act of comparing a work process with that of the best competitor. Through this process one is able to identify what performance measure levels must be surpassed. Benchmarking assists an organization in assessing its strengths and weaknesses and in finding and implementing best practices.

Beneficence   The obligation and duty to promote good, to further and support a patient's legitimate interests and decisions, and to actively prevent or remove harm; that is, to share with the patient risks associated with a particular treatment option.

Beneficiary   An individual eligible for benefits under a particular plan. In managed care organizations beneficiaries may also be known as members (HMO) or enrollees (PPO).

Benefit package   The sum of services for which a health plan, government agency, or employer contracts to provide. In addition to basic physician and hospital services, some plans also cover prescriptions, dental, and vision care.

Benefits   The amount payable by an insurance company to a claimant or beneficiary under the claimant's specific coverage.

Capitation   A fixed amount of money per-member-per-month (PMPM) paid to a provider for covered services. The typical reimbursement method used by HMOs. Whether a member uses the health service once or more than once, a provider who is capitated receives the same payment.

Care management   A healthcare delivery process that helps achieve better health outcomes by anticipating and linking patients with the services they need more quickly. It also helps avoid unnecessary services by preventing medical problems from escalating.

Caregiver   The person responsible for caring for a patient in the home setting. Can be a family member, friend, volunteer, or an assigned healthcare professional.

Carrier   An insurance company or administrator of benefits under an insurance contract.

Carve out   Services excluded from a provider contract that may be covered through arrangements with other providers. Providers are not financially responsible for services carved out of their contract.

Case management   A patient care delivery system that focuses on meeting outcomes within identified timeframes using appropriate resources. Case management follows an entire episode of illness, from admission to discharge, crossing all healthcare settings in which the patient receives care.

Case management plan   A timeline of patient care activities and expected outcomes of care that address the plan of care of each discipline involved in the care of a particular patient. It is usually developed prospectively by an interdisciplinary healthcare team in relation to a patient's diagnosis or surgical procedure.

Case manager   Responsible for coordinating the care delivered to an assigned group of patients based on diagnosis or need. Other responsibilities include patient/family education and outcomes monitoring and management.

Case mix complexity   An indication of the severity of illness, prognosis, treatment difficulty, need for intervention, or resource intensity of a group of patients.

Case mix group (CMG)   Each CMG has a relative weight that determines the base payment rate for inpatient rehabilitation facilities under the Medicare system.

Case mix index (CMI)   The sum of DRG-relative weights of all patients/cases seen during a 1-year period in an organization, divided by the number of cases.

Case-based review   The process of evaluating the quality and appropriateness of care based on the review of individual medical records to determine whether the care delivered is acceptable. It is performed by healthcare professionals assigned by the hospital or an outside agency (e.g., Peer Review Organization [PRO]).

Caseload   The total number of patients followed by a case manager at any point in time.

Catastrophic case   Any medical condition in which total cost of treatment is expected to exceed an amount designated by the HMO contract with the medical group.

Certification   The approval of patient care services, admission, or length of stay by a health benefit plan (e.g., HMO, PPO) based on information provided by the healthcare provider.

Claim   A form that is submitted to an insurance agency requesting payment in return for healthcare services provided to an enrollee. The form contains information such as member/enrollee identification number, provider identification, date of service, type of service, quantity, procedure code, diagnosis code, and place of service.

Clinical pathway   See **case management plan.**

Coding   A mechanism of identifying and defining patient care services/activities as primary and secondary diagnoses and procedures. The process is guided by the ICD-9-CM coding manual, which lists the various codes and their respective descriptions.

Coinsurance   A type of cost sharing in which the insured person pays or shares part of the medical bill, usually according to a fixed percentage.

Comorbidity   A preexisting condition (usually chronic) that, because of its presence with a specific condition, causes an increase in the length of stay by about 1 day in 75% of the patients.

Complication   An unexpected condition that arises during a hospital stay or healthcare encounter that prolongs the length of stay at least by 1 day in 75% of the patients and intensifies the use of healthcare resources.

Concurrent review   A method of reviewing patient care and services during a hospital stay to validate the necessity of care and to explore alternatives to inpatient care. It is also a form of utilization review that tracks the consumption of resources and the progress of patients while being treated.

Consensus   Agreement in opinion of experts. Building consensus is a method used when developing case management plans.

Continued stay   A type of review used to determine that each day of the hospital stay is necessary and that care is being rendered at the appropriate level.

Continuous quality improvement (CQI)   A key component of total quality management that uses rigorous, systematic, organization-wide processes to achieve ongoing improvement in the quality of healthcare services and operations. It focuses on both outcomes and processes of care.

Continuum of care   A range of medical, nursing, and social services and treatments offered in a variety of settings that provide services most appropriate to the level of care required.

Copayment   A supplemental cost-sharing arrangement between the member and the insurer in which the member pays a specific charge for a specified service. Copayments may be flat or variable amounts per unit of service and may be for such things as physician office visits, prescriptions, or hospital services. The payment is incurred at the time of service.

Credentialing   A review process to approve a provider who applies to participate in a health plan. Specific criteria are applied to evaluate participation in the plan. The review may include references, training, experience, demonstrated ability, licensure verification, and adequate malpractice insurance.

Current procedural terminology (CPT)   A listing of descriptive terms and identifying codes for reporting medical services and procedures performed by physicians.

Custodial care   Care provided primarily to assist a patient in meeting the activities of daily living but not requiring skilled nursing care.

Database   An organized, comprehensive collection of patient care data. Sometimes it is used for research or for quality improvement efforts.

Deductible   A specific amount of money the insured person must pay before the insurer's payments for covered healthcare services begin under a medical insurance plan.

Delay in service   Used to identify delays in the delivery of needed services and to facilitate and expedite such services when necessary.

Demand management   Telephone triage and online health advice services to reduce members' avoidable visits to health providers. This helps reduce unnecessary costs and contributes to better outcomes by helping members become more involved in their own care.

Denial   No authorization or certification is given for healthcare services because of the inability to provide justification of medical necessity or appropriateness of treatment or length of stay. This can occur before, during, or after care provision.

Diagnosis-related group (DRG)   A patient classification scheme that provides a means of relating the type of patient a hospital treats to the costs incurred by the hospital. DRGs demonstrate groups of patients using similar resource consumption and length of stay.

Disability case management   A process of managing occupational and nonoccupational diseases with the aim of returning the disabled employee to a productive work schedule and employment.

Discharge criteria   See **discharge outcomes.**

Discharge outcomes   Clinical criteria to be met before or at the time of the patient's discharge. They are the expected/projected outcomes of care that indicate a safe discharge.

Discharge planning   The process of assessing the patient's needs of care after discharge from a healthcare facility and ensuring that the necessary services are in place before discharge. This process ensures a patient's timely, appropriate, and safe discharge and appropriate use of resources.

Discharge status   Disposition of the patient at discharge (e.g., left against medical advice, expired, discharged home, transferred to a nursing home).

Disease management   The process of intensively managing a particular disease across different care settings and levels of care using a population-based complex and sophisticated program that places a heavy emphasis on health risk identification, prevention, and maintenance.

Disenrollment   The process of terminating healthcare insurance coverage.

Distributive justice   Deals with the moral basis for the dissemination of goods and evils, burdens and benefits, especially when making decisions regarding the allocation of healthcare resources.

Durable medical equipment   Equipment needed by patients for self-care. Usually it must withstand repeated use, is used for a medical purpose, and is appropriate for use in the home setting.

Effectiveness of care   The extent to which care is provided correctly (i.e., to meet the patient's needs, improve quality of care, and resolve the patient's problems).

Efficiency of care   The extent to which care is provided to meet the desired effects/outcomes to improve quality of care and prevent the use of unnecessary resources.

Emotional intelligence   The ability to sense, understand, and effectively apply the power and acumen of emotions as a source of energy, information, connection, and influence. It also is the ability to motivate oneself and persist in the face of frustration; control impulse; regulate one's mood; and keep distress from swamping the ability to think, empathize, and hope.

Encounter   An outpatient or ambulatory visit by a health plan member to a provider. It applies mainly to physician's office but may also apply to other types of encounters.

Enrollee   An individual who subscribes for a health benefit plan provided by a public or private healthcare insurance organization.

Enrollment   The number of members in an HMO. The process by which a health plan signs up individuals or groups of subscribers.

Exclusive provider organization (EPO)   A managed care plan that provides benefits only if care is rendered by providers within a specific network.

Fee schedule   A listing of fee allowances for specific procedures or services that a health plan will reimburse.

Fee-for-service (FFS)   Providers are paid for each service performed, as opposed to capitation. Fee schedules are an example of fee-for-service.

First-level reviews   Conducted while the patient is in the hospital, care is reviewed for its appropriateness.

Gag rules   A clause in a provider's contract that prevents physicians or other providers from revealing a full range of treatment options to patients or, in some instances, from revealing their own financial self-interest in keeping treatment costs down. These rules have been banned by many states.

Gatekeeper   A primary care physician (usually a family practitioner, internist, pediatrician, or nurse practitioner) to whom a plan member is assigned. Responsible for managing all referrals for specialty care and other covered services used by the member.

Global fee A predetermined all-inclusive fee for a specific set of related services, treated as a single unit for billing or reimbursement purposes.

Group model HMO The HMO contracts with a group of physicians for a set fee per patient to provide many different health services in a central location. The group of physicians determines the compensation of each individual physician, often sharing profits.

Guidelines See **practice guidelines.**

Health benefit plan Any written health insurance plan that pays for specific healthcare services on behalf of covered enrollees.

Health maintenance organization (HMO) An organization that provides or arranges for coverage of designated health services needed by plan members for a fixed prepaid premium. There are four basic models of HMOs: group model, individual practice association (IPA), network model, and staff model. Under the Federal HMO Act an organization must possess the following to call itself an HMO: (1) an organized system for providing healthcare in a geographical area, (2) an agreed-on set of basic and supplemental health maintenance and treatment services, and (3) a voluntarily enrolled group of people.

Healthcare proxy A legal document that directs the healthcare provider/agency in whom to contact for approval/consent of treatment decisions or options whenever the patient is no longer deemed competent to decide for self.

Home health resource group (HHRG) Groupings for prospective reimbursement under Medicare for home health agencies. Placement into an HHRG is based on the OASIS score. Reimbursement rates correspond to the level of home health provided.

Hospital-issued notice of noncoverage (HINN) A letter provided to patients informing them of insurance noncoverage in case they refuse hospital discharge or insist on continued hospitalization despite the review by the peer review organization (PRO) that indicates their readiness for discharge.

ICD-9-CM International Classification of Diseases, Ninth Revision, Clinical Modification, formulated to standardize diagnoses. It is used for coding medical records in preparation for reimbursement, particularly in the inpatient care setting.

Incentive A sum of money paid at the end of the year to healthcare providers by an insurance/managed care organization as a reward for the provision of quality and cost-effective care.

Indemnity Benefits paid in a predetermined amount in the event of a covered loss. Fee-for-service health insurance plans are often referred to as *indemnity plans.*

Indemnity benefits Benefits in the form of payments rather than services. In most cases after the provider has billed the patient, the insured person is reimbursed by the company.

Independent case management Also known as *private case management* or *external case management*, it entails the provision of case management services by case managers who are either self-employed or are salaried employees in a privately owned case management firm.

Indicator A measure or metric that can be used to monitor and assess quality and outcomes of important aspects of care or services.

Individual practice association (IPA) model HMO An HMO model that contracts with a private practice physician or healthcare association to provide healthcare services in return for a negotiated fee. The IPA then contracts with physicians who continue in their existing individual or group practice.

Informed consent Consent given by a patient, next of kin, legal guardian, or designated person for a kind of intervention, treatment, or service after the provision of sufficient information by the provider.

Inpatient rehabilitation facilities patient assessment instrument (IRF-PAI) The Inpatient Rehabilitation Facilities Patient Assessment Instrument, used to classify patients into distinct groups based on clinical characteristics and expected resource needs. The PAI determines the CMG classification.

Integrated delivery system (IDS) A single organization or group of affiliated organizations that provides a wide spectrum of ambulatory and tertiary care and services. Care may also be provided across various settings of the healthcare continuum.

Intensity of service An acuity of illness criteria based on the evaluation/treatment plan, interventions, and anticipated outcomes.

Intermediate outcome A desired outcome that is met during a patient's hospital stay. It is a milestone in the care of a patient or a trigger point for advancement in the plan of care.

Internet A public, cooperative creation that operates using national and international telecommunication technologies and networks, including high-speed data lines, phone lines, satellite communications, and radio networks.

Justice Maintaining what is right and fair and making decisions that are good for the patient.

Length of stay The number of days that a health plan member stays in an inpatient facility.

Levels of service Based on the patient's condition and the needed level of service, used to identify and verify that the patient is receiving care at the appropriate level.

Liability Legal responsibility for failure to act appropriately or for actions that do not meet the standards of care, inflicting harm on another person.

Licensure A mandatory and official form of validation provided by a governmental agency in any state affirming that a practitioner has acquired the basic knowledge and skill and minimum degree of competence required for safe practice in his or her profession.

Litigation A contest in a court for the purpose of enforcing a right, particularly when inflicting harm on another person.

Living will A legal document that directs the healthcare team/provider in holding or withdrawing life support measures. It is usually prepared by the patient while he or she is competent, indicating the patient's wishes.

Malpractice Improper care or treatment by a healthcare professional. A wrongful conduct.

Managed care A system of healthcare delivery that aims to provide a generalized structure and focus when managing the use, access, cost, quality, and effectiveness of healthcare services. Links the patient to provider services.

Managed competition A state of healthcare delivery in which a large number of consumers choose among health plans that offer similar benefits. In theory, competition would be based on cost and quality and ideally would limit high prices and improve quality of care.

Management service organization A management entity owned by a hospital, physician organization, or third party. It contracts with payers and hospitals/physicians to provide certain healthcare management services such as negotiating fee schedules and handling administrative functions, including utilization management, billing, and collections.

Medicaid A federal program administered and operated individually by state governments that provides medical benefits to eligible low-income persons needing healthcare. The costs of the program are shared by the federal and state governments.

Medical durable power of attorney A legal document that names a surrogate decision maker in the event that the patient becomes unable to make his or her own healthcare decisions.

Medical loss ratio (MLR) The ratio of healthcare costs to revenue received. Calculated as total medical expense/total revenue.

Medical necessity on admission A type of review used to determine that the hospital admission is appropriate, clinically necessary, justified, and reimbursable.

Medically necessary A term used to describe the supplies and services provided to diagnose and treat a medical condition in accordance with nationally recognized standards.

Medicare A nationwide, federally administered health insurance program that covers the cost of hospitalization, medical care, and some related services for eligible persons. Medicare has two parts. Part A covers inpatient hospital costs (currently reimbursed prospectively using the DRG system). Medicare pays for pharmaceuticals provided in hospitals but not for those provided in outpatient settings. Also called *Supplementary Medical Insurance Program*. Part B covers outpatient costs for Medicare patients (currently reimbursed retrospectively).

Minimum data set (MDS) The assessment tool used in skilled nursing facility settings to place patients into RUGs, which determines the facilities reimbursement rate.

Multidisciplinary action plan (MAP) See **case management plan (CMP)**.

Negligence Failure to act as a reasonable person. Behavior is contrary to that of any ordinary person facing similar circumstances.

Network model HMO This is the fastest growing form of managed care. The plan contracts with a variety of groups of physicians and other providers in a network of care with organized referral patterns. Networks allow providers to practice outside the HMO.

Nonmaleficence Refraining from doing harm to others; that is, emphasizing quality care outcomes.

Nursing case management See also **case management**. A process model using the components of case management in the delivery aspects of nursing care. In nursing case management delivery systems, the role of the case manager is assumed by a registered professional nurse.

Outcome The result and consequence of a healthcare process. A good outcome is a result that achieves the expected goal. An outcome may be the result of care received or not received.

Outcome and assessment information set (OASIS) A prospective nursing assessment instrument completed by home health agencies at the time the patient is entered for home health services. Scoring determines the HHRG.

Outcome indicators Measures of quality and cost of care. Metrics used to examine and evaluate the results of the care delivered.

Outcomes management The use of information and knowledge gained from outcomes monitoring to achieve optimal patient outcomes through improved clinical decision making and service delivery.

Outcomes measurement The systematic, quantitative observation, at a point in time, of outcome indicators.

Outcomes monitoring The repeated measurement over time of outcome indicators in a manner that permits causal inferences about what patient characteristics, care processes, and resources produced the observed patient outcomes.

Outlier Something that is significantly well above or below an expected range or level.

Outlier threshold The upper range (threshold) in length of stay before a patient's stay becomes an outlier. It is the maximum number of days a patient may stay in the hospital for the same fixed reimbursement rate. The outlier threshold is determined by the Centers for Medicare and Medicaid Services (CMS), formerly known as the Health Care Financing Administration (HCFA).

Overutilization Using established criteria as a guide, determination is made as to whether the patient is receiving services that are redundant, unnecessary, or in excess.

Panel of providers Usually refers to the healthcare providers, including physicians, who are responsible for providing care and services to the enrollee in a managed care organization. These providers deliver care to the enrollee based on a contractual agreement with the managed care organization.

Payer The party responsible for reimbursement of healthcare providers and agencies for services rendered such as the Centers for Medicare and Medicaid Services and managed care organizations.

Peer review organization (PRO) A federal program established by the Tax Equity and Fiscal Responsibility Act of 1982 that monitors the medical necessity and quality of services provided to Medicare and Medicaid beneficiaries under the prospective payment system.

Per diem　A daily reimbursement rate for all inpatient hospital services provided in one day to one patient, regardless of the actual costs to the healthcare provider.

Performance improvement　The continuous study and adaptation of the functions and processes of a healthcare organization to increase the probability of achieving desired outcomes and to better meet the needs of patients.

Physician-hospital organization　Organization of physicians and hospitals that is responsible for negotiating contractual agreements for healthcare provision with third-party payers such as managed care organizations.

Plaintiff　A person who seeks a lawsuit in court because of a belief that his or her rights have been violated or a legal injury has occurred.

Point-of-service (POS) plan　A type of health plan allowing the covered person to choose to receive a service from a participating or a nonparticipating provider, with different benefit levels associated with the use of participating providers. Members usually pay substantially higher costs in terms of increased premiums, deductibles, and coinsurance.

Practice guidelines　Systematically developed statements on medical practices that assist a practitioner in making decisions about appropriate diagnostic and therapeutic healthcare services for specific medical conditions. Practice guidelines are usually developed by authoritative professional societies and organizations.

Preadmission certification　An element of utilization review that examines the need for proposed services before admission to an institution to determine the appropriateness of the setting, procedures, treatments, and length of stay.

Preauthorization　See **precertification.**

Precertification (prior approval)　The process of obtaining and documenting advanced approval from the health plan by the provider before delivering the medical services needed. This is required when services are of a nonemergent nature.

Preexisting condition　A condition or illness for which a member has received treatment during a specified period before becoming a member/enrollee of a health insurance policy.

Preferred provider organization (PPO)　A program in which contracts are established with providers of medical care. Providers under a PPO contract are referred to as *preferred providers.* Usually the benefit contract provides significantly better benefits for services received from preferred providers, thus encouraging members to use these providers. Covered persons are generally allowed benefits for nonparticipating provider services, usually on an indemnity basis with significant copayments.

Premature discharge　The release of a patient from care before he or she is deemed medically stable and ready for terminating treatment/care (e.g., discharging a patient from a hospital when he or she is still needing further care and/or observation).

Premium　The rate that a plan subscriber pays for coverage of specific health services.

Prepaid health plan　Health benefit plan in which a provider network delivers a specific complement of health services to an enrolled population for a predetermined payment amount (see **capitation**).

Primary care　The point when the patient first seeks assistance from the medical care system. It also is the care of the simpler and more common illnesses.

Primary care provider　Assumes ongoing responsibility for the patient in both health maintenance and treatment. Usually responsible for orchestrating the medical care process either by caring for the patient or by referring a patient on for specialized diagnosis and treatment. Primary care providers include general or family practitioners, internists, pediatricians, and sometimes OB/GYN doctors.

Principal diagnosis　The condition that chiefly required the patient's admission to the hospital for care.

Principal procedure　A procedure performed for definitive rather than diagnostic treatment, or one that is necessary for treating a certain condition. It is usually related to the principal diagnosis.

Prior authorization　See **precertification.**

Prospective payment system　A healthcare payment system used by the federal government since 1983 for reimbursing healthcare providers/agencies for medical care provided to Medicare and Medicaid participants. The payment is fixed and based on the operating costs of the patient's diagnosis.

Prospective review　A method of reviewing possible hospitalization before admission to determine necessity and estimated length of stay.

Protocol　A systematically written document about a specific patient's problem. It is mainly used as an integral component of a clinical trial or research. It also delineates the steps to be followed for a particular procedure or intervention to meet desired outcomes.

Quality assurance　The use of activities and programs to ensure the quality of patient care. These activities and programs are designed to monitor, prevent, and correct quality deficiencies and noncompliance with the standards of care and practice.

Quality improvement　An array of techniques and methods used for the collection and analysis of data gathered in the course of current healthcare practices in a defined care setting to identify and resolve problems in the system and improve outcomes of care.

Quality indicator　A predetermined measure for assessing quality; a metric.

Quality management　A formal process by which an organization measures the extent to which the providers conform to defined standards and, based on the data, improve the process, structure, and outcomes of care.

Quality monitoring　A process used to ensure that care is being delivered at or above acceptable quality standards and as identified by the organization or national guidelines.

Rehabilitation impairment categories (RIC)　Represent the primary cause of the rehabilitation stay. They are clinically homogeneous groupings that are then subdivided into CMGs.

Reimbursement　Payment regarding healthcare and services provided by a physician, medical professional, or agency.

Relative weight An assigned weight that is intended to reflect the relative resource consumption associated with each DRG. The higher the relative weight, the greater the payment/reimbursement to the hospital.

Report card An emerging tool that is used by healthcare providers, purchasers, policymakers, governmental agencies, and consumers to compare and understand the actual performance of health plans and other service delivery programs. It usually includes data in major areas of accountability such as quality, utilization of resources, consumer satisfaction, and cost.

Resource utilization group (RUG) Classifies skilled nursing facility patients into 7 major hierarchies and 44 groups. Based on the MDS, the patient is classified into the most appropriate group, and with the highest reimbursement.

Retrospective review A form of medical records review that is conducted after the patient's discharge to track appropriateness of care and consumption of resources.

Risk Probability that revenues of the insurer will not be sufficient to cover expenditures incurred in the delivery of contracted services.

Risk management A comprehensive program of activities to identify, evaluate, and take corrective action against risks that may lead to patient or staff injury with resulting financial loss or legal liability. This program aims at minimizing losses.

Risk sharing The process whereby an HMO and contracted provider each accept partial responsibility for the financial risk and rewards involved in cost-effectively caring for the members enrolled in the plan and assigned to a specific provider.

Root cause analysis A process used by healthcare providers and administrators to identify the basic or causal factors that contribute to variation in performance and outcomes or underlie the occurrence of a sentinel event.

Sentinel event An unexpected occurrence, not related to the natural course of illness, that results in death, serious physical or psychological injury, or permanent loss of function.

Severity of illness An acuity of illness criteria that identifies the presence of significant/debilitating symptoms, deviations from the patient's normal values, or unstable/abnormal vital signs or laboratory findings.

Skilled care Patient care services that require delivery by a licensed professional such as a registered nurse or physical therapist, occupational therapist, speech pathologist, or social worker.

Staff model HMO The most rigid HMO model. Physicians are on staff with some sort of salaried arrangement and provide care exclusively for the health plan enrollees.

Subacute care facility A healthcare facility that is a step down from an acute care hospital and a step up from a conventional skilled nursing facility intensity of services.

Supplementary medical insurance (SMI) A secondary medical insurance plan used by a subscriber to supplement healthcare benefits and coverage provided by the primary insurance plan. The primary and secondary/supplementary plans are unrelated and provided by two different agencies.

Target utilization rates Specific goals regarding the use of medical services, usually included in risk-sharing arrangements between managed care organizations and healthcare providers.

Telephone triage Triaging patients to appropriate levels of care based on a telephonic assessment of a patient. Case managers use the findings of their telephone-based assessment to categorize the patient to be of an emergent, urgent, or nonurgent condition.

Telephonic case management The delivery of healthcare services to patients and/or families or caregivers over the telephone or through correspondence, fax, e-mail, or other forms of electronic transfer. An example is telephone triage.

Third-party payer An insurance company or other organization responsible for the cost of care so that individual patients do not directly pay for services.

Total quality management See **quality management.**

Transitional planning The process case managers apply to ensure that appropriate resources and services are provided to patients and that these services are provided in the appropriate setting or level of care as delineated in the standards and guidelines of regulatory and accreditation agencies.

Underutilization Using established criteria as a guide, determination is made as to whether the patient is receiving all of the appropriate services.

Utilization The frequency with which a benefit is used during a 1-year period, usually expressed in occurrences per 1000 covered lives.

Utilization management Review of services to ensure that they are medically necessary, provided in the most appropriate setting, and at or above quality standards.

Utilization review A mechanism used by some insurers and employers to evaluate healthcare on the basis of appropriateness, necessity, and quality.

Utilization review accreditation commission (URAC) A not-for-profit organization that provides reviews and accreditation for utilization review services/programs provided by freestanding agencies. It is also known as the American Accreditation Health Care Commission.

Variance Any expected outcome that has not been achieved within designated timeframes. Categories include system, patient, and practitioner.

Veracity The act of telling the truth.

Withhold A portion of payments to a provider held by the managed care organization until year end that will not be returned to the provider unless specific target utilization rates are achieved. Typically used by HMOs to control utilization of referral services by gatekeeper physicians.

Workers' compensation A program that provides medical benefits and replacement of lost wages for persons suffering from injury or illness that is caused by or occurred in the workplace.

REFERENCES

There are many excellent sources for case management–related terminology. The glossary of terms was developed based on the authors' own views and understanding of case management practice and adaptations from other sources, including the following:

American Medical Association Specialty Organization, Inc: *AMSO dot com, managed care terms,* 2001. Available online at http://www.amso.com/terms.htm (accessed 2/11/02).

American Nurses Association: *Healthcare in chaos: will we ever see real managed care?* 1997. Available online at http://www.nursingworld.org/mods/mod3/cemcfull.htm (accessed 2/12/02).

Huntington J: Glossary for managed care, *Online J Iss Nurs* 1997. Available online at http://www.nursingworld.org/ojin/tpc2_gls.htm (accessed 2/12/02).

Integrated Healthcare Association: *Managed healthcare: a brief glossary,* 1997. Available online at http://www.iha.org/gloss.htm (accessed 3/20/02).

Kongstvedt P: *Essentials of managed care,* ed 4, Gaithersburg, Md, 2001, Aspen.

Powell S: *Advanced case management: outcomes and beyond,* Philadelphia, 2000, Lippincott Williams & Wilkins.

Powell S: *Case management: a practical guide to success in managed care,* ed 2, Philadelphia, 2000, Lippincott Williams & Wilkins.

Index

Page numbers followed by a *t* indicate tables; page numbers followed by an *f* indicate figures.